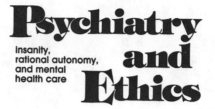

Psychiatry and Ethics

Insanity, rational autonomy, and mental health care

Psychiatry and Ethics

insanity,
rational autonomy,
and mental
health care

edited by
Rem B. Edwards

Prometheus Books

700 East Amherst Street
Buffalo. N.Y. 14215

Health Care and Medical Ethics Series
Marvin Kohl, Editor

Psychiatric ethics.

Published 1982 by Prometheus Books
700 East Amherst Street, Buffalo, New York 14215

Library of Congress Catalog Card Number: 82-62135
ISBN 0-87975-178-9 (Cloth)
ISBN 0-87975-179-7 (Paper)

Printed in the United States of America

For the patients and the staff
of Lakeshore Mental Health Institute

Contents

Preface

One of the greatest strengths of the doctoral program in medical ethics at the University of Tennessee is its ability to give its students considerable clinical exposure in a variety of medical settings. A vitally important part of this is the summer-long clinical practicum at Lakeshore Mental Health Institute in Knoxville, Tennessee. This book is dedicated to Lakeshore's patients and staff. At Lakeshore, students rotate through each unit of the hospital on a weekly basis, spending approximately five hours a day as participant/observers in the clinical process of making value-laden decisions about mental hospital patients. Two seminars per week are held on hospital grounds and attended by students as well as hospital staff in order to report on and analyze the value dimensions of what the students are observing. I developed this practicum during the summer of 1977 with the aid of a grant from the Institute for Human Values in Medicine.

In the early stages of the Lakeshore program, there was an obvious need for curriculum materials that would provide our students with an adequate intellectual background for their clinical experience. During the fall quarter of 1979, I was given released time under our department's National Endowment for the Humanities Developmental Grant in Medical Ethics (ED-32672-78-652) to develop these curriculum materials in the area of ethical and legal issues in mental health care. My time was spent reading through every relevant article I could find in legal, psychiatric, psychological, philosophical, and related journals. By the end of the year I had amassed a large number of articles and an enormous bibliography. Since then, much of my research time has been spent identifying the key issues, organizing information, and culling the presentations to find the very best ones. The present book is the result of those efforts, and I believe it will be of great interest to present and future

13

professionals in the areas of law, psychiatry, psychology, advocacy, social services, chaplaincy, and medical ethics who must comprehend and apply the value dimensions of mental health care.

I found the professionals at Lakeshore Hospital struggling to apply an ethic designed to promote and honor the rational autonomy of their patients; and I found the same ethic at work in many journal articles. The purpose of this book, therefore, is to organize the various attempts to understand and apply such an ethic in relation to the difficult situations in which mental patients find themselves. Interestingly enough, an ethic of rational autonomy is an ideal of moral behavior which persons of diverse philosophical persuasion can agree to adopt, though for reasons peculiar to their own standpoints. Kantians will want to adopt the ideal of promoting and honoring rational autonomy because it is an appropriate expression of the *categorical imperative,* which states that we should treat persons as ends in themselves and never merely as means. Rule utilitarians may adopt the ethic of rational autonomy because they think that if everyone followed the rule "We ought to promote and respect rational autonomy," then the best overall consequences would result. On the other hand, the rule may be adopted by act utilitarians as a rule of thumb for identifying those kinds of acts which will generally have the best consequences. Qualitatively hedonistic utilitarians like John Stuart Mill could adopt this ethic (as Mill did in *On Liberty* and in *Utilitarianism*) as the only effective way to maximize that long-range happiness for the greatest number which is high in both quality and quantity. Those who insist that we adopt our values under ideal rational conditions of freedom, enlightenment, and impartiality can hold that this either presupposes or results in an ethic of rational autonomy. Thus, there are many good reasons for adopting such an ethic, and we need not agree on the reasons in order to agree on the ethic.

I would like to express my sincere appreciation to each of the journals and authors who have given their permission to reprint the essays contained in this volume. No attempt has been made to standardize the systems of notation used in the various articles. I do not believe that retaining notations as given in original sources will create insuperable difficulties for intelligent readers.

Finally, I would like to express my deep appreciation to my editor, Steven L. Mitchell of Prometheus Books, for the able assistance which he has provided in the production of this volume.

1. "Mental Illness" and "Mental Health" Value Dimensions

Introduction

Most of the philosophically minded thinkers who have recently taken a critical look at our concepts of "mental health" and "mental illness" have found them to be inherently value-laden. This is to say that an evaluative component is an inescapable part of their very meaning, which is not to deny that a descriptive element may also be a part of their meaning. We pack our value preferences into these notions. This is true for particular psychiatric diagnostic categories as well as for general notions of mental illness and health. Concepts of physical health and illness are also infected by the values of those who employ them. The deceptive thing is that the evaluative component of such concepts is often hidden, disguised, or unrecognized.

When applied to the third edition of the American Psychiatric Association's *Diagnostic and Statistical Manual of Mental Disorders* (1980), the foregoing remarks mean that both the general definition of "mental disorder" and the particular diagnostic categories would involve both evaluative and descriptive components, whether these are clearly recognized or not. "Mental disorders" are chosen in relation to the disvalues of disability (or dysfunction) and distress (or pain). In these respects, such concepts resemble other paradigm evaluative concepts such as "good" and "bad," which have been closely scrutinized in twentieth-century metaethics. A number of components in our notion of "good" have been recognized. "X is good" is today widely acknowledged to mean: (a) that *someone* (not necessarily the speaker) approves of X, or takes a positive attitude toward it; (b) that X exhibits certain empirical features or "good-making characteristics" which occasion approval; and (c) that X is being commended to others for their approval and choice. Similarly, "bad" involves an expression of approval, grounded in disapproval-generating descriptive traits, and solicitation for avoidance and disapproval by others. In particular cases, one or more of these meaning-use elements may be more prominent than others. The apple grader or used car dealer may separate good from bad apples or cars on the basis of their good-making or bad-making empirical characteristics alone, without taking any particular attitude toward them at all. Yet, *someone* must approve red, juicy, well-shaped, worm-free apples if standards for separating good from bad apples are ever to be established in the first place. It is at the level of initially identifying and establishing the set of descriptive properties which constitute standards for differentiating between good and bad apples, cars, or what have you, that the evaluative elements of meaning—those indicating approval or disapproval—are most essential for value-laden concepts.

We inject our approval or disapproval into our concepts of health and disease, mental no less than physical, and then, often, we promptly forget that we have done so. Our disease concepts are constructed out of those descriptive properties of which we strongly disapprove, either directly or because they are the cause or the effect of those traits which are directly disapproved. Usually, these are inherently distressing or painful properties, properties causing disabilities or incapacities, ones that involve objectionable deformities, or properties resulting in death. Medical professionals often lose track of the evaluative dimensions of their work, like the apple graders who need not assume a negative attitude toward the bad apples they discard. They forget that *someone's* disapproval was essential for the initial identification of the bad-making characteristics.

Logically it is possible to hold that allegedly value-laden concepts like "disease," "health," "normality," "treatment," and others are: (1) purely evaluative, containing no empirical elements; (2) purely descriptive, containing no evaluative elements; or (3) composed of both evaluative and descriptive elements. The selections included in this section represent all of these positions. At least in emphasis, Thomas Szasz usually comes very close to holding position (1), always heavily stressing the evaluative dimension. Christopher Boorse is one of the very few recent theorists subscribing to position (2). And in a variety of different ways, position (3), which is clearly the dominant view today, is presupposed or explicitly developed by Peter Sedgwick, H. Tristram Engelhardt, Jr., and Rem B. Edwards.

Thomas S. Szasz

The Myth of Mental Illness

My aim in this essay is to raise the question "Is there such a thing as mental illness?" and to argue that there is not. Since the notion of mental illness is extremely widely used nowadays, inquiry into the ways in which this term is employed would seem to be especially indicated. Mental illness, of course, is not literally a "thing"—or physical object—and hence it can "exist" only in the same sort of way in which other theoretical concepts exist. Yet, familiar theories are in the habit of posing, sooner or later—at least to those who come to believe in them—as "objective truths" (or "facts"). During certain historical periods, explanatory conceptions such as deities, witches, and microorganisms appeared not only as theories but as self-evident *causes* of a vast number of events. I submit that today mental illness is widely regarded in a somewhat similar fashion, that is, as the cause of innumerable diverse happenings. As an antidote to the complacent use of the notion of mental illness—whether as a self-evident phenomenon, theory, or cause—let us ask this question: What is meant when it is asserted that someone is mentally ill?

In what follows I shall describe briefly the main uses to which the concept of mental illness has been put. I shall argue that this notion has outlived whatever usefulness it might have had and that it now functions merely as a convenient myth.

Mental Illness as a Sign of Brain Disease

The notion of mental illness derives its main support from such phenomena

From the *American Psychologist* 15 (1960):113–118. Copyright © 1960 by The American Psychologist. Reprinted by permission of the publisher and author.

as syphilis of the brain or delirious conditions — intoxications, for instance — in which persons are known to manifest various peculiarities or disorders of thinking and behavior. Correctly speaking, however, these are diseases of the brain, not of the mind. According to one school of thought, *all* so-called mental illness is of this type. The assumption is made that some neurological defect, perhaps a very subtle one, will ultimately be found for all the disorders of thinking and behavior. Many contemporary psychiatrists, physicians, and other scientists hold this view. This position implies that people *cannot* have troubles — expressed in what are *now called* "mental illnesses" — because of differences in personal needs, opinions, social aspirations, values, and so on. *All problems in living* are attributed to physicochemical processes which in due time will be discovered by medical research.

"Mental illnesses" are thus regarded as basically no different than all other diseases (that is, of the body). The only difference, in this view, between mental and bodily diseases is that the former, affecting the brain, manifest themselves by means of mental symptoms; whereas the latter, affecting other organ systems (for example, the skin, liver, etc.), manifest themselves by means of symptoms referable to those parts of the body. This view rests on and expresses what are, in my opinion, two fundamental errors.

In the first place, what central nervous system symptoms would correspond to a skin eruption or a fracture? It would *not* be some emotion or complex bit of behavior. Rather, it would be blindness or a paralysis of some part of the body. The crux of the matter is that a disease of the brain, analogous to a disease of the skin or bone, is a neurological defect, and not a problem in living. For example, a *defect* in a person's visual field may be satisfactorily explained by correlating it with certain definite lesions in the nervous system. On the other hand, a person's *belief* — whether this be a belief in Christianity, in Communism, or in the idea that his internal organs are "rotting" and that his body is, in fact, already "dead" — cannot be explained by a defect or disease of the nervous system. Explanations of this sort of occurrence — assuming that one is interested in the belief itself and does not regard it simply as a "symptom" or expression of something else that is *more interesting* — must be sought along different lines.

The second error in regarding complex psychosocial behavior, consisting of communications about ourselves and the world about us, as mere symptoms of neurological functioning is *epistemological*. In other words, it is an error pertaining not to any mistakes in observation or reasoning, as such, but rather to the way in which we organize and express our knowledge. In the present case, the error lies in making a symmetrical dualism between mental and physical (or bodily) symptoms, a dualism which is merely a habit of speech and to which no known observations can be found to correspond. Let us see if this is so. In medical practice, when we speak of physical disturbances, we mean either signs (for example, a fever) or symptoms (for example, pain). We speak of mental symptoms, on the other hand, when we refer to a patient's *communications about himself, others, and the world about him*. He might state that he is

Napoleon or that he is being persecuted by the Communists. These would be considered mental symptoms *only* if the observer believed that the patient was *not* Napoleon or that he was *not* being persecuted by the Communists. This makes it apparent that the statement that "*X* is a mental symptom" involves rendering a judgment. The judgment entails, moreover, a covert comparison or matching of the patient's ideas, concepts, or beliefs with those of the observer and the society in which they live. The notion of mental symptom is therefore inextricably tied to the *social* (including *ethical*) *context* in which it is made in much the same way as the notion of bodily symptom is tied to an *anatomical* and *genetic context* (Szasz, 1957a, 1957b).

To sum up what has been said thus far: I have tried to show that for those who regard mental symptoms as signs of brain disease, the concept of mental illness is unnecessary and misleading. For what they mean is that people so labeled suffer from diseases of the brain; and, if that is what they mean, it would seem better for the sake of clarity to say that and not something else.

Mental Illness as a Name for Problems in Living

The term "mental illness" is widely used to describe something which is very different than a disease of the brain. Many people today take it for granted that living is an arduous process. Its hardship for modern man, moreover, derives not so much from a struggle for biological survival as from the stresses and strains inherent in the social intercourse of complex human personalities. In this context, the notion of mental illness is used to identify or describe some feature of an individual's so-called personality. Mental illness — as a deformity of the personality, so to speak — is then regarded as the *cause* of the human disharmony. It is implicit in this view that social intercourse between people is regarded as something *inherently harmonious,* its disturbance being due solely to the presence of "mental illness" in many people. This is obviously fallacious reasoning, for it makes the abstraction "mental illness" into a *cause,* even though this abstraction was created in the first place to serve only as a shorthand expression for certain types of human behavior. It now becomes necessary to ask: "What kinds of behavior are regarded as indicative of mental illness, and by whom?"

The concept of illness, whether bodily or mental, implies *deviation from some clearly defined norm.* In the case of physical illness, the norm is the structural and functional integrity of the human body. Thus, although the desirability of physical health, as such, is an ethical value, what health *is* can be stated in anatomical and physiological terms. What is the norm deviation from which is regarded as mental illness? This question cannot be easily answered. But whatever this norm might be, we can be certain of only one thing: namely, that it is a norm that must be stated in terms of *psychosocial, ethical,* and *legal* concepts. For example, notions such as "excessive repression" or "acting out an unconscious impulse" illustrate the use of psychological concepts for judging (so-called) mental health and illness. The idea that chronic hostility, vengeful-ness, or divorce are indicative of mental illness would be illustrations of the use of ethical norms (that is, the desirability of love, kindness, and a stable mar-riage relationship). Finally, the widespread psychiatric opinion that only a mentally ill person would commit homicide illustrates the use of a legal con-cept as a norm of mental health. The norm from which deviation is measured whenever one speaks of a mental illness is a *psychosocial and ethical one*. Yet, the remedy is sought in terms of *medical* measures which—it is hoped and assumed—are free from wide differences of ethical value. The definition of the disorder and the terms in which its remedy are sought are therefore at serious odds with one another. The practical significance of this covert conflict between the alleged nature of the defect and the remedy can hardly be exaggerated.

Having identified the norms used to measure deviations in cases of mental illness, we will now turn to the question: "Who defines the norms and hence the deviation?" Two basic answers may be offered: (*a*) It may be the person himself (that is, the patient) who decides that he deviates from a norm. For example, an artist may believe that he suffers from a work inhibition; and he may implement this conclusion by seeking help *for* himself from a psychother-apist. (*b*) It may be someone other than the patient who decides that the latter is deviant (for example, relatives, physicians, legal authorities, society gener-ally, etc.). In such a case a psychiatrist may be hired by others to do something *to* the patient in order to correct the deviation.

These considerations underscore the importance of asking the question "Whose agent is the psychiatrist?" and of giving a candid answer to it (Szasz, 1956, 1958). The psychiatrist (psychologist or nonmedical psychotherapist), it now develops, may be the agent of the patient, of the relatives, of the school, of the military services, of a business organization, of a court of law, and so forth. In speaking of the psychiatrist as the agent of these persons or organiza-tions, it is not implied that his values concerning norms, or his ideas and aims concerning the proper nature of remedial action, need to coincide exactly with those of his employer. For example, a patient in individual psychotherapy may believe that his salvation lies in a new marriage; his psychotherapist need not share this hypothesis. As the patient's agent, however, he must abstain from bringing social or legal force to bear on the patient which would prevent him from putting his beliefs into action. If his *contract* is with the patient, the psychiatrist (psychotherapist) may disagree with him or stop his treatment; but he cannot engage others to obstruct the patient's aspirations. Similarly, if a psychiatrist is engaged by a court to determine the sanity of a criminal, he need not fully share the legal authorities' values and intentions in regard to the criminal and the means available for dealing with him. But the psychiatrist is expressly barred from stating, for example, that it is not the criminal who is "insane" but the men who wrote the law on the basis of which the very actions that are being judged are regarded as "criminal." Such an opinion could be voiced, of course, but not in a courtroom, and not by a psychiatrist who makes it his practice to assist the court in performing its daily work.

To recapitulate: In actual contemporary social usage, the finding of a mental illness is made by establishing a deviance in behavior from certain psychosocial, ethical, or legal norms. The judgment may be made, as in medicine, by the patient, the physician (psychiatrist), or others. Remedial action, finally, tends to be sought in a therapeutic — or covertly medical — framework, thus creating a situation in which *psychosocial, ethical,* and/or *legal deviations* are claimed to be correctible by (so-called) *medical action.* Since medical action is designed to correct only medical deviations, it seems logically absurd to expect that it will help solve problems whose very existence had been defined and established on nonmedical grounds. I think that these considerations may be fruitfully applied to the present use of tranquilizers and, more generally, to what might be expected of drugs of whatever type in regard to the amelioration or solution of problems in human living.

The Role of Ethics in Psychiatry

Anything that people *do* — in contrast to things that *happen* to them (Peters, 1958) — takes place in a context of value. In this broad sense, no human activity is devoid of ethical implications. When the values underlying certain activities are widely shared, those who participate in their pursuit may lose sight of them altogether. The discipline of medicine, both as a pure science (for example, research) and as a technology (for example, therapy), contains many ethical considerations and judgments. Unfortunately, these are often denied, minimized, or merely kept out of focus; for the ideal of the medical profession as well as of the people whom it serves seems to be having a system of medicine (allegedly) free of ethical value. This sentimental notion is expressed by such things as the doctor's willingness to treat and help patients irrespective of their religious or political beliefs, whether they are rich or poor, etc. While there may be some grounds for this belief — albeit it is a view that is not impressively true even in these regards — the fact remains that ethical considerations encompass a vast range of human affairs. By making the practice of medicine neutral in regard to some special issues of value need not, and cannot, mean that it can be kept free from all such values. The practice of medicine is intimately tied to ethics; and the first thing that we must do, it seems to me, is to try to make this clear and explicit. I shall let this matter rest here, for it does not concern us specifically in this essay. Lest there be any vagueness, however, about how or where ethics and medicine meet, let me remind the reader of such issues as birth control, abortion, suicide, and euthanasia as only a few of the major areas of current ethicomedical controversy.

Psychiatry, I submit, is very much more intimately tied to problems of ethics than is medicine. I use the word "psychiatry" here to refer to that contemporary discipline which is concerned with *problems in living* (and not with diseases of the brain, which are problems for neurology). Problems in human relations can be analyzed, interpreted, and given meaning only within given social and ethical contexts. Accordingly, it *does* make a difference — arguments to the contrary notwithstanding — what the psychiatrist's socioethical orientations happen to be; for these will influence his ideas on what is wrong with the patient, what deserves comment or interpretation, in what possible directions change might be desirable, and so forth. Even in medicine proper, these factors play a role, as for instance, in the divergent orientations which physicians, depending on their religious affiliations, have toward such things as birth control and therapeutic abortion. Can anyone really believe that a psychotherapist's ideas concerning religious belief, slavery, or other similar issues play no role in his practical work? If they do make a difference, what are we to infer from it? Does it not seem reasonable that we ought to have different psychiatric therapies — each expressly recognized for the ethical positions which they embody — for, say, Catholics and Jews, religious persons and agnostics, democrats and communists, white supremacists and Negroes, and so on? Indeed, if we look at how psychiatry is actually practiced today (especially in the United States) we find that people do seek psychiatric help in accordance with their social status and ethical beliefs (Hollingshead & Redlich, 1958). This should really not surprise us more than being told that practicing Catholics rarely frequent birth control clinics.

The foregoing position which holds that contemporary psychotherapists deal with problems in living, rather than with mental illnesses and their cures, stands in opposition to a currently prevalent claim, according to which mental illness is just as "real" and "objective" as bodily illness. This is a confusing claim since it is never known exactly what is meant by such words as "real" and "objective." I suspect, however, that what is intended by the proponents of this view is to create the idea in the popular mind that mental illness is some sort of disease entity, like an infection or a malignancy. If this were true, one could *catch* or *get* a "mental illness," one might *have* or *harbor* it, one might *transmit* it to others, and finally one could get *rid* of it. In my opinion, there is not a shred of evidence to support this idea. To the contrary, all the evidence is the other way and supports the view that what people now call mental illnesses are for the most part *communications* expressing unacceptable ideas, often framed, moreover, in an unusual idiom. The scope of this essay allows me to do no more than mention this alternative theoretical approach to this problem (Szasz, 1957c).

This is not the place to consider in detail the similarities and differences between bodily and mental illnesses. It shall suffice for us here to emphasize only one important difference between them: namely, that whereas bodily disease refers to public, physicochemical occurrences, the notion of mental illness is used to codify relatively more private, sociopsychological happenings of which the observer (diagnostician) forms a part. In other words, the psychiatrist does not stand *apart* from what he observes, but is, in Harry Stack Sullivan's apt words, a "participant observer." This means that he is *committed* to some picture of what he considers reality — and to what he thinks society considers reality — and he observes and judges the patient's behavior in the light of these considerations. This touches on our earlier observation that the notion of mental symptom itself implies a comparison between observer and observed, psychiatrist and patient. This is so obvious that I may be charged with belaboring trivialities. Let me therefore say once more that my aim in presenting this argument was expressly to criticize and counter a prevailing contemporary tendency to deny the moral aspects of psychiatry (and psychotherapy) and to substitute for them allegedly value-free medical considerations. Psychotherapy, for example, is being widely practiced as though it entailed nothing other than restoring the patient from a state of mental sickness to one of mental health. While it is generally accepted that mental illness has something to do with man's social (or interpersonal) relations, it is paradoxically maintained that problems of values (that is, of ethics) do not arise in this process.[1] Yet, in one sense, much of psychotherapy may revolve around nothing other than the elucidation and weighing of goals and values—many of which may be mutually contradictory—and the means whereby they might best be harmonized, realized, or relinquished.

The diversity of human values and the methods by means of which they may be realized is so vast, and many of them remain so unacknowledged, that they cannot fail but lead to conflicts in human relations. Indeed, to say that human relations at all levels—from mother to child, through husband and wife, to nation and nation—are fraught with stress, strain, and disharmony is, once again, making the obvious explicit. Yet, what may be obvious may be also poorly understood. This I think is the case here. For it seems to me that—at least in our scientific theories of behavior—we have failed to *accept* the simple fact that human relations are inherently fraught with difficulties and that to make them even relatively harmonious requires much patience and hard work. I submit that the idea of mental illness is now being put to work to obscure certain difficulties which at present may be inherent—not that they need be unmodifiable—in the social intercourse of persons. If this is true, the concept functions as a disguise; for instead of calling attention to conflicting human needs, aspirations, and values, the notion of mental illness provides an amoral and impersonal "thing" (an "illness") as an explanation for *problems in living* (Szasz, 1959). We may recall in this connection that not so long ago it was devils and witches who were held responsible for men's problems in social living. The belief in mental illness, as something other than man's trouble in getting along with his fellow man, is the proper heir to the belief in demonology and witchcraft. Mental illness exists or is "real" in exactly the same sense in which witches existed or were "real."

Choice, Responsibility, and Psychiatry

While I have argued that mental illnesses do not exist, I obviously did not imply that the social and psychological occurrences to which this label is currently being attached also do not exist. Like the personal and social troubles which people had in the Middle Ages, they are real enough. It is the labels we give them that concerns us and, having labelled them, what we do about them. While I cannot go into the ramified implications of this problem here, it is worth noting that a demonologic conception of problems in living gave rise to therapy along theological lines. Today, a belief in mental illness implies — nay, requires — therapy along medical or psychotherapeutic lines.

What is implied in the line of thought set forth here is something quite different. I do not intend to offer a new conception of "psychiatric illness" nor a new form of "therapy." My aim is more modest and yet also more ambitious. It is to suggest that the phenomena now called mental illnesses be looked at afresh and more simply, that they be removed from the category of illnesses, and that they be regarded as the expressions of man's struggle with the problem of *how* he should live. The last mentioned problem is obviously a vast one, its enormity reflecting not only man's inability to cope with his environment, but even more his increasing self-reflectiveness.

By problems in living, then, I refer to that truly explosive chain reaction which began with man's fall from divine grace by partaking of the fruit of the tree of knowledge. Man's awareness of himself and of the world about him seems to be a steadily expanding one, bringing in its wake an ever larger *burden of understanding* (an expression borrowed from Susanne Langer, 1953). *This burden, then, is to be expected and must not be misinterpreted.* Our only *rational* means for lightening it is *more understanding,* and appropriate *action* based on such understanding. The main alternative lies in acting as though the burden were not what in fact we perceive it to be and taking refuge in an outmoded theological view of man. In the latter view, man does not fashion his life and much of his world about him, but merely lives out his fate in a world created by superior beings. This may logically lead to pleading nonresponsibility in the face of seemingly unfathomable problems and difficulties. Yet, if man fails to take increasing responsibility for his actions, individually as well as collectively, it seems unlikely that some higher power or being would assume this task and carry this burden for him. Moreover, this seems hardly the proper time in human history for obscuring the issue of man's responsibility for his actions by hiding it behind the skirt of an all-explaining conception of mental illness.

Conclusions

I have tried to show that the notion of mental illness has outlived whatever usefulness it might have had and that it now functions merely as a convenient myth. As such, it is a true heir to religious myths in general, and to the belief in witchcraft in particular; the role of all these belief-systems was to act as *social tranquilizers,* thus encouraging the hope that mastery of certain specific problems may be achieved by means of substitutive (symbolic-magical) operations. The notion of mental illness thus serves mainly to obscure the everyday fact that life for most people is a continuous struggle, not for biological survival, but for a "place in the sun," "peace of mind," or some other human value. For man aware of himself and of the world about him, once the needs for preserving the body (and perhaps the race) are more or less satisfied, the problem arises as to what he should do with himself. Sustained adherence to the myth of mental illness allows people to avoid facing this problem, believing that mental health, conceived as the absence of mental illness, automatically insures the making of right and safe choices in one's conduct of life. But the facts are all the other way. It is the making of good choices in life that others regard, retrospectively, as good mental health!

The myth of mental illness encourages us, moreover, to believe in its logical corollary: that social intercourse would be harmonious, satisfying, and the secure basis of a "good life" were it not for the disrupting influences of mental illness or "psychopathology." The potentiality for universal human happiness, in this form at least, seems to me but another example of the I-wish-it-were-true type of fantasy. I do not believe that human happiness or well-being on a hitherto unimaginably large scale, and not just for a select few, is possible. This goal could be achieved, however, only at the cost of many men, and not just a few being willing and able to tackle their personal, social, and ethical conflicts. This means having the courage and integrity to forego waging battles on false fronts, finding solutions for substitute problems — for instance, fighting the battle of stomach acid and chronic fatigue instead of facing up to a marital conflict.

Our adversaries are not demons, witches, fate, or mental illness. We have no enemy whom we can fight, exorcise, or dispel by "cure." What we do have are *problems in living* — whether these be biologic, economic, political, or sociopsychological. In this essay I was concerned only with problems belonging in the last mentioned category, and within this group mainly with those pertaining to moral values. The field to which modern psychiatry addresses itself is vast, and I made no effort to encompass it all. My argument was limited to the proposition that mental illness is a myth, whose function it is to disguise and thus render more palatable the bitter pill of moral conflicts in human relations.

NOTE

1. Freud went so far as to say that: "I consider ethics to be taken for granted. Actually I have never done a mean thing" (Jones, 1957, p. 247). This surely is a strange thing to say for someone who has studied man as a social being as closely as did Freud. I mention it here to show how the notion of "illness" (in the case of psychoanalysis, "psychopathology," or "mental illness") was used by Freud — and by most of his followers — as a means for classifying certain forms of human behavior as falling within the scope of medicine, and hence (by *fiat*) outside that of ethics!

REFERENCES

Hollingshead, A. B., & Redlich, F. C. *Social class and mental illness.* New York: Wiley, 1958.

Jones, E. *The life and work of Sigmund Freud.* Vol. III. New York: Basic Books, 1957.

Langer, S. K. *Philosophy in a new key.* New York: Mentor Books, 1953.

Peters, R. S. *The concept of motivation.* London: Routledge & Kegan Paul, 1958.

Szasz, T. S. Malingering: "Diagnosis" or social condemnation? *AMA Arch Neurol. Psychiat.,* 1956, 76, 432–443.

Szasz, T. S. *Pain and pleasure: A study of bodily feelings.* New York: Basic Books, 1957.   (a)

Szasz, T. S. The problem of psychiatric nosology: A contribution to a situational analysis of psychiatric operations. *Amer. J. Psychiat.,* 1957, 114, 405–413.   (b)

Szasz, T. S. On the theory of psychoanalytic treatment. *Int. J. Psycho-Anal.,* 38, 166–182.   (c)

Szasz, T. S. Psychiatry, ethics and the criminal law. *Columbia law Rev.,* 1958, 58, 183–198.

Szasz, T. S. Moral conflict and psychiatry, *Yale Rev.* [1960, 49, 555–566.]

Christopher Boorse

What a Theory of Mental Health Should Be

Among mental-health professionals there is wide agreement that the concept of mental health is a web of obscurity. One growing body of opinion, ably led by Szasz (1961, 1963, 1970a, 1970b), Sarbin (1967, 1969), and the behaviour-modification theorists, maintains that the whole idea of mental illness has out-lived its usefulness and become both "scientifically worthless and socially harmful" (Szasz, 1961, p. ix). This remains a minority view; but those writers who continue to believe in mental health disagree sharply about what it is and even about how one might find out. At the bottom of this impasse, I think, are two causes. One is the lack of "a completely acceptable supertheory on which psychiatry can . . . rest its work" (Redlich & Freedman, 1966, p. 79). Until general psychology can achieve the broad theoretical consensus characteristic of other sciences, deep controversies over mental health seem inevitable. But these controversies are likely to remain irresolvable until a second obstacle is removed as well. I refer to the unwillingness of mental-health theorists to take physiology as a paradigm.

Reluctance to require any analogy between mental and physical health tends to cripple clinical discussion, from high-level theory to the analysis of particular conditions like homosexuality (e.g., Stoller et al., 1973). The reason is that mental-health theory and practice have not sprung up in a vacuum. On the contrary, they originally rose within physiological medicine, a mature and fairly well-articulated body of thought. From this established discipline they borrowed both the root notion of health and the many unspoken assumptions

From *Journal of the Theory of Social Behavior,* 6:1 (April 1976). Copyright © 1976 by Basil Blackwell. Reprinted by permission of the publisher and the author.

that surround it: that health is worth promoting, for example, and that well-informed observers ought in principle to agree on the norms of the healthy personality. We are by now so familiar with the "medical model" that any use of the term "health" brings these and other assumptions irresistibly in its train. In consequence, I think, there are only two terminological options consistent with clarity and social responsibility. One may abandon the medical vocabulary altogether, as Szasz and the behaviour modifiers have urged, and found clinical psychology and psychiatry on something other than the model of health and disease. Or one may continue to use the health vocabulary in the same way in which it is used in physiological medicine — and accept the implications of such use in the psychological domain.

To explore and defend the second option is the purpose of this essay. In the first section I shall argue that the functional idea of health in physical medicine applies as straightforwardly to the mind as to the body. Section II examines accepted procedures for obtaining mental-health ideals, and concludes that all of them are inappropriate to a theory of health. Despite this methodological failure, section III suggests that current clinical criteria may have something to tell us about mental health after all.

I

Most discussions of the "medical model" of mental illness are vitiated by confusion about what this model involves.[1] One reason for this confusion is that physical medicine itself has never felt the need to produce any clear philosophical analysis of its notions of health and disease. I am going to presuppose the results of my own attempt at such an analysis, which might be summarized as follows:

> An organism is *healthy* at any moment in proportion as it is not diseased; and a *disease* is a type of internal state of the organism which:
> (i) interferes with the performance of some natural function — i.e., some species-typical contribution to survival and reproduction — characteristic of the organism's age; and
> (ii) is not simply in the nature of the species, i.e. is either atypical of the species or, if typical, mainly due to environmental causes.[2]

The crucial points about this analysis are two. First, diseases are interferences with natural functions. Second, since the functional organization typical of a species is a biological fact, the concept of disease is value-free. Whether or not an organism is diseased can be settled in principle by the methods of natural science. The popularity of the opposite view is, I think, due to a failure to distinguish between the idea of a disease and the much narrower idea of an illness. Diseases become illnesses only when they satisfy certain further, and normative, conditions:

A disease is an *illness* only if it is serious enough to be incapacitating, and therefore is

(i) undesirable for its bearer;

(ii) a title to special treatment; and

(iii) a valid excuse for normally criticizable behaviour. (Boorse, 1975)

Thus we must distinguish, as Szasz and others usually do not, between two questions: whether "mental illness" makes sense, and whether "mental disease" makes sense. I shall consider only the latter question here.[3]

The analysis of health just given, though derived from physiology, shows no obvious partiality to body over mind. Physical health is simply the special case obtained by focusing on the functions of physiological processes. Mental health, then, would be the special case obtained by focusing on the functions of mental processes; and so there is such a thing as mental health if there are mental functions. For this, two conditions must be satisfied. First, some mental processes must play a causal role in action. Since philosophers are divided over whether mental events can be causes, the issue cannot readily be treated here. I agree with Davidson (1963) that the arguments against mental causation are weak and will conduct the discussion on that assumption. The second condition required for mental health is that mental processes contribute to action in a sufficiently species-uniform way to have natural functions. This thesis also seems plausible. Freud aside, the work of Chomsky and Piaget suggests that there are complicated patterns of mental functioning invariant in the species. No doubt it is generally assumed, outside the orbit of learning theory, that the human mind has *some* characteristic organization and operation. It is something of a historical accident that the term "biological function" calls to mind sex and excretion rather than intelligence and drive; Darwin, for one, was deeply interested in the evolution of the human mental apparatus. If certain types of mental processes perform standard functions in human behaviour, it is hard to see any obstacle to calling unnatural obstructions of these functions mental diseases, exactly as in the physiological case. So far the analogy between physical and mental health is unproblematic.

One source of disanalogy is that we may expect normal psychological functions to be somewhat less specific than their physiological counterparts. The outstanding feature of human mentality is its plasticity. There is an enormous range of physical and cultural environments to which the human mind can adapt its functioning. This adaptability, as a characteristic of the individual as well as of the group, is without parallel in the biological kingdom. Even so, however, and without relying on any controversial psychological theory, it is easy to draw some of the outlines of human mental functioning. Perceptual processing, intelligence, and memory clearly serve to provide information about the world that can guide effective action. Drives serve to motivate it. Anxiety and pain function as signals of danger, language as a device for cultural co-operation and cognitive enrichment, and so on. If these and other mental processes play standard functional roles throughout the species, we seem to have everything requisite for the possibility of mental health. Why then do Szasz and Sarbin reject this possibility?

These authors object to the idea of mental health on two grounds. One is that it involves Cartesian dualism; the other is that it involves explaining behaviour causally as due to disease entities in this immaterial soul, rather than explaining it by a "rule-following" or "communication" or "social systems" model. As one would expect from this compressed description, Ryle and Peters are the philosophical mainstays of this line of criticism of the medical model in psychiatry. Sarbin writes:

> The basic Galenic model was not rejected by psychiatry and its immediate antecedents. Microbes, toxins, and growths, which were material and operated according to mechnical principles, were appropriate "causes" for diseases of the body. They were *inside* the body. The appropriate causes for abnormal *behavior* had to be sought along different lines. Since the dualistic mind-body concept was everyone's heritage, the hypothesis could be entertained that the causes of abnormal conduct, conduct already considered as nonsomatic disease, were *in the mind.* . . .
>
> Through historical and linguistic processes, the postulation was reified. Contemporary users of the mental illness concept are guilty of illicitly shifting from metaphor to myth. Instead of maintaining the metaphorical rhetoric "it is as if there were states of mind" and "it is as if such states of mind could be characterized as sickness," the contemporary mentalist conducts much of his work as if he believes that minds are "real" entities and that, like bodies, they can be sick or healthy (1969, pp. 15, 19).

Sarbin's discussion, though fascinating, is not an accurate reconstruction of the origin of the mental-illness concept. In many respects Freud is the beginning of the tradition Sarbin is criticizing, but he was far from being a Cartesian. Instead he seems to have anticipated a full physiological reduction of his theoretical apparatus.[4] As we have seen, the part of everyone's heritage on which the mental-illness idea depends is not Cartesian dualism, but just the mentalistic framework of beliefs, perceptions, wishes, fantasies, dreams, etc. One need not be a Cartesian to believe that people have such mental states as these, and Sarbin is surely not questioning their existence in questioning the reality of the mind. Rather, he is disputing whether they are states of an incorporeal substance, and further whether they can be causes of behaviour. We can agree that the mental-health concept stands or falls with mental causation. The interesting question is why Sarbin supposes that dualism is the only mind-body view that can support such a notion of mental health. I suspect the answer is that he implicitly accepts the following argument. If mental states are states of the body rather than of a soul, then mental diseases must be diseases of the brain or nerves. In that case there is no need for a concept of mental health distinct from physical health, and we are back with pre-Freudian neuropathology. This reasoning is defective, and I shall now explain why.

Consider the relation between mental and physical health according to one familiar variant of the identity theory, which is a fusion of ideas of Putnam and Davidson.[5] This view holds that every mental event is a physical event. Taking mental states as degenerate mental events, consisting merely of the persistence of some psychological property over time, a parallel claim can be made about states. Every mental state is a physical state. But the states thus claimed identical are to be particulars, i.e. dated conditions of specific persons, rather than universals, i.e. types of conditions. Not *the* desire for a lobster dinner, but *Smith's* desire for a lobster dinner as felt between 4 and 5 p.m. on 13 February 1975, is claimed to be identical to his being in some neural configuration during this period.[6] The distinction is crucial, for if types of mental states are defined by their functional properties, type-type identity statements are unlikely to hold. If Smith's current neural state is a desire for a lobster dinner, that is probably not because of any anatomical feature, such as its containing a lobster-shaped nerve net. Rather, on the view we are considering, it is because of the motivational role this state plays in producing a search for seafood restaurants or other lobster-obtaining behaviour. Now the same motivational role might be played by quite different neural configurations in different people. Hence the neural state in Smith that is his desire for a lobster dinner may bear no anatomical resemblance to the neural state in Jones that is his desire for a lobster dinner. And so there may be no set of anatomical properties that could define the mentalistic term "desire for a lobster dinner"; the mentalistic vocabulary, even for a materialist, may not be neurologically definable.

My purpose in rehearsing this view is to show why it is in no way obvious that psychiatrists who reject Cartesian dualism thereby destroy the autonomy of their discipline. On the version of the identity theory just summarized, they must concede that any particular person's mental disease is a physical state. But this is a very limited admission. It is not the same as saying that every mental disease is a physical disease. Diseases, e.g. tuberculosis or cancer or schizophrenia, are essentially universals rather than particulars. They are types of states which are instantiated in particular patients. But there is no guarantee that a mentalistically defined disease-type will coincide with any physiologically defined disease-type. Suppose, for example, that a type of mental disorder is marked by ambivalent feelings toward the patient's father. As in the lobster case, there may be no anatomical criterion by which one could examine the patient's brain and discover the idea of the father. The brains of the various patients who share this disorder may show no distinctive neural similarity. Thus mental diseases, in spite of being everywhere instantiated by neural states, may fail to be physical diseases by failing to be physiologically definable.

Further support for this suggestion emerges if one asks what makes a patient's condition a mental disease in the first place. It is not the presence of mental symptoms. Pain, delirium, and depression are mental symptoms that occur in many physical diseases. Nor does it seem to be true that a disease is classed as a mental illness when it has mental symptoms and is assumed to have a physical aetiology currently unknown. "Mental illness" is not just a short-hand for "obscure brain disease," since various conditions with obscure neural bases — dyslexia, aphasia, retardation — are not usually called mental illnesses. Rather, a mental disturbance gets classed as "mental illness" when some accepted explanation of it refers not to the patient's physiology but to his feelings, beliefs, and experiences. The defining property of mental disease is mental causation.[7] Now on the version of the identity theory just discussed, the causal chain of mental events leading to a disease condition must be equally a chain of physical events. But this chain figures in a causal *explanation* only in so far as it can be brought under causal laws (Hempel, 1965, pp. 347 ff.). If the mentalistic vocabulary is not neurologically definable, there will be no way to reduce causal laws of the mind to causal laws of the body. If so, the distinction between conditions that receive one kind of causal explanation and those that receive the other may be a permanent one, justifying an autonomous science of mental health.

In practice the issue of materialism tends to be confused with the separate issue of how to treat mental diseases. If mental states are brain states, it is assumed that mental diseases must yield to such physical methods as drugs and surgery. This conclusion is doubly unfounded. In the first place, according to our version of the identity theory, it is as unreasonable as expecting a computer expert called in for consultation on a botched program to locate the trouble by going into the machine with a flashlight and a screwdriver. Whether and how a computer program, or a mental state, is dysfunctional need not be evident from any of its physical properties. In the second place, physical medicine itself includes conditions, e.g. partial paralysis of a limb following nerve damage, that can be treated only by molar like exercise. Of course, nothing that I have said proves that physical medicine *cannot* find an explanation and treatment for familiar mental disorders; what I am arguing is that materialism *per se* gives no guarantee that it can. A psychiatrist who rejects dualism can consistently regard mental diseases as a theoretical category distinct from physical diseases and calling for unique molar treatment, e.g. psychotherapy. What threatens the concept of mental disease is not materialism, but the denial of mental causation.

II

So far we have seen that given a few plausible assumptions, the idea of mental health not only makes perfect sense but generates an autonomous field of clinical theory. We now encounter a striking paradox. It is quite likely that there is such a thing as mental health; yet the majority of "mental-health" theorists use methodologies that offer no assurance of finding out the first thing about it. They do not set out to investigate the normal functional organization of the human mind, as they ought to do if their subject is mental health. Instead they arrive at their mental-health criteria by one of three unsatisfactory routes.

The first route is to select some set of personality traits that are highly valued, either by the theorist or by our culture, and call them "mental health." The view that health judgments are at bottom nothing but value judgments has in fact come to be a sort of orthodoxy among clinicians.[8] But it is a mistaken view. In physical medicine the health of a body is not at all the same as its worth. One does not expect physicians to call anything they dislike about a person's body, e.g. its ugliness, a disease and proceed to shape it to their own standards. Whether the subject is disease or illness, all judgments of physical health involve factual claims about the conformity of the individual to the species design, i.e., to the inherited adaptive organization which is the basic subject matter of biology (Boorse, 1975). The doctrines of physiology about this functional design rest on empirical evidence and are either true or false. Where this factual component is wholly lacking, then, as in much psychological and psychiatric discussion, we do not have a *health* concept at all but one of moral acceptability or the good life for man.[9]

It is easy to notice that a mental-health theorist's criteria rests on nothing but a personal affirmation of values when one disagrees with the values. The Victorian flavour of such a statement as the following now inspires amusement:

> Wholesome-minded people are not averse to frank consideration of sex under proper conditions and right motives, but they do not enjoy having it dragged into prominence on every possible pretext and occasion. Dignity and decency are the marks of successful sex adjustment.[10]

But we might not be so quick to realize that we have a right to ask for evidence for the claim that

> the crucial consideration in determining human normality is whether the individual is an asset or a burden to society and whether he is or is not contributing to the progressive development of man.[11]

No doubt most people, like Adler, admire individuals who contribute to the development of man more than individuals who do not. But that in itself gives us no reason whatever to suppose that individuals who do not are unhealthy, i.e. suffer from psychological dysfunction.

Even no less an authority than Karl Menninger leaves room for similar worries about the provenance of his idea of health:

> Let us define mental health as the adjustment of human beings to the world and to each other with a maximum of effectiveness and happiness. Not just efficiency, or just contentment — or the grace of obeying the rules of the game cheerfully. It is all of these together. It is the ability to maintain an even temper, an alert intelligence, socially considerate behavior, and a happy disposition. This, I think, is a healthy mind. (1930, 2)

I would not suggest that Menninger has no evidence that he has correctly described the healthy mind. Nevertheless the opening phrase and inspirational tone of this proposal, as well as its position at the beginning of his discussion, tend to obscure the fact that what the healthy mind is like is an empirical question that can be answered correctly or incorrectly. We are no more free to define mental health as the constellation of qualities we most admire than we would be for physical health. Mental health must be a constellation of qualities displayed in the standard functional organization of members of our species. Only empirical inquiry can show whether normal human beings have an even temper, engage in socially considerate behaviour, and advance the species — or make love with "dignity and decency." Some animals are naturally irascible and treat their peers with unbroken hostility. Most copulate with utter abandon. Perhaps we are not so constituted; perhaps we are. The point is that a theory of health should be a description of how we are constituted and not how we would like to be.

Besides the affirmation of values, a second popular route to mental-health criteria is to abstract them from a set of agreed instances of disease. Presupposing that some class of mental conditions, e.g. psychoses, are unhealthy, the theorist looks for their common features and takes these as a negative definition of mental health. A good illustration is Kubie's view that mental health consists in a low level of unconscious motivation:

> The implicit ideal of normality that emerges . . . is an individual in whom the creative alliance between the conscious and preconscious systems is not constantly subject to blocking and distortion by the counterplay of preponderant unconscious forces . . . (1954, p. 187).

Kubie presents this view as a general account of mental health. His title confirms, however, that the core class of instances from which he has abstracted it is the neuroses. To see some practical difficulties with this abstraction route, one needs only ask whether, say, character disorders are unhealthy. Some character disorders are not marked by psychic conflict; thus by Kubie's criterion one would not be inclined to call them diseases. On the other hand, one could equally well abstract other criteria from Kubie's class of instances — e.g., capacity for accurate empathy for others — by which these character disorders *would* count as unhealthy. Any class of agreed instances may have various common features that imply different verdicts on problematic cases outside the class. And this first problem is intensified by two more. From a class of cases all defective in some quality, one cannot tell how much of the quality would be required in a healthy specimen. If psychotics are alike in, say, a lack of self-knowledge, how much self-knowledge is required for health? The abstraction method is incapable of giving any answer. Worst of all, the class of disorders on which almost all mental-health theorists would agree is severely limited. At best it includes psychoses and fairly spectacular neuroses, psychopathic personalities, etc. Certainly persons whom Kubie would call neurotic and therefore unhealthy, such as compulsively ambitious politicians, would not be called unhealthy by everyone. One writer's character neurosis is another writer's model of successful adjustment. Not surprisingly, then, the abstraction method invariably fails in practice to produce any wide consensus.

From the theoretical standpoint, an equally telling objection to the abstraction route is its presupposition that any given cases are unhealthy ones. As Szasz insists, the fact that a condition involves incapacitation and suffering is no proof that it is an illness.[12] It is even less obvious that every neurosis or character disorder is a defect of health. Conceptually speaking, neuroses could easily be what biologists call facultative adaptations to life circumstances, like the calluses on a workman's fingertips. That there is adaptive value in unconscious processes seems evident enough, from dreams to the syntax of spoken language and the symphonies of Mozart. Why then should we think that the unconscious motivation of the neurotic deviates from species design? No doubt we would be more creative, more flexible, and happier without our neuroses; but would we be healthier? However we may disvalue neurosis and seek to eradicate it, we cannot call it unhealthy until we know that the mind is not supposed to work that way. It is in no way obvious, and requires empirical support, that what clinicians see in their offices are usually cases of biological dysfunction.

It is surely in part a desire to avoid the hazards of these first two routes that leads many mental-health theorists to follow the third one. The opening move in this final strategy is to discard mental processes altogether in favour of behaviour. The aim of providing criteria of mental health is replaced by the aim of providing criteria of normal behaviour. Redlich and Freedman justify this move as follows:

> In older texts and in current lay parlance, psychiatry is often defined as the science dealing with mental diseases and illnesses of the mind or psyche. Since these are terms reminiscent of the metaphysical concepts of soul and spirit, we prefer to speak of behavior disorder. Behavior refers to objective data that are accessible to observation, plausible inference, hypothesis-making, and experimentation. The term disorder, although vague, is descriptive of malfunctioning of behavior without specifying etiology or underlying mechanism (1966, p. 2).

This quotation, like the earlier one from Sarbin, suggests the misconception that a true "mental disease" would have to be a sort of gangrene on the Cartesian ego. It does not have to be, as we have seen; it need only be a psychogenic disturbance of mental functions. But the great popularity of this behavioural approach merits continued analysis.

Health in physiology is primarily a feature of the internal state of an organism rather than of its behaviour. One can imagine extending the concept to label behaviour itself as healthy or unhealthy. Behaviour as well as internal processes may have a biological function (cf. Roe & Simpson, 1958), as long as the behaviour is uniform in the species. Indeed, it is *via* their contributions to behaviour that internal processes have functions. One might call behaviour healthy or unhealthy, then, accordingly as it is biologically functional or dysfunctional. This new concept would apply most clearly to the fixed motor patterns studied by animal ethologists; whether anything of interest to clinicians would emerge in the human case is open to question. But an immediate problem is that this resort to behaviour does nothing to mark off a domain of "mental" health as distinguished from physical health (Macklin, 1972, p. 342). If something we might call biologically dysfunctional behaviour can result from psychosis, it can certainly also result from multiple sclerosis or epilepsy or blindness. Unless one wishes psychiatry to swallow up medicine, therefore, some criterion must be given to distinguish those "behaviour disorders" that fall within the province of psychiatry from those that do not. The most natural suggestion is unavailable: that psychiatry studies behaviour disorders that are produced by disfunctional mental processes. Avoiding mental processes was the motivation for the behavioural approach in the first place. As soon as they are reinstated, it is not more obvious why mental disease has to show up in overt behaviour than physical disease. The proper domain of psychiatry will then consist of disorders of the mind rather than disorders of behaviour, and we will return to square one.

Given that one is determined to avoid mental processes, the best move might be to hold that psychiatry deals with dysfunctional behaviour in which there is no physiological abnormality. This position is not the one adopted by theorists of our third group. Instead they almost universally make a fatal error: they desert biological dysfunction in favour of social deviance. Redlich and Freedman have this to say about the term "behaviour disorder":

> Defying easy definition, the term refers to the presence of certain behavioral patterns — variously described as abnormal, subnormal, undesirable, inadequate, inappropriate, maladaptive, or maladjusted — that are not compatible with the norms and expectations of the patient's social and cultural system (1966, p. 1).

Since deviant behaviour can result from physical disease, presumably the intended view is that psychiatry deals with those behavioural patterns deemed deviant by society which are not physiologically explainable.

This move to social deviance makes Szasz's criticisms quite unanswerable. As long as the physiological paradigm is to be given any weight at all, society can have no title to decree what states of organisms are unhealthy. Tuberculosis and epilepsy are diseases not because society disvalues them, but because they are cases of biological malfunction. They would not cease to be disease if some culture developed an admiration for epileptics or consumptives; like anything else, diseases can be assigned to a high social status. Within the realm of physiology social judgments of illness are no more infallible than social judgments of the shape of the earth or the number of planets, for they involve claims about the biological constitution of man. When, therefore, psychiatric theorists discard this biological constitution altogether in favour of the norms of a "social and cultural system," it seems fair to say that they have stopped talking about health. To reject the straightforward extension of the health vocabulary to the psychological domain, while giving it instead a new meaning grossly disanalogous to its established use, is hardly a responsible terminological policy.

One can indeed admit the conceptual gulf between biologically dysfunctional behaviour and socially disvalued behaviour and nevertheless assume that the two happen to coincide. In other words, one can hold it to be an *empirical* fact that behaviour is healthy only if society approves of it. But as an empirical hypothesis the view seems most implausible when clearly understood. It is true that man is a social animal. Our biological design, both mental and physical, seems to be adapted to life in a social group. But which social group? When judgments of deviance are made, the usual reference class is society at large. By this standard homosexuals, drug addicts, women's liberationists, Vietnam protesters, and fornicators are among the paradigm American deviants. But it is notorious that these and other non-conformists can flourish within non-conforming subcultures. As long as a person's behaviour is consistent with adjustment to *some* social group, one cannot call it unhealthy on the grounds that man is a social animal. As ordinarily understood, then, behavioural deviance seems too wide to be a sufficient condition of mental disorder. A narrower notion of deviance would count behaviour deviant only when it is considered deviant by all social groups. But this account will be clinically unsatisfactory for the opposite reason. Psychotics may be thoroughly accepted by their fellow patients in a psychiatric hospital, but they are surely not thereby healthy. Deviance from every conceivable standard is not a necessary condition for mental disorder.

Whether or not there is some middle ground, finally, seems irrelevant simply because deviants are not usually wholly ostracized even from the group that considers them deviant. Neither sexual swingers nor unwed mothers nor radical feminists are biologically incompetent in the sense of being totally excluded from the group way of life. They are merely disapproved of. And it would be fantastic to suggest that biological normality requires complete approval by one's peers, rather than just enough approval to satisfy whether needs of ours involve the medium of a group. It is not as though existing social structures reward conforming members with ideal opportunities for human fulfilment. Social agitation of a sort that is unpopular and even illegal is often morally justified; and there is no reason to suppose that the moral sensitivity and individual autonomy which can drive such behaviour is unnatural to the species. So Wootton's comments on "adjustment," i.e. social acceptance, again seem right on target:

In the literature of mental health generally, this concept of adjustment is particularly prominent. Fine phrases cannot, however, obscure the fact that adjustment means adjustment to a particular culture or to a particular set of institutions; and that to conceive adjustment and maladjustment in medical terms is in effect to identify health with the ability to come to terms with that culture or with those institutions — be they totalitarian methods of government, the dingy culture of an urban slum, the contemporary English law of marriage, or what I have elsewhere called the standards of an "acquisitive, competitive, hierarchical, envious" society.[13]

There is in the end so little evidence for any general connection between social deviance and biological dysfunction that one is tempted to class the "behaviour disorder" view as one more affirmation of values on the part of some conservative clinicians.

Thus Redlich and Freedman, along with the many other psychiatric authors who take the social-deviance route, are in fact doing what the behaviour modifiers are doing more openly. They are *abandoning* the "medical model," i.e. the model of health and disease. In this charge Szasz is perfectly correct. Since social deviance does not define any health concept, it would be preferable to introduce a new vocabulary. For example, one might speak with Ullmann and Krasner of "maladaptive behaviour":

> Maladaptive behavior is behavior that is considered inappropriate by those key people in a person's life who control reinforcers (1966, p. 20).

This definition suggests a refreshing lack of pretense that non-conformity is sickness. However, the value of the new terminology depends on our constantly remembering — as behaviour-modification theorists often do not — that "maladaptive" so defined cannot be used interchangeably with "pathological" or "abnormal" or any other term meaning "unhealthy." It is both dishonest and dangerous to throw the health concept out at the front door and then let it in at the back. If one wishes to avoid the theoretical inconveniences of the medical model, one must constantly relinquish its practical implications as well. There is no objection to advocating the use of techniques like behaviour modification on clinical populations. But if the aim of such techniques is to be "adaptive behavior" rather than mental health, one should candidly admit that many of our assumptions about health — in particular, its desirability — may not carry over to adaptive behaviour at all.

III

We have been directing heavy criticism upon the three main sources of contemporary mental-health criteria: affirmations of values, abstraction from established diagnostic classes, and social judgments of behaviour. We have seen that there is no reason, in principle, why any of these methods that mental-health theorists typically follow should generate an accurate account of mental health. It is time for some conciliatory remarks.

Apart from the inherent difficulties of all psychological research, there are several reasons why theorists overlook their obligation to describe the system of normal mental functions in which mental health must consist. One reason is that the functional conception of health in physiological medicine has gone largely unrecognized, both by philosophers and by physicians. A second reason is that contemporary biology has not, for the most part, continued Darwin's interests in the adaptive functions of mental abilities (Montague, 1962). Psychologists influenced by a narrowly physiological view of biology will tend to discount any possibility of transferring its functional model to the mental domain.

Perhaps a third reason, however, is the most important of all. Early physical medicine itself undoubtedly began with a primitive notion of illness lacking all reference to natural physiological functions. Patients were presumably classified as ill by a criterion of observable suffering or incapacitation alone. In time, with the rise of empirical thinking, supernatural explanations of these conditions were gradually replaced by the idea of internal malfunction. Contemporary psychiatry has not yet reached the stage of agreement on a substantive theory of the mind. In default of such a theory, it has, not unnaturally, reverted to the primitive conception of illness, although it must be said that it has also immeasurably extended its scope. Once again medical professionals are calling people "ill" without any thought of internal malfunctioning, but solely on the grounds of emotional turmoil or social maladjustment.

The trouble with this procedure, however understandable, is that it is two thousand years too late. Physiological medicine has in the interim undergone a particular historical development. That development has culminated in the functional conception of disease with which we are thoroughly familiar. Not everyone is willing to assume that psychiatry can follow the same course of development, which is the assumption we defended earlier in connection with the functional notion of mental health. But to revert at this point to the archaic usage of the health vocabulary is to invite unbearable cognitive strain. My proof for this statement is simply the opacity of current controversies over mental health. In the interests of conceptual clarity, psychiatry must either conform its usage of "health" to the functional paradigm or else devise new ways of speaking of the conditions with which it deals. And my final suggestion is that in spite of the methodological defects of current mental-health theory, it would be a mistake for the clinical disciplines to follow Szasz et al. in discarding mental health. Regardless of the origin of existing clinical criteria, there is reason to take many of them seriously as hypotheses about the normal human design. I will conclude with a series of points in defence of this suggestion.

Consider first some broad categories of traditional psychopathology. It seems certain that a few of the recognized mental disorders are genuine diseases, whether mental or physical. Even without any knowledge of the relevant functional systems, one can sometimes infer internal malfunction immediately from biologically incompetent behaviour. Functions in physiology are species-typical contributions of a part to survival and reproduction. Some mental patients, e.g. catatonic schizophrenics, are clearly incompetent with respect to these biological goals and would remain so under almost any circumstances. Whatever the detailed functional organization of the human mind and body may be, then, these people depart from it and so are authentically unhealthy.

Of course, the class of conditions that supports this kind of inference is only a fraction of the domain of standard clinical theory. Even some psychotic people, as well as the great mass of those with neuroses and character disorders, function successfully at the minimal level required for basic biological goals. Since different cultures achieve these goals by an astonishing variety of life-styles anyway, any further defence of established clinical categories seems to require some specific functional assumptions about the mind.

One should not underestimate the mileage that can be got out of elementary functional assumptions that are scarcely controversial. We may surely assume, for example, that the main function of perceptual and intellectual processes is to give us knowledge of the world. The imperfection of this cognitive apparatus is obvious. Since there are limits both to human intelligence and to the evidence on which it works, it would be wrong to suppose that every false belief is a functional abnormality. Nevertheless, one could plausibly suggest that the perceptions and beliefs of a healthy mind must at least show, in Jahoda's words, "relative freedom from need-distortion" (1958, 51). That is, if my cognitive functions are disrupted to a highly unusual degree by my wishes, it seems safe to call my condition an unnatural dysfunction, i.e. a disease. By this standard schizophrenia and all other psychoses with thought disorders look objectively unhealthy. Moreover, if one accepts the traditional analytic description of the neurotic process, very limited functional assumptions will suffice to construe serious neurosis as a disease. Since opposite desires are common in human beings, there must be some normal mechanism for resolving them without permanent and paralysing conflict. If some of the neurotic's strongest desires remain locked in combat without freely releasing their motivational force in behaviour, it is not an implausible hypothesis that the conflict-resolution mechanism is functioning incorrectly.

These arguments show that some elementary functional claims about the species, together with a small body of widely accepted descriptive information about the mental processes of psychotics and neurotics, may give good grounds for provisionally calling these conditions pathological. Any stronger vindication of current clinical categories would require a detailed and well-confirmed theory of the functions of a normal human mind. But a further reason for clinical professionals to cast their lot with mental health is that a well-developed example of the right kind of theory is already in the field. Formally speaking, psychoanalytic theory is the best account of mental health we have. It closely follows the physiological model by positing three mental substructures, the id, ego, and superego, and assigning fixed functions to each. It is not entirely clear that the mental functions psychoanalysts describe are functions in the biological sense. One sometimes has the impression in psychoanalytic writing that the function of a mental process is the gratification it can secure for the id.[14] From the biological standpoint, the function of a mental process is its contribution, not to our pleasure, but to our behaviour; pleasure itself has a function in producing behaviour. But it would not be difficult to construe psychoanalytic theory as a set of theses about biological functions of the mind. On this view the id might emerge as a reservoir of motivation, the ego as an instrument of rational integration and cognitive competence, and the superego as a device for socialization.[15] One could then give a straight-forward argument that neurosis is disease by appealing to its disturbance of the integrative and motivational functions of the ego and the id. In any case, it is this sort of structural detail that is necessary to raise claims about psychopathology above the level of plausible conjecture.

I am recommending psychoanalytic theory as our best model, apart from physiology, of what a theory of mental health should be. Hence I will also mention a recurrent failure in its exposition. This is the uncritical assumption that neurosis is always unhealthy. Freud was willing to call religion a "universal neurosis" (1927, p. 44). It is also often suggested that a mild childhood neurosis is a typical developmental stage. This evidence does not lead psychoanalytic writers to abandon the assumption. For example, Hartmann writes:

> Typical conflicts are a part and parcel of "normal" development, and disturbances in adaptation are included in its scope. . . . Here health clearly includes pathological reactions as a means to its attainment.[16]

Although I am not sure what Hartmann means here, it is hard to imagine how a standard developmental stage can be pathological. The normal functional organization for an organism is always relative to its age. If the functional organization of children of a certain age includes neurotic conflict, the correct conclusion is that neurosis is not always unhealthy. In general, according to the analysis I gave at the outset, a nearly universal condition can be unhealthy only if it can be viewed as an environmental injury. It is just possible that Freud had environmental injuries in mind when he said that "a normal ego . . . is, like normality in general, an ideal fiction" (1937, p. 235). But it seems more likely that he was employing the same rigorous standard Ernest Jones uses as a definition of health: "the fullest possible development of the organism" (1932, p. 80).

What these quotations reveal is a clear tendency among psychoanalytic writers to make of the concept of health something more grandiose than it is in physical medicine. To have a healthy heart or biceps, I need not subject them to their fullest possible development. Health never requires ideal functioning, but only the functioning of each part at a species-normal level unimpeded by atypical or environmentally induced obstructions. Apart from the trivial injuries of a hostile environment, a normal biceps is far from an "ideal function." Along with many other writers, some psychoanalytic theorists are confusing the healthy personality with the *ideal* personality—a much more demanding goal—and presenting their notions of "vital perfection" (Hartmann, 1964, p. 5) or the good life for man as if they were norms of health. It would be better to admit that what is undesirable, including neurosis, is not necessarily pathological. If it standardly happens that the child ego is presented with impulses it is too immature to master, that is surely a design defect in the species rather than a disease. How strong or lasting a neurotic process must be to be a disease is a question I cannot discuss here. But it seems evident that psychoanalysts could prevent considerable misunderstanding by avoiding such claims as that "we have no experience of a completely normal mind" (Jones, 1932, p. 81), when what is meant is that we have no experience of a completely non-neurotic mind or a mind subjected to its fullest possible development. The hypothesis that neurosis is always abnormal seems to be contradicted by psychoanalytic doctrine itself.[17]

Although it seems to me a model theory in its broad outlines, psycho-analysis is far from general acceptance. Hence I wish to make one final point in defence of the continued relevance of the mental-health concept. Jahoda's milestone survey (1958) of criteria of mental health in current clinical practice reveals a bewildering variety of proposals. This is not surprising, if only because the human mind has a bewildering variety of tasks and abilities. To mention each criterion and assess the likelihood that it objectively describes the human personality design would require lengthy discussion. But it is striking how many of Jahoda's criteria could be subsumed, with some plausibility, under the heading of *maturity*. It is an empirical fact that the usual course of human development shows a growth in knowledge of self and world, informed self-acceptance and sense of identity, unification of life goals, tolerance for stress and frustration, autonomy of thought and action, and various kinds of environmental mastery. At any rate, adults tend to have more of these qual-ities than children. To whatever extent the increase in these traits can be shown part of a normal developmental sequence, it is correct to call them requirements of health in an adult. Freud is sometimes accused of confusing morals with medicine in taking his "genital type" to be a health ideal.[18] I have just suggested that this confusion is not unknown among psychoanalysts, but the mere idea of a developmental disease, i.e. arrest or retardation of normal growth, is not a case of it. What is controversial is that Freud's oral, anal, phallic, and genital stages are a genuine series of normal stages of develop-ment. It is not controversial that a failure to traverse normal stages is unhealthy.

This point should scarcely be seen as a full vindication of the various cri-teria just mentioned. Considerable argument would be required to show that the emergence of, say, accurate self-knowledge is objectively a feature of nor-mal human growth in the same way as permanent teeth or secondary sex char-acteristics. As recent controversy over Piagetian theory illustrates, the notion of a developmental stage is itself in need of detailed analysis. Furthermore, the bare observation that most adults have more self-knowledge than children does not show how much self-knowledge, or of what kind, is a necessary condition of objective maturity. At most, the correlation between existing mental-health criteria and observable maturity provides some evidence that these criteria would remain in a theory free of the methodological deficiencies discussed in section II.

Thus I continue to maintain that the methods used by most theorists of "mental health" are essentially indefensible. Psychiatrists and psychologists who employ the notion of health must swallow what for some will be a bitter pill. Apart from a theory of the structure and functions of the human mind, virtually all assertions about mental health are either misuses of language or flatly conjectural. It is true that many of the disorders traditionally recognized in clinical theory, e.g. psychoses and serious neuroses, seem likely to be mental diseases in the literal sense. What this means is simply that past confusion about the health concept may not have led clinicians too wide of the mark in practice. But the time has now arrived when the clinical disciplines face a parting of the ways. With Szasz and the behaviourists, they may decide that mental health is not what they are interested in after all and adopt something else, e.g. happiness or social adjustment, as their official aim. Alternatively, they may retain the concepts of health and disease and pursue substantive theories of mental functioning of the psychoanalytic variety.[19] I have tried in this essay to clarify the choice, and to argue that the second option deserves serious inquiry.

NOTES

Support from the Delaware Institute for Medical Education and Research and the National Institute of Mental Health (grant RO₃ MH 24621) is gratefully acknowledged.

1. Critics of the "medical model" have some very different interpretations of it (Macklin, 1973). It may or may not be thought to include any of the following assumptions: that individual therapy is the best mode of treatment; that all treatment should be done by physicians; that drugs are better than psychotherapy; that there are classical disease entities in psychology; and that all mental diseases are physical diseases. Interestingly, none of these five theses entails any of the others. In this essay I defend only the basic view that the idea of mental health is coherent and clinically useful.

Apropos of the second of the five listed theses, I should also say that I have longed in vain for a brief term covering all mental-health professionals at once: psychiatrists, clinical psychologists, social workers, counsellors, etc. Specific terms like "psychiatric" in the text are usually a stylistic convenience with no disciplinary implications.

2. This summary includes the main features of the analysis in my forthcoming essay "Health as a theoretical concept." It omits a number of details that also have repercussions for mental health. Further defence of a functional analysis of health in physiology, as well as of the thesis that physiological medicine should be viewed as the paradigm health discipline, can be found in Flew (1973).

3. For the second question, cf. Boorse (1975). The distinction between disease and illness there argued for is one feature that separates my position from that of Flew (1973). I take the term "disease" to be a technical term belonging to medical theory, and I use it in the textbook sense to cover any and all unhealthy conditions. This broad usage should be kept in mind below in the discussion of mental diseases. In my view "illness" belongs instead with the institutions of medical practice; hence the analysis just given aims to capture a sort of professionalized ordinary usage.

4. See, for example, Freud (1915), p. 175: "Our psychical topography has *for the present* nothing to do with anatomy; it has reference not to anatomical localities, but to regions in the mental apparatus, wherever they may be situated in the body" (italics original). Holt (1965) has an illuminating critical discussion of Freud's physiological presuppositions.

5. Putnam (1960) defends the view that mental states are functional states. Davidson (1966) argues for an ontology of event-particulars and applies it to mental events (1970). A connected account of functionalism can also be found in Fodor (1968, ch. 3). The term "functionalism" itself

is perhaps uniquely unfortunate for present purposes. It is the mathematical sense of "function" that seems suggested by Putnam's original discussion; but Fodor's automotive examples allow an alternative interpretation in terms of contributions to goals. Without pursuing this conceptual tangle any further, let me simply state that my claim that mental states have biological functions is entirely independent of the functionalist solution to the mind-body problem.

6. For convenience I ignore the distinction in Smart (1959) between a desire and the having of a desire.

7. Usage of "mental illness" does not invariably conform to this description. But if physical diseases can have mental symptoms, it is hard to imagine any other basis for distinguishing mental from physical health besides the contrast between mental and physical aetiology. On any account the specialty of psychiatry, as defined by its textbooks, includes some physical diseases, e.g. brain syndromes due to infections, tumours, or alcohol poisoning. It is also worth noting that the scope of "mental disease" may vary according to one's conception of the mark of the mental.

8. Some endorsements of this view by clinicians and by philosophers are quoted and discussed in Boorse (1975).

9. Concerning the prevalence of the normative route to mental-health criteria, Wootton writes: "It must, however, be admitted that most of the current definitions of mental health . . . with their visions of 'inner harmonious adjustment,' of 'trustfulness' and of 'socially considerate behavior' — not to mention happy family life, successful sex adjustment, training for citizenship, economic independence and freedom from industrial unrest — most of them are clearly attempts to formulate conceptions of the ideal, under the guise of the healthy, man. They express the personal value-judgments of their authors, rather than scientifically established facts . . ." (1959, 216).

10. Howard and Patry, quoted by Wootton (1959), p. 214.

11. This is a summary by Mowrer (1948) of Alfred Adler's (1939) position. It seems fairly accurate, except for being more specific than any of Adler's own formulations. It is possible that Adler's views should be represented as derived by the second method discussed below, the abstraction route, rather than by pure evaluation.

12. This point is eloquently argued by Szasz (1961); see also Schofield (1964, pp. 22–3).

13. Wootton (1959), p. 218. London (1969) also has a perceptive discussion of the adjustment ideal.

14. Cf. Alexander (1953): "The function of the ego consists in finding ways and means for the gratification of the subjective needs by adequate behavior."

15. Hallowell (1965), an evolutionary biologist, gives an interesting treatment of ego and superego functions in the cultural context. It has become commonplace to draw a sharp distinction between biology and culture on the grounds that culture is not genetically inherited. This difference should not obscure the fact that cultural environments play a role in natural selection. Because of this effect, the psychological endowments that allow individuals to succeed within cultures are a biological phenomenon.

16. Hartmann (1964), p. 7. Further discussion of the healthiness of unconscious conflict occurs in the responses to Redlich and Hartmann by Kubie (1954).

17. In connection with these issues, cf. Eidelberg (1968, p. 273): "From a practical point of view, most analysts agree that an individual who is able to love, to be loved, and to work may be considered normal. While it is true that the presence of repressed infantile wishes interferes with mental health, the decisive factor in determining whether an individual is normal and healthy is the quantitative evaluation of the blocked, repressed mental energy." What I suggest is that something like this out to be true of theoretical as well as practical health on the psychoanalytic model. Some discussion of more demanding accounts of health than the functional view I defend is contained in my "Health as a theoretical concept" (forthcoming).

18. Margolis (1966, pp 75 ff); see also Macklin (1972, p. 354).

19. Family therapists often adopt a position that seems to fall between these two options. This position retains the concepts of health and disorder but applies them to the family instead of to the individual. Families are called healthy or disturbed in a sense held not to be reducible to the individual health of their members. It is interesting that from the biological standpoint for which I

have argued, there is no difficulty in viewing a family as a functionally organized unit in its own right. The idea is as old as Darwin. But apart from all objections to such a significant alteration in the health concept as application to a group entails, it seems unlikely that family therapists would find the biological approach congenial. It would appear that their use of the family as a unit reflects simply a conviction about therapeutic strategy, together with some distaste for traditional depth psychology. Source material on family therapy may be found in Sager & Kaplan (1972).

REFERENCES

Adler, A. (1939). *Social Interest: A Challenge to Mankind.* Trans. Linton and Vaughan. New York: G. P. Putnam's Sons.

Alexander, F. (1953). 'The therapeutic applications of psychoanalysis.' In Roy Grinker, ed., *Mid-Century Psychiatry* (Springfield, Ill.: Charles C. Thomas, 1953).

Boorse, C. 'Health as a theoretical concept.' Forthcoming.

Boorse, C. (1975). 'On the distinction between disease and illness.' *Philosophy and Public Affairs,* Fall 1975.

Davidson, D. (1963). 'Actions, reasons, and causes.' *The Journal of Philosophy* 60, 685–700.

Davidson, D. (1966). 'The logical form of action sentences.' In Nicholas Rescher, ed., *The Logic of Decision and Action* (Pittsburgh: University of Pittsburgh Press).

Davidson, D. (1970). 'Mental events.' In Lawrence Foster and J. W. Swanson, eds., *Experience and Theory* (Amherst: University of Massachusetts Press), pp. 79–101.

Eidelberg, L., ed. (1968). *Encyclopedia of Psychoanalysis.* New York: The Free Press.

Flew, A. (1973). *Crime or Disease?* New York: Barnes and Noble.

Fodor, J. A. (1968). *Psychological Explanation.* New York: Random House.

Freud, S. (1915). 'The Unconscious.' In James Strachey, ed., *The Standard Edition of the Complete Psychological Works of Sigmund Freud.* (London: The Hogarth Press, 1961), vol. 14, pp. 166–215.

Freud, S. (1927). *The Future of an Illusion.* In Strachey, vol. 21, pp. 5–56.

Freud, S. (1936). *Analysis Terminable and Interminable.* In Strachey, vol. 23, pp. 216–53.

Hallowell, A. I. (1965). 'Hominid evolution and culture.' In de Reuck and Porter, eds., *Transcultural Psychiatry* (Boston: Little, Brown, 1965).

Hartmann, H. (1939). 'Psychoanalysis and the concept of health.' In *Essays on Ego Psychology* (New York: International Universities Press, 1964), pp. 1–18.

Hempel, C. G. (1965). *Aspects of Scientific Explanation and Other Essays in the Philosophy of Science.* New York: The Free Press.

Holt, R. R. (1965). 'A review of some of Freud's biological assumptions and their influence on his theories.' In Norman S. Greenfield and William C. Lewis, eds., *Psychoanalysis and Current Biological Thought* (Madison, Wisc.: University of Wisconsin Press, 1965), pp. 93–124.

Jahoda, M. (1958). *Current Concepts of Positive Mental Health.* New York: Basic Books.

Jones, E. (1932). 'The concept of a normal mind.' In Samuel D. Schmalhausen, ed., *Our Neurotic Age* (New York: Farrar and Rinehart, 1932), pp. 65–81.

Kubie, L. (1954). 'The fundamental nature of the distinction between normality and neurosis.' *Psychoanalytic Quarterly* 23, 167–204, including discussion by Redlich and Hartmann.

London, P. (1969). 'Morals and mental health.' In Stanley C. Plog and Robert B. Edgerton, eds. *Changing Perspectives in Mental Illness* (New York: Holt, Rinehart and Winston, 1969), pp. 32–48.

Macklin, R. (1972). 'Mental health and mental illness: some problems of definition and concept formation.' *Philosophy of Science,* 39, 341–65.

Macklin, R. (1973). 'The medical model in psychoanalysis and psychotherapy.' *Comprehensive Psychiatry* 14, 49–69.

Margolis, J. (1966). *Psychotherapy and Morality.* New York: Random House.

Menninger, K. A. (1930). *The Human Mind.* New York: Knopf.

Montagu, M. F. A., ed. (1962). *Culture and the Evolution of Man.* New York: Oxford University Press.

Mowrer, O. H. (1948). 'What is normal behavior?' In L. A. Pennington and Irwin A. Berg, eds., *An Introduction to Clinical Psychology* (New York: Ronald, 1948). Omitted from later editions.

Putnam, H. (1960). 'Minds and machines.' In Sidney Hook, ed., *Dimensions of Mind* (New York: New York University Press, 1960), pp. 138–64.

Redlich, F. C. & Freedman, D. X. (1966). *The Theory and Practice of Psychiatry.* New York: Basic Books.

Roe, A. & Simpson, G. G., eds. (1958). *Behavior and Evolution.* New Haven: Yale University Press.

Sager, C. J. & Kaplan, H. S. (1972). *Progress in Group and Family Therapy.* New York: Brunner-Mazel.

Sarbin, T. (1967). 'On the futility of the proposition that some people be labeled "mentally ill".' *Journal of Consulting Psychology* 31, 447–53.

Sarbin, T. (1969). 'The scientific status of the mental illness metaphor.' In Stanley C. Plog and Robert B. Edgerton, eds., *Changing Perspectives in Mental Illness* (New York: Holt, Rinehart and Winston, 1969), pp. 9–31.

Schofield, W. (1964). *Psychotherapy: The Purchase of Friendship.* Englewood Cliffs, N.J.: Prentice-Hall.

Smart, J. J. C. (1959). 'Sensations and brain processes.' *The Philosophical Review* 68, 141–56.

Stoller, R. J., et al. (1973). 'A symposium: should homosexuality be in the APA nomenclature?' *American Journal of Psychiatry* 130: 1270–16.

Szasz, T. S. (1961). *The Myth of Mental Illness.* New York: Hoeber-Harper.

Szasz, T. S. (1963). *Law, Liberty, and Psychiatry.* New York: Macmillan.

Szasz, T. S. (1970a). *Ideology and Insanity.* Garden City, N.Y.: Doubleday.

Szasz, T. S. (1970b). *The Manufacture of Madness.* New York: Harper and Row.

Ullmann, L. P. & Krasner, L. (1966). *Case Studies in Behavior Modification.* New York: Holt, Rinehart and Winston.

Wootton, B. (1959). *Social Science and Social Pathology.* London: George Allen and Unwin.

Peter Sedgwick

Illness — Mental and Otherwise

What Is "Illness"?

What, then, is "illness"? It will be recalled that critical theory in psychiatry has tended to postulate a fundamental separation between mental illnesses and the general run of human ailments: the former are the expression of social norms, the latter proceed from ascertainable bodily states which have an "objective" existence within the individual. One critic of psychopathological concepts, Barbara Wootton, has suggested that the expurgation of normative references from psychiatry is at least a theoretical ideal, though one immensely difficult of achievement:

> . . . anti-social behavior is the precipitating factor that leads to mental treatment. But at the same time the fact of the illness is itself inferred from the behavior. . . . But any disease, the morbidity of which is established only by the social failure that it involves, must rank as fundamentally different from those of which the symptoms are independent of the social norms . . . long indeed is the road to be travelled before we can hope to reach a definition of mental-cum-physical health which is objective, scientific, and wholly free of social value judgments and before we shall be able, consistently and without qualification, to treat mental and physical disorders on exactly the same footing.[1]

Wootton's view has stimulated at least one attempt to begin the task of purging all cultural norms — with their inconvenient variability from one society to

From Peter Sedgwick, *Psycho Politics* (Harper & Row, 1982), pp. 28–42, by permission of the publisher and the author. Originally published in Hastings Center Studies 1:3 (1973).

another—from the diagnosis of mental illness: Dr. Joseph Zubin has reported some work on "culture-free" assessments of schizophrenia which involve the analysis of reaction-times, responses to electrical stimulation, and the like, among schizophrenic patients.[2] It would be fair to say that research in the refinement of psychiatric categories has been mounted with a similar perspective in mind, straining towards the physical-medicine ideal of a set of symptom-descriptions "independent of the social norms." Value-judgments and cultural stereotypes are seen as one form of "error" coming between the investigator and his desired data, and the ultimate standard sought in the description of illness is taken to be a socially inert, culturally sterile specification of facts and processes which are grounded in the bacteriology, bio-chemistry, physiology or perhaps some variety of cybernetic systems-theory.

But this enterprise, tending constantly towards the microscopic and molecular analysis of the "objective" substrate of behavior, forms only one of the ways in which we might begin to place mental and physical illnesses "on exactly the same footing." If we examine the logical structure of our judgments of illness (whether "physical" or "mental") it may prove possible to reduce the distance between psychiatry and other streams of medicine by working in the reverse direction to Wootton: not by annexing psychopathology to the technical instrumentation of the natural sciences but by revealing the character of illness and disease, health and treatment, as social constructions. For social constructions they most certainly are. All departments of nature below the level of mankind are exempt both from disease and from treatment—until man intervenes with his own human classifications of disease and treatment. The blight that strikes at corn or at potatoes is a *human intervention,* for if man wished to cultivate parasites (rather than potatoes or corn) there would be no "blight," but simply the necessary foddering of the parasite-crop. Animals do not have diseases either, prior to the presence of man in a meaningful relation with them. A tiger may experience pain or feebleness from a variety of causes (we do not intend to build our case on the supposition that animals, especially higher animals, cannot have experiences or feelings). It may be infected by a germ, trodden by an elephant, scratched by another tiger, or subjected to the aging processes of its own cells. It does not present itself as being *ill* (though it may present itself as being highly distressed or uncomfortable) except in the eyes of a human observer who can discriminate illness from other sources of pain or enfeeblement. Outside the significances that man voluntarily attaches to certain conditions, *there are no illnesses or diseases in nature.* We are nowadays so heavily indoctrinated with deriving from the technical medical discoveries of the last century-and-a-half that we are tempted to think that nature does contain diseases. Just as the sophisticated New Yorker classes the excrement of dogs and cats as one more form of "pollution" ruining the pre-established harmony of pavements and gardens, so does modern technologized man perceive nature to be mined and infested with all kinds of specifically morbid entities and agencies. What, he will protest, are there no diseases in nature? Are there not infectious and contagious bacilli? Are there not definite and objective lesions in the cellular structures of the human body? Are there not fractures of bones, the fatal ruptures of tissues, the malignant multiplications of tumorous growths? Are not these, surely, events of nature? Yet these, as natural events, do not—prior to the human social meanings we attach to them—constitute illnesses, sicknesses, or diseases. The fracture of a septuagenarian's femur has, within the world of nature, no more significance than the snapping of an autumn leaf from its twig: and the invasion of a human organism by cholera-germs carries with it no more the stamp of "illness" than does the souring of milk by other forms of bacteria.[3] Human beings, like all other naturally occurring structures are characterized by a variety of inbuilt limitations or liabilities, any of which may (given the presence of further stressful circumstances) lead to the weakening or the collapse of the organism. Mountains as well as moles, stars as well as shrubs, protozoa no less than persons have their dates of expiry set in advance, over a time-span which varies greatly over different classes of structure but which is usually at least roughly predictable. Out of his anthropocentric self-interest, man has chosen to consider as "illnesses" or "diseases" those natural circumstances which precipitate the death (or the failure to function according to certain values) of a limited number of biological species: man himself, his pets and other cherished livestock, and the plant-varieties he cultivates for gain or pleasure. Around these select areas of structural failure man creates, in proportion to the progress of his technology, specialized combat-institutions for the control and cure of "disease": the different branches of the medical and nursing profession, veterinary doctors, and the botanical specialists in plant-disease. Despite their common use of experimental natural science, these institutions operate according to very different criteria and codes; the use of euthanasia by vets, and of ruthless eugenic policies by plant-pathologists, departs from most current medical practice with human patients. All the same, the fact that these specialisms share the categories of disease and illness indicates the selective quality of our perceptions in this field. Children and cattle may fall ill, have diseases, and seem as sick; but who has ever imagined that spiders or lizards can be sick or diseased? Plant-diseases may strike at tulips, turnips, or such prized features of the natural landscape as elm trees: but if some plant-species in which man had no interest (a desert grass, let us say) were to be attacked by a fungus or parasite, we should speak not of a disease, but merely of the competition between two species. The medical enterprise is from its inception value-loaded; it is not simply an applied biology, but a biology applied in accordance with the dictates of social interest.

It could be argued that the discussion of animal and plant pathology deals in cases that are too marginal to our central concepts of health and illness to form a satisfactory basis for analysis. Such marginal instances are of course frequently used by logicians in the analysis of concepts since their peripheral character often usefully tests the limits within which our ideas can be seen to be applicable or inapplicable. However, a careful examination of the concept of illness in man himself will reveal the same value-impregnation, the same dependency of apparently descriptive, natural-scientific notions upon our norms of what is desirable. To complain of illness, or to ascribe illness to another person, is not to make a descriptive statement about physiology or anatomy. Concepts of illness were in use among men for centuries before the advent of any reliable knowledge of the human body, and are still employed today within societies which favor a nonphysiological (magical or religious) account of the nature of human maladies. Our own classification and explanation of specific illnesses or diseases is of course tremendously different from the categories that are current in earlier ages or in contemporary tribal societies, but it is implausible to suppose that the state of illness itself has no common logical features over different types of society. Homer's sick warriors were tended by magical incantations as well as by herbs and other primitive technical remedies, but the avowal and ascription of illness in Homer does not set up a distance between his characters and ourselves but rather (like his descriptions of bereavement or of sexual attraction) a powerful resonance across the ages.[4] Similarly, the meaning of illness among primitive peoples is usually sufficiently close to our own to enable them to take advantage of modern medical facilities when these are made accessible within their territories: tribesmen and peasants do not have to be indoctrinated into Western physiological concepts before they can accept help from physicians and nurses trained in advanced societies. Sickness and disease may be conceptualized, in different cultures, as originating within bodily states, or within perturbations of the spirit, or as a mixture of both. Yet there appears to be common features in the declaration or attribution of the sick state, regardless of the causal explanation that is invoked.

Valuation & Explanation

All sickness is essentially deviancy. That is to say, no attribution of sickness to any being can be made without the expectation of some alternative state of affairs which is considered more desirable. In the absence of this normative alternative, the presence of a particular bodily or subjective state will not in itself lead to an attribution of illness. Thus, where an entire community is by Western standards "ill," because it has been infected for generations by parasites which diminish energy, illness will not be recognized in any individual except by outsiders.[5] The Rockefeller Sanitary Commission on Hookworm found in 1911 that this disease was regarded as part of normal health in some areas of North Africa.[6] And in one South American Indian tribe the disease of dyschromic spirochetosis, which is marked by the appearance of colored spots on the skin, was so "normal" that those who did not have them were regarded as pathological and excluded from marriage.[7] Even within modern urbanized nations we cannot assume that aches, pains and other discomforts are uniformly categorized as signs of illness among all sections of the community. Although little work has been done on social-class variations in the construction of what constitutes "health" and "sickness,"[8] the example of tooth-decay is suggestive: among millions of British working-class families, it is taken for granted that children will lose their teeth and require artificial dentures. The process of tooth-loss is not seen as a disease but as something like an act of fate. Among dentists, on the other hand, and in those more-educated sections of the community who are socialized into dental ideology, the loss of teeth arises through a definite disease-process known as caries, whose aetiology is established.[9] Social and cultural norms also plainly govern the varying perception, either as essentially "normal," or as essentially "pathological," of such characteristics as baldness, obesity, infestation by lice, venereal infection, and the presence of tonsils and foreskins among children.

Once again it can be argued that these cultural variations apply only to marginal cases of sickness and health, that there are some physical or psychological conditions which are *ipso facto* symptomatic of illness, whether among Bushmen or Brobdignagians, duchesses or dockworkers. But there is no reason to believe that the "standardized" varieties of human pathology operate according to a different logic from the "culturally dependent" varieties. The existence of common or even universal illnesses testifies, not to the absence of a normative framework for judging pathology, but to the presence of very wide-spread norms. To be ill, after all, is not the same thing as to feel pain, or to experience weaknesses, or to fail to manifest this or that kind of behavior. Rather it is to experience discomfort (or to manifest behavioral failure) in a context of a particular kind. Consider the imaginary conversations between physician and client:

(a) *Client*: Doctor, I want you to examine me, I keep feeling terrible pains in my right shoulder.
Doctor: Really? What are they like?
Client: Stabbing and intense.
Doctor: How often do they happen?
Client: Every evening after I get home from work.
Doctor: Always in the same spot?
Client: Yes, just in the place where my wife hits me with the rolling-pin.
(b) *Client*: (Telephoning Doctor). Doctor, I haven't consulted you before but things are getting desperate. I'm feeling so weak, I can't lift anything heavy.
Doctor: Goodness, when does this come on you?
Client: Every time I try to lift something or make an effort. I have to walk quite slowly up the stairs and last night when I was packing the big suitcase I found I couldn't lift it off the bed.
Doctor: Well, let's have some details about you before you come in. Name?
Client: John Smith.
Doctor: Age?
Client: Ninety-two last February.

In the first example, the "patient's" pain is not an illness because we expect pain as a normal response to being hit in tender places; indeed, if he did *not* feel pain when he was hit or prodded he would be taken to be suffering from some disease involving nerve-degeneration. In the second example, the patient's infirmity would usually be ascribed not to the category of "illness" but to that of "aging." (If he had given his age as "twenty-two" the case would be different.) In our culture we expect old people to find difficulty in lifting heavy weights, although it is easy to conceive of a culture in which mass rejuvenation among the aged had been perfected (perhaps by the injection of hormones, vitamins or other pep-pills into the water-supply) and where, in consequence, a dialogue of the type recounted would lead to a perfectly ordinary referral for medical treatment. The attribution of illness always proceeds from the computation of a gap between presented behavior (or feeling) and some social norm. In practice of course we take the norm for granted, so that the broken arm or the elevated temperature is seen alone as the illness. But the broken arm would be no more of an illness than a broken fingernail unless it stopped us from achieving certain socially constructed goals; just as, if we could all function according to approved social requirements within any range of body-temperature, thermometers would disappear from the household medical kit.

This is not to say that illness amounts to any deviancy whatsoever from social expectations about how men should function. Some deviancies are regarded as instances not of sickness but of criminality, wickedness, poor upbringing or bad manners (though not all cultures do in fact draw a firm line between illness and these other deviations, e.g., primitive societies for whom illness is also a moral flaw and modern liberal circles for whom drug-addiction is categorized in medical as well as moral terms). Looking over the very wide range of folk-concepts and technical ideas about illness which exist in the history of human societies, one finds it difficult to discern a common structural element which distinguishes the notion of illness from other attributions of social failure. Provisionally, it is possible to suggest that illness is set apart from other deviances insofar as the description (or, at a deeper level, the explanation) of the sick state is located within a relatively restricted set of causal factors operating within the boundaries of the individual human being. One may become ill as the result of being infected by germs, or through being centered by evil demons, or visited by a curse from the Almighty. Each culturally specific account of illness must involve a theory of the person, of the boundaries between the person and the world "outside" him, and of the ways in which adverse influences can trespass over these limits and besiege or grip him. If the current theory of the person is positivistic and physical, the agencies of illness will be seen as arising from factors within (or at the boundaries of) his body; in cultures with an animistic tradition, the invasion will be one of the spirit or soul. But, however variously the nature of illness is specified from culture to culture, the attribution of illness appears to include a *quest for explanation,* or at least the descriptive delimiting of certain types of causal factor, as well as the normative component outlined above. It is indeed likely that the concept of illness has arisen in close parallel with the social practice of therapy, i.e., with the development of techniques to control those human afflictions which can be controlled at the boundaries of the individual person. It is hard to see how the category of illness, as a distinct construction separate from other kinds of misfortune, could have arisen without the discovery that some varieties of pain and affliction could be succored through individual specialized attention to the afflicted person. In traditional societies, of course, the institution of medicine is not crystallized out as an applied branch of natural science: "Therapy" for the Greeks was simply the word used for looking after or tending somebody, and, in Greece as well as elsewhere, a great deal of therapy goes on either in the patient's household or in conjunction with religious and magical specialisms. A specifically "medical" framework of treatment is not necessary to provide the link between illness and practical action.

Practice and concept continue their mutual modification over the ages. In a society where the treatment of the sick is still conducted through religious ritual, the notion of illness will not be entirely distinct from the notion of sinfulness or pollution. Correspondingly, with the growth of progressively more technical and more autonomous specialisms of therapy, the concepts of disease and illness themselves become more technical, and thereby more alienated from their implicit normative background. Thus we teach the position of the present day where any characterization of an "illness" which is not amenable to a diagnosis drawn from physiology or to a therapy based on chemical, electrical, or surgical technique becomes suspect as not constituting, perhaps, an illness at all. Such has been the fate of mental illness in our own epoch. It has been much easier for societies with an animistic theory of the person (and of his boundaries and susceptibilities to influence) to view mental disturbances on a par with bodily ailments. Ceremonies of ritual purgation and demon-expulsion, along with primitive "medical" methods of a herbal or surgical type, are used indifferently by traditional healers on patients with a mental or with a bodily dysfunction. Fever and madness, the broken limb or the broken spirit are situated within the same normative frame, within the same explanatory and therapeutic system. Even the development of a technical-physiological specialism of medicine, such as emerged with the Hippocratic tradition which runs in fits and starts from antiquity to modern times, does not impair the possibility of a unitary perspective on physical and mental illness, *so long as a common structure of valuation and explanation applies over the whole range of disorders of the person*. The medicine of the seventeenth and eighteenth centuries in Western Europe, for instance, was able to interpret our present-day "mental" disorders as a group of illnesses inhabiting the embodied person on much the same plane as other sorts of malady: the insane or the emotionally disturbed patient was suffering from a fault of "the vapors," "the nerves," "the fluids," "the animal spirits," "the spleen," "the humors," "the head," or the forces and qualities of the body.[10] This unitary integration of human illnesses was of course only achieved at the cost of a stupendously inaccurate and speculative physiology. But an integrated theory of illness, whether achieved within a unitary-animistic or a unitary-physicalistic doctrine of the person, has one singular advantage over a more fragmentary perspective: it is not beset by the kind of crisis we now have in psychotherapy and psychiatry, whose conceptual and moral foundation has been exploded now that "illness" has acquired a technical-physical definition excluding disorders of the whole person from its purview. Animistic and unitary-physicalistic accounts of illness both dealt in the whole embodied individual, but the medical technology of the nineteenth century and onwards has succeeded in classifying illnesses as particular states of the body only. Psychiatry is left with two seeming alternatives: either to say that personal, psychological, and emotional disorders are really states of the body, objective features of the brain-tissue, the organism-under-stress, the genes or what have you; or else to deny that such disorders are illnesses at all. If the latter, then the way is open to treat mental illnesses as the expression of social value-judgments about the patient, and psychiatry's role will not belong to the disciplines of objective, body-state medicine. Instead, it will be analogous to the value-laden and non-medical disciplines of moral education, police interrogation, criminal punishment or religion (depending on how low or how lofty a view one takes of the values inherent in psychiatric practice).

This dilemma will perhaps seem somewhat to dissolve if we recapitulate what was previously said about the nature of illness as a social construction. *All* illness, whether conceived in localized bodily terms or within a larger view of human functioning, expresses both a social value-judgment (contrasting a person's condition with certain understood and accepted norms) and an attempt at explanation (with a view to controlling the disvalued condition). The physicalistic psychiatrists are wrong in their belief that they can find objective disease-entities representing the psychopathological analogues to diabetes, tuberculosis, and post-syphilitic paresis. Quite correctly, the anti-psychiatrists have pointed out that psychopathological categories refer to value-judgments and that mental illness is deviancy. On the other hand, the anti-psychiatric critics themselves are wrong when they imagine physical medicine to be essentially different in its logic from psychiatry. A diagnosis of diabetes, or paresis, includes the recognition of norms or values. Anti-psychiatry can only operate by positing a mechanical and inaccurate model of physical illness and its medical diagnosis.

In my own judgment, then, mental illnesses can be conceptualized just as easily within the disease framework as physical maladies such as lumbago or TB.

The Future of Illness

There are several misunderstandings that might arise, or indeed have arisen, from my declarations of this position: let me try to remove these misapprehensions at once. In the first place, it does not follow from my statement that the existing "official" diagnostic categories of mental illness are the most useful or truthful ones that we can reach. I believe, for example, that "psychopathy" represents no more than an attempt at social labelling, for control purposes, by psychiatrists working in tandem with the judicial authorities. It is likely, also, that "schizophrenia" is a pretty useless dustbin category for a variety of psychic ills which have little logically or biologically in common with one another. Equally, though, I have no doubt that many current diagnostic categories in physical medicine will disappear in the next century or so, and be replaced by others apparently (and provisionally) more adequate. I can see that, for example, by the year 2072 nobody will be classed as having diabetes or asthma, though they will undergo feelings of discomfort similar to those experienced by present-day diabetics and asthmatics. In the future development of our species, we can anticipate *either* that some conditions now classified as illnesses will be re-allocated to a different framework of deviancy (or, more drastically, become regarded as essentially normal and non-deviant), *or* that, on the contrary, conditions which are nowadays viewed in a non-illness category of deviancy (as sins, perhaps, or as consequences of aging or excessive effort) will be re-grouped into the range of the illnesses or diseases. The latter prospect — the progressive annexation of not-illness into illness — seems at the moment much more likely to happen than the former, especially since the stupendous achievements of medical technology make it more and more difficult for doctors to sign death certificates under the rubric "died of natural causes." The natural causes of death are becoming, more and more, causes that we can control: so that the terminally ill, and their relatives, will be putting strong pressures on the medical profession to redefine the natural (and inevitable) causes of fatality, rendering them into medical (and hence controllable) pathologies which require the services of a doctor rather than of a mortician. *The future belongs to illness*: we just are going to get more and more diseases, since our expectations of health are going to become more expansive and sophisticated. Maybe one day there will be a backlash, perhaps at the point when everybody has become so luxuriantly ill, physically or mentally, that there will be poster-parades of protest outside medical conventions with slogans like ILLNESS IS NOT SO BAD, YOU KNOW? or DISEASE IS THE HIGHEST FORM OF HEALTH. But for the moment, it seems that illness is going to be "in"; a rising tide of really chronic sickness. Even despite the Canutes of deviancy-sociology.

Secondly and much more importantly, nothing in my argument confirms the technologizing of illness; the specialized medical model of illness is not the only possible one, as I have already indicated. As Dubos points out in his fundamental work *The Mirage of Health* (to which this paper is merely more or less a vulgarized addendum), the greatest advances in the control of diseases have often come about through non-medical measures, and in particular through social and political change. The insertion of windows into working-class houses (with the consequent beneficial influx of sunlight), or the provision of a pure water-supply and an efficient sewage-disposal, did more to clear up the plagues of modern epidemic infection than did the identification of particular microbes or the synthesis of "medical discoveries" like the various antibiotics and antitoxins. There are some authorities, notably Siegler and Osmond,[11] who argue that, since the category of illness is infinitely preferable from the standpoint of the mentally deranged, to any other variety of deviancy, we have to concentrate entirely on a narrow medical model for explaining diseases and curing them; in their view, social explanations for the onset of illnesses like schizophrenia and drug-addiction are incompatible with any illness-model, and so should be ruthlessly jettisoned. But we do not need to technologize illness beyond the point at which we decide that it is helpful to do so; even with physical illness, the concept of a "social disease" is indispensable in the understanding and treatment of, for example, tuberculosis. Preventive medicine and public medicine are bound to invoke social explanations and social measures, to occupy a space which occurs, in short, at the intersection of medicine and politics. My case points, not to the technologizing of illness, to the medicalization of moral values (so obvious in the practice of psychiatry that it needs no fresh rehearsal here): but, on the contrary, to the politicization of medical goals. I am arguing that, without the concept of illness — including that of mental illness since to exclude it would constitute the crudest dualism — we shall be unable to *make demands* on the health-service facilities of the society that we live in.

Those labelling theorists who like to yearn for the Lost Territories of deviancy now occupied by the invading armies of medical diagnosis, are committing a *sociological irredentism* quite as offensive as the better-known bogey of Psychiatric Imperialism. Assemblies of deviancy-experts remind me of nothing so much as the sad, morale-boosting reunions of Sudeten Germans in the Federal Republic: they appear dangerous to the Czechs, but basically such gatherings are those of the devotees of a lost cause, joining in old songs and refurbished regional accents in order to maintain a losing identity against the harsh world which offers many rival opportunities for re-socialization. The "demands" of the Sudeten Germans are, in 1972, a ritual, even if they were not so in 1938. The demands of the sociological revisionists of mental illness are not very obvious even as ritual: they appear to want more money for their own research, and one or two of their allies want to be left undisturbed to carry on rewarding private psychoanalytic practices.[12] But theirs is a passive irredentism; after all, the sociologists never actually lived in the territories that the psychiatric colonizers have now taken over, so there cannot be very much energy in their grumbles. This very passivity is, however, highly dangerous in the present historical period when the amount of public money available for investment in the health services is so grossly inadequate. The voice of labelling sociology, including a good many of the "immanentist" theoreticians, chimes in with the cautious, restrictive tones of the cheese-paring politician who is out to deny the priority of resource-allocation for the public psychiatric services (at the same time as he budgets lavishly for the military). Public psychiatry, as the result of the onslaughts of Szasz, Goffman and Laing and — to a smaller extent — of the other academic "anti-psychiatrists," has become thoroughly unpopular with the general reading public. And since this middle-class public forms the great reservoir of candidates from which the officer-class of possible pressure-groups gets selected, the unpopularity of public-health psychiatry is an important factor which prevents the crystallization of a vocal and determined lobby for the provision of intensive psychiatric facilities on a mass scale. Mental illness, like mental health, is a fundamentally *critical* concept: or can be made into one provided that those who use it are prepared to place demands and pressures on the existing organization of society. In trying to remove and reduce the concept of mental illness, the revisionist theories have made it that bit much harder for a powerful campaign of reform in the mental-health services to get off the ground. The revisionists have thought themselves, and their public, into a state of complete inertia: they can expose the hypocrisies and annotate the tragedies of official psychiatry, but the concepts which they have developed enable them to engage in no public action which is grander than that of wringing their hands. Of course they do it beautifully. But the tragic stance of labelling theory and anti-psychiatric sociology cannot be taken seriously as a posture which is "above the battle" for the priorities of spending within our bureaucratized and militarized capitalism. It is *in* the battle, on the wrong side: the side of those who want to close down intensive psychiatric units and throw the victims of mental illness on to the streets, with the occasional shot of tranquilizer injected in them to assure the public that something medical is still happening.

I have caught, in some discussions of a draft of this paper, a certain pervasive anxiety among my audience, an anxiety which is afraid lest psychiatry may, in the service of our abominable social and economic order, succeed in "adjusting" the mentally ill to its goals. It is as though people believe that there is only a finite pool of grievances and maladjustments available in this society, for radicals to work with: the fear is that psychiatry, with its tranquilizers, hospitals, and what-not, may succeed in mopping up this limited supply of miseries, discharging its patients into the hell of the factory and the purgatory of the home as permanently "cured" and adjusted robots. Once again; if capitalism could really "adjust" people, through psychiatry or any other technology, who would want to quarrel with it? I myself am perfectly happy to see as many mentally-ill persons as possible treated, fully and effectively, in this society; for no matter how many maladjustments may become adjusted through expert techniques, the workings of capitalism will ever create newer and larger discontents, infinitely more dangerous to the system than any number of individual neuroses or manias. Some people have seemed to me to be wanting to hoard the existing supply of neuroses and insanities, by leaving them untreated as long as possible, in the conviction that these are the best grievances we have got, and once they have gone, where will we get any more? I can suggest plenty more alternative sources of maladjustment, within our present-day society. But I forebear from doing so; for there is no arguing with people who will not read the newspapers.

NOTES

1. Barbara Wootton, *Social Science and Social Pathology* (London, 1959), p. 225.

2. J. Zubin, "A Cross-Cultural Approach to Psychopathology and Its Implications for Diagnostic Classifications," in *The Classification of Behavior Disorders,* ed. by L. D. Eron (Chicago, 1966), pp. 43–82.

3. The above discussion is heavily indebted to René Dubos' masterly *The Mirage of Health* (New York: Harper & Row, 1971), especially pp. 30–128.

4. See the excellent account of Homeric medicine in P. Lain Entralgo, *The Therapy of the World in Classical Antiquity* (New Haven: Yale Univ. Press, 1970).

5. I have taken this observation from Dr. L. Robbins' discussion in Eron (ed.), *The Classification of Behavior Disorders.*

6. Cited by A. L. Knutson, *The Individual, Society and Health Behavior* (New York: Russell Sage, 1965), p. 49.

7. Cited by Mechanic, *Medical Sociology,* p. 16.

8. Knutson, *The Individual, Society and Health Behavior,* p. 48, quotes one New York study showing lower-class indifference to the need for medical attention for such conditions as ankle-swelling and backache. But these should still have been regarded as illnesses by the respondents, who could have had their own reasons (such as lack of cash) for refusing to consider medical treatment.

9. There is now some doubt among dental experts as to whether "caries" is a genuine disease-entity or an artifact of diagnostic labelling.

10. See Foucault, *Madness and Civilization,* pp. 119, 121, 123, 129, and 151ff. Entralgo, in *The Therapy of the Word in Classical Antiquity,* has similar explanations collected from ancient Hippocratic medicine.

11. Miriam Siegler and Humphry Osmond, "Models of Madness," *British Journal of Psychiatry* 112 (1966), 1193–1203; "Models of Drug Addiction," *International Journal of the Addictions* 3 (1968), 3–24. See also "The Sick Role Revisited," in this issue, especially footnote 5.

12. The whole literary oeuvre of Szasz and Leifer is an attempt to justify one important way in which they earn their living: they are both psychoanalysts in private practice, accepting fees, sufficient to compensate them for the loss of time they might be spending in other work, from people who are in agony. Like any other intellectual, each of them has to justify what he is doing. They have to say: "Well, at least it's better than what other people (e.g., psychiatrists in the community health services) are doing." They also have to say: "There is something rather important and special about this private fee-paying relationship: for example, it guarantees confidentiality and the responsibility of the therapist to the client alone, in a way which the psychiatrists in a publicly financed and organized health service, with their necessarily divided loyalties, cannot manage." Hence their imperative need to destroy, intellectually (they cannot of course do it in practice, and would probably feel guilty if they could) the public mental-health service through attacking its main ideology, the category of "mental illness." There are of course serious problems, of the kind they adeptly stigmatize, in the bureaucratized psychiatric professions; divided loyalties are a fairly common fact of everyday life, but not everybody with a division of loyalties is a traitor. A psychiatrist or counselor in a publicly financed institution is expected to be something of a double agent who can of course lay himself open to accusations of betrayal from either cause that he serves, i.e., from the institution or from the client. But being a double agent can be a perfectly honorable profession, at least before the court of honor which is the agent's own conscience. Whether other people believe that a person with divided loyalties is honorable or treacherous is, of course, a matter of *their* judgment alone.

H. Tristram Engelhardt, Jr.

Psychotherapy as Meta-ethics

It is almost fashionable to draw attention to ethical presuppositions in psychotherapy and allege that psychotherapy involves an ethic or is even an "applied
ethics." But it is one thing for psychotherapy to forward freedom or autonomy
vis-à-vis control by unconscious drives or unacknowledged forces, and another
thing to forward a particular set of actions or endorse a particular set of goals.
The difference is between allowing one to choose the good and telling one what
the good is. This distinction can be understood in terms of levels of language
as suggested by Bertrand Russell; though psychotherapy may often advance a
particular ethic, it is more properly involved in making certain meta-ethical
assertions about the possibility of any ethic whatsoever. Examining the nature
of the distinction between ethical and meta-ethical propositions and assertions
allows a clearer understanding of the nature of the values ingredient in psychotherapy and is consonant with themes in Freud's works. Interestingly, it shows
that the goals of psychotherapy are similar to those of medicine in general
rather than unique in forwarding a particular ethic. Both seek to remove hin-
drances and augment a patient's freedom.

"Cure" is always a liberation from some hindrance and what counts as a
significant hindrance is, at least to some extent, socially determined and is a
value-infected concept. Treatment is, thus, an activity directed toward a certain value. But, in psychotherapy, basic values are addressed, even the question
of valuing a common reality. For example, autism, as Bleuler pointed out, is a
logic that allows one to act according to fantasy and, thus, to withdraw from our

From *Psychiatry* 36 (1973):440–445. Copyright © 1973 by The William Alanson White Psychiatric
Foundation, Inc. Reprinted by permission of the publisher and the author.

common reality.[1] It is also, though, a question of values. Psychotherapy aims at getting one to value reality, to cathect its objects. It also aims at freeing one from drives and forces that encumber free action. Not all psychiatrists, obviously, would agree with this portrait of psychotherapy, but it is sufficient for the purpose of this essay that some would. By stipulation, psychotherapy will refer to a broadly, psychologically conceived enterprise of current mental illnesses. This essay will allege that such an enterprise involves one in a question of values, but not in a particular ethic. Rather, it involves a meta-ethical issue. The term "meta-ethics" is used here to refer to propositions concerning ethical propositions as such and involves Bertrand Russell's notion of levels of language (Russell, p. xxii). One level, for example, is ethical and states that certain actions are good or bad and certain things are to be done or avoided. Another level, "meta" to, or referring to the first, states what is involved in ethics, its structure and language.[2] A possible meta-ethical proposition would be, "ethics involves a choice between goods or duties and, therefore, involves the general value of responsible choice or *free* choice." In this case, "being free" or "making autonomous choices" concerns the possibility of any ethics. "Freedom" is advanced as a necessary condition and ingredient of any particular ethic. One could say it is a meta-value. Of course, a particular ethic can also advance "freedom" as a value (e.g., "One should not constrain the freedom of others"). But, in holding the thesis that psychotherapy involves a meta-ethics, one is not asserting that psychotherapy is a process of lobbying for a particular ethic. Rather, psychotherapy is setting the stage for the possibility of ethical decisions. This is the meta-ethical activity of psychotherapy: the therapist seeks to aid the patient in integrating his mental life so that he can come to effective terms with his impulses and his external environment. Values again enter, packed into the term "effective." It conceals a dedication to a value, "the freedom or autonomy of the individual," which precedes any particular ethics. Psychotherapy is directed toward liberating the patient from the control of unconscious drives and unacknowledged forces. These allegations will now be examined.

At the end of his fourth lecture on psychoanalysis, Freud described this treatment as a form of education for the "overcoming of the residues of childhood" (Vol. 11, p. 48). These residues were to be overcome because they entailed a withdrawal from reality: ". . . we find that the withdrawal from reality is [not only] the main purpose of the illness but also the main damage caused by it" (p. 49). Freud could have said more generally, in fact, that disease is a failure to adapt or come to terms with reality. He is suggesting that one "come to terms with reality" and achieve independence from otherwise inadequately acknowledged natural forces. This involves the judgment that one must face reality in order to be "normal." Indeed, why should one prefer "common unhappiness" to "hysterical misery" (Freud, Vol. 2, p. 305), if facing reality does not itself involve an overriding value? This presupposition about reality and the value of an autonomous stance vis-à-vis reality can be appreciated as more than a particular ethic. Surely it says something about what man should be, and, in that sense, it is normative. It is normative in respect of human conduct and as a result has been characterized as an "applied ethics." In a recent issue of *Psychiatry,* Peter Breggin says, for example: "The discovery of the importance of values in psychoanalysis and in therapy in general has led to a radical possibility: that psychotherapy is, in fact, applied ethics. The notion that certain ethics 'tainted' Freud's treatment methods would be replaced by recognition that values and the modification of values are at the root of psychotherapy" (p. 60). Perhaps, most would be inclined to agree that psychotherapy does, indeed, involve an ethic. It would not be startling to find that such an activity as psychotherapy, involved with value-charged activities such as sex and aggression, should subtly promote certain values. But what is especially interesting is that the goal of autonomy precedes particular ethical propositions. This is very important in understanding how coming to terms with reality is a basic value.

To examine this, three statements by Breggin will be used as points of departure. They suggest ways in which psychotherapy defines man's relationship to reality and *a fortiori* to the domain of values:

(1) "The normal man brought increasing aspects of his self under the rule of the ego" (p. 62). The force of the position would seem to be: the healthy, "normal man" comes to grips (a) with his inner impulses and (b) with outer reality considered generally. A certain personal autonomy or personal integrity is embraced as a *summum bonum.* Psychotherapy is engaged in augmenting the autonomy of the self.[3]

(2) "The mature man had left behind much of his narcissism; he invested his libido more in others than in himself. This concept of narcissism was core to Freud's ethical concerns, for he used it as clinicians do today, as a label of opprobrium upon persons who concentrated their energies too much on themselves. Thus, in Freud's writing, numerous somewhat 'inferior' people are at one time or another said to have a considerable amount of narcissism compared to the mature male: schizophrenics, homosexuals, children, mob leaders, women" (p. 63). This theme can be seen to specify one dimension of what it means to come to terms with external reality. The mature *good* self is one that comes to terms with reality in general, and other persons in particular. Apart from investing its libido in reality, the ego remains one-sided, incomplete, and abstracted from a potentially concrete life of ethical decisions. In short, apart from this "erotic" involvement in reality, the autonomy of the self is restricted. Investing itself in reality makes the self-control of the ego significant. This second point is, therefore, a lemma to the first, telling in greater detail what is meant by autonomy.

(3) "Freud saw mature man as having insight and a comparatively greater degree of consciousness. Mature man was honest about himself and realistic about life; he accepted the *reality principle*" (p. 63). This completes the specification of the correct relation to reality — the acceptance of its exigencies in order to come to terms with it. Accepting this stance entails, though, a greater prospect of controlling reality and oneself in reality than would the rejection of the

reality principle. Again, the value of personal autonomy is prominent. Psychotherapy is urging that one recognize the parameters of reality so that one can best chart his own course. Mental health then describes a state in which, amongst other things, one is willing to recognize the demands of reality and to come to terms with them—and, consequently, better come to terms with oneself.

In summary, Breggin offers an interesting suggestion—that psychotherapy encourages an "ethic" of autonomy. He sees this implicit in psychotherapy in general as well as Freud in particular. "The overall impression of Freud's ethic is that man must tame his instincts. . . . Man, for Freud, should move from an other-domesticated animal to a self-domesticated animal. He becomes autonomous, but if he's mature, according to Freud, he will not take rash, dangerous, antisocial actions" (p. 63). But, it is necessary to notice that this "ethic" is not specific and would, as such, countenance various particular varieties of ethics. Autonomy appears, rather, as a general presupposition for realizing any particular, "wholesome" ethic. In this sense, the restriction is meta-ethical in defining what, indeed, counts as properly ethical without specifying any particular ethical system. Rather one supports freedom as a positive value and subvenes its development so that choices can be made. To also quote Freud: ". . . this involves a temptation for the analyst to play the part of prophet, saviour and redeemer to the patient. Since the rules of analysis are diametrically opposed to the physician's making use of his personality in any such manner, it must be honestly confessed that here we have another limitation to the effectiveness of analysis; after all, analysis does not set out to make pathological reactions impossible, but to give the patient's ego *freedom* to decide one way or the other" (Vol. 19, p. 50n).

The considerations that have been reviewed lead to a particular adumbration of psychotherapy—one that stresses one aspect of this activity, namely, its support of personal autonomy. "Personal autonomy" within this context is an explication of "mental health" and specifies the goal of psychotherapy. The goal is presented as a successful mediation between one's impulses on the one hand and the limitations imposed by reality and society on the other. The last enters in two guises—one overt, explicit and fully voluntary, the other as an internalization of one's encounter with significant others—as a conscience. The goal of psychotherapy is to achieve a satisfactory adjustment to one's needs and to the limitations upon one's needs so that one can effect an adaptation that allows one "to choose" between alternatives. This is underscored by the peculiar educative or meta-educative functions of psychotherapy often indicated by Freud. "We serve the patient in various functions, as an authority and a substitute for his parents, as a teacher and educator; and we have done the best for him if, as analysts, we raise the mental processes in his ego to a normal level, transform what had become unconscious and repressed into preconscious material and thus return it once more to the possession of his ego" (Freud, Vol. 23, p. 181). In short, Freud is interested in establishing a normal attitude, one "which takes account of reality" (Vol. 23, p. 202).

Thomas Szasz has dramatized, isolated, and emphasized this dimension of therapy and, consequently, provides a rather illuminating example. For Szasz, the aim of psychotherapy is "to extend the control of the ego over certain areas of the id, as they (the Freudians) put it, or to augment the client's capacity for self-determination and making choices, as I prefer to put it" (p. 6). "The purpose of psychoanalysis is to give patients constrained by their habitual patterns of action greater freedom in their personal conduct" (p. 18). For Szasz, this represents the historical development of a paradigm singularly appropriate for psychotherapy. It is for him the emergence of the recognition of the individual, particularly by psychiatry. "Pre-Freudian psychotherapies were characteristically repressive; they tended to abridge the patient's freedom of feeling, thought, and action. Freud's great contribution lies in having laid the foundations for a therapy that seeks to enlarge the patient's choices and, hence, his freedom and responsibility" (p. 16).

In this sense, psychotherapy offers no particular advice, nor does it forward a particular ethic. It advances, rather, a general possibility, a precondition for any particular way of handling one's life, any particular ethic. Szasz characterizes this as "meta-education" or "meta-advice." In other words, psychotherapy does not entail conveying particular bits of advice (or at least not as such, though it is often diverted into being supportive and, indeed, directive). It augments the patient's ability to educate himself, to gain insight. It catalyzes his self-education, his ability to advise himself.

> Education, in this special sense, means meta-advice. Much of the teaching and learning in analysis belongs to this class. For example, through the analyst's decoding of the patient's symptoms and dreams, the patient learns about his unacknowledged ("unconscious") transferences; the patient obtains an inventory of his major interpersonal strategies, their origins, and aims. In all these ways, the analytic teacher (therapist) gives more to his student (patient) than does the therapist who gives advice. And yet, in a sense, he also gives less, for he requires the student to work his own way from meta-advice to advice.
>
> Psychoanalytic insight or understanding may be put to various uses; the choice rests with the patient. Once more, this is like giving a tourist a map of a strange city: the analytic traveler may, with a map, orient himself, but not find out where he *should* go. [Szasz, pp. 51–52]

Talking about psychotherapy as meta-education specifies what is meant by meta-ethics. Any particular education as training in a way of life imparts an ethic. In contrast, psychotherapy is embarked upon in order "to liberate the patient" (Szasz, p. 16), specifically so that he can effect a way of life that is not imposed on him either by impulse or guilt but by a clear assessment of reality. The paradigm of psychotherapy is, thus, specified as: (1) a form of meta-ethics, (2) having a particular goal—liberation of the patient so that he can more effectively engage in interpersonal relations.

This paradigm clearly goes beyond, though it does not necessarily exclude, the medical model. Perhaps, it would be best to say that it is more encompassing.

Szasz would make the medical and analytic therapies exclusive, particularly in terms of a division of roles. An analyst should not as a practical matter, according to Szasz, attempt to do both medical and analytic therapy. Such a position, though, does not preclude psychotherapy as uniquely supplementing or complementing the rest of medicine. In this sense, medicine's goal of liberating mankind from the limitations of disease is instanced in the analysand's attempt to liberate himself from the limitations of his personal development through the instrumentality of the analyst. The implicit "personal" goals of medicine (i.e., liberating a person from disease) become explicit in focusing directly on personal autonomy. Szasz, though, fails to realize that his model is more encompassing than exclusive and represents the goal of all medical therapy — the increase of autonomy. It is only that in the case of psychotherapy the themes of personal autonomy are more explicit. All medicine seeks to liberate man from his afflictions; psychotherapy, though, focuses on making that liberation significant, on increasing the possibility of free choice. The focus is directly upon the precondition or presupposition of any ethics, and it concerns the nature of any ethics insofar as ethics presupposes free choice. But it is not itself a particular ethic, a particular choice of values or of a lifestyle. In fact, free choice could be used to embrace a loss of freedom. Though Szasz fails to clearly recognize that forwarding autonomy does not involve psychotherapy in a particular ethic,[4] unlike Breggin he suggests a distinction between forwarding a particular ethic and advancing autonomy, a value presupposed for any ethic. The distinction is crucial. Involvement in a particular ethic would make psychotherapy a form of ethical tyranny, not a step toward personal autonomy.[5]

In summary, it has been argued that certain aspects of psychotherapy can be better understood if psychotherapy is construed as a form of meta-ethics. In particular, it has been asserted that psychotherapy's commitment to aiding the patient's self-control can only be understood in terms of a certain presupposition — the value of autonomy from unconscious drives and unacknowledged forces. This value, though, does not involve any particular set of actions and is, therefore, best termed a meta-ethical commitment. It is a precondition of any particular ethic or free choice of conduct. Psychotherapy is not "applied ethics" in the sense of offering particular suggestions about how to live life, but rather, teaches (or "meta-teaches") certain strategies that allow one to act more autonomously. In short, the paradigm of psychotherapy is one in which the "therapy" or "cure" is effected through language, by meta-education toward the goal of self-reliance. The disease addressed is characterized as a state of being coerced by one's impulses, feelings of guilt, and misapprehensions of reality. Health, the goal of the cure, is personal autonomy in the sense of an effective mediation between one's impulses and reality. The picture is a value-laden one, but the enterprise of effecting the "picture of health" is meta-ethical — it is an applied meta-ethics, not the application of a particular ethic.

NOTES

1. "In the same way as autistic feeling is detached from reality, autistic thinking obeys its own special laws. To be sure, autistic thinking makes use of the customary logical connections insofar as they are suitable, but it is in no way bound to such logical laws. Autistic thinking is directed by affective needs; the patient thinks in symbols, in analogies, in fragmentary concepts, in accidental connections. Should the same patient turn back to reality, he may be able to think sharply and logically" (Bleuler, p. 67).

2. The term "meta-ethical" must be used broadly to encompass not only remarks concerning the general syntax of ethical statements but, also, the general substance of ethical statements. Statements concerning what can be substantially or materially ethical are not themselves on the same level of discourse as ethical statements and are not a part of any particular ethical system. Further, a non-normative meta-ethical endeavor may be impossible in that the exclusion of syntactically deviant statements itself involves one in certain normative positions; see R. C. Solomon.

3. If it were not for Freud's interest in psychical determinacy, one could without ambiguity say Freud forwarded personal freedom or freedom for the self or Ego. But, in assessing Freud in this regard, it should be noted that Immanuel Kant saw no difficulty in reconciling strict universal determination with freedom. The first was a presupposition for science, the second for ethics, or for treating men as persons. It is in this second mode, considering patients explicitly as persons, that psychotherapy forwards autonomy as a supreme value for the self. See Immanuel Kant, *Critique of Pure Reason,* A 554-B 582, A 555-B 583.

4. Szasz says for example, "Yet I contend that, as psychotherapy, psychoanalysis is meaningless without an articulated ethic" (p. 17). Although this assertion is qualified by subsequent statements, failure to explicitly address the distinction between levels of value suggests a possible confusion.

5. This distinction is implicit in Avery Weisman's notion of existential responsibility, which responsibility is not a particular responsibility but an ongoing project prior to particular responsibilities (esp. pp. 5 and 11).

REFERENCES

Bleuler, Eugen. *Dementia Praecox or the Group of Schizophrenias,* trans. J. Zinkin; Internat. Univ. Press, 1966.

Breggin, Peter Roger. "Psychotherapy as Applied Ethics," *Psychiatry* (1971) 34:59–74.

Freud, Sigmund. *Complete Psychological Works*; Hogarth: "Studies on Hysteria," Vol. 2, 1955; "Five Lectures on Psychoanalysis," Vol. 11, 1957; "The Ego and the Id," Vol. 19, 1961; "An Outline of Psychoanalysis," Vol. 23, 1964.

Russell, Bertrand, "Introduction," in L. Wittgenstein, *Tractatus Logico-Philosophicus*; Routledge and Kegan Paul, 1963.

Solomon, R. C. "Normative and Meta-Ethics," *Philosophy and Phenomenological Research* (1970) 31: 97–107.

Szasz, Thomas S. *The Ethics of Psychoanalysis*; Basic Books, 1965.

Weisman, Avery. *The Existential Core of Psychoanalysis*; Little, Brown, 1965.

Rem B. Edwards

Mental Health as Rational Autonomy

It has often been noted that psychiatric labeling has grave moral consequences, i.e. consequences which seriously affect the moral standing, rights,
and quality of life of other people. In the name of supposedly scientific and
objective medicine, it legitimatizes the enormous power which psychiatrists
and mental institutions have over other people, especially the weaker and
more vulnerable members of society. Psychiatric labeling is a form of moral as
well as medical behavior which has clear disadvantages as well as clear advantages. On the debit side, it serves to isolate socially those persons to whom
labels of lunacy are applied; and it often generates enormous mistrust and
alienation between them and their family and friends. It permanently stig-
matizes those so characterized and negatively affects for years to come their
opportunities for such basic amenities as self respect, employment, promotion, housing, education, marriage, and general social trust and acceptance. It
dehumanizes and degrades those to whom it is applied, allowing us to regard
and treat the mentally ill as slightly less than human. Nevertheless, it may still
be a rationally acceptable and justifiable mode of inter-personal interaction,
despite its obvious moral liabilities. Recognizing that psychiatric labeling of
individual persons may have grave consequences, we should also acknowledge
that the very act of defining and providing a range of application for such concepts as "mental health" and "mental illness" is itself a moral act which greatly
affects the lives of others.

There is both an evaluative and a descriptive dimension to our concepts of

From *The Journal of Medicine and Philosophy*, 6 (1981): 309–322. Copyright © 1981 by D. Reidel
Publishing Co. Reprinted by permission.

"mental health" and "mental illness." The latter term applies to describable mental and/or behavioral deviations of which we strongly disapprove. In addition to statistical abnormality, the disapproval element is a necessary condition for applying the term; for there are many "healthy" minority deviations of which we strongly approve, such as the rare but precious intellectual genius, creativity and sensitivity of our most outstanding artists, writers, scientists, philosophers, and moral and religious leaders. It is a great but often made mistake, however, to allow statistical deviation and the disapproval element to be sufficient conditions for applying the notion of "mental illness," for then we must allow every peculiar mental/behavioral process of which we disapprove to count as a mental illness. To avoid the excesses into which so much of psychiatry has lapsed in recent years, we must allow the notion to be applied only to a small sub-class of disapproved psychic processes, distresses, and behaviors. The issue is: do we wish to medicalize the whole of life, or do we wish instead to recognize and preserve other evaluative realms of discourse such as that of intrinsic value and disvalue, as well as distinctive moral, political, and religious norms?

Our present problem is not merely of academic interest, for there is a powerful tendency to work in modern secular, scientific society to allow older religious and moral values simply to fade away and to medicalize the whole sphere of moral, political, and religious deviation. When confronted by conditions and behaviors of which we disapprove, so many of us no longer use such ethico-religious terms as "ungodly," "sinful," and "immoral," or even such political terms as "unjust" or "undemocratic." Instead we apply such highly evaluative pseudo-scientific terms as "sick," "unhealthy," "immature," "a sad case," etc. We often do not realize that this whole way of talking tends to put ministers, political activists, and even serious-minded moralists as such out of business. Physicians and psychiatrists become the secular priests and final arbiters of what we should value and disvalue—in the name of "empirical" medicine. Many recent authors such as René Dubos, Ivan Illich, Nicholas Kittrie and Thomas Szasz have condemned such creeping medical imperialism and totalitarianism for a variety of reasons. Some protestors do so simply because they wish to make a place for moral, political, and religious norms and deviations which should not be confused with or collapsed into an all embracing domain of "mental health" and "mental illness." This may involve recognizing and respecting other intrinsic, moral, social, political, and religious values and disvalues in their own right. E. Fuller Torrey was doing this when he criticized as follows the 1977 report of President Carter's Commission on Mental Health, which equated mental illness with the unhappiness which results from social injustice, discrimination, and poverty:

> Certainly poverty and discrimination are terrible injustices that cause widespread anguish and unhappiness. But anguish and unhappiness are not mental illness, and herein lies the confusion. Poverty and discrimination are no more "mental health" problems than famine and war. They are human problems and should be

attacked as such, with all the governmental and private resources at our disposal: jobs must be created; opportunities equalized; housing built; food supplies fairly distributed. Labeling them mental-health problems not only obscures their true importance but also creates the illusion that they can be "cured" if we will only put enough mental-health professionals into positions of power (Torrey, 1977, p. 10).

Resisting medical imperialism in psychiatric labeling may also involve an awareness of the grave moral consequences of psychiatric name-calling, or an appreciation of the horrendous physical and psychic consequences of much that passes for "therapy," or a sense of the desirability of protecting the integrity of language itself. Economic considerations also are very much involved in any decision to expand or restrict our notion of "illness," even of "mental illness." If a condition gets classified as an illness, insurance companies and government agencies such as Medicare and Medicaid will be expected to pay the bills in many cases; and if the condition is not so classified, these agencies will not pay. There are many good reasons for wanting to limit the scope of application for the notion of "mental illness," rather than allow it to swallow up *all* those states of mind, distresses, and deviant behaviors of which we disapprove. Surely things have gotten way out of hand when a psychoanalyst such as Fine (1967, p. 95) tells us, "neurosis is defined in the analytic sense as distance from the ideal; then it can be said to affect 99 percent of the population. Thus, the essential thesis of this paper emerges: The ultimate goal of psychoanalysis is the reform of society."

I shall now make a conservative proposal for the proper limitation of the very notion of "mental illness" which until recently has been a presupposition of our entire legal system, which is very close to what I have found many mental health professionals actually using in their work in mental hospitals, and which is also very close to what the term traditionally meant before the advent of the sort of medical imperialism which Kittrie (1971, pp. 340–410) has called "the therapeutic state," or which Illich (1976, pp. 31–60) has called "the medicalization of life." There is nothing final about this proposal. It is merely an attempt to generate a discussion of the proper limits of "mental illness," *recognizing that the lives of many people will be greatly affected by where we draw the line.*

Definition: "Mental illness" means only those undesirable mental/behavioral deviations which involve primarily an extreme and prolonged inability to know and deal in a rational and autonomous way with oneself and one's social and physical environment. In other words, madness is extreme and prolonged practical irrationality and irresponsibility. Correspondingly, "mental health" includes only those desirable mental/behavioral normalities and occasional abnormalities which enable us to know and deal in a rational and autonomous way with ourselves and our social and physical environment. In other words, mental health is practical rationality and responsibility. A number of other theorists such as Breggin (1974, 1975), Engelhardt, Jr. (1973), Fingarette (1972), and Moore (1975), have arrived at similar views.

There is much here that needs explaining. By "mental/behavioral" I mean thinking, willing and feeling which may manifest itself in publicly observable bodily alterations and activities. By "autonomy" I mean having and freely actualizing a capacity for making one's own choices, managing one's own practical affairs and assuming responsibility for one's own life, its station and its duties. Before defining "rationality," and specifying its relevant realm of application, let us first recognize that there is a large domain of human belief which falls quite legitimately into the category of contested beliefs and unanswered questions, and which should be regarded as only peripherally relevant to the identification of madness. Most of our political, philosophical, and religious beliefs, many scientific and factual beliefs, and many questions of value and practice belong to the class of contested beliefs and unanswered questions. There is no clear answer to what it is and what it is not rational to believe in these areas. I keep telling my colleagues in philosophy that in such matters, there is very little difference between being around a mental hospital and being around a department of philosophy! Political, philosophical, and religious beliefs especially should never provide us with *primary* grounds for diagnosing mental illness. If that restriction had been observed, attempts would not have been made to have Mary Baker Eddy declared insane and institutionalized involuntarily for being a Christian Scientist. Nor would Ezra Pound have been institutionalized for political dissent. Irrationality and irresponsibility with respect to knowing and dealing with oneself and one's social and physical environment should be the primary focus for defining and diagnosing mental illness. We cannot declare a Christian Scientist mentally ill for believing that a broken bone has been miraculously healed if indeed no fractures show up any longer on X-rays. However, if anyone for any reason insists that healing has occurred when the fractures are still showing up, or if a woman insists that she has a million children and spends all her time looking for them, or if someone insists that they no longer need to eat since they died yesterday and are now in Heaven, then questions of sanity may be very legitimately raised and would be so raised even by Christian Scientists. True, there will be some tough marginal cases such as that of the sociopath; but some cases will be clear enough. Situations will also arise in which philosophical and religious beliefs impinge upon personal, empirical, and social realities, but mental illness should not be diagnosed unless it manifests itself in these practical areas.

Are we all just a little bit crazy, as some psychotherapists and much of our popular wisdom and humor insinuate? This depends in part on whether we are willing to call *any* momentary lapse into irrationality and irresponsibility a form of "mental illness," or whether we wish to reserve the term only for extreme and persistent forms of such. Because of the grave consequences of psychiatric labeling, it seems morally desirable to limit it to the latter, and I am offering a moral argument for a very limited and conservative conception of "mental illness." As for the factors of duration and degree, there is no *precise* answer to the question of "how long?" or "how extreme?" But it seems both socially undesirable and linguistically unconventional (at least prior to our recent medicalization of the whole of life) to count momentary and relatively superficial confusions, lapses of memory, emotional traumas and perceptual errors, etc. as indications of mental illness. A moment of confusion does not count as a mental illness any more than a single sneeze counts as a respiratory disease. The concept of duration belongs in our definitions of all diseases. On my analysis, mental illness will be a matter of degree of both time and severity of impairment and as such will be on a continuum with the whole of life; and there will be a grey area of controversial borderline cases. But some instances of it will be unmistakable in their duration and degree. If we take the duration factor seriously, there will be no such thing as temporary insanity, but this has never been anything more than a legal fiction invented for excusing certain persons when no other legal rationale for doing so could be found. It is important that we understand that only relatively extreme forms of such mental/behavioral malfunctions count as mental disorders. Though the question is worth exploring, we should be wary of altering this to mean that any such malfunction which is *capable* of taking an extreme form is a mental illness, for then we would be right back to the medicalization of the whole of life. It should also be noted that the factual claim that extreme mental/behavioral malfunctions are grounded in some "underlying pathology," located in the brain, the unconscious, the enduring structure of the mind itself, or what have you, has not been built into our definition of mental illness. This is a hotly contested issue, especially between behaviorally oriented psychologists and their adversaries; and such a consideration can be introduced only when it has been confronted head-on and found to be justified. All the data are not in on this one yet.

Now, what is meant by "rational"? Whatever it is, mental disorders are shortcomings or departures from it, and only those disorders which involve the absence of it are to count as mental disorders. Other undesirable mental/behavioral deviations should be classified in other ways, such as intrinsically bad, immoral, criminal, irreligious, etc. There are a number of defining elements in our common notion of "rationality." This is an important word in our living languages, not a technical word invented by philosophers. But philosophers may contribute to its clarification, and there is widespread agreement among both philosophers and non-philosophers that rationality involves (1) being able to distinguish means from ends and being able to identify processes and manifest behaviors which likely will result in the realization of consciously envisioned goals; (2) thinking logically and avoiding logically contradictory beliefs; (3) having factual beliefs which are adequately supported by empirical evidence, or at least avoiding factual beliefs which are plainly falsified by experience; (4) having and being able to give reasons for one's behavior and beliefs; (5) thinking clearly and intelligibly, and avoiding confusion and nonsense; (6) having and exhibiting a capacity for impartiality or fair mindedness in judging and adopting beliefs; (7) having values which have been (or would be) adopted under conditions of freedom, enlightenment, and impartiality. Rationality is a function of how we know, not of what we know. Ignorance is not insanity, but irrationality is. Stupidity, the deliberate choice of self-defeating ends, is also not insanity.

I am fully aware that many books could be and have in fact been written explicating all the complications of and full conceptual significance of these seven defining features of "rationality," but I do not have space here to rewrite such books. I do think that the last element is so difficult to apply that it should never be used in diagnosing insanity, though it has very legitimate philosophical uses. For purposes of defining "mental illness," I hope that enough has been said to indicate the sort of direction in which the notions of "rationality" and "irrationality" as deviations from such, have been traditionally understood. Of course, there are all sorts of degrees in the development of our human capacity for rationality, and it is only fairly extreme and persistent departures from some of our seven defining features of rationality which count as mental illness. Only a few of these factors need be involved in any particular case. Most people are not *very* rational, but most people are nevertheless sane. *Extreme* departures from sanity are not as difficult to identify in practice as some skeptical critics, especially lawyers and philosophers who have never spent any time around mentally disturbed persons, would have us to believe. Cases on the borderline of such extremities are the ones which understandably give headaches to mental health professionals, but such professionals can also cite many clear-cut cases involving extreme and prolonged incompetence and self-defeating performances in selecting effective means to avowed ends, of radically inconsistent practical belief systems, items of which are plainly controverted by empirical facts, of inability to cite reasons for belief and behavior, of persisting and pervasive conceptual confusions, and of intrenched inabilities to adopt fair-minded perspectives on either factual or valuational beliefs.

Since being rational involves having and acting upon factual beliefs supported by common experience and avoiding beliefs clearly at odds with common experience, it is easy to understand how persisting hallucinations and perceptual distortions contribute to irrationality. They involve loss of contact with our common world and generate beliefs about and behaviors directed toward things that are just not there. To the extent that unconscious conflicts, powers, and processes interfere with the functioning of conscious rational autonomy, they too are relevant for diagnosing mental illness.

No account of underlying pathology in the brain or in a Freudian psyche has been built into the definition here proposed of mental illness as loss of practical rational autonomy. Neither has the attempt to correlate mental illness with such pathology been excluded by such an analysis. Indeed, I wish to encourage an exploration of possible connections between mental illness so conceived and current concepts of and research on organic brain pathology, the standard functional psychoses and neuroses, and mental retardation. My suspicion is that standard (and desirable) brain structure, function, and chemistry can be correlated with all manifestations of rational autonomy, even if the precise relation between them always remains shrouded in metaphysical mystery. Though we do not know precisely how conscious thought and decision processes are related to brain function, we might still find that predictable correlations can be made between consciousness and brain. We might discover, and to some extent have actually found, that physical therapies such as psychotropic drugs, electroshock, and even carefully controlled psychosurgery have predictable connections with restoration to rational autonomy and mental health. True, drugs *may* be used as "chemical strait jackets." They may also be used to correct an imbalance in the dopamine circuit of the brain of the schizophrenic. A renewal of rational autonomy may thus be correlated experimentally with a return to more normal brain chemistry. The medical model is not included in our concept of mental illness/health, but its relevance is not excluded either. In this area much work remains to be done.

The problem of placing proper limits on the notion of mental disorder becomes especially acute when it is allowed to range over the whole spectrum of disapproved mental/behavioral phenomena, including those which have little or nothing to do with breakdowns of rational autonomy, but which still might be disapproved on moral, legal, or religious grounds. It is not very difficult to see that schizophrenics, paranoids, and manic depressives, etc. are irrational and have lost control; but many people certainly have great difficulty seeing that irrationality has much to do with many other conditions which are often classified as mental disturbances. An example of such a highly controversial classification would be homosexuality uncomplicated by distress, which was listed in 1968 as a mental disorder in the American Psychiatric Association's *Diagnostic and Statistical Manual of Mental Disorders, II,* but which is not listed in the new *DSM-III* in 1980. Has Anita Bryant persuaded us that this is really an ethico-religious problem after all, or have we been convinced that it is really no problem at all? In the 19th century, masturbation was regarded as a manifestation of madness and treated with the harshest of imaginable "therapies," but few persons even disapprove of it these days, much less classify it as madness. *DSM-III* includes caffeinism and excessive smoking as mental disorders. Will these have the same ultimate fate as masturbation? Anyone who has read Szasz (1972) knows that alcoholism and drug addictions are very debatable categories of mental illness. As he puts it, "Bad habits are not disease: a refutation of the claim that alcoholism is a disease." Is alcoholism a mental or a moral problem? My own view is that alcohol abuse begins as a moral problem and ends as a mental disease as it gradually becomes physically addictive, deprives the individual of much rational autonomy, and in some cases (Korsakov's psychosis) turns the brain to mush. I shall not attempt to work through *DSM-II* or *DSM-III* in detail to see which diagnostic categories might involve a confusion of irrationality with immorality or irreligion. Let the A.P.A. do that! I wish only to assert that not every disapproved mental/behavioral phenomenon should count as mental illness, that we should make a concerted effort to disentangle legitimate psychiatric valuations from moral and religious ones, and that we should attempt to put a screeching halt to the rampant proliferation of psychiatric diagnostic categories because of the grossly detrimental effects of the very act of psychiatric labeling if for no other reason. I am convinced that psychiatric labeling does have legitimate uses, but it also has illegitimate ones, and it will be the mark of the wise psychiatrist, psychologist, and philosopher to be able to distinguish the two.

No doubt, many psychologists and psychiatrists will want to reject the definitions of "mental illness" and "mental health" here proposed. This is not a great embarrassment, however, for there is *no* definition of these terms anywhere in the literature that many psychologists and psychiatrists would not want to reject. One of the truly embarrassing aspects of this field of medicine is that there is so little agreement on theoretical fundamentals. This always adds fuel to the fire of those who insist that the "medical model" has no legitimate application to mental/behavioral disorders. Why should anyone want to reject the conservative definition of "mental illness" in terms of impairment of rational autonomy here being proposed? I am confident that most objections will be based upon the tendency inherent in all medical imperialism to engulf all disapproved mental/behavioral conditions and processes under the label of "sick," and to recognize no separate domains of intrinsic, social, moral, political, legal, and religious values and disvalues.

The same imperialistic tendency is at work when we come to positive conceptions of "mental health." The tendency in so many cases is to equate this with *everything* desirable, not simply with the desirability of rational autonomy. *Every* desirable mode of experience, activity, self-realization, happiness and social organization are packed into imperialistic conceptions of "mental health." Consider and analyze for yourself the intrinsic, social, moral, religious, legal, etc. values which are packed into the following definitions.

1. "Health is a state of complete physical, mental and social well-being and not merely the absence of disease or infirmity" (The World Health Organization, 1978, p. 89).

2. "The crucial consideration in determining human normality is whether the individual is an asset or a burden to society and whether he is or is not contributing to the progressive development of man" (Alfred Adler as summarized by O. H. Mower in Boorse, 1976, p. 69).

3. "Let us define mental health as the adjustment of human beings to the world and to each other with a maximum of effectiveness and happiness. Not just efficiency, or just contentment—or the grace of obeying the rules of the game cheerfully. It is all of these together. It is the ability to maintain an even temper, an alert intelligence, socially considerate behavior, and a happy disposition. This, I think, is a healthy mind" (Karl Menninger in Boorse, 1976, p. 69-70).

4. "Mental health in the humanistic sense, is characterized by the ability to love and to create, by the emergence from the incestuous ties to family and nature, by a sense of identity based on one's experience of self as the subject and agent of one's powers, by the grasp of reality inside and outside of ourselves, that is by the development of objectivity and reason. . . . The mentally healthy person is the person who lives by love, reason and faith, who respects life, his own and that of his fellow man" (Fromm, 1955).

5. ". . . here we have to deal with those persons who fall ill as soon as they pass beyond the irresponsible age of childhood, and thus never attain a phase of

health—that of unrestricted capacity in general for production and enjoyment"
(Freud equating mental health with his "genital phase" of personality development, in Rickman, 1957, p. 66).

6. "True Sanity entails in one way or another the dissolution of the normal
ego, that false self competently adjusted to our alienated social reality; the emergence of the 'inner' archetypal mediators of divine power, and through this death a
new kind of ego-functioning, the ego now being the servant of the divine, no
longer its betrayer" (Laing, 1967).

Many wonderful things other than rational autonomy are mentioned in
the foregoing imperialistic definitions of mental health, and we should realize
that the judgment that they do not belong in such a definition is not by any
means the same as the judgment that they are not wonderful! Nor is it the
same as the judgment that we never need help and counseling in achieving
these wonderful things. It simply recognizes that those who do such counseling
should more honestly be termed applied axiologists, moral educators, spiritual
mentors, political activists, etc. Szasz (1974, p. 262) has a point in condemning
"mental illness" as a myth *where values other than those of rationality and autonomy are
involved* in the therapist-patient relationship. *Beyond that point,* psychotherapists
are dealing with what he terms "personal, social, and ethical problems in living." *Up to that point,* however, they are dealing with real insanity, which Szasz
fails to see. The rationally autonomous person may *choose for himself* just how
much value he will attach to social conformity and adjustment, productivity,
pleasure, heterosexuality, socially considerate behavior, love, faith, creativity,
introspection, mysticism, and all such good things. The rationally
autonomous person may still need value education in such matters, and it may
be a perfectly legitimate function of psychotherapists and mental hospitals to
provide such, though not in the name of treating mental illness or under the
guise of *medical* expertise.

We should acknowledge that two great and interrelated goods have been
built into our very conception of sanity—rationality and autonomy. It is quite
possible, however, to agree that these are great goods without agreeing upon
precisely what kind of goods they are, and for most practical purposes it is not
even necessary to agree upon the latter. Philosophers distinguish intrinsic
goods, things worth having, experiencing, doing, preserving for their own
sake from instrumental goods, things required for the actualization of other
values beyond themselves. Are rationality and autonomy intrinsic ends in
themselves? Are they merely indispensable means to other intrinsic goods such
as enjoyment or long range happiness defined in terms of enjoyment? Is their
actualization inherently enjoyable in itself, so that they become an integral
part of our happiness, as John Stuart Mill suggested? We need not agree upon
such abstruse philosophical questions in order to agree that rationality and
autonomy are great and indispensable human goods, and that life is so greatly
impoverished that it merits the labels "insanity" or "mental illness" where these
functions are significantly diminished.

Rationality and autonomy are controversial goods, not universally prized, however. Blind faith and obedience to external authority are greatly preferred by many (but not all) religious thinkers and by totalitarian political regimes everywhere. A well functioning democracy must be heavily populated by citizens exemplifying a significant degree of rational autonomy, and in that sense there is a political dimension to our definitions of mental health and mental illness. And though *we* may conceive of rational autonomy as the very essence of moral agency, we should not forget that many religious and non-democratic political perspectives regard rational autonomy with dismay and insist that *their* ideal moral agents renounce it, or better yet never develop it, for blind, unthinking, inherited or emotionally induced devotion to unquestioned authority. In Russia, it is the rationally autonomous person who is involuntarily institutionalized in mental hospitals! Thus, it may not be possible to separate *completely* the values of mental health as rational autonomy from *all* political, moral, and religious values. We can separate them from *most* such values, i.e. all the others, however; and it is necessary in a democratic society so to do.

Finally, we should realize that the value dimensions of how we conceive of "mental illness" and "mental health" are relevant to the practice of medicine in a mental hospital. If a mental hospital declares (as one with which I am acquainted has done) that "The goal of the institute is to restore its patients to an optimum level of social, intellectual, emotional, and vocational functioning in the community," we need to ask whether this is a realistic goal and just what it implies practically for patients. My own view is that "optimum" is much too strong a word to use here, just as "complete" was much too strong in the World Health Organization definition of "health." As a general affirmation of charity toward all and malice toward none, such formulations have a legitimate place. But as an avowal of realistic goals, such a statement is surely too strong. *All* the institutional and social arrangements and efforts of society and all the energies of the individual are required for the *summum bonum,* whatever that might be conceived to be; and no medical institution should claim or aspire to have the power and the resources required for its achievement. Reaching the *summum bonum* should certainly not be a prerequisite for discharge from such a hospital, for no one would ever be discharged! In that sense such a goal is not a realistic one, especially for involuntarily committed patients. It would be much more sensible for mental hospitals to aim at a restoration to minimal sanity in the present conservative sense of the term, i.e. a degree of rational autonomy which is minimally sufficient for "making it" in society, recognizing that even this is relative to what any given society or functional segment thereof expects of its members and provides by way of support.

Although care for and cure of mental illness should be the primary functions of a mental hospital, they certainly need not be its sole legitimate functions, any more than the physical care for and cure of disease need be the sole legitimate function of general hospitals and other medical practitioners. Medical professionals both within and without mental hospitals may also willingly and legitimately accept the additional tasks of relieving and preventing pain even where there is no hope of a cure, of assisting in social adaptation, giving moral counsel, and even being religious mentors (chaplains have a place) if they find that their patients are willing to ask and pay voluntarily for such services, or that society is willing to provide such services for those who want them but cannot pay. My only concern is that they recognize and admit what they are doing and not confuse treating mental illness with every form of aiding in the pursuit of justice and happiness.

NOTE

Writing of this paper was supported by a N.E.H. Development Grant in Medical Ethics, ED-32672-78-652.

REFERENCES

Breggin, P. R.: 1974, 'Psychotherapy as applied ethics', *Psychiatry* 34, 59–74.

Breggin, P. R.: 1975, 'Psychiatry and psychotherapy as political processes', *American Journal of Psychotherapy* 29, 369–382.

Boorse, C.: 1976, 'What a theory of mental health should be', *Journal for the Theory of Social Behavior* 6, 61–84.

Engelhardt, Jr. H. T.: 1973, 'Psychotherapy as meta-ethics', *Psychiatry* 36, 440–445.

Fine, R.: 1967, 'The goals of psychoanalysis', in Alvin R. Mahrer (ed.), *The Goals of Psychotherapy*, Appleton-Century-Crofts, New York, pp. 73–98.

Fingarette, H.: 1972, 'Insanity and responsibility', *Inquiry* 15, 6–29.

Fromm, E.: 1955, *The Sane Society*, Fawcett Publications, Greenwich, Conn., pp. 180–181.

Illich, I.: 1976, *Medical Nemesis, The Expropriation of Health*, Bantam Books, New York, pp. 31–60.

Kittrie, N.: 1971, *The Right to be Different: Deviance and Enforced Therapy*, The Johns Hopkins Press, Baltimore, pp. 340–410.

Laing, R. D.: 1967, *The Politics of Experience*, Ballantine Books, New York.

Moore, M. S.: 1975, 'Some myths about "Mental Illness"', *Archives of General Psychiatry* 32, pp. 1483–1497.

Rickman, J. (ed.): 1957, *A General Selection from the Works of Sigmund Freud*, Doubleday & Co., Garden City, New York, p. 66.

Szasz, R. S.: 1972, 'Bad habits are not diseases: A refutation of the claim that alcoholism is a disease', *The Lancet* 2, 83–84.

Szasz, T. S.: 1974, *The Myth of Mental Illness*, Harper & Row, New York.

Torrey, Fuller E.: 1977, 'Carter's little pills', *Psychology Today* 11, 10–11.

World Health Organization: 1978, 'A definition of health', in R. Beauchamp, and Le Roy Walters (eds.), *Contemporary Issues in Bioethics*, Dickenson Publishing Co., Encino, California, p. 89.

Suggestions for Further Reading

Value and Descriptive Dimensions
of "Mental Illness" and "Mental Health"

Bibliography of Society, Ethics and the Life Sciences. Hastings-on-Hudson, New York: The Hastings Center, 1979–80. A general source.

Boorse, Christopher. "On the Distinction between Disease and Illness." *Philosophy and Public Affairs* 5 (1975):49–68.

———. "What a Theory of Mental Health Should Be." *Journal for the Theory of Social Behavior* 6 (1976):61–84.

Braginsky, Dorothea D., and Braginsky, Benjamin M. "The Mentally Retarded: Society's Hansels and Gretels." *Psychology Today* 7 (March 1974):18ff.

———. "Psychologists: High Priests of the Middle Class." *Psychology Today* 7 (December 1973):15ff.

Brody, Baruch A., and Engelhardt, H. Tristram, Jr., eds. *Mental Illness: Law and Public Policy*. Boston: D. Reidel, 1980.

Brown, Robert. "Physical Illness and Mental Health." *Philosophy and Public Affairs* 7 (1977):17–38.

Caplan, Arthur L., et al., eds. *Concepts of Health and Disease: Interdisciplinary Perspectives*. Reading, Massachusetts: Addison-Wesley, 1981.

Cassimatis, Emmanuel. "Mental Health Viewed as an Ideal." *Psychiatry* 42 (August 1979):241–254.

Engel, G. L. "A Unified Concept of Health and Disease." *Perspectives in Biology and Medicine* 3 (960):459ff.

Engelhardt, H. Tristram, Jr. "The Concepts of Health and Disease." In Engelhardt, H. T., Jr. and Spicker, S. F., eds. *Evaluation and Explanation in the Biomedical Sciences*. Dordrecht-Holland: D. Reidel Publishing Co., pp. 125–141.

————. "Ideology and Etiology." *Journal of Medicine and Philosophy* 1 (September 1976):256–268. A critique of Boorse.

Engelhardt, H. Tristram, Jr., and Spicker, Stuart F. *Mental Health: Philosophical Perspectives.* Boston: D. Reidel, 1978.

Fabrega, Horacio, Jr. "Concepts of Disease: Logical Features and Social Implications." *Perspectives in Biology and Medicine* 15 (1972):583ff.

————. *Disease and Social Behavior: An Interdisciplinary Perspective.* Cambridge, Massachusetts: The MIT Press, 1974.

————. "The Position of Psychiatry in the Understanding of Human Disease." *Archives of General Psychiatry* 32 (December 1975):1500–1512.

Farina, Amerigo, et al. "Some Consequences of Changing People's Views Regarding the Nature of Mental Illness." *Journal of Abnormal Psychology* 87 (1978):272–279.

Gaylin, Willard. "In Matters Mental or Emotional, What's Normal?" *The New York Times Magazine* (April 1, 1973):14, 54, 56, 57.

Goleman, Daniel. "Who's Mentally Ill?" *Psychology Today* 11 (January 1978): 34ff.

Jahoda, Marie. *Current Concepts of Positive Health.* New York: Basic Books, 1958.

Leifer, Ronald. *In the Name of Mental Health.* New York: Science House, Inc., 1969.

London, Perry. *The Modes and Morals of Psychotherapy.* New York: Holt, Rinehart, and Winston, 1964.

Macklin, Ruth. "Mental Health and Mental Illness: Some Problems of Definition and Concept Formation." *Philosophy of Science* 39 (September 1973): 341–365.

————. "Values in Psychoanalysis and Psychotherapy: A Survey and Analysis." *The American Journal of Psychoanalysis* 33 (1973):133–150.

Mahrer, Alvin R., ed. *The Goals of Psychotherapy* New York: Appleton-Century-Crofts, 1967.

Margolis, Joseph. "The Concept of Disease." *Journal of Medicine and Philosophy* 1 (September 1976):269–280. A critique of Boorse.

"Mental Health" and "Mental Illness" in Reich, Warren T., ed. *Encyclopedia of Bioethics* Vol. III. New York: The Free Press, 1978, pp. 1059–1071, 1089–1108.

Mischel, Theodore. "The Concept of Mental Health and Disease: An Analysis of the Controversy between Behavioral and Psychodynamic Approaches." *The Journal of Medicine and Philosophy* 2 (1977):197–219.

Plog, Stanley C., and Edgerton, Robert B., eds. *Changing Perspectives in Mental Illness.* New York: Holt, Rinehart and Winston, Inc., 1969.

Sedgwick, Peter. "What Is Illness?" *The Hastings Center Studies* 1 (1973):19–58.

Skinner, B. F. "The Ethics of Helping People." *Criminal Law Bulletin* 11 (1975): 623–636.

Spitzer, Robert L., and Klein, Donald F. *Critical Issues in Psychiatric Diagnosis* New York: Raven Press, 1978, Parts 1 and 2.

Torrey, E. Fuller. *The Mind Game, Witchdoctors and Psychiatrists.* New York: Emerson Hall Publishers, 1972.

Rational Autonomy and Mental Health

Beauchamp, Tom L., and Childress, James F. *Principles of Biomedical Ethics.* New York: Oxford University Press, 1979, Ch. 3.

"Behavior Control." In Reich, Warren T., ed. *Encyclopedia of Bioethics* Vol. I. New York: The Free Press, 1978, pp. 85–101.

Breggin, Peter R. "Psychiatry and Psychotherapy as Political Processes." *American Journal of Psychotherapy* 29 (1975):369–382.

———. "Psychotherapy as Applied Ethics." *Psychiatry* 34 (1971):59–74.

———. "Psychotherapy as Applied Utopian Ethics." *Mental Health and Society,* 1972. (Proceedings of 4th International Congress on Social Psychiatry in May, 1972).

Dworkin, Gerald. "Autonomy and Behavior Control." *Hastings Center Report* 6 (February 1976):23–28.

Ellis, Albert. *Humanistic Psychotherapy: The Rational Emotional Approach.* New York: Julian Press, 1973.

Ellis, Albert, and Grieger, Russell, eds. *Handbook of Rational-Emotive Therapy.* New York: Springer Publishing Co., 1977.

Ellis, Albert, and Harper, Robert A. *A New Guide to Rational Living.* Englewood Cliffs, New Jersey: Prentice-Hall, 1975.

Engelhardt, H. Tristram, Jr. "Psychotherapy as Meta-ethics." *Psychiatry* 36 (November 1963):440–445.

Furlong, F. W. "Determinism and Free Will: Review of the Literature." *American Journal of Psychiatry* 138 (April 1981):435–439.

Glasser, William. *Reality Therapy, A New Approach to Psychiatry* New York: Harper & Row, 1975.

Glover, Jonathan. *Causing Death and Saving Lives.* New York: Penguin Books, 1977, Ch. 5.

Gruen, Arno. "Autonomy and Compliance: The Fundamental Antithesis." *Journal of Humanistic Psychology* 16 (1976):61–69.

Lodenson, Robert F. "A Theory of Personal Autonomy." *Ethics* 86 (October 1975):30–48.

McCarley, Tracey. "Issues of Autonomy and Dignity in Group Therapy." *Psychiatric Annals* (December 1975):35ff.

Mischel, T. "Concerning Rational Behavior and Psychoanalytic Explanation." *Mind* 74 (1965):71–78.

Mullane, Harvey. "Psychoanalytic Explanation and Rationality." *Journal of Philosophy* 68 (July 22, 1971):413–426.

Szasz, Thomas S. "The Moral Dilemma of Psychiatry: Autonomy or Heteronomy?" *American Journal of Psychiatry* 121 (1964):521–528.

———. "Our Despotic Laws Destroy the Right to Self-Control." *Psychology Today* (December 1974):19ff.

Medical Imperialism

Callahan, Daniel. "The WHO Definition of Health." *Hastings Center Studies* 1 (1973):77–87.

Carlson, Richard J. *The End of Medicine.* New York: John Wiley & Sons, 1975.

Dubos, René. *The Mirage of Health: Utopian Progress and Biological Change.* New York: Anchor Books, 1959.

Fox, Renee C. "The Medicalization and Demedicalization of American Society." *Daedalus* 106 (Winter 1977):9–23.

Friedson, Eliot. *Professor of Medicine: A Study of the Sociology of Applied Knowledge.* New York: Dodd, Mead & Co., 1970, Part III.

Gross, Martin L. *The Psychological Society.* New York: Random House, 1978.

Horrobin, David F. *Medical Hubris: A Reply to Ivan Illich.* Quebec: Eden Press, 1980.

Illich, Ivan. *Medical Nemesis: The Expropriation of Health.* New York: Bantam Books, 1976, Ch. 2.

Kittrie, Nicholas N. *The Right to Be Different: Deviance and Enforced Therapy.* Baltimore: The Johns Hopkins Press, 1971, Chs. 8 and 9.

Szasz, Thomas S. *Ideology and Insanity.* Garden City, New York: Doubleday & Co., 1970.

————. *The Manufacture of Madness.* New York: Harper and Row, 1970.

Torrey, E. Fuller. "Carter's Little Pills." *Psychology Today* 11 (December 1977): 10ff.

Zola, Irving Kenneth. "Medicine as an Institution of Social Control." *The Sociological Review,* New Series 20 (1972):487–504.

2. The Ethico-Medical Model and Mental Health Care

Introduction

Our modern Western view of mental illness as a *medical* problem is a relatively recent historical development. Prior to the eighteenth-century Enlightenment, the insane were not usually thought of as sick. Instead they were regarded as sinners, criminals, witches, or possessed by demons; and society responded to them with condemnation, execution, imprisonment, ostracism, torture, and exorcism. Institutions for the social isolation, confinement, degradation, and torture of the mentally ill were created in a number of countries as early as the sixteenth century. Bedlam in England had been established in the thirteenth century. But it was the Enlightenment which gave birth to several far-reaching ideas: that these unfortunates were sick and entitled to all the benefits and privileges of the "sick role," that medical science could and should provide therapy for the relief of their condition, and that they were entitled to humane living conditions even in mental institutions. It was the Enlightenment which transformed mental institutions into medical hospitals, insisting that society adopt an ethico-medical model to deal with the mentally deranged. As any historian of medicine knows, the Western World was painfully slow in adopting and implementing such enlightened ideas; and, to this day, critics of mental asylums insist that these ideas have never been properly implemented in most places. Even since the eighteenth century, the record of our attempts to deal with the mentally ill gives us little of which to be proud. Indeed, it is still one of the many hidden disgraces of Western Civilization.

There has been a profound ethical dimension to the so-called "medical model" from its very inception, prompting the suggestion here offered that we should call it the "ethico-medical model." Philippe Pinel, the great French Enlightenment medical reformer of mental institutions, wrote that "The mentally ill, far from being guilty persons who merit punishment, are sick people whose miserable state deserves all the consideration due to suffering human-ity." In insisting on humane treatment as an integral part of medical care, the Enlightenment accentuated the ethical dimension of the medical model in mental health care. Today our society has, and is continuing to refine, an awareness of the ethical dimension of the doctor-patient relationship in all of medicine; but it is perhaps most obvious in the conferring of the "sick role" and all that this involves. In the first selection, Robert Veatch gives special empha-sis to this aspect of the medical model, along with many other of its evaluative and empirical features.

In spite of the acknowledged good intentions of the reformers who first insisted that we apply a medical model to mental disturbances, many contem-porary critics of today's mental institutions insist that it was all a mistake from the beginning. Applying the medical model to mental illness involves both egregious conceptual confusion and unacceptable moral consequences, we are told by a whole chorus of contemporary critics led by Thomas Szasz but involving other antipsychiatric psychiatrists such as Peter Breggin, Fuller Tor-rey, R. D. Laing; by sociologists and social psychologists such as Erving Goff-man, Benjamin and Dorothea Braginsky, Robert Perrucci, T. J. Scheff, Theodore R. Sarbin; and by judges, lawyers, and civil libertarians such as Bruce Ennis, Richard Emery, and—believe it or not—Chief Justice Warren Burger himself (as Michael Moore points out).

In spite of the vagueness of the term, those who wish to deny that the medi-cal model applies to mental illness usually interpret the model as having the following features:

1. Genuine disease concepts are purely *descriptive* concepts.
2. Diseases exhibit *physical manifestations and symptoms.*
3. Diseases involve *physical abnormalities.*
4. Diseases have (known?) *physical causes.*
5. Diseases are properly *treated* by *physical interventions.*
6. *Physicians* are the *proper authorities* to deal with diseases.
7. The *fee-for-service* private practice model insures the primary *loyalty* of the physician to the client.
8. Patients assigned to the "sick role" by physicians are *not responsible* for their condition and/or behavior and should be:
   a. *released* for their normal duties and
   b. *excused* from blame and punishment.

Critics insist that the medical model does not properly apply to the "mythical" concept of "mental illness" because:

1. Spurious mental disease concepts are purely *normative* concepts.
2. Mental illnesses exhibit *only behavioral* manifestations and symptoms.
3. Mental illnesses involve *only behavioral* abnormalities.
4. Mental illnesses do *not* have (known?) *physical causes.*

5. Mental illnesses should *not* be *treated* by any *physical interventions*.
6. *Physicians* are *not* the proper authorities to deal with mental illnesses.
7. Once the individualistic fee-for-service model is abandoned, mental health professionals are *"double agents"* who *betray their clients*.
8. Mental patients should *not* be assigned the "sick role" because in reality they are fully responsible for their conditions and/or behavior and should not be:
   a. released from any normal duties and
   b. excused from blame and punishment.

It is very doubtful that a single feature of this absolutistic contrast between the medical model as applied to physical illness and mental illness will actually survive critical scrutiny. In the following essays, Robert M. Veatch is highly critical of purely physicalistic, non-normative conceptions of the medical model; he nevertheless rejects the relevance of the model to mental illness because the latter is "psychological" instead of "organic" in nature. Although the term "medical model" is not used in his essay, Michael Moore does a superb job of showing why most of the arguments which have been used to support any sort of absolutistic contrast are unsuccessful, including the one emphasized by Veatch. A better understanding of what physical and mental illnesses really involve will inevitably lead to the conclusion that the ethico-medical model applies just as legitimately to the former as to the latter. Our concept of the "ethico-medical model" should incorporate the most basic features of what is actually there in the practice of physical medicine, not what some simplistic view mistakenly claims to be there in the practice of physical medicine.

Robert M. Veatch

The Medical Model: Its Nature and Problems

With few exceptions addiction to morphine and heroin should be regarded as a manifestation of a morbid state.

British Rolleston Committee, 1926

Addiction should be regarded as an expression of mental disorder, rather than a form of criminal behavior.

Brain Committee, 1961

. . . the addict should be regarded as a sick person . . . and not as a criminal, provided he does not resort to criminal acts.

Brain Committee, 1965

. . . according to the prevalent understanding of the words, crime is not *a disease. Neither is it an illness, although I think it* should be!

Karl Menninger, 1968

Ultimate policy control of the programs as well as day-by-day supervision must be securely lodged in medical *rather than political, probation, parole, or police hands.*

Consumer Union Report on Licit and Illicit Drugs, 1972

In sociological parlance, a model is a complex, integrated system of meaning used to view, interpret, and understand a part of reality; and one of the most

From *Hastings Center Studies* 1 (1973):59–76. Copyright © 1973 by the Hastings Center. Reprinted by permission of the publisher and the author.

deeply rooted such systems in our rationalistic and scientifically oriented Western society is the medical model. A pervasive and complex instrument for interpreting a wide range of behavior, the medical model has served well as a means of organizing our attidues and actions toward a variety of human abnormalities. In fact, it has served so well that attempts are continually being made to expand its boundaries to include forms of abnormal behavior which had previously been interpreted within other models.

Today an entire series of behaviors are doubtful candidates for the category of illness, that is, for interpretation in the medical model: narcotic addiction, mental deviancy, unwanted pregnancy, alcoholism, homosexuality, unwanted folds in the facial skin, and virtually all criminal behavior. At least some members of our society view all or some of these conditions as most meaningfully understood in the medical model, as part of the health-illness complex in some sense or another. Some generations ago, other forms of abnormality were in a similar position as dubious illnesses: tuberculosis, leprosy, epilepsy, psychosis from lead poisoning. The fact that we have a history of expanding the medical model to include an ever widening circle of forms of human variant behavior previously interpreted as resulting from moral, religious, or political aberration is sometimes used as an argument from precedent, i.e., with further enlightenment (i.e., scientific understanding) we shall see how the presently ambiguous variant behaviors also fit into the medical model.

What, then, is the nature of the medical model, its basic elements, and its implications for society? Before outlining what I see as the basic characteristics of the medical model, however, we must first examine the nature of illness as one among many forms of socially constructed deviancy. Having done this, we can then consider what I see as four essential characteristics of the medical model. Finally, we shall conclude by exploring the implication of the medical and other models for marginal forms of deviancy.

I. Illness as a Socially Constructed Deviancy

A. The Social Construction of Deviancy

In the past two decades the sociology of medicine and the sociology of knowledge have together made great progress in gaining insight into the human interpretation of human behavior. Individuals who are ill, according to our ordinary understanding, are in possession of biological attributes seen as abnormal in some sense. While we are all familiar with concepts of psychogenic and psychosomatic illness, the man on the street normally conceives of illness as a biological aberration. Beginning, however, with Parsons' work in the 1950s, it became apparent that the process of being labelled as ill was much more complex. Illness is a socially assigned category given meaning from society to society by social intepretation and evaluation of the biologically abnormal characteristics. Thus Freidson argues that two kinds of imputed deviance figure in the notion of illness: biological and social.[1]

It is clear that biological aberration alone is not enough to make a person ill. The seven-foot tall basketball player is hardly ill. He is admittedly grossly abnormal—and rewarded for it. Thus some kinds of biological aberration are deviant (both socially and biologically), yet positively evaluated. Still other kinds of biological deviance are not positively evaluated, but are not negatively valued either—sporadic dense pigmentation of the skin called "freckles," for instance. In the sociology of deviance, normally the term deviance is limited to *negatively* evaluated deviance. However, it is possible to possess a negatively evaluated attribute which is clearly biological in nature and still not have the condition interpreted in the medical model. In a racist society, for instance, which evaluates generally distributed black pigmentation negatively, possessors of that biological characteristic will encounter discrimination but are not considered sick.

All forms of deviancy have in common the fact that they are necessarily social constructions. Freidson argues, "Human, and therefore social, *evaluation of what is normal, proper, or desirable is as inherent in the notion of illness as it is in notions of morality.*"[2] We should not lose sight of the fact that all understandings of reality are socio-cultural constructions. Working with perceptual raw data, which are nothing more than an endless series of impressions, human beings, as members of social groups, construct categories and systems of meaning and value which make sense out of an otherwise meaningless stream of existence.[3] This is true even for such fundamental systems of meaning as the Western scientific world view. But it is more obviously true for the socially constructed patterns by which types of deviancy are evaluated and for the establishment of roles which organize the life of the deviant.

To claim that all understandings of reality are socio-cultural is emphatically not the same as saying that all meanings and values are culturally relative. It is simply to say that *understandings* and *systems* of meaning which are used by human beings to interpret experience are necessarily products of a culture. Certainly language is a critical element in interpretation and understanding of experience, and language is a cultural construction. Likewise world views, underlying systems of meaning and value, are the products of a culture. But in making this claim we are purposely leaving open the question of whether there may be "in reality" values and meanings upon which our socio-culturally constructed systems of understanding are based, and which could give rise to meaningful debate about whether or not such social constructions are "constructed properly."[4]

To have one's body invaded by bacterial organisms which produce fever, nausea, and vomiting is not the same as being sick. Animals quite ordinarily may have the former characteristics, but it is not until social interpretation is given to those characteristics that the affected one is "sick." To be sick is to have aberrant characteristics of a certain sort which society as a whole evaluates as being bad and for which that society assigns the sick role.[5] According to the Parsonian formulation, the sick role includes two exemptions from normal responsibilities and two obligations or new responsibilities.[6] First, the person in the sick role is exempt from normal social responsibilities. Second, the person in the sick role is exempt from responsibility for his condition and cannot be expected to get well by an act of decision or will; he cannot be expected to "pull himself together." The third characteristic of the sick role is that it is itself undesirable. There is an obligation to want to get well.[7] Finally, one in the sick role has an obligation to "seek technically competent help."

No matter how unusual, "unnatural," or even death-inducing a set of characteristics may afflict him, the individual is not "sick," and thus exhibiting behavior interpreted in the medical model, until a social judgment is made. Among other things, that social judgment must include a negative evaluation. That is true for *any* class of deviant behavior no matter what its origin.[8]

This critical point should not be lost throughout the remainder of this discussion. Even organic sickness in the most narrow and traditional sense as interpreted in the medical model necessarily contains a socially bestowed negative evaluation. Sedgwick and others are thus on the right track in attacking Szasz, Leifer, Goffman, and other critics of treating mental illness in the medical model, when they base their argument on the assumption that mental illness differs from organic illness. These critics claim that while organic illness refers to biological conditions which are objective and exist independent of any human value judgments, mental illness is a social, value-laden category.[9] I shall later disagree with Sedgwick's conclusion that because organic and mental illness share in common a socially constructed negative evaluation which is in either case a value judgment, mental deviation should, therefore, be classified as an illness. That shall be argued later, but at this level Sedgwick is certainly correct and reflects sound thinking in the sociology of knowledge and the sociology of medicine. If one refuses to place mental deviation in the same "illness" category as organic illness, it must be done on grounds other than that the former involves social value judgments and the latter supposedly does not.

B. The Differentiation of Social Deviances

Having identified all illness as a type within the broader category of social deviance, it is now important to differentiate it from other types and to trace the history of that differentiation and the study of it. Nowadays it is a commonplace to recognize that in an earlier age deviances were not well differentiated. The ill person, the criminal, the possessed, the religiously inspired were not well separated into different roles. Likewise the functionaries with special roles were not differentiated. In many societies, the medical practitioner, law enforcer, psychologist, and priest were combined in one role, that of the medicine man-priest. One of the primary characteristics of "higher" civilization, however, according to this school of functional analysis, is the differentiation of different functionary roles.

Talcott Parsons again has provided the definitive analysis of the differentiation of the medical model from other major forms of deviancy which he saw as important conceptual models in societies.[10] Parsons differentiated deviancies on two major axes.[11] First, he separated those deviancies which involve disturbances in commitments to norms and values (giving rise to the deviancies of crime and sin respectively) from those deviancies attributed to "the exigencies of the situation in which the person must act" (deviancies of disloyalty and illness). The second axis of differentiation separates those deviancies of the person as a whole from those which involve only a problem of accepting particular obligations. Disturbances of particular obligations (disloyalty and crime) are differentiated from disturbances of the total person (immorality and illness). When these two variables are crossed as the major axes of differentiation, illness is thus separated from immorality in being situational rather than normative in focus; from disloyalty by being a disturbance of the total person rather than of particular obligations; and from crime or illegality on both of the axes.

In less sophisticated analyses, the polarity is erroneously reduced to the extremes of crime and illness. For example, the title of an important study, formulating policy for two major relevant professional groups on the subject of drug addiction, poses the question—"Drug Addiction: Crime or Disease?"[12] It is little wonder that the authors had difficulty reaching a conclusion. Once again the origins of the study suggest that the *Sitz im Leben* may be important for the understanding of the theoretical categories for classifying negatively evaluated deviancies and the unique interests and perspectives of the professional groups in the debate. The study was conducted by the professional associations representing the cadres of experts in the two models posed as alternatives for interpretation of drug addiction: the American Bar Association and the American Medical Association. One wonders what the alternative models would have been if the study had been sponsored by associations of priests, behavioral psychologists, or sociologists.

For understanding the medical model and the disputes currently arising about doubtful illnesses such as narcotic addiction, it is crucial to realize the nature of the primary axes of major differentiations of types of deviancy. At the level of the Parsonian differentiation, if a deviance is to be seen as situational (rather than normative) and total (rather than particular), the only category available is "illness." Since one of the primary motives (functions) for classifying a doubtful illness as illness is to gain these characteristics, it may be that we are in need of more than one category with such characteristics, and that only failure to carry the analysis far enough has left but one appropriate category, that of illness. Much of the difficulty about classifying doubtful illnesses may rest here.

The task of model differentiation has been carried somewhat further by the work of Siegler and Osmond. Working with a series of questionable forms of negatively evaluated deviancies (schizophrenia, alcoholism, drug addiction) they have constructed a series of models of interpretation now numbering eight: the medical, moral, psychoanalytic, social, family interactional, impaired, psychedelic, and conspiratorial models.[13]

The classification of marijuana use may well rest at this level of debate. If it is the case that marijuana is relatively harmless to the physical health of the self and to others, it is still possible to argue that it is wrong to use it—on the grounds that it would lead to a life style which is incompatible with the value system of those doing the disapproving. On the other hand, proponents of marijuana's legitimacy would simply reply by arguing that its use is consistent with a better set of values. Independent of whether a deviancy is included in the medical model, one must still deal with the social value judgment that the deviancy is evaluated negatively rather than positively. Thus it would be possible to have a deviancy which clearly fit the characteristics of the medical model and to still reject that this medical deviancy is negatively evaluated. For the use of drugs or any other deviant behavior to be a medical problem, the behavior must first of all be considered bad.

II. The Characteristics of the Medical Model

Having argued that the medical model is a systematic mode of interpretation of a type of social deviance and that it, therefore, incorporates negative evaluations of the deviancy, we must now move on to specify the characteristics of the medical model—those elements which differentiate this model from other models of interpretation of deviancy. It is our thesis that a negatively evaluated deviancy will be perceived as fitting the medical model to the extent it conforms to these characteristics.

We have identified four characteristics which seem to be essential. A deviancy will be placed within the medical model if it is seen as (a) non-voluntary and (b) organic, if (c) the class of relevant, technically-competent experts is physicians, and if (d) it falls below some socially defined minimal standard of acceptability. A negatively evaluated deviancy will be perceived as fitting the medical model to the extent that it conforms to these characteristics. Every example of negatively evaluated deviancy which is a doubtful illness and therefore only ambiguously included in the medical model can be shown, we believe, to be questioned on at least one of these grounds.

A. Non-Voluntariness

Probably the most central characteristic of the medical model is incorporated in the second exemption from the sick role. As Parsons defined it, the person in the sick role is exempt from responsibility for his condition. A sinner or criminal or morally irresponsible person would be seen as deficient in character to the extent that he has brought on his condition; the person in the sick role is not. More significantly, one in the sick role is not expected to use will power or self control to overcome his condition. This is a crucial dimension of the medical model and one of the reasons for its attractiveness. The other major candidates for models of interpretation — especially the criminal, moral, and sinner models — normally suggest deficiency of the will of the deviant person. In the Parsonian major axes of differentiation, all of the other forms of deviancy are probably voluntary forms of deviancy. The one exception would be some interpretations of the sinner role, especially in a Calvinistic form of double predestination where, logically at least, the sinner is predestined to his sinner role by the decree of God and, therefore, is not responsible for his condition. Needless to say, the doctrine of double predestination is not very viable in contemporary society, and if an individual is to be considered non-culpable for his actions, another model of interpretation must be found.[14]

It seems clear that one of the primary functions of the medical model is to remove culpability. The attempt to place narcotic addiction, violence associated with rage, and larceny and assault by children into the medical model is in large part a move to remove blame by removing attribution of voluntary control of the action. We think there is sound empirical and moral reason for efforts to remove culpability from many forms of deviance. Nevertheless, there are serious problems in using the medical model to do this.

First, we believe it is reductionistic to force all forms of blameless deviance into the medical model. We have already seen that there are forms of non-culpable religious deviance for which the individual is in no way to be blamed. There are, at least at the theoretical level, many other types of non-voluntary deviancy which should not be forced into the medical model. This will be discussed more fully in the next section.

Second, increasing scientific study of biology and medicine has jeopardized the notion of blamelessness for even some of the human conditions most traditionally classified in the medical model. Certainly a heart attack is partially preventable, and an individual who fails to watch diet, exercise, and standards for physical examination may be seen as blameworthy if he has a coronary. Exposure to bacteria may be willful, through failure to observe sanitary and innoculation precautions known or thought to be effective. A parent may be blamed and feel guilty if his child suffers an attack of a preventable disease. The elaborate precautions taken by parents of the previous generation to avoid contact with children with polio suggests the extremes to which traditional illnesses can be culpable. Even cancer is now subject to the norms of the "seven danger signals." Genetic counseling and screening is moving rapidly to make even genetic disease a culpable event albeit culpable at the parental level. This suggests that the notion of non-responsibility in the sick role is in jeopardy although the assumption that one cannot get well by an act of the will alone certainly remains central to all of these illnesses. The medical model may be less functional for the removal of culpability in the future than it has been in the past.

Third, the *utility* of attributing non-culpability is most recently being challenged. Over the past century there has been increasing enlightenment about the implausibility and injustice in assigning blame to individuals who are quite possibly acting in a non-voluntary manner. The medical model served this purpose well. Very recently, however, the virtue of culpability is being rediscovered, especially by radical groups of mental patients, minors, political radicals, and advocates of alternative life styles. They recognize that to place an individual in the medical model is to remove blame, but to remove blame is to remove responsibility, and to remove responsibility is to challenge the dignity of the individual and the validity of the values he claims to be acting upon. Removing culpability by means of the assumption that the act is non-voluntary is thus not without its price. Those who place great significance on the values of diversity, autonomy, and individual freedom and dignity will accordingly be very cautious in assigning a deviant behavior to the medical model.[15]

This, of course, is a discussion of the functional status of the medical model in removing culpability. In the end, assigning a deviancy to the medical model or to models which imply voluntarism (and, therefore, praiseworthiness and blameworthiness for actions) depends at least in part on the ontological status of the concept of individual free will. The question of whether there really is such a thing as free will is one of the classic debates in philosophy and probably will not be resolved definitively in the near future. Those who opt (or are determined) for the deterministic interpretation of man's nature will be more inclined to the medical model, while those who are determined (or opt) for a position more supportive of the free will position will be more cautious.

It is important to realize, however, that Western society in general and the United States in particular is heavily committed to the voluntarist tradition. The victories of the political voluntarists combine with the victories of the Arminian and anti-predestinarian theological forces to make American society probably the most heavily committed to voluntarism of any society in history. This reality is manifested even in the Skinnerian claim that we must *choose* to use the correct conditioning techniques for the correct ends if our society is to survive in an age beyond freedom and dignity. Such an extreme commitment to voluntarism probably predisposes us to abandon the medical model in its classical form as scientific and technological breakthroughs rationalize and routinize illness. We may well be coming to the day when all illness will be divided into two classes: those blameworthy at the individual level when some individual preventive actions could have been taken and were not, and those blameworthy at the national level where the National Institutes of Health will be blamed for failure to develop scientific explanation and cure. This possible trend toward the decline of the medical model as an interpretation of deviance stands directly in opposition to Parsons' suggestion that American value predispositions to "activism," "instrumentalism," and "worldliness" lead us to place selectively high emphasis on the health-illness complex.[16]

I have argued that many questionable forms of deviancy may be brought into the medical model in order to remove culpability and imputation of blame by removing the attribution of voluntary choice. There are good functional and philosophical reasons, I believe, for continuing to hold that many of these forms of deviancy (narcotic addiction, alcoholism, other erratic behavior) really are based on an element of voluntary choice. Probably the man in the street is really not convinced that the alcoholic, the addict, the "criminal," are really acting from some drive or determining force independent of voluntary control. So long as that belief remains, it will be impossible to incorporate these deviancies into the medical model in any complete way. Let us now turn, however, to those deviancies which are assumed, according to the belief system of the society, to be non-voluntary.

B. Organicity

1. Sub-System Theories of Determinism.

In order to differentiate different types of non-voluntary, negatively evaluated deviancy, it is perhaps most helpful to use a standard classification of the total realm of human behavior. The division of behavior into organic, psychological, social, and cultural sub-systems is helpful in clarifying and codifying different levels of action.[17] The cultural sub-system includes the systems of symbol, value, belief, and meaning. It can in turn be differentiated into the language system, the basic philosophical assumptions organizing conceptions of reality with a system of belief and meaning (philosophy and theology), and the basic values of the culture. The social system encompasses the basic institutions of the society which include the economic, the familial, the political, and the religious forms of organization. Both the cultural and the social sub-systems are clearly super-personal in character. On the other hand the psychological and organic sub-systems are more often seen as intra-individual. This internal-external dichotomy is particularly important, but the somatic-psychological dichotomy, sometimes represented in the body-soul duality in the history of philosophy, is also crucial.

A total realm of human action may be interpreted with any one of these sub-systems as the primary reference point. In fact, reductionistic philosophies specifically expressing deterministic or non-voluntary causation have focussed on each. Somatic (organic, biochemical, or physical) determinisms have been contemplated by every college philosophy student. But the psychological deterministic theory of Skinnerian behaviorism is also well known. Social sub-system determinisms are less clearly represented; but with the emergence of the social sciences, they also have had their impact. Their view is best illustrated by the notion that a ghetto child involved in a crime is not guilty of willful wrong-doing, but is determined by racial, economic, and political factors to a role in life which forces him into his particular act. Cultural level determinisms are probably best illustrated by variants of predestination theories in which divine forces control man's every action, but also include sophisticated linguistic theories dealing with the ways in which language organizes behavior and in turn controls the individual.

It is clear that a total explanation of the universe can originate from any one of these sub-systems. Taken exclusively, any one of these theories of causation is reductionistic. In the end, the only theory which adequately accounts for man's total experience is one which works simultaneously with several causation theories as well as a doctrine of free will.

2. *Stages of Sub-system Analysis*

The notion of organicity as an essential element of the medical model becomes even more confusing when we realize that there are many different points of analysis. Every human action is organically related in the sense that a heavy dose of barbiturate (from a blow dart if necessary) will probably modify every conceivable human behavior. While clear-cut traditional diseases are conceived of as somatic, all of the doubtful illnesses also are related in some way to a somatic component. I shall propose four different stages for subsystem analysis: the deviant behavior itself, the response (treatment), the proximal cause, and the ultimate cause.

a. *Behavioral Stage*. Taking narcotic addiction as our model, we shall see that the confusion about organicity (and, therefore, about the appropriateness of the medical model) begins at the level of the deviant behavior itself. What is the behavior (symptom) which arouses our interest in narcotic addiction? On the one hand, there are clearly organic symptoms experienced by the addict in withdrawal—nausea, vomiting, dilated pupils, diarrhea, elevated heart rate and blood pressure—which are negatively evaluated. In this dimension narcotic addiction is not very different from invasion of an influenza virus. Yet narcotic addiction also produces psychological symptoms—euphoria, craving, feelings of dependency. Perhaps the social and cultural impact arouses the most interest, however. The narcotic addict's symptoms, albeit derivatively, include social impact which is economic and political and a life style (e.g. that of the stereotype opium den) which probably are the major worries of the public. Thus even at the behavioral level there is confusion about the subsystem classification. It appears, however, that some addicts, maintained on maintenance heroin, survive and behave quite normally. William Halsted, one of the four founders of Johns Hopkins School of Medicine and a practicing physician, continued to function effectively for roughly half a century as an addict.

b. *Response Stage*. At another stage, that of response to the deviant behavior, narcotic addiction may also be classified as organic.[18] The addict may be maintained on maintenance doses or brought down on gradually declining doses of narcotics. He may have his behavior blocked by blocking agents such as N-allylnormorphine, or he may be conditioned away from his addiction using succinylcholine. The same may be said for alcoholism and nicotinism. But other forms of response are possible to these doubtful illnesses, including jail, social and psychological manipulation, preaching, moral exhortation, and peer group pressure. On the other hand, clearly non-somatic forms of social deviancy can be controlled by the use of organic agents as a response, especially if one includes conditioning agents. I believe that organicity of the response, like organicity of the deviant behavior itself, should not be sufficient to classify the behavior within the medical model. A problem is created here because if the response is organic (a drug, a surgical procedure, or a physio-logically acting device) it may require an "organicity expert" (a physician) to administer the response. This necessarily brings the deviancy closer to the medical model, but physicians will be among the first to reject their function-ing as societal control agents for types of deviant actors whom physicians clas-sify as other than ill. The most dramatic example of the situation requiring an "organicity expert" for response, although the situation cannot be adequately interpreted in organic categories alone, is probably the abortion chosen because of, say, high parity and low socio-economic status. The condition which is to be controlled (the pregnancy) and the method of response (dilation and currettage, saline injection, or hysterectomy) are clearly organic in every conceivable way. Yet it is only with the greatest effort (and then probably for pragmatic political purposes and not very effectively) that abortion for socio-economic reasons is forced into the medical model.

c. *Proximal Cause Stage.* The contrast between an abortion for socio-economic reasons and one for "medical" reasons such as a cancerous uterus indicates the third stage of sub-system analysis. In the abortion for the cancer-ous uterus the cause of the "problem" is also organic. In narcotic addiction the cause of the deviant behavior may also be seen as organic. There certainly are organic changes in the body when one is addicted.

On the other hand, other theories of addiction deal with immediate causes of the behavior which are more psychological. The notion of "needle addiction" probably suggests a psychological causation model. We need to dis-tinguish between the immediate causes of addiction, which are at least par-tially organic in character, from earlier causes. Let us use the terms proximal and ultimate causes.[19]

d. *Ultimate Cause Stage.* Even if the proximal or immediate cause of addic-tive behavior is organic, which it may well be, it is still an open question whether the earlier or "ultimate" cause is organic. There are at least three addiction theories proposed today.[20] The psychological theories are based on the belief that there are "addiction prone personalities." Through childhood or other personality structuring, the individual acquires a behavioral pattern which is served by addiction; the appropriate response would requiring restructuring of the psychological make-up of the addict. Sociological theories place causation in the surrounding environment of the addict. Racial, eco-nomic, and political conditions, according to this view, predispose the individ-ual to addiction. A third theory of causation is biochemical. While holders of all theories are willing to concede that the proximal cause of addiction has a biochemical component, holders of the biochemical causation theory place organic chemical factors in a much more central place. One version of the theory holds that the morphine molecule causes physical changes which are permanently coded in the nervous system of the individual, perhaps changes in the receptor site. This, however, from our perspective would still not be an ultimate biochemical causation theory. If, however, one were to argue that there are anatomical or biochemical predisposing factors which lead certain individuals to addiction—say by the presence of aberrant enzymes or biochemical ratios—then organic causation would be ultimate in the sense in which we are using the term. There are analogous causation theories for homosexuality and schizophrenia. Narcotic addiction is organic at the level of ultimate cause only according to the biochemical causation theory.

The confusion over the placing of narcotic addiction into the medical model on the dimension of organicity is thus seen. It is only ambiguously organic at each of the four stages of analysis: behavior, response, proximal, and ultimate cause. No wonder there is doubt about the appropriateness of the medical model.

3. *Organicity in Other Doubtful Diseases.*

Other "illnesses" also raise confusion about the dimension of organicity. A heart attack, for instance, is clearly organic or somatic at the level of the behavioral symptom which is the origin of concern. Likewise, the treatment may be primarily organic, as is the proximal cause. But at the stage of the ultimate cause, there is more doubt. Certainly social factors predispose to heart attack. The sedentary life or poor social patterns may increase risk, but then more narrowly organic factors might do so also.

Cystic fibrosis may be the prototypical organic disease. Its symptoms are somatic, as is the intervention with vasodilators and respiratory aids. The genetic origin, which is not clearly understood and not diagnosable prenatally, leads us to believe that the causation is somatic and little can be done to modify the disease process. At all four stages, it is plausible to believe that the somatic component dominates.

In contrast, alcoholism seems to be heavily somatic in its symptomatology, but the response may be organic (as in succinylcholine "therapy") or social (as with Alcoholics Anonymous). The immediate cause of the behavior of the alcoholic is clearly organic, and we know precisely what the chemical is; but an organic theory of an ultimate cause must share a place with psychological, social, and cultural level causal theories. Alcoholism's organic proximal cause, behavior, and possible treatment do not make alcoholism as clearly an organic disease as is the case of cystic fibrosis.

Homosexuality lends itself to organic interpretation primarily at the causal level with research on andosterone/estrogen ratios suggesting abnormal balances in homosexuals. Treatment, however, has tended to be psychological. It appears that the more clearly the deviance is associated with organicity at the four stages we have identified, the more neatly it fits the medical model.

The relationship between organicity and non-voluntariness is important. There is quite clearly an association between a belief in organicity and non-voluntariness. If behavior is "in the chemistry," we are convinced it is not in the control of the will. For the most part this association tends to be borne out, but there are enough instances where behavior which is clearly non-organic at all four stages is non-culpable and, on the other hand, instances of behavior which is organic yet culpable, that the correlation is not perfect. When these inconsistencies arise, the appropriateness of the medical model is questioned.

The World Health Organization's definition of health as "complete physical, mental, and social well-being, and not merely the absence of disease or infirmity" is an innovative definition in which an attempt is made to stretch the concept of health and illness beyond the organic metaphorically to the non-organic. Whether or not this reforming definition will lead to a change in the meaning of the term is not to be decided here. The reason for this move, however, is apparent. Proponents of this definition are attempting to gain the virtue of non-culpability for non-organic forms of negatively evaluated deviancy as well as to mobilize the imperatives which have been associated with health and illness, i.e., the right to health and the obligation to give its attainment high priority. I believe there are great dangers in this expansionistic conception of health. Rather it seems preferable to make clear the missing categories — namely, non-culpable deviancy caused psychologically, socially, and culturally, for example, by the lack of various forms of psychological, social, and cultural welfare. The case can then be made that such psychological, social, or cultural support, too, is fundamental to man's existence, at least as fundamental as health in the somatic sense.

If it is the case that deviancies can be meaningfully differentia.ed as organic and non-organic as well as voluntary and non-voluntary, then we must disagree with Sedgwick in the conclusion he draws in his argument against Szasz, Laing, Goffman, and others. Earlier I indicated that Sedgwick was correct in his claim that both organic and mental deviancies require social evaluations. Merely establishing, however, that the two phenomena are not to be differentiated on *this* dimension does not establish the positive argument that therefore "mental illness *is* illness." Against Sedgwick, I would argue that even though they are the same in both being negatively evaluated social deviancies, they diffei in that one is organic while the other is in the psychological realm. This, we shall argue, has important practical as well as theoretical implications.

Thus far, I have focussed on the primarily analytical argument, claiming that the medical model, at least in its original and pure form, applies to non-voluntary and organic deviations from the norms established by a society. Let us now turn to the practical implications. By far the most important practical consequence of the limitation of the medical model refers to the professional cadre who will become involved depending upon the model employed. Before taking up that point in the next section of the paper, however, I wish to consider a question growing out of the alternative role models implied in the different sub-systems.

In a theoretical discussion of types of roles, Lemert distinguishes between primary and secondary deviant roles.[21] This distinction, also reflected in Parsons' axis of differentiation between total and partial deviance, is between roles which totally reorganize one's life and roles which permit one to continue in other roles with minimal impact. Freidson applies this distinction to the medical model and argues that there are really different types of deviant roles in the health-illness complex.[22] Minor medical difficulties, of which the cold is the type case, produce only a primary role. The individual with a cold does not normally fully adopt the sick role with its new exemptions and responsibilities. On the other hand, the person with a major disease such as polio clearly adopts all of the characteristics of the role. The sick role, or at least the patient role, is thus a secondary role, while minor forms of deviancy in the medical model (a cold, a cut finger, a headache) generate only a new primary role actor.

Now the question arises if there is a precisely parallel pattern in deviancies which, according to our philosophy of causation, are best understood as non-organic. There is no theoretical reason why that would be the case. There may well be something uniquely associated with organicity which would lead to the development of a secondary deviant role. The notions of contagion, the need for rest for bodily repair, the effectiveness of special technical instruments and procedures for "healing" the sick person may generate pressures to remove the (organically) sick individual from his normal roles in favor of the sick role which are far greater than for the non-organically caused deviancy. People interpreted as being psychologically deviant may be more likely to continue in their normal primary roles. Those with deviancies thought to be socially caused are quickly put in the criminal role, but the role implies voluntary deviance in the social realm. The concept of non-voluntary socially determined deviancy is a newer concept and one for which virtually no one is assigned a secondary role. To collapse the different sub-systems may well have a serious impact on the development of primary and secondary deviant roles.

C. The Physician as the Technically Competent Expert

The third characteristic of the medical model is that the technically competent expert is the physician (often supported by a cadre of associates and assistants). The sick role includes an obligation to seek technically competent help appropriate to the need of the sickness. Parsons goes on specifically to state that the technically competent expert is "in the most usual case" the physician. This seems to be one of the most clearly established characteristics of the medical model. One of the important ideological implications of the sick role as Parsons states it is that in addition to removing the sick one from the realm of responsible actors it places him under the control of the medical professional.

The physician has authority; he gives "doctor's orders." More than this, the medical professional has first claim to jurisdiction in labelling of illness.[23] When a case is unambiguously within the medical model, it may well be appropriate for the medical professional to have the primary responsibility for labelling of a specific illness. Thus, when one has a small growth on the skin and wants to know whether it is cancer, a boil, or a normal bump, it is appropriate to turn to a physician. That, it seems to us, is where the authority must stop. It is not appropriate, for instance, for the medical professional to carry out the social evaluation of the badness or the goodness of the cancer (granted that the naming and diagnosing function of the physician must include telling the "seriousness" of the medical condition, the prognosis under various alternatives).

All too often, however, doubtful or ambiguous illnesses are placed into the medical model for the purpose of determining whether or not they are indeed illnesses rather than other forms of deviancy. This is fundamentally different from approaching a physician to determine whether or not a lump is a cancer. Let us grant that the experts in any form of deviancy, if they exist at all, have authority to diagnose the presence of deviancies which are clearly within their realm. But that does not mean that they have authority to arbitrate a dispute about whether an identified but marginal deviancy is within their model.

The British have been particularly guilty of this in the handling of narcotic addiction. In 1924 the British wanted to know whether narcotic addiction should be dealt with in the medical model or some alternative (the criminal being the most viable alternative). To resolve this they turned to the Rolleston Committee, a committee of distinguished physicians. It never seems to have been realized that precisely at that point was the decision made—by the public—to place narcotic addiction into the medical model. The conclusion of the group of physicians—that narcotic addiction was an illness—was anti-climactic and theoretically unsound.

If the question is to determine whether a deviancy is in one model or another, the methodology must involve, as a minimum, not only the acceptance of the deviancy by the experts of one model, but also the rejection of the deviancy by the experts of all the other relevant models. Thus, one might use the Siegler-Osmond list of models and insist that the opinion of functionaries in each model be obtained. Since the moral model has the entire public as the expert class, in effect it is the public which must make the decision to classify a deviancy within or without a model. Turning to the experts within the medical model for this function is a theoretically confused move.

The behavior under consideration is non-organic, non-culpable, but negatively evaluated deviancies. The question is whether such types of behavior should be within the medical model. Recognizing that the medical model not only specifies the obligation to seek technically competent help, but also specifies that those experts are medical professionals, i.e. physicians, the implication is clear. Medically trained professionals are to be placed in control of such behavior and its correction if it is placed on the medical model. This seems to me both dangerous and unjustified in the light of the training and skills of such professionals. It is shocking to realize that, using the basic sub-systems as differentiation points, the psychiatrist is the only professional in Western society who receives his primary training in one of the sub-systems yet practices primarily in another.

The World Health Organization definition of health as encompassing total well-being means that, in effect, the medical professional is the one to turn to for technically competent help in such failures in well being as marriage problems, poverty, and unanswered prayers. This will require either radical retraining and redefinition of the medical professional or, more practically, the development of clearer categories of deviant roles.

In the medical model the early generation of a secondary deviant role places the deviant (ill) one under the control of the medical professional and removes control from the layman. We should, therefore, be careful not to extend this removal of individual freedom and dignity into non-organic forms of behavior too hastily. If the ratio of primary and secondary roles may be different in organic and non-organic deviancy, it may well be that the creation of technically competent experts in these non-organic realms may not follow the same patterns either. Perhaps we will be unable to produce such technically competent experts at all, or we may not be able to differentiate sub-specialties in the same way. The expansion of the medical model to cover such categories could only be dangerous.

D. Restoration of a Minimal Standard of Health

There is a fourth characteristic of the medical model, one which is probably the most difficult to grasp. I argued, in the first section of this paper, that even illness in the most traditional (i.e., non-culpable and organic) sense requires a social evaluation which is negative. The sick role is a socially disapproved, though legitimate, role. This is true by definition. One would not be sick but simply either unusual or super-healthy if he were abnormal in a manner which was not socially disapproved. We have purposely bracketed until now the question of the nature of the norm from which the deviant deviates in the medical model. Whatever it is, it is clear that the name for the norm is "health." Based on the previous discussion we would define health in a preliminary way as an organic condition of the body judged by the social system of meaning and value to be good.

Health, however, is an abstract norm, and abstractions in the human cultural symbol system function on at least two levels. On the one hand, in the abstract form, health exists as an ideal, a norm in the sense of being the highest or ideal type. Health in this meaning would be the organic condition of the body judged by the social system to be the best possible organic condition for a body. Abstract nouns also function in language to refer to some minimal standard, often, but not always, associated with a statistical mean or mode. In this sense, healthiness may be only a condition of the body judged by the social system of meaning and value to be better than a minimal standard. Thus, it is quite meaningful to say of two individuals that they are both healthy, but one is healthier. That statement would be impossible unless we could use the term in both senses simultaneously. "Healthy" refers simply to the minimal societal standard, but the "health" to which the word "healthier" refers is an ideal such that one individual approaches that ideal more closely. This dual function of abstract nouns in language is not unique to the concept health, but applies to all such abstract concepts.

In the medical model the most narrow reference seems to be to the minimal standard of healthiness. A deviancy fits most clearly in the medical model when it is perceived as falling below a minimal standard of healthiness. However, in the broader and more ambiguous sense, the problem of improving someone's health beyond the minimal standard to approach the ideal is only with difficulty assimilated to the medical model.

Our conceptualizations are frequently determined by the formulation of polarizations. Thus, the public health movement has posed the poles of restoring and preserving health. Both functions are clearly within the medical model in the more restricted sense. But this formulation often makes one lose sight completely of the possibility of an option to improve health beyond the normal. A number of somatic improvements are conceivable and perhaps technically feasible. They might include reduction of normal amounts of sleep needed, equipping the body to manufacture amino acids which now need to be obtained from animal protein, elimination of the menstrual cycle, and elimination of baldness. Would such activities be classed within the medical model? I think only with difficulty. They fit the medical model imperfectly and are analogous to other conditions which fit some, but not all, of the characteristics of the medical model.

While there is no necessary reason why medical practitioners should be limited to restoring and preserving minimal, socially defined standards of health, at least in Western medicine, the priority of these tasks seems well established. Even the normative principles of medical ethics reflect this orientation. At least according to one major strand of professional medical ethics, the primary moral principle is "first of all do no harm." This maxim differs in a significant way from classical utilitarianism even if it were applied solely with reference to the patient. The "don't harm rather than maximize the good" maxim is built on the same notion of a theoretical, socially defined minimal standard or base line. It gives rise to a philosophical problem which we might call the "baseline problem." The idea of normalcy from which one can measure health and illness, benefit and harm, commission and omission of an act, ordinary and extraordinary means, or positive and negative incentives, is not well explored in the philosophical literature — and should be. In any case, it seems to have been incorporated into the medical as well as the legal and normative ethical tradition. An action is less ambiguously included in the medical model when it is an effort to restore or preserve that baseline of minimally accepted health rather than to improve health beyond that baseline to an ideal.

III. The Medical Model and Marginal Deviancies

In the last section of this paper, I traced what I see as four essential defining characteristics of the medical model. For a type of deviant behavior to be interpreted as falling clearly within the medical model, it must first of all be negatively evaluated. Then it must be seen as (1) non-voluntary, (2) organic, (3) within the province of the medical professional, and (4) falling below some societally defined minimal standard of health. To the extent that the deviancy fits all of those characteristics, it will clearly be within the medical model. It is, however, when the behavior fails to meet one or more of these characteristics, or is called into question on one or more of them, that the medical model begins to seem less appropriate. The difficulty with such doubtful illnesses as narcotic addiction is thus apparent. For many, addiction remains a voluntary choice which sufficient will power could overcome. The testimonies of former addicts about how difficult the habit was to overcome only support this view. For many, addiction is non-organic at the stages of behavior, response (treatment), proximal or ultimate cause. In part because of these factors, these doubters may (but not necessarily will) reject the physician as the appropriate technical professional to respond to addiction. While addiction is clearly statistically aberrent, it may not always be considered below a minimal standard of health and may, especially in the case of marijuana, not be negatively evaluated as an alternative life style at all. With doubts at all of these levels, it is hardly surprising that narcotic addiction and similar deviancies are disputed in classification.

I believe that the bulk of the problem comes from reductionistic tendencies to polarize deviancy between the extremes of crime and illness and the use of the single category of illness to cover all non-voluntary deviancy. If all of the variables mentioned in this paper were cross tabulated, 48 models would result (voluntary/non-voluntary x organic/psychological/social/cultural x technical expert/no technical expertise x restoring health/preserving health/improving health). If differentiation within categories such as the social and cultural subsystems were included, the figure would be that much higher. I feel that the expansion of the medical model to cover the other models is dangerous when unique characteristics exist for the other models and treating such deviancies as unique entities would be more realistic.

Particularly interesting and troublesome will be the models which combine the assumed need for technically competent biomedical experts with the characteristics of the other three dimensions which tend away from the medical model. We have seen that in relation to each of the characteristics of the medical model, there may be conditions requiring medical expertise for the resolution of perceived problems which are not considered to be unambiguously within the medical model. The clearest example may arise on the sub-system dimension. There are (or at least theoretically may be) deviancies which are considered non-organic in ultimate and proximal cause as well as in behavior, yet susceptible to chemical, surgical, or other medical "treatment" (response). We know, with a degree of certainty, that amygdalotomy will control violent behavior while we may not be certain that the "cause" of the behavior is somatic. We know chemical agents can condition avoidance of alcohol even if we are not sure the cause of alcoholism is biochemical. Likewise, we know that voluntarily induced somatic complaints are amenable to treatment by a physician. Recent discussion of hair implants has raised the question whether such procedures are sufficiently medical to justify tax deduction. This and other procedures may be medical in all senses except that they improve the bodily condition beyond societal standards of minimal acceptability. These cases will raise serious conflict for the medical professional as well as for the tax collector.

These ambiguous categories (voluntarily induced somatic complaint; non-voluntary, non-organic complaint; and somatic complaint requiring extension beyond societal standards of minimal acceptability) are frequently labelled "elective" in contrast to "therapeutic" procedures. The term applies equally well to abortions for serious social reasons or "cosmetic" surgery which is considered beyond the minimal standards of physical health. These terms are terribly imprecise and probably misleading. In fact, in a country where free choice is valued, all medical procedures are elective for the patient (except in the case of incompetents where guardians elect medical treatments of, if necessary, courts will appoint a new guardian for the purposes of election). On the other hand, if "therapeutic" means simply "corrective" it might apply equally to non-somatic as well as somatic complaints provided the fourth criterion of intervention necessary to produce a minimal standard established by society is met. It might be better to abandon these terms, recognizing instead that, increasingly, medically trained experts will be called upon to provide response to conditions which are not clearly in the medical model or are clearly not in the medical model.

This will be confusing and frustrating for professional and layman alike, but is a necessary concomitant to increasing biomedical technology which gives ever greater power to control, increasing sophistication about non-organic theories of causation, and expanding horizons about what is possible over and beyond that which is minimally acceptable. Nevertheless, the mere usefulness of intervention by technically competent medically trained individuals should not be a sufficient condition to place the deviancy into the medical model. Instead we would reserve that model for conditions which more nearly meet all four of the characteristics outlined here. Even deviancies clearly within the medical model rest upon a social judgment that the condition is unacceptable, so any such categorization cannot be used to isolate an "objective" value-free zone; but it can make clear our philosophical presuppositions about free will and determinism, our theories of causation linked to sub-systems, or judgments about distinctions between restoring, preserving, and improving health, and differentiation in the role of the relevant technically competent professional as well as in the role of the actor whose behavior is in question.

NOTES

1. Eliot Friedson, *Profession of Medicine* (New York: Dodd, Mead, 1971), p. 211.
2. Ibid., p. 208. Italics in the original.

3. See Peter L. Berger and Thomas Luckmann, *The Social Construction of Reality* (Garden City, N.Y.: Doubleday, 1966).

4. In fact, it is our position that there are "absolute and objective" values and meanings upon which one may properly or improperly construct a socio-cultural understanding, but to argue this point, just as to argue the point of whether or not there are in fact real physical objects in reality to which our natural scientific sense impressions should correspond, is to lead into the realm of metaphysics and theology. I have made such arguments elsewhere (*Hastings Center Studies* 1 [Number 1, 1973], pp. 50-65), but would claim that the present discussion is independent of these debates about the nature of the transcendent. For a similar position see Peter L. Berger, "Appendix II. Sociological and Theological Perspectives," in *The Sacred Canopy* (Garden City, N.Y.: Doubleday, 1967), pp. 179-88.

5. Of course, it may be, at least for a holder of the view that real values and meanings exist in the transcendent world of objectivity, that some individuals have characteristics which ought to be seen and treated by a society and yet are not — or, on the other hand, are seen and treated by society as sick but ought not to be. The fact is however that one really is sick in the sense of living the sick role if and only if the social judgment is made by society or some portion of it.

6. Talcott Parsons, *The Social System* (New York: The Free Press, 1951), pp. 428-79. This chapter is probably the most significant in (and the origin of) contemporary sociology of medicine. It grows out of an earlier field study of medical practice conducted by Parsons. It is important to realize that not only sociology of medicine, but some important categories in theoretical sociology, especially the sociology of the professions and the sociology of deviance, grow out of this medical context. We would suspect that the use of the medical model as the paradigm for study of these more general issues has generated the expansionist tendencies for the medical model, the sick role and related theoretical constructs, the use of the model to cover all legitimated, non-culpable forms of deviancy, and the transfer of the obligation to seek technically competent help to the obligation to use medical personnel. Other sociological interpretations of illness as a form of legitimated deviancy can be found in David Mechanic, *Medical Sociology* (New York: The Free Press, 1968); Robert N. Wilson, *The Sociology of Health* (New York: Random House, 1970); Stanley H. King, "Social Psychological Factors in Illness," in Howard E. Freeman, Sol Levine, and Leo G. Reeder (eds.), *Handbook of Medical Sociology* (Englewood Cliffs, N.J.: Prentice-Hall, 1963), pp. 99-121, especially p. 112; and Robert N. Wilson, "Patient-Practitioner Relationships," in ibid., pp. 273-95, especially pp. 276-77.

In addition there are now several examples in the literature of authors who begin with the notion of illness as socially constructed deviancy and build this into a critical commentary on the incorporation of major forms of deviancy into the medical model. These include Erving Goffman, *Asylums* (Garden City, N.Y.: Doubleday, 1961); Thomas Szasz, *The Myth of Mental Illness* (New York: Harper & Row, 1961), and *The Manufacture of Madness* (New York: Harper & Row, 1970).

7. There is some disagreement about whether the person in the sick role has an obligation to "want" to get well or only to "try" to get well. Normally desires or wants are not obligated. Robert N. Wilson in *The Sociology of Health* (New York: Random House, 1970), p. 17, claims simply that there is "an obligation to 'get well' and to cooperate with others to this end." If, however, the sick role is by social definition undesirable, probably Parsons' formulation of the obligation to "want to get well" is appropriate. Parsons in "Definitions of Health and Illness in the Light of American Values and Social Structure," in E. G. Jaco (ed.), *Patients, Physicians and Illness* (New York: The Free Press, 1958), p. 176, says the sick person has an "obligation to try to 'get well.'"

8. Classifying illness as one among many types of socially defined deviant behavior which are disapproved does not mean that blame is imputed. The literature distinguishes between "legitimated" and "nonlegitimated" forms of social deviancy.

9. See the article by Peter Sedgwick in this issue. (See this book, pp. 49-60).

10. Talcott Parsons, "Definitions of Health and Illness in the Light of American Values and Social Structure," pp. 165-87.

11. Ibid., p. 173.

12. *Drug Addiction: Crime or Disease?* Interim and Final Reports of the Joint Committee of the American Bar Association and the American Medical Association on Narcotic Drugs (Bloomington:

Indiana University Press, 1961). In a newly published volume, Anthony Flew, *Crime or Disease?* (New York: Macmillan, 1973), creates the same polarization for the opposite motive in a discussion of the nature of mental disorder. He finds the removal of responsibility implied in the "disease" model a threat to individual dignity and is thus critical of its application to criminal behavior.

13. Miriam Siegler and Humphry Osmond, "Models of Madness," *British Journal of Psychiatry* 112 (1966), 1193-1203; "Models of Drug Addiction," *International Journal of Addictions,* 3 (No. 1, 1968), 3-24; and "The Impaired Model of Schizophrenia," *Schizophrenia* 1 (No. 3, 1969), 192-202; and Miriam Siegler, Humphry Osmond, and S. Newell, "Models of Alcoholism," *Quarterly Journal of the Study of Alcoholism* 29 (No. 3, 1968), 571-91. Unfortunately, the authors in this series do not devote much attention to the theoretical distinctions responsible for the differentiation of their interesting list of models.

14. We shall sometimes use the term non-culpable in place of non-voluntaristic. Technically, however, an important difference should be noted. A deviancy such as marijuana smoking may be viewed as voluntary and yet non-culpable if one simply challenges the negative evaluation. Culpability thus implies simultaneously willful control and negative evaluation.

15. See Goffman, *Asylums,* pp. 153-54.

16. Parsons, "Health and Illness," pp. 178ff.

17. Talcott Parsons, et al. (eds.), *Theories of Society: Foundation of Modern Sociological Theory* (New York: The Free Press, 1961).

18. Treatment is a term which probably could be applied to this level, but in some contexts implies a medical model metaphor. This is possibly not always true—crops are treated with insecticide—but we prefer to use the more neutral term "response."

19. Ultimate is clearly a relative word. The Western notion of causation often implies an infinite regress. I, however, shall consider a cause ultimate at the level of the individual to be organic if the first entry into the human organism in the causation chain is organic.

The British Rolleston Committee documented its use of the distinction between organic and non-organic causation models when it defined drug addiction as the use of a drug for purposes other than the relief of symptoms of an organic disease.

20. Edward M. Brecher and the Editors of Consumer Reports, *Licit and Illicit Drugs* (Boston: Little, Brown and Company, 1972), pp. 67-68, offers a brief summary.

21. Edwin Lemert, *Social Pathology* (New York: McGraw-Hill, 1964).

22. Freidson, *Profession of Medicine,* p. 231-34.

23. See ibid., p. 251.

Michael S. Moore

Some Myths About "Mental Illness"

The concept of mental illness has had a long and interesting history in man's thoughts about himself, his nature, and his responsibility. It stands at one junction of law, morals, and medicine, with the result that lawyers, psychiatrists, and philosophers have long shared a concern for the nature of the concept. This shared concern has not given rise to any consensus, however, and the debates, particularly between lawyers and psychiatrists, have often been acrimonious and unfruitful. Since the advent of "radical psychiatry," the theoretical justification of which is to be found notably in the works of Thomas Szasz, the battle lines have been redrawn somewhat along other than professional lines, but the result has not been added clarity about the nature of the concept of mental disease or its moral and legal relevance.

Indeed, quite the reverse has occurred, so that essentially ethical and political questions about psychiatric practices or legal doctrines with regard to the mentally ill are increasingly answered by the trundling out of the contemporary shibboleth that mental illness is a myth rather than in terms of the ethical and political arguments necessary to answer such questions. There is a disturbing tendency to regard complicated legal issues, notably the proper place of mental illness in various legal tests (of insanity in criminal trials, of incompetency to perform various legal acts or to stand trial, the tests for civil commitment), as solved by the new truth that mental illness is but a myth anyway. Equally disturbing is the apparent belief that problems of social policy and social justice, such as what in fact society should do with dangerous persons

From *Archives of General Psychiatry*, 32 (December 1975):1483–1497. Copyright © 1975 by American Medical Association. Reprinted by permission of the publisher and the author.

who have not committed any criminal acts, are satisfactorily resolved if legislatures would but recognize mental illness for the sham that it is.

If mental illness were a myth, acceptance of such a truth would provide straightforward answers to such legal, ethical, and political questions. One would not have to muddle along in the grubby details of comparing awful prisons with almost as awful hospitals for the criminally insane. One would not have to grapple with difficult policy issues, such as the rationale for punishment generally and its relation to those found to be not guilty by reason of insanity, for it would be instantly clear that those we call mentally ill should be punished just like anyone else if they commit a criminal act; that they should have all the rights of an accused criminal if society should seek to deprive them of their liberty no matter how the proceeding or the place of confinement might be named; that legal tests should abolish the phrase; and, easiest of all, that psychiatrists should mind their own business and leave the law to the lawyers.

The problem is that mental illness is not a myth. It is not some palpable falsehood propagated among the populace by power-mad psychiatrists, but a cruel and bitter reality that has been with the human race since antiquity. This is such an obvious truism that to have stated it 20 years ago would have been an embarrassment. Since the advent of radical psychiatry and its legal entourage, however, such truths need restatement. Even more, they need restatement in a form specifically addressed to the various senses in which mental illness has been thought to be a myth. Since on my reading of the radical psychiatrists there seem to be five distinguishable points they have in mind in thinking of mental illness as a myth, the discussion will proceed by considering them seriatim.

THE MYTHOLOGY OF RADICAL PSYCHIATRY

The Myth as a Question of Ontological Status:
There Is No Such Thing as Mental Illness Because
There Is No Referent of the Phrase

Mental illness is a myth because, as quoted by the present Chief Justice of the United States Supreme Court, "there is neither such a thing as 'insanity' nor such a thing as 'mental disease.' These terms do not identify entities having separate existence. . . ."[1] (p. 859) As was more formally stated:

> It is a term without ostensive referent [sic], and lacking any, it cannot even be said to have outlived its usefulness, because there is no reason to think that it ever had any.[2] (p. 184)

Szasz and his psychiatric and legal followers are suspicious of mental illness as an entity or thing; when looking into their ontology, they see no such thing. The following three points require discussion here:

1. If the argument is that entity-thinking *as such* is to be regarded with suspicion, as Szasz at times suggests, then the critique is radical indeed. As Quine has noted, "we talk so inveterately of objects that to say we do so seems almost to say nothing at all; for how else is there to talk?"[3] (p. 1) Thing-theory is implicit throughout our ordinary and scientific speech, and it is simply wrong to regard it as some primitive form of speech that is replaced with a more sophisticated mode of talk with the maturity of a science. Thus, Szasz's statement that "Entity-thinking has always preceded process-thinking"[4] (p. 1) is not an accurate characterization of the development of modern science. In fact, higher order theoretical statements characteristic of advancing science *increase* the number of entities we admit into our ontology, not decrease it. Forces, fields, and electrons are obvious examples.

2. If the argument is that entity-thinking is scientifically legitimate, but only about those entities referred to by terms capable of ostensive reference, such as "Nixon," or "St. Elizabeth's Hospital," the radical psychiatrists have a radically impoverished ontology — a nominalist ontology that would not admit the "thinghood" of abstract entities such as the number two, squareness, shape, zoological species, or, more to the point perhaps, psychological states. Such a restricted ontology is characteristic neither of science nor of common understanding.

Indeed, in such a restrictive ontological system physical illnesses would not exist either. The names of physical illnesses do not refer to concrete entities, for "Diseases are not *things* in the same sense as rocks, or trees, or rivers. Diseases . . . are not material."[5] Although diseases might be *caused* by the presence in the body of some such entity (as a cold may be caused by a virus), and although they might be associated with *symptoms* that are concrete entities (e.g., the fluid present in the sinuses), a physical illness is not (identical with) either its causes or its symptoms. The only thing one can fix as the reference of the names of various physical illnesses are states the ill are in, abstract entities incapable of being pointed at in some ostensive definition.

3. In any case, most of the things people have wanted to say about mental illness can be said without making ontological commitments to any entity, concrete or abstract, referred to by the phrase, and thus any criticism of its use based on its lack of a referent, ostensive or otherwise, is misconceived. In his essay on Sense and Reference Frege made famous the distinction between the sense of a term, and its reference.[6] The important corollary for our purpose is that words may be used significantly (make good sense) and yet *not refer*. As Quine has elaborated, "Being a name of something is a much more special feature than being meaningful." Even "[a] singular term need not name to be significant."[7] (pp. 9, 11)

This is particularly evident in our use of predicates. We can say "some dogs are white" or "some houses are red," without making ontological commitments to (without presupposing there are such things as) whiteness or redness. Similarly, we can say that "some persons are mentally ill" without making ontological commitments to any *thing* referred to by "illness." More colloquially, the denial of the existence of any thing called mental illness hardly entails a denial of the existence of *persons* who are mentally ill.

In addition to describing people as being mentally ill, we also often wish to explain their behavior as being due to their mental illness. While such statements as "He did it because of his mental illness" appear to require an entity referred to by the phrase "mental illness," in fact such explanations mean nothing more than is conveyed by "He did it because he is mentally ill"—another use of the predicate, "is mentally ill" that does not require a reference to be significant.

To the extent that common and psychiatric discourse about mental illness can be paraphrased so as to avoid the hypostasis of an entity named by the phrase, then any criticism that complains that there is no such thing as mental illness is beside the point; for orthodox psychiatry and common understanding can happily agree, but still use the phrase to make significant (albeit nonreferring) statements. We often make use of the names of states, attributes, properties, and traits as if they named some things in our ontology, for economy of speech is often gained by so doing. To be sure, if someone (such as Szasz) makes an issue of the ontological commitments involved in our uses of "redness," or "illness," the burden is of course on us to paraphrase or retract.[3] (p. 100) However, if we can paraphrase the usage into the noncommitting use of "ill," then the phraseology is a harmless but convenient mode of speaking, against which the "ontological discovery" of radical psychiatry is irrelevant.

For my own part, I think this detour into ontology is a red herring. The lack of any thing one can point to as the referent of the phrase "mental illness" does not do orthodox psychiatry the damage Szasz and his followers suppose; if mental illness is a myth in this sense, it is in the good company of many other words and phrases useful in science and everyday life that have either no reference or a reference only to abstract entities. That this herring is constantly being dragged across our path is doubtless due to the immense popular appeal the denial-of-existence idiom has when used in the hands of a skillful polemist. It makes the study of mental illness *sound* about as useful as the study of unicorns.

Once one perceives that ontological status is not really an issue here, then other types of arguments must be marshalled in favor of eliminating "mental illness" from our vocabulary.

The Myth as an Empirical Discovery: No One Is in Fact Mentally Ill

Often mental illness is said to be a myth, not just in the sense that it does not exist, but also in the sense that no one is in fact mentally ill. The claim, in other words, denies not just that "mental illness" is a name of some thing, but that "mentally ill" is ever truly predicable of a person. The claim is that no one is really mentally ill.

This claim that mental illness is a myth is put forward as an empirical discovery—all of these people that have been thought to be mentally ill (i.e., irrational) are in fact just as rational as you and I. Szasz makes this claim when he argues that "insane behavior, no less than sane, is goal-directed and motivated . . ." and concludes from this that we should regard "the behavior of the madman as perfectly rational from the point of view of the actor. . . ."[8] (p. 123) Braginsky and co-workers purport to have made the same "discovery" regarding schizophrenics:

> The residents who remain in 'mental hospitals' are behaving in a perfectly rational manner to achieve a personally satisfying way of life—often the most satisfying of which they are capable . . . in a certain sense an individual *chooses* his career as a mental patient; it is not thrust upon him as a consequence of his somehow becoming 'mentally ill.' But in just what sense does the individual 'choose' his career? In our view, having and maintaining the status of a mental patient is the outcome of *purposive* behavior. Furthermore, given the life circumstances of most of the persons who become and remain residents of mental hospitals, their doing so evinces a realistic appraisal of their available alternatives; it is, in short a *rational choice*.[2] (p. 171)

The central thrust of this form of the argument is not to claim that "mental illness" or "mentally ill" are meaningless—their meaning is assumed to be closely connected with that of "irrational"—but to dispute as a factual matter that there are persons who fit the agreed-upon definition of mental illness (irrationality). In fact, however, what has been done here is not to present a discovery of new facts, overlooked by orthodox psychiatrists because of their own self-interest or whatever, but rather to stretch our concepts of "rationality" and "purposive behavior" to accommodate within their criteria facts well-known to orthodox, as well as to radical, psychiatrists. The facts—the behavior of patients—are often undisputed. What is disputed is the precise nature of the criterion to be applied in judging the behavior as rational or not.

As the above quotations from Szasz and Braginsky et al. make clear, the notion of rationality relevant here is linked to the actor having reasons (purposes, motives) for his actions. A more precise account of the relationship between an agent being thought to be rational and his acting for reasons may perhaps best be brought out by the following schema of reason-giving explanations. When we explain an action by giving the actor's motive, the following premises are involved:

1. Agent X wants result R to obtain.
2. X believes that in situation S, action A will cause R to obtain.
3. X believes that he is in situation S.
4. If X believes that he is in situation S and believes that in S action A will cause R to obtain, and if X wants R to obtain, then, ceteris paribus, X will do A.
5. Ceteris paribus.

With these premises, it follows that X will do A.

In ordinary English, in order to make out a motivational explanation we need to know what the agent wanted and what he believed about the situation and his abilities to achieve through action what he wanted. In addition, we need to know that he is a rational creature in the fundamental sense of "rational" defined by the fourth premise, that is, one who, other things being equal, will act so as to further his desires in light of his beliefs; and we need to know that other things are in fact equal, namely, that the agent does not have desires and beliefs that conflict with the desires and beliefs on which he is about to act.

The actions of the mentally ill may be nonrational or irrational in any of five following corresponding senses: (1) R may be an unintelligible thing to want, such as soaking one's elbow in the mud for its own sake; (2) the belief that A will lead to R may be an irrational belief (e.g., a belief that saying "storks" instead of "stocks" will make one a mother); (3) the belief that one is in situation S may also be irrational (e.g., a belief that one is being persecuted by spirits); (4) there may be no set of beliefs and desires, no matter how bizarre, by virtue of which one can make out the action as the rational thing to do; or (5) the beliefs and desires of the particular practical syllogism may be inconsistent with other standing beliefs and desires.

The rationality of an *agent* is a function of the rationality of his actions over time. The more irrational behavior we observe of an individual in any of these five senses, the less rational we will judge him as an agent to be.

By and large, the empirical version of the myth argument is only intended to show that the behavior of the mentally ill is rational in the fundamental sense defined by the fourth premise above, i.e., there is *some* set of beliefs and desires (no matter how bizarre) furthered by the act in question. The crunch for even this limited attempt at making out the behavior of the mentally ill as rational, comes in making more precise the nature of the beliefs and desires of mental patients in terms of which their actions are to be so adjudged. More specifically, the fudge occurs with the use of *unconscious* beliefs and desires to fill in where we all know that mental patients did not consciously guide their actions to achieve such goals in light of such beliefs. Braginsky and colleagues are explicit about this: "It is obvious that rational goal-directed behavior does not guarantee that the individual appreciates what he is up to."[2] (p. 171) Szasz is particularly transparent in his glossing over of this distinction:

In describing this contrast between lying and erring, I have deliberately avoided the concept of consciousness. It seems to me that when the adjectives "consciously" and "unconsciously" are used as explanations, they complicate and obscure the problem. The traditional psychoanalytic idea that so-called conscious imitation of illness is "malingering" and hence "not illness," whereas its allegedly unconscious simulation is itself "illness" ("hysteria"), creates more problems than it solves. It would seem more useful to *distinguish between goal-directed and rule-following behavior on the one hand, and indifferent mistakes on the other* . . . In brief, *it is more accurate to regard hysteria as a lie than as a mistake.* People caught in a lie usually maintain that they were merely mistaken. The difference between mistakes and lies, when discovered, is chiefly pragmatic. From a purely cognitive point of view, both are simply falsehoods.[4] (pp. 142, 143)

The fudge occurs in the shift from our judgments of rationality being based on the agent's conscious beliefs and objectives to a notion of rationality by virtue of which we adjudge an action at least minimally rational if we can posit any set of beliefs or objectives with which we can explain the action. The problem is that it is notoriously easy to posit beliefs and desires to explain any finite sequence of the behavior of anything. Simply pick a consequence of the behavior and label it the objective, pick a set of beliefs by virtue of which it would appear likely that such a consequence would indeed ensue as a result of the behavior, and one is then in a position to adjudge the behavior as rational, relative to that objective and that set of beliefs. The shedding of leaves by a tree, the falling of stones, the pumping of blood by the heart, and the most chaotic word-salad of a schizophrenic are all "rational" activities judged by such a standard. The "action" of a tree in shedding its leaves is rational if we suppose that it desires to survive the coming winter, and believes that the only way to do this is to lower its sap level, thereby killing off its leaves. The same analysis can be applied to stones, hearts, and schizophrenics.

The reason such explanations are so easy to manufacture is because without the requirement that an agent be conscious of the beliefs and the desires by which we (and he) judge his action as rational, there is no means of fixing the nature of such beliefs or wants independently of the behavior to be explained and adjudged. Behavior is by itself inherently ambiguous as a criterion for such matters. If we know by some independent means that an agent believes that action A will lead to result R, and he does A, we have good grounds for attributing to him a desire for R; if we know that he desires R, and does A, we have equally good grounds for supposing that he believes that A will lead to R. However, if we know neither his beliefs nor his desires, but only that he does A and that A does result in R being the case, we have no means of singling out R as his motive, for any other consequence of A would do as well. "There is nothing in a pure behaviorist theory to prevent us from regarding each piece of behavior as a desire for whatever happens next."[9] (p. 108)

Szasz can thus ignore the conscious/unconscious distinction only at the price of significance. What he fails to realize is that any behavior can be seen as rational (or as in accordance with rules of a game, or as furthering certain goals — Szasz's substitute criteria for consciousness), if one allows oneself the freedom to *invent* the beliefs and desires in terms of which the behavior is to be so viewed.

It may be objected that good sense at least seems to be made in the use of unconscious beliefs and unconscious desires in explaining human action, even in orthodox psychoanalysis, and thus that the foregoing must be an inadequate account of motivated action and hence, of rational action. As Stuart Hampshire[10] and Dilman[11] have pointed out, unconscious beliefs and unconscious desires can make good sense, so long as they are used in a way that ties them to consciousness. One may have the same independent grounds for ascribing beliefs and desires to an agent if his first person statements of his *memory* of them are accorded the same authority as are his normal, first person, present tense reports of them. When in successful psychoanalytic therapy the patient comes to know his motives or beliefs, he comes to know them in the same noninferential, nonobservational way as we all normally know our own motives, and in such cases it makes sense to grant the usual authority to his sincere avowals of what they are. As long as the nature of such beliefs or desires is dependent on authoritative statements of the agent who himself remembers them (as opposed to inferring them from observing his own behavior or acceding to the authority of his analyst), significant explanations of his behavior can be formed using such unconscious motives.

So restricted, how much of the behavior of the mentally ill can even be said to be unconsciously motivated? Are there sets of beliefs and desires, conscious *or* unconscious, that explain the peculiar string of words and sounds sometimes uttered as a kind of word-salad by the mentally ill? Can one give such an explanation of the actions-by-omission of the vegetating catatonic, or of the violent actions against self-interest such as beating one's head against the wall? Note that the question is not whether one can or cannot come up with legitimate *causal* hypotheses about why the patient is in the state he is in. Nor is the question whether or not one can *invent* some set of beliefs and desires which, *if* the patient had them, would render his action rational. Rather, the question is whether such patients are performing an action for reasons which they either recognize, or if sufficient effort were made, could come to recognize as an action *they* were doing for reasons *they* found sufficient. Put this way, much of the behavior by which the more extreme forms of mental illness are diagnosed remains unmotivated and hence nonrational.

In any case, such behavior of the mentally ill as can be legitimately explained by reference to unconscious beliefs or unconscious desires is not fully rational. By hypothesis, such behavior is minimally rational because motivated. It is typically *irrational,* however, in each of the several other senses of "rationality" mentioned earlier—the desires may be unintelligible, the beliefs about means irrational (or at least the means/end calculation grossly inefficient), the beliefs about the situation in which the actor finds himself irrational, or the beliefs and desires inconsistent with standing beliefs and desires. Since these aspects of the irrationality of unconscious motive explanations have been explored by others,[12-15] they need not be pursued further here.

On occasion, the empirical version of the myth claim is put forward without any extensive reliance on some supposed unconscious beliefs or desires of the mentally ill. Laing in particular explicitly disavows[16] (p. 26) use of unconscious beliefs or desires in reaching his well known conclusions that "*without exception* the experience and behavior that gets labeled schizophrenic is *a special strategy that a person invents in order to live in an unlivable situation.*"[17] (pp. 114, 115) Nonetheless, such studies do not show schizophrenics to be as rational as everyone else, for the conscious beliefs such patients admittedly do have are themselves irrational beliefs; and actions that are predicated on irrational beliefs, and actors who hold them, are, in common understanding, irrational.

This is quite clear with regard to many of Laing's reported patients. The woman who avoids crowds may be rational in so doing, *given* her belief that "when she was in a crowd she felt the ground would open up under her feet."[16] (p. 131) Similarly many of the peculiar actions of one who believes that "she had an atom bomb inside her"[16] (p. 75) may be rational, *given* such a belief. But the beliefs themselves are irrational, with the result that neither the agent nor the action they explain can be said to be rational. To be sure, Laing's studies of the "social intelligibility" of schizophrenic symptoms do not end with the discovery of such obvious beliefs; Laing often attempts to go further and explain how such beliefs could be formed by an individual in the patient's situation. The explanation Laing typically gives—the patient "adopts" the symptom as the only response to an intolerable situation—involves reference to further beliefs that are also irrational.

A convenient example is the case of "Joan," a catatonic woman who was not one of Laing's patients but whose case Laing believed to afford "striking confirmation" of his views regarding schizophrenia. Joan's own subsequent avowals were used by Laing in attributing to her catatonic withdrawal a rational basis. She recalled that when she was catatonic, she "tried to be dead and grey and motionless." She thought that her mother "would like that," for "she could carry me around like a doll." She also felt that she "had to die to keep from dying. I know that sounds crazy but one time a boy hurt my feelings very much and I wanted to jump in front of a subway. Instead I went a little catatonic so I wouldn't feel anything."

Laing finds in such statements the two typical motives for catatonic withdrawal. First, "there is the primary guilt of having no right to life . . . and hence of being entitled at most only to a dead life." Since Joan's parents had wanted a boy, and since "she could not be anything other than what her parents wanted her to be," she sought to be "nothing," i.e., a passive catatonic. Secondly, Joan's withdrawal was viewed by Laing as a defensive mechanism to avoid the loss of identity (Joan's metaphorical "dying") with which she was threatened by any normal relationship with others:

One no longer fears being crushed, engulfed, overwhelmed by realness and aliveness . . . since one is already dead [by the catatonic withdrawal]. Being dead, one cannot die, and one cannot kill. The anxieties attendant on the schizophrenic's phantastic omnipotence are undercut by living in a condition of phantastic impotence.[18] (p. 176)

None of this would convince us that Joan or others like her were rational in effective catatonic withdrawal (even if we were convinced that at least in her case the withdrawal was an *action* she performed for reasons at all, a conclusion contrary to that reached by the original reporters of her case[19]). Her action is

based on a series of beliefs that are irrational, including her belief in a dis-
embodied self, a belief in her parents' complete determination of her worth,
and a belief in her own omnipotence and impotence.

It is sometimes believed that the rationality of beliefs is not a matter that
can be objectively judged and that calling them irrational is simply a pejorative way of saying that they are false. The conclusion in the present context
would be that people like Joan are thus as rational as the rest of us, only mistaken about certain facts. While the topic of rational belief is a difficult one,
prima facia the most obvious way to differentiate beliefs that are irrational
from those that are merely false is by looking at the influence relevant evidence
would have on the holder of the belief. It is characteristic of irrational beliefs
that their holder maintains them despite countervailing evidence or despite
inconsistencies with other beliefs he has. There is a fixed or frozen nature
about such beliefs, in the sense that they are not correctable by relevant evidence. Irrational beliefs are held with a strength (relative to other beliefs the
actor has) disproportionate to the evidence known to the actor. Thus the man
"who believes very strongly that his brother is trying to poison him (in spite of
appearances) and who believes, rather weakly by comparison, that Boston is
north of New York is likely to be flying in the face of evidence and the claims
that the evidence renders likely"[20] (p. 33)—he is likely, in other words, to be
irrational in his belief of his imminent poisoning.

The empirical version of the myth argument fails because it is empirically
false. By our shared concept of what it is to be rational, the mentally ill are not
as rational as the rest of the population. Only by muddling the concept of
rationality have the radical psychiatrists appeared to call into question this
obvious truth. Only by attributing unconscious beliefs and desires to the mentally ill for which there is no evidence, or only by referring to beliefs that are
themselves irrational can motives be found for the peculiar behavior symptomatic of mental illness. Neither of these moves satisfies what we usually mean
by "rational" as applied to actions and agents. One may, of course, like Humpty
Dumpty, choose to make a word like "rationality" mean what he pleases, but
surely it is unhelpful when one does so to then present the manufactured
match between the facts and the new criteria for the word, as a discovery of
new facts, previously overlooked because of the willful blindness of self-
interested psychiatrists or whatever. To do so is to create one's own myths.

The Myth as a Category Mistake: Mental Illness is Not a Physical Cause

In *The Concept of Mind*,[21] Ryle made popular the notion of a category mistake. His motive for using this notion was to avoid having to take a position on
the ontological status of mental entities. The dualism attributed to Descartes,
i.e., the two-worlds view that there are minds and there are bodies, each in
their own species of existence, is untenable for all of the reasons Ryle recounts
throughout the whole of the book. Yet neither form of monism—that there are

only minds (idealism) or there are only bodies (physicalism) — seems to do justice to the way we speak of ourselves as human beings. We do use mental terms such as "belief," "desire," "pain," etc., in apparently significant discourse, and yet when one attempts to say something about the entities to which such terms ostensibly refer, one is baffled. How does one describe a belief? What properties can one give it? Does it have physical extension? And if it has no such properties, what sort of a thing is it anyway?

Ryle wants to avoid answering these questions about the ontological status of mental entities. One kind of question we do not have to answer is a question that is not meaningful. Ryle wants to say that the question "Are there bodies and minds?" is not meaningful, because a category mistake has been made in conjoining a term in one category ("bodies") with a term in another ("minds"). It is like conjoining hopes, the tide, and the average age of death to say (in the same logical tone of voice) that all three are *rising*. Ryle explicitly avoids the snare of saying that there are two species of existence (dualism); he is operating on the level of language only, claiming that we use the word "exists" in two different senses when we speak of bodies and when we speak of minds.[21] (p. 23) Hence, a difference of linguistic categories for Ryle does not imply a difference in ontological status (nor does it exclude it).

One of the particular category mistakes that Ryle is at pains to correct throughout his book is the assumption that "there are mechanical causes of corporeal movements and mental causes of corporeal movements."[21] (p. 22) For Ryle, this statement contains a category mistake because it is a conjunction of words in different categories — specifically, the names of the candidates for mental causes, such as "belief," "desire," "volition," and the like, are in a different category from the kinds of words we use to label mechanical causes. Ryle later brings out this difference: he likens mental words, such as "desire" or "motive," to dispositions and contrasts them with mechanical causes. His well-known example is the broken window; one sense of explaining the shattering of a window is because a rock hit it; another sense of explaining this breaking is because the glass was brittle, i.e., because it had a tendency to break when hit by a hard object. The first form of explanation is to refer to a mechanical cause and the second to a dispositional property. Ryle construes motive words such as "vanity" or "greed" similarly to words such as "brittle" or "soluble"; such words do not cite a cause, but a tendency of persons or objects to behave in certain sorts of ways.

By his examples, vocabulary, and explicit citation, Szasz makes it clear that he has read Ryle with approval. He begins, for example, part 1 of *Law, Liberty, and Psychiatry* with a quote from Ryle on the nature of myths:

> A myth is, of course, not a fairy story. It is the presentation of facts belonging in one category in the idioms belonging to another. To explode a myth is accordingly not to deny the facts but to re-allocate them.[22] (p. 11)

"Mental illness" is a myth, then, in the same way that other mental terms are myths — it is as improper to place mental illness in the same category with real illnesses (read as physically caused illnesses) as it is to treat "belief," "desires," "perception," etc., as the names of mechanical or paramechanical causes.

There are, in fact, a number of distinguishable uses of the doctrine of categorical differences made by Szasz in his attack on mental illness as a myth, which include the following: (1) his primary use is to focus on "mental" in the phrase "mental illness" and to argue that mental illness is a myth because mind is a myth (and hence a sick mind is a myth). (2) He also focuses on "illness," to argue that the latter term necessarily refers to physiochemical goings-on in the body; thus, saying that a mind could be ill is absurd because only physical bodies can be ill (in the ordinary meaning of "ill"). (3) Szasz also utilizes the doctrine of category difference to inveigh against any use of the names of particular mental diseases, such as "schizophrenia," "hysteria," etc.; the argument here is that the names of particular illnesses illicitly conjoin words referring to behavioral tendencies with words referring to physiological happenings in the brain, as well as with words whose only reference is to mental experience—a clear example, for Szasz, of a category mistake. (4) Fourthly and finally, because of the categorical differences between mind words and brain words, Szasz appears to believe that it is logically impossible to establish correlations between the mental and behavioral-based syndromes we call mental illnesses, and the brain events that may cause them; hence, the scientific aspirations of psychiatry, and the medical treatment of mental illness, are forever condemned to frustration because the aspirations themselves are logically absurd.

It should be noted that the first two of these arguments deal with "mental illness" in general and the second two deal with the names of particular illnesses. For clarity, it helps to keep these two discussions separated, even though they are obviously related. Thus, I shall proceed to discuss Szasz's use of the doctrine of categorical differences in the four-part order set forth above. The ultimate conclusion of all of them, it is worth emphasizing, is that mental illness, and mental illnesses, are myths.

1. What is a sick mind? Surely a large part of the appeal of the myth argument stems from the difficulty one has in answering this question. One may indeed be tempted by the radical psychiatrists' reply that only bodies can be sick and that minds are not the sorts of things that can be either healthy or ill. Yet a good deal of the attraction of this argument should be eliminated once it is realized that the difficulty we have in saying anything very intelligible about what a sick mind is stems directly from the difficulty we have in saying anything very intelligible about what a mind is. For, unless one is prepared to jettison our talk about minds in toto (as Szasz plainly is not), merely pointing out that "mental illness" has no clearer reference than does "mind" itself is hardly a sufficient basis for labelling it a myth.

Fixing the reference of "mind" and mental words generally is notoriously difficult, yet in fact we can leave the question of reference open, and still see that in no pejorative sense is a sick mind a myth. One may adopt any nondualistic position on the ontological status of mental entities (the popular ones presently being logical behaviorism, which asserts that minds are hypothetical constructs from behavior; materialism, which asserts that minds are (identical with) an as yet unknown set of physiological phenomena; functionalism, which contends that minds are functional states of physical systems; or Ryle's own position, that one may avoid the question because it cannot be meaningfully framed.) Perhaps "mind" and other mental terms are not even referential in character, as has also been suggested,[23] so that we need not worry about what sorts of things minds are. Whichever of these positions one adopts about what minds are, he is immune to the kind of criticism Ryle directed against Cartesian dualism (criticisms that Szasz and others would redirect against the supposedly dualistic assumptions inherent in "mental illness"); in none of them does one presuppose the existence of some funny, nonmaterial mind substance. In none of them need one who speaks of mental illness be committed to "paramechanical myths" about ghostly mind-things being "injured" in some nonspatial way. "Mental illness" can make perfectly good sense — as much so as 'mind' and mind words generally — no matter which of these general positions one takes as to the reference of mental terms, even if the position adopted should be that none of them refer to anything.

The question, "What is a sick mind?" can be left aside in favor of a more useful question — "Does 'mental illness' have as significant a descriptive/explanatory use as other mental expressions?" If it does not, then "myth" is as good a pejorative label as any; but if the phrase does have a significant use, then no amount of Rylean exorcism as to the phrase's supposedly ghostly referents can be a sufficient reason to eliminate it from our vocabulary.

Our mentalistic vocabulary may conveniently be divided between experiential terms and those terms that we use to describe and explain human actions. Thus, when we predicate "is in pain," "is feeling tired," or "is seeing an orange afterimage" of another, we are ascribing mental experiences to him; when we predicate "is murdering," "is hiding," "is intending to hide," or "is desiring a yacht" of another, we describe his doings as actions and explain such actions by his (mental) intentions, desires, beliefs, motives, etc. Since the concept of mind is intimately connected with our concept of what it is to be a person, predicating mental experiences, actions, and intentions to another being is not only necessary before we will say that he has a mind, but also before we will think of that being as a person.

"Mental illness" is used to deny that all of the mind words can be properly predicated of another. Specifically, it is used to deny that the action/intention predicates are as regularly or as properly applicable to the mentally ill as they are to more normal persons. This is merely a corollary of saying that the mentally ill are not as rational as the rest of us, in the senses of "rational" discussed earlier. For those senses of rationality are all linked to our usage of the action/intention predicates. If an individual is irrational in the sense that his desires are unintelligible, or that his beliefs are irrational, or that the set of his beliefs or desires are inconsistent, then the action/intention mode of explanation begins to break down. If the individual is so far gone that for some of his actions we are unable to make out any set of beliefs or desires, no matter how bizarre or inconsistent, then this mode of explanation breaks down entirely. Although no one would deny that the mentally ill have mental experiences (indeed, they typically have something of a surplus), the diminished rationality of the mentally ill does entail a diminished applicability of the other part of our mentalistic vocabulary, the action/intention predicates.

If we observe enough behavior of the same individual for which we are unable to apply the action/intention predicates, we will come to regard that individual differently than most of our fellows, differently, because we lack *the* form of description/explanation of his behavior by virtue of which we understand ourselves and others in daily life. To make out another being as a person fully like us, we need rather regularly to be able to see his actions as promoting desires we find intelligible in light of beliefs we find rational.

A "sick mind" is thus properly predicated of an individual when we are unable to presuppose his rationality to the same extent as we do for others. A sick mind is an incapacity to act rationally, which, in the senses of "rational" here used, means an incapacity to act so as to further intelligible desires in light of rational beliefs.

In so using "mental illness," one is thus committed to no funny, nonmaterial substances that are in some nonspatial way injured or impaired. "Mind" and other mind-terms may not refer to such paramechanistic myths, but then, "mental illness" doesn't either. To say that someone's mind is ill is only to say that his capacity for rational action is diminished, that the subject himself is irrational. Since "mind" in Ryle's own analysis is the name of all such capacities for intelligent performances, a lack of some of them may as properly invoke mind words as may the possession of them. To the extent that one is willing to say of another, "he has a mind" (or "he is a person"), then to the same extent should one be willing to say, "his mind is defective" (or "he is not wholly a person"), if he in fact lacks the relevant capacities.

2. Of course, if "illness" meant "deviation from an anatomical or physiological norm,"[8] (p. 167) as Szasz believes, then *mental* illness would still make no sense, for how can a mind (or capacities for intelligent performances) deviate from physical norms? Minds cannot be normal or abnormal vis-à-vis such physiological norms, and, Szasz argues, beliefs to the contrary are simply category mistakes.

Does "illness" properly predicated of a person mean that the person's bodily structure is abnormal in comparison with other people's bodily structure? The first thing one wants to say is that "illness" was a word in the English language long before anyone knew very much about anatomy or physiology, and thus, the meaning of the word cannot be a matter of statistical deviation from a physiological or anatomical norm (else the word would have had no use prior to knowing of such norms and such deviations). Still, one might think that our ancestors had a different concept of illness than we do. So, to press on to contemporary examples, consider the following two: first, imagine an individual possessed of a cubical stomach. This stomach, while abnormal in its physical structure, functions perfectly efficiently in digesting food, etc.; it thus allows its owner as long a life as people with normal stomachs. Suppose further, it causes him no discomfort and that it allows him to eat and drink the variety and quantity of foods and beverages available in his society. Despite the presence of an abnormal physical condition, no one would call this individual ill.

Next, imagine an individual who possesses a small gland common to all mankind. As with everyone else, this gland causes him pain, increases his chance of early death, and prevents him from eating a large number of foods. Despite the fact that this physiological condition (until corrected by surgery) is universal, no one would hesitate to label the state caused by it an illness, similar to tonsillitis or appendicitis.

What these examples show is that being ill, even physically ill, is not the same as being in a certain state, even if that state deviates widely from what is normal for human beings. Being ill is not a state in which one's bodily structure deviates from a statistical norm, as Szasz argues throughout his work.[8] (p. 167), [24] (pp. 19, 23) Such deviance from a physiological norm is in itself neither a necessary nor a sufficient condition to being ill. It is simply irrelevant.

While to say what "illness" does not mean is considerably easier than specifying what it does mean, being ill seems to involve something like being in a state of pain or discomfort, which, if not removed, may lead to premature death, and which, for its duration, incapacitates the patient from certain activities thought normal in our society. One might assume that such states are physically caused; but such assumptions are irrelevant to what we mean by "illness." There are presumably physical causes for us being in all kinds of states, such as being a thousand miles from Paris, or for being alert or angry, etc. *Whether* there are physical causes for such states, and if so, *whether* they are manifested by abnormal physical structures, is irrelevant to whether or not one is ill, alert, angry, or a thousand miles away from Paris. Merely discovering a physical deviation in no way tells us that the person whose body it is that deviates is ill. To properly predicate "illness" of another we instead need to know such things as whether he is in pain, is incapacitated, or is dying.

The reason this has been so well camouflaged by the radical psychiatrists is because the names of *particular* illness, such as "polio," "pneumonia," etc., do involve knowledge of physical causes (as will be discussed at the end of this section). Whether one has polio or pneumonia is determined in part by knowledge of the virus involved. Yet whether one is ill (in general) is *not* determined by such causes; whether one is ill in general is determined by wholly different criteria, seemingly connected with pain, incapacitation, or a hastened death.

Once one appreciates this, then the propriety of terming hysterics (mentally) ill is also evident. The activities for which one is incapacitated by a paralyzed arm differ not a whit, no matter if the paralysis is anatomical or hysterical. In either case, one cannot, for example, play baseball or tend after one's father effectively, etc. The admittedly sincere reports of pain of an hysteric throat irritation are as good as evidence that the hysteric feels pain, as are such reports of one whose C fibers are really jingling with physiological pain signals due to a physically caused throat irritation. More generally, those whose capacity to act rationally is diminished because their memory, perception, reasoning abilities, or other mental faculties are impaired, are incapacitated from a normal life in our society no less, e.g., than is the chronic alcoholic whose short-term memory banks have been physically damaged by his long-term drinking habits (Korsakoff syndrome).

Being in a state properly called "ill," then, does not depend on one's knowing, or even in the first instance of there being, any particular physiological condition. It depends on one's being in a state characterized (roughly) by pain, incapacitation, and the prospect of a hastened death. There is nothing mythical about such states, whether they be due to a broken leg or a broken home.

3. If mental illness is not a myth, that is not yet to say that psychiatry is the scientific way to go about studying it. The claim of orthodox psychiatry to scientific expertise, in other words, rests not only on there being a nonmythical subject of study (mental illness), but also on there having been acquired some scientific knowledge about it. Such knowledge as there is is by and large to be found in the diagnostic categories of orthodox psychiatry.

It is for this reason that it has been important for radical psychiatrists to attack the validity of the traditional diagnostic categories. Szasz's version of the attack is based on the categorical differences of Ryle. Szasz's primary use of the doctrine of category difference here is as a reminder that "schizophrenia," "hysteria," etc., do not presently refer to known events in physiology that cause behavior, but this is undisputed, and provides no grounds for saying that "schizophrenia," "hysteria," etc., are mere myths, or for denying that such words have a significant use. Understanding that "schizophrenia" is on a par with some of our other mental-conduct terms, in that it does not presently refer to any set of mechanical or paramechanical causes, is not to eliminate it from our vocabulary but to "reallocate it," in the language of Ryle quoted earlier. The syndromes we call "schizophrenia" and other such syndromes may currently explain behavior only in a way analogous to explanations in terms of character traits, that is, in terms of dispositions themselves implied from the pattern of a person's prior behavior, and not by reference to any set of physiological conditions. However, as Ryle points out, we engage in the same construct-building when we explain the breaking of glass or the dissolution of salt by citing the dispositional properties of brittleness or solubility. Significant, explanatory (albeit nonmechanistic) truths can be framed with all such terms, and no one goes around writing books on "the myth of brittleness" or "the myth of greediness."

Szasz, however, presses the argument to claim that "schizophrenia," and other such terms, are logically absurd in ways that, e.g., "brittleness" is not. There seem to be two versions of the category-mistake argument here — the first is the juxtaposition of behavioral symptoms and brain symptoms in the same classificatory scheme:

> Consider, for example, general paresis. This diagnosis refers to a physio-chemical phenomenon. The term does not describe any particular behavioral

event. How then can we hope to bring it into a meaningful relation with other psychiatric diagnoses that refer only to behavioral events, such as hysteria, reactive depression, or situational maladjustment? . . . It is as if, in the periodic table of elements, we would find coal, steel, and petroleum interspersed among items such as helium, carbon, and sulfur. This is the main reason the taxonomic system known as psychiatric nosology does not work. . . .[22] (p. 25)

Secondly, Szasz in other points in his works makes the rather curious argument that psychiatrists cannot classify human behavior because human beings react to the classificatory labels placed upon them, whereas stones, plants, stars, etc., do not. This error is "not due to any lack of humane feeling in psychiatrists, but rather to the fallacy of thinking in terms of natural science." This approach ignores "the differences between persons and things and the effects of language on each." In the orthodox account of mental disease, Szasz asks,

'What is the status of human action . . . ?' The answer is: 'None.' There is no such thing as action to attain a goal — only behavior determined by causes. Herein lies the fundamental error of the medical and mechanomorphic approach to human behavior and to psychiatric classification.[24] (pp. 191–196)

The first of these two additional attacks on the classificatory scheme is mistaken for the reasons discussed in the following subsection — there is no logical error in supposing that mental incapacities can be *correlated* with brain events to form composite aggregations of symptoms even if minds are not *identical* with brains. Discussion of this will be deferred briefly. The second of Szasz's arguments here obviously has nothing to do with "the logic of classification," as Szasz sometimes terms his Rylean weaponry. The blunt fact of the matter is that in everyday life and in social science we do classify human behavior all the time, and the fact that those labelled "patriotic," "ambitious," "greedy," or "schizophrenic" may not care for the label has nothing whatsoever to do with their propriety for descriptive or explanatory purposes. One might have *ethical* qualms about *telling* the subjects they are being so classified, particularly if one has the authority of a psychiatrist in a mental hospital to make the label stick; such ethical qualms, or their associated therapeutic concerns, are totally beside the point if one is judging psychiatric classifications of behavior by their logical or scientific methodology. The error, if any there be, is more akin to that of a nuclear physicist working on the atomic bomb — a mistaken sense of personal value, perhaps, but hardly a mistake in the scientific methodology of nuclear weapons.

There are questions that might be raised about the diagnostic categories of psychiatry, but they are not questions of category difference. The aggregation of symptoms associated with hysteria, schizophrenia, etc., form inductive claims whose nature is clear — as clear as the nature of the claim that people who tend to look in the mirror often also tend to feel pleased when flattered, avoid conversations in which others are praised, etc. (Ryle's partial unpacking of the character trait of vanity). There is nothing logically suspect about the inductive process by which we classify familiar, as well as bizarre behavior, into character traits and mental diseases.

4. The heaviest burden placed by Szasz on the category mistake version of the myth argument comes in another of his uses of it — his attempt to construct a logical chasm out of Ryle's categorical differences. For Szasz not only asserts that "schizophrenia" and other terms are not presently to be explained by reference to mechanical causes, but appears to insist that such explanations cannot be given, no matter what medical discoveries might be made; unlike physical illnesses, those syndromes we call mental illnesses cannot be caused by some set of physiological events. In this logical claim he is surely in error.

What Szasz has in mind here are the distinctions R. S. Peters (building on Ryle and Wittgenstein) drew between actions and movements and between reasons and causes.[25] Physical bodies, including the physical bodies of human beings, move through space in a manner describable by physical descriptions in terms of velocities, accelerations, spatial coordinates, directions, etc. According to Peters, such movements of the human body constitute *actions,* however, only if they are seen in the light of human conventions — the physical movements of the arm and fingers in moving wooden figures on a checkered board only constitute the action of "castling his king" in light of an intelligent agent following the rules of chess. Further, on the Peters view, it is only physical movements that can be explained by the mechanical causes provided by the laws of physics, whereas for actions, only reasons (purposive rule-following) are appropriate. One neither explains the orbiting of the planets by reference to their motives nor does one explain why another human being castled his king by reference to his synaptic firing patterns.

While I do not believe that Peters' (or Szasz's) rule-following analysis is adequate as a general account of human action, but rather represents an analysis of one species of *complex* actions, it does not matter for present purposes. For Szasz and Peters do have hold of part of a very important and far-reaching result of the analytic philosophy of the last 25 years — embedded in our language are two fundamentally dissimilar ways of describing and explaining things in the world, variously polarized as the language of actions vs. that of movements, of reasons vs. that of causes, of teleology vs. that of mechanism. Intentional idioms vs. the nonIntentional, intensional talk vs. extensional, the language used to describe meaningful behavior vs. that used to describe the inanimate, those claims known with certainty vs. those claims supported only by fallible, inductive inferences, as in science. In numerous ways philosophers have sought to capture the striking fact that the words we apply to describe and explain the doings of *persons* differ significantly from the words we use to describe and explain natural phenomena. The even more striking result of this work has been to revive (with some dissent) Brentano's irreducibility thesis, which holds that one cannot reduce our "person-talk" to the language of physical science. We not only have two dissimilar modes of speaking, but we are stuck with them for we have no way to paraphrase the idiom of one to that of the other.

If one accepts none of this, then of course it is no mistake to believe that mental illness may be physically caused. Even if one grants the existence of this fundamental cleavage in one's speech, and its irreducibility, however, that does not mean (contra Peters and Szasz) that the various mental illnesses may not be explained by reference to physiological events or any other mechanical causes; this, for two reasons—(1) what the irreducibility thesis entails is that one cannot identify mental entities such as beliefs, desires, pains, etc., with physical events, either behavioristic or physiological. One of the reasons for this is the idea that Szasz quotes[4] (p. 171) from Peters: movements "cannot be characterized as intelligent or unintelligent, correct or incorrect, efficient or inefficient." One may only describe *actions* with such adjectives.[25] (p. 15) Since one of the principal requirements of using the identity sign is that the expressions referring to the same thing be substitutable for one another without change of truth value, one cannot identify action with movements, but this argument goes only against *identifying* mental entities with physical ones; it says nothing about correlating the two and calling one the cause of the other, for there is no substitutivity requirement for the names of effects and their causes. More generally, the irreducibility thesis does not entail that one may not *correlate*, e.g., the mental experience of pain, with certain physiological events (the stimulation of C fibers in the brain). Nor does it entail that, e.g., schizophrenia may not be correlated with some sorts of events in the brain.

As importantly, "mental illness" does not seem to share just those features of mental concepts that differentiate them from the concepts used in physical science. Specifically, (*a*) "mental illness" and its subspecies are not the names of mental experiences, as are "pain," "wish," etc.; the names of the various forms of mental illness are more like the names of character traits, such as "stupidity" or "greed," that is, inductively built up from overt behavior alone. (*b*) The names of the various forms of mental illness do not imply intelligent, purposive behavior, as do *some* character traits. Like "stupidity" and "violent character," but unlike "greed," "schizophrenia," and like terms do not presuppose goal-directed behavior. Rather, the names of the various mental illnesses negate the assumption of rationality, which is in some cases to negate the goal-directed nature of the behavior. (*c*) Like character traits, but unlike mental experiences and intentional actions, mental illness is known to the subject only by the usual inferential processes of scientific thinking. One knows what action he is performing, or that he is in pain, without evidence or observation; he knows that he is mentally ill only on the basis of evidence (that is often brought to his attention by others).

Hence, even if such correlations were logically impossible for most other mental-conduct terms, it would be possible to correlate schizophrenia and like terms with events in physiology without significant change in meaning of the terms. One could only support this assertion with a detailed review of the various arguments given against such a thesis in general, and by demonstrating how each such argument fails to apply to the nonintelligent, nonexperiential, fallibly known syndromes we call mental illnesses. Since in any event, there is no logical reason for denying causal correlations in the first place, one need not pursue this line of argument here.

None of this is to say that such correlations between the syndromes we label as mental illnesses of various kinds and physiology do exist — for one cannot tell in advance what slices of behavior can be correlated with what slices of physiology (this is true no matter how strictly one subscribes to determinism). It is a question for empirical discovery, and logical arguments either way are not determinative. The correlations between the disposition to bleed profusely and certain chemical states of the blood (hemophilia); violent character and XYY genetic makeup; and certain addictions (dispositions to act in certain ways) and the events in physiology that cause them are all suggestive examples. Whether similar correlations can be found between schizophrenia and certain happenings in physiology is a matter calling for painstaking research, not for the armchair guess-work more frequently found in philosophy than in medicine.

It might be argued that it is illegitimate of psychiatrists to anticipate such discoveries before they are made by use of implicitly causal disease words such as "schizophrenia" or "kleptomania." Szasz argues, for example, that it is "faulty reasoning for it makes the abstraction 'mental illness' into a cause of, even though this abstraction was originally created to serve only as a short-hand expression for, certain types of human behavior."[24] (p. 15) Yet as Hilary Putnam has shown,[26, 27] this is done all the time in "real" medicine as well as in psychiatry. Clusters of symptoms are thought to be due to an underlying condition, named and treated as illnesses, well before one could identify the cause of such symptoms. Polio was a disease before one discovered its virus origin. Moreover, we say that such diseases are (causally) responsible for the cluster of symptoms; even in the absence of knowing the cause, and knowing only the behavioral symptoms, we still do not mean that, e.g., polio *is* just the symptoms by which we diagnose it. If we had meant this prior to knowing the causes of polio, no doctor could have "ever said (and many did) 'I believe this may not be a case of polio,' knowing that all of the text-book symptoms were present . . ."[27] (p. 5) By "polio" we mean *whatever* was responsible for the symptoms doctors observed, assuming that in time scientific research would tell us what the "whatever" might be.

Unless one can show that there is some good reason to suppose that the symptoms of the various mental illnesses may not be caused by some kind of events in physiology (which I have attempted to show cannot be done, at least on logical grounds), then schizophrenia and other such afflictions are no more myths because of the lack of any presently known physical cause than was polio a myth in the absence of similar knowledge.

The Myth as a Deduction From Epistemological Relativity:
We Are Equally Mad From the Epistemological
Point of View of Those We Label Mad

"The quality of myth," Quine tells us, "is relative; relative . . .to the epistemological point of view."[7] (p. 19) Mental illness is a myth on the interpretation here discussed, because our current epistemology, in which we have concepts like "mental illness," is a myth—judged of course from another epistemological point of view, not from our own. If one subscribes to the view that there is no judging between such basic points of view, then the argument of Laing and others—that from the point of view of those we label insane we are insane—has some sting. Attribute to those we label as mentally ill an epistemology; grant that although it differs from ours, the relative merits cannot be judged; then our labelling of others as mentally ill is a myth because it presupposes what it cannot have, namely, a standard of judgment applicable to those judged as well as to those judging.

One can dress up the argument a bit by likening the word-salads of schizophrenics or the somatic symptoms of hysterics to forms of intelligent communication: "the problem of hysteria is more akin to the problem of a person speaking a foreign tongue than it is to that of a person having a bodily disease."[4] (p. 11) Add the Wittgensteinian argument that we cannot even detect what patterns are *speech* patterns to the creatures who speak radically foreign tongues, e.g., perhaps, lions; or stir in a smidgen of the later Quine (any translation of a radically foreign language is necessarily indeterminate, there being no one uniquely correct translation); and the attribution of anything so portentous as an epistemology to those we label mentally ill becomes somewhat less troublesome.

It seems to me that this position, and epistemological relativity in general, stem from a simple failure to take one's own epistemology seriously. Free as we might like to think we are in our most speculative moments to shop among competing epistemologies, ontologies, geometries, logics, like so many wares in the store window, we are in fact limited to small purchases at any one time—limited by the high prices of even small purchases. This is not, however, a tidy issue that needs resolution here.

The Myth as an Evaluation Masquerading as an Explanation:
The Abuse of the Normative Connotations of "Mental
Illness" by Orthodox Psychiatry

Sensitivity to the normative connotations of the concepts of "mental health" and "mental illness" is, I suspect, rather widespread. When one of the psychiatrists at the annual meeting of the American Psychiatric Association (APA) some years ago loudly diagnosed a women's-libber who was disrupting the meeting, as a "stupid, paranoid bitch," something other than a value-neutral explanation of her behavior was intended. The same suspicions are engendered when psychiatrists label homosexuals as mentally ill, or when "mental health" is used as a synonym for whatever way of life is adjudged good. The radical psychiatrists build on these kinds of examples to argue that "mental illness" and the predicate "mentally ill" are used *only* to make evaluations of others' behavior, and that these terms are particularly effective as evaluations because they are paraded as value-neutral, scientific explanations: "while allegedly *describing* conduct, psychiatrists often *prescribe* it."[22] (p. 18)

> The masquerading of promotive assertions in the guise of indicative sentences is of great practical significance in psychiatry. Statements concerning "psychosis" or "insanity" . . . almost always revolve around unclarified equations of these two linguistic forms. For example, the statement "John Doe is psychotic" is ostensibly indicative and informative. Usually, however, it is promotive rather than informative . . .[4] (p. 131)

It may seem curious to claim that "mental illness" is used like "bad" or "wrong" or "ugh"—that is, used to pass moral evaluations—when by our shared notions of moral responsibility we use the same phrase to *excuse* those who are mentally ill. To attribute a harmful action to the actor's mental illness, then, cannot always be exactly the same as attributing it, say, to his "murderous personality." What Szasz sometimes has in mind in saying that "mental illness" is used prescriptively or promotively is not that moral judgments are made with such use; rather, psychiatric usage of the phrase is often promotive, etc., in the quite different sense that the capability of being morally responsible is denied. "Mental illness" for Szasz and others is evaluative often only in the sense that it denies the "personhood" of those to whom it is applied:

> What better way is there . . . for degrading the culprit than to declare him incapable of knowing what he is doing. . . . This is the general formula for the dehumanization and degradation of all those persons whose conduct psychiatrists now deem to be "caused" by mental illness.[8] (pp. 122, 123)

Although needlessly stated in inflammatory terms (as if orthodox psychiatry were universally motivated by a desire to degrade the mentally ill), Szasz here suggests a very important feature of mental illness. "Insanity" and "mental illness" mean, and have historically meant, "irrational"; to be insane, or to be mentally ill, is not to act rationally often enough to have the same assumption of rationality made about one as is made of most of humanity; and absent such an assumption of rationality, one cannot be fully regarded as a person, for our concept of what it is to be a person is centered on assuming rationality in the senses introduced earlier. Unless we can perceive another being as acting for intelligible ends in light of rational beliefs, we cannot understand that being in the same fundamental way that we understand each other's actions in daily life. Such beings lack an essential attribute of our humanity. It is thus easy to appreciate that historically the insane have been likened to young children, the intoxicated, and wild beasts; for absent the assumption of rationality, the mentally ill are, as Bleuler said of his schizophrenic patients, stranger to us than the birds in our gardens.

Such statements are of course offensive to the ears of those concerned about the moral claims and legal rights of mental patients. However, unless radical psychiatry and its lawyerly following can show, as I have argued earlier in this article it has not, that those we label mentally ill are just as rational as everyone else, part of our fundamental explanatory scheme and part of our fundamental notion of personhood are not applicable to the mentally ill. This includes notions about their lack of responsibility and their lack of an ability to choose and act upon their own conception of their good. If one believes (contra Szasz and followers) that there are in fact people who do not act rationally often enough for us to make the same assumption of rationality for them as we do for most of our fellows, then this "evaluative" feature of the phrase "mental illness" is accurate enough in its reflection of how the mentally ill fit into our fundamental conceptual scheme.

Szasz, at other times, seems to have in mind a second kind of normative use we do on occasion make of "mentally ill" in everyday expressions such as, "That was an insane thing to do," or "That's crazy!" In such usages we do seem to be expressing disapproval of the agent's ends and his actions, recommending that one ought not to do such things or seek such ends, etc. Thus Szasz is also accurate in noting that at times, "mentally ill" or "insane" can be used as terms of general disapproval: "The difference between saying 'He is wrong' and 'He is mentally ill' is not factual but psychological."[22] (p. 205) Other examples with which we began this section were the women's libber's diagnosis and the use of "mental health" as if it were synonymous with "good" by some psychoanalysts, e.g., Erich Fromm.

To the extent that orthodox psychiatry uses these words in this way it is plainly abusing them. The phrase "mental illness" and its companions are so abused, not by being applied to those who are in fact irrational, but by being applied to persons whose actions are often rational but of whose ends prevailing psychiatric opinion does not approve. An action that is fully rational in each of the senses examined earlier cannot, without ignoring the meaning of the words, be said to be insane or due to mental illness, no matter how deviant may be the end pursued. The fact that homosexuals have a preference for a sexual relationship not shared by most of the populace is hardly a ground (as the APA with strong dissent implicitly recognized recently in its deletion of homosexuality as an illness) for labelling that preference irrational (ill). Homosexuals may (sometimes, often, or always) be mentally ill, if their capacity for rational action is significantly diminished below our expectations; such irrationality is hardly shown, however, by their unpopular sexual desires alone if those ends are pursued on the basis of rational and consistent beliefs, without conflict with other strong desires, and by relatively efficient means.

The mistake of radical psychiatry is to assume that mental illness is a myth just because the phrase can be so abused. The mistake is to assume that because words such as "murder," "greediness," "mental illness," or even "good" can be used to express attitudes, kindle emotions, pass evaluations, and the like, they cannot also be used at the same time as a legitimate form of explanation and/or description, or at different times only as a description/explanation. Those moral philosophers who have raised another logical gulf between evaluative and

descriptive statements insufficiently stress the fact that words used in evaluations can also be used to express descriptions. Merely because a woman may
call the doctor who through surgical error kills her husband a murderer, despite
the fact that one of the main criteria for that term's proper use is not met (viz.,
intentional killing), is not sufficient to show that the term "murderer" cannot
have legitimate descriptive and explanatory uses.

To the extent that one views mental illness as a myth solely because of its
evaluative connotations, one makes the same mistake. I do not believe one can
accuse Szasz himself of this error because he conjoins this point with one of the
preceding four points; mental illness is a myth because it has no descriptive
meaning (take your pick of any of the first four myth arguments) *and* because
it can be and is sometimes used to pass moral judgment on those so labelled.
If, however, one rejects the first part of this thesis, the second is an insufficient
basis on which to label mental illness a myth. "Mental illness" is perhaps a dangerous term because its normative connotations make possible the kind of
abuse mentioned earlier; but then the same can be said of many of the terms
with which we describe and explain human action, such as "greedy," "stupid,"
"murder," "manipulative," etc.

SOME LEGAL IMPLICATIONS

The disease that radical psychiatry has contracted (and which appears to
be contagious, at least for those lawyers who always knew that psychiatry was
pseudoscience anyway) is the temptation to regard complex legal, social, ethical, and conceptual problems as solved once it administers a sufficient amount
of antimyth antidote. In Szasz's case in particular, it is an attempt to use the
therapeutic tools of modern philosophy to dissolve the problems, not to solve
them.

If indeed one believes that there is no such thing as mental illness, that
those we call mentally ill are fully as rational as anyone else only with different
aims, that the only reason anyone ever thought differently was because of
unsophisticated category mistakes or because of their adherence to the epistemology of a sick society, and that the phrase accordingly is only a mask used
to disguise moral judgments in pseudoscientific respectability—one who in
other words accepts the myth theses—will necessarily also believe that he
wields an Alexandrian sword with which to cut through the knotty legal problems surrounding the treatment of the mentally ill. For once one subscribes to
these versions of the myth argument, a number of radical consequences for the
present treatment of the mentally ill are self-evident truths to all but the unini-
tiated: either the insanity defense should be abolished and those we call mentally ill punished like anyone else, or at the least the phrase should play no part
as a separate defense; the incompetency plea should either be abolished or
highly limited; those we call mentally ill should be sued for breach of contract

like anyone else, not excused from their contractual obligations because of supposed incapacity to contract; no one should be civilly committed for mental illness, for the mentally ill know their own good and have the capacity to act in accordance with such conception no less than anyone else, the state thus having no parental role to play here; anyone inside or outside of a mental hospital should have the full civil rights of any citizen because he is just like any citizen. In short, one who subscribes to the myth argument will believe "that we abolish the problem of mental illness by abolishing the concept of mental illness."[28]

Unfortunately, the mentally ill and their attendant problems will not go away this easily. Unlike some of the conceptual problems against which the analytic philosophy on which Szasz relies has been directed in this century, there are no logical or methodological shortcuts by which one can dissolve the ethical, legal, and medical problems presented by the mentally ill. Belief that there are such shortcuts only impedes the search to solve these problems in a manner consistent with the accepted values of our society.

It is beyond the scope of this article to document in any complete way the impact that the myth argument has had on the legal issues mentioned above. I shall content myself with one example, the proposal to abolish the insanity defense. For there the conclusions of the myth argument are both clear and disturbing. The myth argument seems to have led in two related directions here.

1. The conclusions that some lawyers have drawn from one or more variants of the myth argument has been more limited than a complete abolition of the insanity plea. Rather, the conclusion drawn has been that the defense could be retained but any use of such allegedly meaningless phrases as "mental defect," "mental illness," "mental disease," or the like, be omitted. Thus, for example, Hardisty[29] has reached this conclusion explicitly because of the "mythical nature of the phrase 'mental illness'. . . ." Hardisty, relying on Szasz and a sprinkling of the other radical psychiatrists or sociologists, is much impressed that there are no "definite referents" of the phrase "mental illness," that it is "a phrase without a denotation," and, accordingly, that the "ontological conception of mental disease as a thing present or not present in the individual is an erroneous, medieval, and premedieval concept . . .";[29] (p. 757) further, that "the reification of 'mental illness' in the irresponsibility test is a fiction" serving a number of "hidden functions." He further notes that "mental illness" is neither the name of a cause of incapacity ("legalists have a confused conception of 'mental illness,' believing it accurately describes a cause for the incapacity, when actually it is more nearly a vague and value-loaded synonym for incapacity"), nor the name of a state of the organism that might be correlated with physical causes. Hardisty further assumes that "people employ 'mental illness' for its rhetorical power," that psychiatrists still employ the words "mental illness" but do so not to describe a medical condition but rather to achieve social purposes," and that the functions of the phrase may now be entirely outside its validity as a descriptive term."

The reliance on various versions of the myth argument should be apparent. From such premises, the conclusion intended does indeed follow, for no

one would knowingly frame legal tests employing terms with such characteristics. As the present Chief Justice of the United States once said,

> No rule of law can possibly be sound or workable which is dependent upon the
> terms of another discipline whose members are in profound disagreement about
> what those terms mean.[1] (p. 860)

Citing and quoting Szasz among others, (now) Chief Justice Burger also
adopted the view that "[mental] 'disease' . . . has no fixed, agreed or accepted
definition in the discipline which is called upon to supply expert testimony, . . ."
and that accordingly it was "a tenuous and indeed dangerously vague term to
be a critical part of a rule of law on criminal responsibility."[1] (pp. 861, 862)

If "mental illness" were indeed in a sorry state depicted by the radical
movement in law and psychiatry, its use should be discontinued. Yet it is not,
for the reasons set forth in the body of this article, and the proposals to eliminate the phrase from legal tests of insanity, are as erroneous as the premises on
which they are based.

2. The more radical conclusion to be drawn from the myth arguments is
that the insanity defense should be abolished and that those presently excused
by the defense should be dealt with like any other offenders, viz., punished.
This is the conclusion Szasz himself correctly perceives to be entailed by his
myth arguments, and he unflinchingly endorses it: "mental illness should
never be accepted as a release from criminal responsibility. . . ."[22] (p. 228)

Such a result does real violence to our notions of fairness. No one merits
society's condemnation or punishment unless they are morally blameworthy,
and no one is blameworthy if he acts as he does because of his mental disease.
Szasz's conclusion is reminiscent of the Erewhonian practice of punishing the
ill, and evokes in most of us the same distaste.

Szasz is not unaware of this fundamental objection. Rather than softening
the argument, however, as many of his lawyerly admirers are inclined to do,
he proclaims that indeed the mentally ill *deserve* to be blamed and punished like
any criminals. This follows axiomatically from an unswerving adherence to
that version of the myth argument that claims as a matter of fact that the mentally ill are really as purposive, as rational, as the rest of us. Thus,

> Insofar as men are human beings, not machines, they always have some choice in
> how they act—hence, they are *always* responsible for their conduct. There is
> method in madness, no less than in sanity.[22] (p. 135)

Just as those who act in ignorance of the law are not excused but expected to
learn it, so those ignorant of themselves (the mentally ill), being fully purposive beings, are expected to educate themselves.

> Just as the recognition of ignorance and its correction are the responsibility of the
> adult citizen, so also are the recognition of mental illness and its correction.[22] (p. 133)

Ultimately, we should abolish the insanity defense—"this crime against humanity"[24] (p. 112)—because "by treating offenders as responsible human beings, we offer them the only chance . . . to remain human."[22] (p. 137) (Szasz is referring to the denial of the status of a person which is involved in using "insanity").

The problem with this response is the problem with the basic argument on which it rests, examined earlier—despite the mental gymnastics Szasz would lead us through, the purposive idioms are not as often applicable to explain the doings of the mentally ill as they are to explain the actions of most people; the mentally ill are not as rational as most people. Hence, to say that the mentally ill engage in criminal conduct for purposes sufficient to themselves, like any other criminals, or worse, that they should correct their condition just as the normal citizen is expected to correct any ignorance he may have about the law, is an erroneous, (and in this instance, cruel) distortion of the facts.

For lawyers, perhaps the most persuasive of the Szaszian arguments for either of the two conclusions regarding the insanity defense—that either the concept of mental disease or the entire defense should be abolished—has been the third version of the category mistake argument—"mental illness" is not the name of a mechanical cause, and, as set forth earlier, it is not. "Mental illness" and its subspecies, "schizophrenia," and other terms are not the names of physiological events that cause criminal actions. Thus, when Szasz attacks[22] (pp. 133-135) [31] (p. 191) the Durham decision[30] as "unadulterated nonsense" because in its explicitly causal language (the criminal act must be the *product* of mental disease) there has been committed a category mistake, he seems to have pointed to a serious defect.

The conclusion that is supposed to follow from this insight in the present context is that mental illness should not excuse; mental illness is only a pseudo-cause of the criminal behavior of the mentally ill. Once one sees through this myth, then he can see that that behavior is as uncaused as that of the rest of us; and with such contra-causal freedom comes responsibility. The softer version of this argument is that other conditions usually present in those we call mentally ill—compulsion, ignorance, or lack of mens rea—do excuse such persons without reference to the supposed causal agency of some entity called mental illness.[32,33] (pp. 985, 986) The heroic line is Szasz's—such persons should not be excused at all.

The mistake common to both positions is to be found in the assumption that it is only because "mental illness" was believed to name a mechanical cause that anyone ever thought it itself could be an excusing condition. This is indeed a popular misconception about the role of mental illness vis-à-vis our shared conceptions of responsibility. Yet that it is a misconception can be seen from the fact that, even if "mental illness" were the name of known, mechanical causes, it would not excuse because of such reference.

To believe that mental illness can excuse because it is or could be correlated with as yet unknown mechanical causes would be both to allow one's judgments of responsibility to depend entirely on speculative hypotheses about causes and to accept whole-hog the thesis that any mechanistic explanation of human action ipso facto excuses the actor from responsibility for that action. These two assumptions, however, would be sufficient to eliminate responsibility altogether as a viable concept. For if one is a determinist (which is likely if one believes in the existence of the requisite sorts of correlations between mental diseases and physiology), and if one allows the possibility of any kind of mechanical cause, known or unknown, to vitiate responsibility, then little seems to be left for particular excuses, such as mental illness, to do. One need only see the general implications of these same assumptions to see that everyone is already "excused" by an assumed, but yet unknown, mechanistic science of human behavior. The assumption that underneath the behavioral manifestations of disease there is a physiological explanation is not the source of our excusing the mentally ill from responsibility, no matter how popular the notion that that is the basis for our moral sentiments here.

As I[34] and others[35-38] have argued elsewhere in more detail, the reason it has been a century's-old and fundamental feature of our collective conscience that the mentally ill, who cause injurious results, are nonetheless not morally blameworthy is because, as set forth earlier, one who is mentally ill is not as rational as the rest of us in the senses of "rational" introduced earlier. If we cannot assume the rationality of another being, we cannot think of him as being morally responsible; for this assumption "is a precondition of any moral stance, and if it is jeopardized . . . the notion of moral responsibility is jeopardized in turn."[38] (p. 169) The presupposition of rationality is a necessary condition of taking any moral attitude toward another because it is a necessary condition for understanding that other in human terms, that is, in the idioms of practical reasoning, beliefs, motives, intentions, desires, and the like. Absent from such explanations we cannot understand another in the same fundamental way in which we understand our fellows in daily life, as set forth earlier. It is only beings that we understand in this way that we regard as moral agents.

Since mental illness negates our assumption of rationality, we do not hold the mentally ill responsible. It is not so much that we excuse them from a prima facie case of responsibility; rather, by being unable to regard them as fully rational beings, we cannot affirm the essential condition to viewing them as moral agents to begin with. In this the mentally ill join (to a decreasing degree) infants, wild beasts, plants, and stones — none of which are responsible because of the absence of any assumption of rationality. True, primitive people sometimes do hold such beings responsible, but then such peoples also invariably regard these things as purposive beings, i.e., rational. A widespread attribution of responsibility to infants, animals, and natural objects goes hand in hand with primitive animism or some other anthropomorphic view of the world.

Our intuitive feeling that the mentally ill should not be blamed (and, not being the subject of moral blame, excused from criminal liability), thus survives any insights about category mistakes lawyers or others might make in thinking of mental disease as a mechanical cause. Mental illness is not a mechanical cause of behavior, but then the assumption that it is or could be is not why we feel that the mentally ill should be excused to begin with.

CONCLUSION

Radical psychiatry has a good deal to say that should be of interest to those concerned with the legal status or psychiatric care of the mentally ill, even if its arguments are often stated in oversimplified and polemical terms. Its insights are not limited to the various arguments that mental illness is a myth, and do not all depend on such assumptions. As Wittgenstein once said of Freud, however, one must read Szasz critically if one is to learn anything of value. It has been the central purpose of this article to demonstrate that a critical reading of Szasz in terms of the philosophers on which he relies leaves "the myth of mental illness" as itself a myth, useful perhaps as a battle cry but hardly as the starting point for serious consideration of the legal status or medical treatment of the mentally ill.

The hoped for result of such a critique would be to channel the contemporary discussion of the insanity defense, civil commitment, the civil rights of the mentally ill, etc., away from the notion that mental illness is a myth and away from the methodological and philosophical grounds that allegedly support the myth conclusion. There may be strong arguments, e.g., that we in effect punish the insane anyway by involuntary detention in hospitals hardly worthy of the name, or that it is unjust for society to deprive anyone of his liberty absent either a violation of the law or a demonstrated dangerousness to others. These kinds of arguments do not depend on mental illness being nothing but a myth, and are the kinds of arguments genuinely relevant to the issues. Such arguments assume their proper role, however, only if one thinks more in terms of, say, Mill on liberty, than in terms of Szasz on myths.

REFERENCES

1. *Blocker vs. United States,* 288 F 2d 853, 1961.
2. Braginsky BM, Braginsky OD, Ring K: *Methods of Madness: The Mental Hospital as a Last Resort.* New York, Holt, Rinehart & Winston Inc., 1969.
3. Quine WV: *Ontological Relativity and Other Essays.* New York, Columbia University Press, 1969.
4. Szasz TS: *The Myth of Mental Illness.* New York, Harper & Row, Publishers Inc., 1961.
5. King LS: What is disease? *Philos Sci.* 21:193–203, 1954.
6. Frege G: Uber Sinn und Bedeutung: Zeitschrift Fur Philosophie Und Philosophische Kritik, in Geach PT, Black M (eds.): *The Philosophical Writings of Gottlob Frege.* Oxford, England, Blackwell Scientific Publications, 1960.
7. Quine WV: *From a Logical Point of View.* New York, Harper & Row Publishers Inc., 1963.
8. Szasz TS: *The Manufacture of Madness.* New York, Harper & Row Publishers Inc., 1970.

9. Kenny A: *Action, Emotion and Will.* London, Routledge & Kegan Paul Ltd., 1963.

10. Hampshire S: Disposition and memory. *Int. Psychoanal.* 43:59–68, 1962.

11. Dilman I: Is the unconscious a theoretical construct? *Monist* 56:313–342, 1972.

12. Alexander P: Rational behaviour and psychoanalytic explanation. *Mind* 71:326–341, 1962.

13. Mischel T: Concerning rational behaviour and psychoanalytic explanation. *Mind* 74:71–78, 1965.

14. Mullane H: Psychoanalytic explanation and rationality. *J. Philos.* 68:413–426, 1971.

15. Audi R: Psychoanalytic explanation and the concept of a rational action. *Monist* 56:444–464, 1972.

16. Laing RD, Esterson A: *Sanity, Madness, and the Family.* Baltimore, Penguin Books Inc., 1970.

17. Laing RD: *The Politics of Experience.* New York, Ballantine Books Inc., 1967.

18. Laing RD: *The Divided Self.* Baltimore, Penguin Books Inc., 1965.

19. Hayward ML, Taylor JE: A schizophrenic patient describes the action of intensive psychotherapy. *Psychiatr. Q.* 30:211–248, 1956.

20. Ackermann RJ: *Belief and Knowledge.* New York, Doubleday & Co. Inc., 1972.

21. Ryle G: *The Concept of Mind.* London, Hutchinson & Co. Ltd., 1949.

22. Szasz TS: *Law, Liberty, and Psychiatry.* New York, Collier Books, 1968.

23. Dennett DC: *Content and Consciousness.* New York, Humanities Press Inc., 1969, pp. 3–18.

24. Szasz TS: *Ideology and Insanity.* New York, Doubleday & Co. Inc., 1970.

25. Peters RS: *The Concept of Motivation.* London, Routledge & Kegan Paul Ltd., 1958.

26. Putnam H: The meaning of "meaning." *Minn. Stud. Philos. Sci.,* to be published.

27. Putnam H: Brains and behavior, in Butler RJ (ed.): *Analytical Philosophy: Second Series.* Oxford, England, Oxford University Press, 1965.

28. Gerbode FA: Book review. *Santa Clara Lawyer* 13:616–622, 1973.

29. Hardisty JH: Mental illness: A legal fiction. *Washington Law Rev.* 48:735–762, 1973.

30. *Durham vs. United States,* 214 F 2d 862, 1954.

31. Szasz TS: Psychiatry, ethics, and the criminal law. *Columbia Law Rev.* 58:183–198, 1958.

32. Goldstein J, Katz J: Abolish the insanity defense—why not? *Yale Law J.* 72:853–880, 1963.

33. *United States vs. Brawner,* 471 F 2d 969, 1972.

34. Moore MS: Mental illness and responsibility. *Bull. Menninger Clin.* 39:308–328, 1975.

35. Feinberg J: What is so special about mental illness? in *Doing and Deserving.* Princeton, NJ, Princeton University Press, 1970, pp. 272–292.

36. Fingarette H: *The Meaning of Criminal Insanity.* Berkeley, Calif., University of California Press, 1972.

37. Fingarette H: Insanity and responsibility. *Inquiry* 15:6–29, 1972.

38. Dennett DC: Mechanism and responsibility, in Honderich T (ed.): *Essays on Freedom of Action.* London, Routledge & Kegan Paul Ltd., 1973, pp. 159–184.

Suggestions for Further Reading

Critics of the Medical Model

Adams, Henry. "'Mental Illness' or Interpersonal Behavior?" *American Psychologist* 19 (March 1964):191–197.

Brady, John P., and Brodie, H. Keith, eds. *Controversy in Psychiatry*. Philadelphia: W. B. Saunders, Co., 1978, Chs. 1, 2 and 25.

Braginsky, Benjamin M., Braginsky, Dorothea D., and Ring, Kenneth. *Methods of Madness: The Mental Hospital as a Last Resort*. New York: Holt, Rinehart and Winston, Inc., 1969.

Breggin, Peter R. "Psychotherapy as Applied Ethics." *Psychiatry* 34 (February 1971):59–74.

Ennis, Bruce J., and Emery, Richard D. *The Rights of Mental Patients*. New York: Avon Books, 1978.

Goffman, Erving. *Asylums*. Garden City: Doubleday & Co., 1961.

Halleck, S. L. "The Medical Model and Psychiatric Training." *American Journal of Psychotherapy* 30 (April 1976):218–235.

Laing, R. D. *The Divided Self*. Baltimore: Penguin Books, Inc., 1965.

———. *The Politics of Experience*. New York: Ballantine Books, 1967.

Perrucci, Robert. *Circle of Madness: On Being Insane and Institutionalized in America*. Englewood Cliffs: Prentice-Hall, Inc., 1974.

Sarbin, Theodore R. "On the Futility of the Proposition that Some People Be Labeled "Mentally Ill." *Journal of Consulting Psychology* 31 (1967):447–453.

———. "Schizophrenia Is a Myth, Born of a Metaphor, Meaningless." *Psychology Today* 6 (1972):18ff.

———. "The Scientific Status of the Mental Illness Metaphor," in Plog,

Stanley C., and Edgerton, Robert B., eds. *Changing Perspectives in Mental Illness.* New York: Holt, Rinehart & Winston, 1969, pp. 9–31.

Scheff, T. J. *Being Mentally Ill: A Sociological Theory.* Chicago: Aldine Publishing Co., 1966.

―――. *Labeling Madness.* Englewood Cliffs: Prentice-Hall, Inc., 1975.

Szasz, Thomas S. "Repudiation of the Medical Model." In Sahakian, W. S., ed., *Psychopathology Today.* Itasca, Ill.: F. E. Peacock, 1970, pp. 47–53.

Torrey, E. Fuller. *The Death of Psychiatry.* Radnor, Pa.: Chilton Book Co., 1974, Part I.

Veatch, Robert M., "The Medical Model: Its Nature and Problems." *Hastings Center Studies* 1 (1973):59–76.

Defenders of the Medical Model

Adler, David A. "The Medical Model and Psychiatry's Tasks." *Hospitals and Community Psychiatry* 32 (June 1981):387–392.

Begelman, D. A. "Misnaming, Metaphors, the Medical Model, and Some Muddles." *Psychiatry* 34 (February 1971):38–58.

Brady, John P., and Brodie, H. Keith, eds. *Controversy in Psychiatry.* Philadelphia: W. B. Saunders Co., 1978, Chs. 1, 2 and 25.

Brown, Robert. "Physical Illness and Mental Health." *Philosophy and Public Affairs* 7 (1977):17–38.

Dumas, Frank M. "Medical, Nonmedical, or Antimedical Models for Mental Health Centers." *American Journal of Psychiatry* 131 (August 1974):875–878.

Engle, George L. "The Need for a New Medical Model: A Challenge for Biomedicine." *Science* 196 (April 1977):129–136.

Gove, Walter R. *The Labelling Theory of Deviance: Evaluating a Perspective.* New York: Halstead Press, 1975.

―――. "The Stigma of Mental Hospitalization: An Attempt to Evaluate Its Consequences." *Archives of General Psychiatry* 28 (April 1973):494–500.

Grob, Gerald N. "Rediscovering Asylums: The Unhistorical History of the Mental Hospital." *Hastings Center Report* 7 (August 1977):33–41.

Klerman, Gerald L. "Mental Illness, the Medical Model, and Psychiatry." *The Journal of Medicine and Philosophy* 2 (1977):220–243.

Ludwig, Arnold M. "The Psychiatrist as Physician." *Journal of the American Medical Association* 234 (November 1975):603–604.

Macklin, Ruth. "The Medical Model in Psychoanalysis and Psychotherapy." *Comprehensive Psychiatry* 14 (1973):46–69.

Moore, Michael S. "Some Myths About 'Mental Illness'." *Archives of General Psychiatry* 32 (December 1975):1483–1497.

Shagass, Charles. "The Medical Model in Psychiatry." In Sachar, Edward J., ed. *Hormones Behavior and Psychopathology.* New York: Raven Press, 1976.

Sigler, Miriam, and Osmond, Humphrey. *Models of Madness, Models of Medicine.* New York: Harper and Row, 1976.

Stevenson, Leslie. "Mind, Brain and Mental Illness." *Philosophy* 52 (January 1977):27–43.

Trotter, Robert J. "Psychiatry for the 80's." *Science News* 119 (May 30, 1981): 348–349.

Physical Grounds for Psychiatric Disorders

Frazier, Alan, and Winokur, Andrew, eds. *Biological Bases of Psychiatric Disorders.* New York: Spectrum Publications, 1977.

Glaser, Gilbert H., ed. *EEG and Behavior.* New York: Basic Books, 1963.

Gottlieb, J., and Frohman, C. "The Biochemistry of Schizophrenia." In Arieti, S, ed. *Handbook of Psychiatry.* 2nd ed., 1974.

Gross, Martin L. *The Psychological Society.* New York: Random House, 1978, Ch. 4.

Ho, Beng T., and McIsaac, William M. *Brain Chemistry and Mental Disease.* New York: Plenum Press, 1971.

Mandel, Arnold J., et al. "The Search for the Schizococcus." *Psychology Today* 6 (October 1972):68ff.

Restack, Richard M. *The Brain: The Last Frontier.* Garden City, N.Y.: Doubleday, 1979.

———. "Brain Potentials: Signaling Our Inner Thoughts." *Psychology Today* 12 (March 1979):42ff.

Sachar, Edward J., ed. *Hormones, Behavior and Psychopathology.* New York: Raven Press, 1976.

Shagass, Charles, et al., eds. *Psychopathology and Brain Dysfunction.* New York: Raven Press, 1977.

Snyder, Solomon H. "Mending Shattered Minds." *Science Year.* Chicago: World Book-Childcraft International, 1981, pp. 128–139.

Solomon, Philip, and Patch, Vernon D., eds. *Handbook of Psychiatry.* 3rd ed. Los Altos, California: Lange Medical Publications, 1974, especially part II.

Spitzer, Robert L., and Klein, Donald F. *Critical Issues in Psychiatric Diagnosis.* New York: Raven Press, 1978, parts 3 and 4.

Spitzer, Therese. *Psychobattery, A Chronical of Psychotherapeutic Abuses.* Clifton, N.J.: The Humana Press, 1980.

Torrey, E. Fuller. *The Death of Psychiatry.* Radnor, Pa.: Chilton Book Co., 1974, Ch. 10.

———. "Schizophrenia: Sense and Nonsense." *Psychology Today* 11 (November 1977):157.

———. "Tracking the Causes of Madness." *Psychology Today* 12 (March 1979): 78ff.

Tsuang, Ming T., and Vander Mey, Randall. *Genes and the Mind: Inheritance of Mental Illness.* New York: Oxford University Press, 1980.

Wender, Paul H., and Klein, Donald F. "The Promise of Biological Psychiatry." *Psychology Today* 15 (February 1981):25–41.

Williams, Moyra. *Brain Damage, Behavior and the Mind.* New York: John Wiley & Sons, 1979.

Wolf, S. "Disease as a Way of Life: Neural Integration in Systemic Pathology." *Perspectives in Biology and Medicine* 4 (1961):288ff.

3. Therapist-Patient Relationships and Rights

Introduction

Professional codes of ethics and formulations of the rights of both patients and staff attempt to give moral guidance to practitioners in addition to informing patients and staff about their moral rights, many of which are also in the form of concurrent legal rights. Moral rights are generated by moral ideals; their content may differ depending upon which ideal ethical theory one accepts. Legal rights are those which have been enacted into positive law and may differ from one society to another. The general concept of a right was probably as well defined by John Stuart Mill in Chapter 5 of his *Utilitarianism* as by anyone: "When we call anything a person's right, we mean that he has a valid claim on society to protect him in the possession of it, either by the force of law or by that of education and opinion. If he has what we consider a sufficient claim, on whatever account, to have something guaranteed to him by society, we say that he has a right to it." For short, "To have a right, then, is . . . to have something which society ought to defend me in the possession of." A right is the reverse side of an obligation or duty. Although there may be duties without corresponding rights (e.g., charity), rights cannot exist where there are no corresponding duties. Thus, "X has a right to y" means that others have a duty or obligation either to refrain from obstructing X's pursuit of y if he chooses to pursue it (negative rights), and/or in some cases to provide X with y if he so chooses (positive rights). A *moral* right is such a societal, professional, or personal obligation that is in accord with the dictates of an "enlightened conscience" and that ideally ought to be recognized even where it is not. A *legal* right is an obligation that has actually been codified into positive law and thus is already legally protected or provided. A right is considered *absolute* when it is binding in *all* conceivable circumstances and should never be overridden. A *prima facie* right is one which is binding under normal circumstances but may be occasionally over-ridden by more important considerations. Moral philosophies frequently differ over such questions as whether there are any absolute rights at all and what types of circumstances would be required to justify over-riding prima facie rights. Unfortunately, neither philosophers nor medical professionals have arrived at any agreement on the answers to these questions, though we may hope for progress through continuing dialogue and debate.

In the following general overview of the ethical dimensions of the therapist-patient relationship in psychotherapy, Toksoz B. Karasu gives special attention to the patient's right to confidentiality while considering possible conflicts between moral stances taken in professional codes of ethics and recent legal decisions. He also explores the patient's right to freedom from sexism and sexual exploitation. His recognition of "authoritarian" and "egalitarian" models of the therapist-patient relationship could stand a bit of elaboration, however. Each model acknowledges that ideal modes of distributing power between patient and practitioner are built into the way in which the relationship is conceived from the very outset. On a therapist-centered version of the authoritarian model, all power and responsibility are ideally vested in the practitioner and none in the patient. Under this model, the practitioner would make not only the technical medical decisions about the most effective means to therapeutic ends or goals but he would also decide upon the goals themselves, with no input from the patient. On such a model, the "good patient" would be totally passive and would always "follow doctor's orders" even to the extent of allowing the doctor or therapist to decide upon the values to be realized through the relationship. Since he is the only acting moral agent, the therapist assumes full responsibility for all that happens. The patient would never have the right to say "no," and there would be no such thing as a right to refuse medical treatment or to express his or her own value preferences. The doctor or therapist would "always know best." Karasu might profitably have recognized a patient-centered authoritarian model in which the doctor merely explains the medical options to the patient and then simply carries out the wishes of the patient. This would be the case even when the patient's expressed wishes run counter to the therapist's knowledge of what will be medically effective or to the latter's most deeply held values, whether they be moral, religious, or what have you. Here the patient alone decides and assumes full responsibility for all that happens. In the "egalitarian" model explored by Karasu, ideally, patient and practitioner negotiate a contract with one another at the beginning of the relationship with respect to goals and the means designed to achieve them. These are mutually acceptable to each party, both of whom recognize in advance the fact that each of them is a responsible moral agent with agreed upon rights and obligations. Each party would have the right to veto suggested courses of treatment wherein fundamental rights or values might be transgressed. The application of such a model to mental patients would often be complicated by considerations of competence, however, since only competent moral agents are entitled to make contracts. Society must protect and defend the basic rights of mental patients even in cases where these patients are not capable of negotiating courses of treatment for themselves.

Specific rights of mental patients and staff are explored in our second and third selections. Recognized rights of mental patients are spelled out in some detail in the selection entitled "Assuring Patients/Clients of Their Rights" from the 1978 report of the President's Commission on Mental Health. In the final essay, Robert W. Gibson insists that staff members have rights also, and that ideally these harmonize with the rights of patients. In reading the Gibson article, ask yourself if some of the rights he ascribes to the staff might not be classified more properly as duties.

Toksoz B. Karasu

The Ethics of Psychotherapy

In 1978, Spiegel (1) suggested that we have evolved from an Age of Anxiety to an Age of Ethical Crises. Progressive loss of faith in traditional institutions and the erosion of authority are now being met with the increasing challenge of existing standards and widespread concern for safeguarding human values and rights. Today's growing climate of antiestablishment, antiprofessional, and antirational sentiment has direct implications for the roles and responsibilities of the psychotherapist. Growing skepticism about the sanctity of science, medicine, and psychiatry means that these fields are no longer above rebuke or exempt from active moral review by their recipients, professional peers, and others outside of their practice, such as third-party payers. The psychotherapist, once left relatively undisturbed in the private confines of his or her office, has now been besieged from within (2) and without (3). The siege from within reflects psychiatry's own members and critics, who extol widely different models and criteria of mental illness and its treatment, which are confusing and divisive to the field and its future. The siege from without reflects the public voice and confusion regarding the functions, procedures, and powers of the psychotherapist. There is an increasing expectation and demand for accountability, i.e., that the patient be granted, indeed is owed, health as a right and greater participation in determining and assessing the goals and activities as well as the outcome of treatment. Simultaneously, social, political, and personal pressures oblige the psychotherapist (under the prospect of national health insurance) to assess and review his or her practices.

From *The American Journal of Psychiatry* 137 (1980):1502–1512. Copyright © 1980 by the American Psychiatric Association. Reprinted by permission of the publisher and the author.

Michels (4) attributed the failure of the profession itself to stave off this challenge and criticism to four factors: 1) a fundamental disappointment with the limitations of science and reason in answering the problems of mankind, 2) an antielitism that aims to mitigate the power of professionals as symbolic representations of the inequitable distribution of resources in society, 3) the compounding of the antiprofessional stance by members of the profession who have failed and then have turned against it in response to exclusion from membership, and, most relevantly for the morality issue in psychotherapy, 4) the fear of overgeneralization of the authority of the professional from scientific to ethical arenas.

The Interface Between Science and Ethics in Psychotherapy

The issue of the relationship of science to ethics in psychotherapy may be considered the conceptual heart of the matter. *Webster's New World Dictionary* defines "ethics" as "the system or code of morality of a particular person, religion, group or profession," "morals" as "relating to, dealing with, or capable of making the distinction between right and wrong in conduct," and "science," which psychotherapy presumes to be, as "a branch of knowledge or study concerned with establishing or systemizing facts." Theoretically, science and ethics have been viewed as two distinct and separate entities, almost antithetical: science as descriptive, ethics as prescriptive; science as resting on validation, ethics as relying on judgment; and science as concerned solely with "what is," ethics as addressing "what ought to be" (5). The lines become less sharply drawn, however, when the complexities of social reality are brought into the picture, when the psychotherapist is obliged to act as a "double agent" (6) to accommodate conflicts of interest posed between patient and therapist and by third parties to whom the therapist holds allegiance, such as family members and school, hospital, and military authorities (7). The lines become even less clear as the therapist confronts the ambiguity between the science and the art of psychotherapy, dual attitudes of the psychotherapist's identity that differ in degree and quality (8). In fact, there is still a question of whether psychotherapy is a science at all, in that it deals with hermeneutics rather than explanation, is humanistic rather than mechanistic, seeks private rather than public knowledge—in all, in that it is not a science but a body of knowledge with a special status, which frees it from obligations that other sciences share (9).

In addition, although the distinction between the principles of science and those of ethics may more readily hold for the researcher inside his or her laboratory, it is simply less applicable to the clinician in daily practice (10). Lifton (6) highlighted this point in describing his work with Viet Nam veterans, which required him to combine sufficient detachment to make psychological evaluations with involvement that expressed his own personal commitments and moral passions. (He had taken an active antiwar advocacy position during the Viet Nam conflict and expressed profound interest and concern for Hiroshima survivors.) Lifton aptly concluded, "I believe that we [therapists] always function within this *dialectic between ethical involvement and intellectual rigour.*" He went even farther to recommend that "bringing our advocacy 'out front' and articulating it makes us more, rather than less, scientific. Indeed, our scientific accuracy is likely to suffer when we hide our ethical beliefs behind the claims of neutrality and that we are nothing but 'neutral screens.'"

With the above in mind, we may say that it is inevitable for the boundaries between science and ethics to become blurred. To the extent that the therapist implicitly, if not explicitly, cares about "what ought to be" as well as "what is," ethical issues will inhere in virtually all of his or her work. In the broadest terms, then, there has been a growing recognition that subjective commitment (unconscious as well as conscious) places inevitable constraints on the presumed purity and verity of objective treatment. More specifically, the idyllic notion of psychotherapy (and the psychotherapist) as value-free is now widely accepted as a fallacy (11). This is supported by current research demonstrating many contradictions in expressed belief versus reported practices in psychotherapy (12). Buckley and associates (12) hypothesized the presence of a "two-tier" system: one, the ideal or correct (i.e., value-free, nonsuggestive); the other, the practical or applied view (i.e., direct suggestions, encouragement of specific goals), which loosens the adherence to a value-free frame of reference. In brief, when actually applied, psychotherapy represents neither pure science nor pure ethics but a branch of the healing profession that resides somewhere in between. Therefore, Erikson (13) concluded that psychotherapy can find its ethical place only by locating a legitimate and unique area between the two ideological extremes of being an objectively applied true science and representing an ideology of healthy conduct.

Concern with the interface of science and ethics or healthy conduct and with the place of values in treatment is certainly not new to the field of psychotherapy. A major controversy has long pivoted on the degree to which psychoanalysis inherently propounds any particular value system. Some believe it does not do so (14). Others imply that it is political and repressive by definition (15, 16), that it favors particular cultural values, especially biases toward certain social classes over others (17), and that its basic tenets are inherently biased against women (18). Still others, although they accept that psychotherapy cannot be value-free and even believe that in its overall goals it should not be (19), see the fundamental issue as whether the imposition of such values are "deliberate and avowed" or "unrecognized and unavowed" (13).

On a more concrete level, Freud can be credited with the discovery and longtime recognition of the unique power and intensity of the transferential relationship (both to cure and to be resisted) and the inevitable influence of the therapist and his or her values in treatment. This has been classically dealt with in great depth in analytic attempts to maintain the purity of the therapeutic relationship (transference) through the technical neutrality of the therapist, and, when inadvertently violated, the full exploration and understanding of the therapist's countertransference. Freud certainly held an ethical ideal about the conduct of psychotherapy when he wrote, "One must not forget that the relationship between analyst and patient is based on a love of truth, that is, on the acknowledgment of reality, and that it precludes any kind of sham or deceit" (20, p. 248).

The Goals of Psychotherapy

The Principles of Medical Ethics of the American Medical Association (21), first adopted in 1847, set down the standards of practice for physicians. Although psychiatrists are assumed to have the same goals as all physicians, APA added to the *Principles Annotations Especially Applicable to Psychiatry* (22). The rationale for these annotations was that "there are special ethical problems in psychiatric practice that differ in coloring and degree from ethical problems in other branches of medical practice (22). These annotations made no alterations whatever in the original AMA standards.

Section 3 of the AMA *Principles* was the only one not annotated for psychiatry. It states that a physician (and therefore a psychiatrist) "should practice a method of healing founded on a scientific basis; and he should not voluntarily associate professionally with anyone who violates this principle." In the annotation to section 6 of the *Principles* the psychiatrist is advised that "he/she should neither lend the endorsement of the psychiatric specialty nor refer patients to persons, groups, or treatment programs with which he/she is not familiar, especially if their work is based only on dogma and authority and not on scientific validation and replication."

Fisher and Greenberg (23) suggested that the question of the scientific credibility of Freud's theory and therapy, despite extensive exploration, has not been decisively settled in the minds of psychiatrists themselves, although their hearts may tell them otherwise. Moreover, the proliferation of well over 100 supposed schools of psychotherapy,[1] each with its own, albeit overlapping, theory of mental illness and health, therapeutic agents, overall goals, and specific practices (24), reflects the massive nature of investigating therapeutic efficacy and the complexity of establishing scientific guidelines. Given the stunning diversity of therapeutic forms now being offered to potential patients, how does one ethically equate the goals encompassed in a screaming cure (Janov's primal therapy), a reasoning cure (Ellis' rational therapy), a realism cure (Glasser's reality therapy), a decision cure (Greenwald's direct decision therapy), an orgasm cure (Reich's orgone therapy), a meaning cure (Frankl's logotherapy), and even a profound-rest cure (transcendental meditation)? For example, Leo (25) quoted Slavson's assessment of "feeling therapy, nude therapy, marathon therapy, and other new remedies of the ailing psyche." Slavson concluded that "these activities [are] untested, theoretically weak, and potentially very dangerous." More specifically, he asserted that "latent or borderline psychotics with tenuous ego controls and defenses may, under the stress of such groups and the complete giving up of defenses, jump the barrier between sanity and insanity." However, the data on the efficacy of these practices are not yet in. Does the psychotherapist have an ethical responsibility to force closure on these events, especially if his or her judgments are premature?

Such tremendous confusion in the state of the art has led to a virtual identity crisis for psychiatry and the psychotherapist (26–28), highlighted negatively (29) in the recent growth of the antipsychiatry movement, which makes it possible for a psychiatrist to be a psychiatrist by training, accreditation, affiliation, and status but at the same time an antipsychiatrist in ideology and action. (All this under one ethical psychiatric roof.) Indeed, the goals and responsibilities of the psychotherapist are now so broadly and vaguely defined that Raskin (30) said ours is a profession without a "role-specific function" and Vispo (31) said our practices run the gamut from "science to social revolution." Redlich and Mollica (7) described the quandary of whether the practical purpose of psychiatry and the psychotherapist as its agent is "to diagnose, treat, and prevent a relatively defined number of psychoses? to perform this task on a number of neurotics? to make unhappy and incompetent persons happy and competent? or to tackle poverty and civil and international strife?" Although these are not beyond the legitimate concern of psychotherapists in their quest to improve the psychological welfare of their patients, there is a question as to whether these goals are beyond their legitimate competence. Where does one draw the line?

Although broadly recognized goals can include Freud's love and work and variants of growth and maturation, self-realization, self-sufficiency, and security and freedom from anxiety — all of which may be noble aspirations — ethical issues inhere in the practices that are conducted in their name. Across a spectrum of possibilities have been posed questions of freedom to change or not to change versus coercion, helping and healing versus shaping and imposing the therapist's influence, and issues of "cure" of illness versus positive growth. Szasz (32), probably the most prolific and vocal propounder of an antipsychiatry position, views conventional therapy by definition as "social action, not healing" and as "a series of religious, rhetorical, and repressive acts." The basis of the controversy is the medical model's designation of "patient," which presupposes restrictive conceptualizations of normality and health.

One of the most fundamental ethical dilemmas directly related to the goal of therapy is whether to encourage the patient to rebel against a repressive environment or to adjust to his or her condition (33). This issue is illustrated by psychiatry's standard definition and traditional treatment of homosexuals. "Homosexuality" as a "sexual deviation" (*DSM-II*) and its implications have been ardently challenged by advocates for gay rights, and sufficient pressure was brought to bear on APA that the official designation was changed to "sexual orientation disturbance." A review of the psychotherapy and behavior therapy literature indicates that therapists generally regard homosexuality as undesirable, if not pathological (34). On the less theoretical plane of actual treatment goals, the therapist may be obliged to take a position, implicitly if not explicitly, as to whether a heterosexual orientation is a valid ultimate goal for the patient or the patient should maximize the quality of his or her life adjustment as a homosexual. The latter stance, often unpopular, was subject to debate when a behavior therapist treating a man who was sexually attracted to boys provided the patient with methods to transfer that attraction to men, not women (11, 35, 36). Obviously, definition of goals not only vary between therapists but changes with the times as definitions of normality evolve.

Another ethical dilemma in establishing therapeutic goals pertains to the dual allegiance of the therapist to the patient and to society's representatives. This was placed in bold relief in the role of psychiatrists who were treating soldiers in Viet Nam (6). Lifton stated that in such instances the therapist is forced to tread the thin line between advocacy and corruption. With adjustment to the military as the goal of therapy, the psychiatrist most likely "helped" the troubled soldier to remain on military duty. This meant that the soldier had to continue the commission of war crimes, which is what he was expected to do in Viet Nam. Thus psychiatry served unsuspectingly "to erode whatever capacity [the soldiers] retained for moral revulsion and animating guilt" (6), and the goals of psychotherapists became inseparable from those of military authority.

Aside from conflictual goals in psychotherapy posed by the individual versus the larger society, Hadley and Strupp (37) found that a major area of negative effects of psychotherapy according to a survey of practitioners and researchers in the field was "undertaking unrealistic tasks or goals." These authors listed false assumptions concerning the scope and potency of therapy's purported goals first among tendencies in the conduct of treatment that have profound ethical implications. Misleading impressions may be imbued by therapists when their need to instill hope in the patient and the omniscience endowed them (by themselves and/or the patient) become intertwined. Although some degree of positive expectation or hope is regarded as requisite for producing therapeutic effects in all psychotherapies (38), the patient may get the erroneous impression that therapy and the therapist can solve everything. This can perpetuate unrealistic expectations and goals that are ultimately deleterious to the patient. Such tendencies are often compounded by the failure to discuss, describe, or even acknowledge the reality of goals during treatment or when the stated goals are too broad or obscure.

Special technical problems with ethical implications also arise when goals explicitly or implicitly exceed the patient's capabilities, which fosters false hopes of speedy progress that cannot be realized if the patient actually requires longer treatment. Another problem occurs when the patient has accomplished certain goals but the therapist alters the goals to prolong treatment because he or she is unwilling to terminate it. Greenson (39) aptly warned that any form or aspect of therapy that makes the patient an addict to therapy and to the therapist is undesirable.

Therapists are obliged to ask themselves, How ethical is it to have limited goals when the needs of the patient may change or evolve as the therapy progresses, or when the patient is in need of long-term treatment but either financial or administrative expediencies will not permit it? Can superficial interpretations, made in the interests of time, shortchange patients? Where does one draw the line in serving long-term goals? For example, psychotherapists tend not to prescribe medication for moderate insomnia, anxiety, or depression, the presumed justification being the potentially motivating aspect of discomfort and suffering for psychological work. If this is the case, has the patient been informed of the means and ends of the therapist?

In summary, the issue of the goals of psychotherapy is complex and subtle, including professional versus personal, long- versus short-term, nonspecific versus specific, and overt versus covert goals. It is the latter that is ethically the most problematic and the one most under the therapist's and the patient's control.

The Therapeutic Relationship

The therapeutic relationship or special power relationship that exists between doctor and patient constitutes psychotherapy's strength as well as its weakness. The duality inheres in the concept of authority, which may be defined in many ways (40). In its purist sense, it refers to an individual who is a specialist in his or her field and is entitled to credit or acceptance on this basis; in another sense, it refers to power that requires submission. Different types of therapeutic relationships have been formed with different therapies (24) or at different times in the process of the same therapy (41). A common ethical problem for psychotherapy pivots on the degree to which the therapeutic relationship is authoritarian versus egalitarian, or, more specifically, to what extent the pervasive power of the therapeutic transference relationship, which offers the therapist a unique vehicle for exercising enormous influence over another human being, is balanced by a true "therapeutic alliance" (39) or "therapeutic partnership" (42). Redlich and Mollica (7) pointed out that in general psychiatry "the fiduciary system, in which a patient puts his trust in the physician's ability and willingness to make crucial decisions, is being replaced by a contractual system." This trend applies as well to the current psychotherapies.

An egalitarian therapeutic relationship is gaining in prominence and is considered more humanitarian and facilitative of free exchange between patient and therapist than the traditional medical model (i.e., doctor-to-patient) or the behavioral model (i.e., teacher-to-student) (24). Might some aspects of this model, however, have negative implications for the therapeutic endeavor in general? Parsons (43), in his analysis of social structure and the dynamic process, identified certain requirements of the doctor-patient relationship necessary for successful treatment. One of the most essential was the "social distance" between practitioner and client. In their study of human organization Burling and associates (44) concluded, "We are coming to understand that faith in the doctor is a necessary element in cure, [and] that he will not be able to exercise therapeutic leverage if we, as patients, regard him in too prosaic a light" (p. 71). These authors suggested that the therapist's power to claim the patient's confidence and the therapist's effectiveness will be impaired by growing familiarity. Where, then, does one draw the line between the good use of power in the traditional model and its abuse? Where do the new boundaries of partnership end and those of "real" familiarity and friendship begin? More important for the times, will there be new ethical dilemmas in the egalitarian relationship between therapeutic partners?

Goldberg's exposition of the equitable "therapeutic partnership" (42) suggests that it is not only the nature of the therapeutic alliance (i.e., its power distribution) that is critical but the degree to which it is made explicit. Often within its nonexplicit nature lies the ethical rub of psychotherapy. Goldberg recommended that a therapeutic contract establish a mutually agreed on and explicitly articulated working plan (comparable to the medical model's treatment plan), the essence of which is how each agent will ultimately use or restrict his or her use of power. This should consist not only of agreed on goals but established means, evaluation of therapeutic work during its course, and methods of addressing dissatisfactions in the working alliance. Articulating in practice what one intends in theory, however, is an admirable but not easily accomplished task. In addition to goal ambiguity, noted earlier, the distinction between theory and practice has also been a criticism of newer modalities like encounter group therapy (45, 46). Despite appearances of therapeutic virtues like openness, autonomy, and mutuality, encounter group therapy often gives little attention to the specificity of individual participants' psychological needs (45), and treatment is often started without defining what the patient wants or expects to be the result of the encounter (46).

How the therapeutic relationship is manifested also relates to one of the most prominent negative effects of the traditional therapeutic relationship, according to a 1976 survey (37): its insufficient regard for the patient's intentionality or will. This can be exacerbated in many ways. For example, in the analyst's fervent search for unconscious determinants the therapy may soon become an end in itself and the therapist may assume priority over all other people in the patient's life. This can occur in an even more extreme form in the newer, "spiritual" therapies, which encourage pious belief in the therapist that overrides the realities of life itself (witness the tragedy of Guyana). In either event, the therapist's power is greatly exaggerated for reasons that may have more to do with the therapist's needs than those of the patient.

Dependency, nonetheless, is one of the most common characteristics of all patients and allows for the early establishment of the helper-helpee relationship. Other relationships (e.g., transference and a working alliance) that help to play out that dependence and ultimately aid the therapist in encouraging independence in the patient develop in the process of treatment. Some patients, however, need lifelong supervision of their lives even after much of the psychotherapy work is done; often they may take action themselves and terminate treatment. It is also possible that a therapist, because of lack of experience or for less benign reasons (e.g., financial or pathological needs) perpetuates the dependency and unresolved transference of the patient. Although most often viewed within the arena of a technical problem of treatment, the question remains, When does this technical problem in therapy become an ethical issue as well?

Confidentiality

The issues of confidentiality and privileged communication in psychotherapy have had national implications in the last decade, exemplified by the Watergate scandal and the attempt to steal Daniel Ellsberg's records from his psychiatrist's office, but these issues are generally more subtle in everyday psychotherapeutic practice. Although psychotherapists need be concerned here with the ethical rather than the legal aspects of confidentiality, the subject is often complicated by the specter of legal sanction.

The sanctity of confidentiality for the psychotherapeutic endeavor is crucial because of the inherently personal nature of its communications, which plumb the depths of the patient's innermost thoughts, fantasies, and feelings. A number of states, in fact, have statutes that grant the relationship between psychiatrist and patient the same absolute protections from public policy as are accorded to the relationship between husband and wife and attorney and client, to grand jurors, and to secrets of state (47). Indeed, the most elaborate clause of APA's *Annotations* to *The Principles of Medical Ethics* (section 9) (22) relates to this subject. It calls for extreme care in matters of both written and verbal communications, especially in instances of consultation with other professionals, with clinical notes and records, and in case presentations and other use or dissemination of confidential teaching materials. In addition, Redlich and Mollica (7) warned against the more insidious dangers of "gossip" between therapists that might inadvertently prove detrimental to the patient and the therapeutic relationship.

Having to meet current demands for detailed record-keeping in anticipation of the requirements and wishes of third-party payers and peer review organizations means that the confidential boundaries of the traditional dyadic relationship between therapist and patient have greatly enlarged and eroded. Both the domain for potential communication (i.e., who is privy to confidential information) and the risk of violation of confidentiality have geometrically increased. Plaut (48) has said that an escalating conflict exists between the right to secrecy and the right to information because of 1) increasing government involvement in areas that were previously considered private affairs, 2) the electronic revolution in data collection, storage, and retrieval, and 3) the prevailing atmosphere of high suspiciousness between individuals and government authorities, for whom knowledge has always meant power.

In view of these new outside pressures, the major questions of confidentiality in psychotherapy are, Whose agent is the psychotherapist (the patient's?

the family's? society's? the law's?)? What are the goals of divulging confidential material (better treatment? evaluation? consensual validation? support?)? What are the risks? (Will the therapeutic relationship be jeopardized? Will the patient terminate treatment?) Conversely, will rigid adherence to a rule of confidentiality between therapist and patient blind the therapist to worse fates for the patient—the risk of danger to self or others?

Sometimes the confusion of the therapist's allegiance inheres in the nature of the psychotherapy he or she is conducting—individual-, family-, or society-oriented. Although individual-oriented psychotherapy may limit itself to the more orthodox dyadic goals within the private framework of the patient's inner thoughts and feelings, other goals may be more society-oriented and may use the information communicated between therapist and patient to influence the patient's social milieu. A serious question that often arises is the therapist's role and responsibility to the family of the patient. In general, the less healthy the patient, the more important this issue can become. With relatively stable and independent individuals, there is usually no need to contact family members, nor would the therapist encourage any communication from them. Should the latter occur, it is usually in the patient's best interests that he or she be promptly informed of the family contact and that the contact become material for the sessions themselves, grist for the mill of the psychotherapeutic treatment. However, more disturbed patients may not only need the support of the family; they may involve family members with the therapist as an extension of their disturbance. In such circumstances, each communication with the family not only complicates the treatment but also raises serious ethical questions about breaches of confidentiality and whose interests the therapist is serving. In family therapy, whose purported goal is "to treat the family as the patient" (49), the situation may be reversed in that an individual's confidences may be subverted in the therapeutic service of the marital unit or family.

Thus whether a therapist adheres to an individual or a family orientation may determine not only the goals of treatment but also the nature of its treatment of the individual within each mode. How does the therapist determine whether it is in the individual patient's best interests to be seen alone or within the context of the family unit? How ethical is it to impose a systems approach in treatment (e.g., husband and wife, parents and children) because one views the problem as stemming from the family or marriage? On the other side of the coin are instances in which dynamic psychotherapists so strongly believe in utmost confidentiality and individual privacy of the dyadic relationship that they fail to divulge confidences or share information with family members that may prove vital to the welfare of the patient.

Indeed, the only exception to the overall rule of confidentiality between therapist and patient is that of "dangerousness" to others. This concept was legally stipulated by the famous *Tarasoff* decision (50), which enunciated the maxim that "protective privilege ends where public peril begins." According to this decision, therapists must warn authorities specified by law as well as potential victims of possible dangerous actions of their patients. (The legal case involved a young man's confidential announcement to his therapist that he intended to kill his girlfriend. After the therapist had consulted with two psychiatrists and notified the police that the man was dangerous, the young man was detained. However, he was released when he denied such violent intentions. Simultaneously, in response to his therapist's breach of confidence, he broke off treatment. Two months later he murdered his girlfriend. The therapist and his psychiatrist-supervisor were then sued by the woman's parents for failing to warn them of her peril.)

The case, while highly unusual, places in bold relief the dilemmas of therapists in balancing the rights to confidentiality of individuals with the protection of society from danger. Several psychotherapists (51, 52) have been antagonistic to the decision because of its conceptual and practical flaws and its negative implications for psychiatry. Roth and Meisel (51), for example, stated that the decision assumes a degree of expertise in predicting violence or danger that the psychiatrist simply does not possess; that the result will be a confusion and lowering of the threshold of dangerousness for issuing warnings to intended victims, which can compromise the patient's right to confidentiality and possibly his or her treatment; that the psychiatrist is liable not only if he or she fails to warn but also for invasion of privacy or defamation of the patient if the threat of harm does not materialize; and, finally, as actually happened in the *Tarasoff* case, the patient's dangerousness was probably increased because of his sense of betrayal at the therapist's commitment attempt and the patient's premature termination of the very treatment he needed. On a more conceptual level, Gurevitz (52) stated that the *Tarasoff* decision erroneously "defines and reenforces a social control function for psychiatry" by allying the psychotherapist "more with the goal of protecting society than with that of healing patients." It is not, Gurevitz pointed out, that psychiatrists reject the need to balance these functions; in fact, most psychiatrists attempt to fulfill both responsibilities. However, they have done so with procedures that have not mandated them to routinely perform a duty that is "counter to their power of prescience."

Despite the *Tarasoff* decision, and no doubt because of it, alternative courses of action that can be taken by psychotherapists short of actual warning have been recommended. For example, due to their very strong convictions about the importance of confidentiality in the doctor-patient relationship, in no instance have Roth and Meisel (51) directly warned a potential victim without first obtaining the patient's permission. Since actual violence is relatively rare, they stated that it is prudent to "rely on odds and not warn." In addition, they suggested that therapists should inform the patient of the boundaries and limits of confidentiality. Even when danger seems imminent, the therapist should consider a number of social or environmental manipulations to reduce dangerousness before he or she makes the decision to compromise confidentiality. When confronted with a potentially violent patient, the therapist has options that include 1) continued therapeutic management of the patient, 2) involuntary hospitalization, 3) notifying the police, and 4) notifying the potential victims. Each of these choices of action places a differing weight on the competing values of confidentiality versus protection of the social order (or protection from "public peril").

There is also the question of the more private peril of the patient's danger to himself or herself. The following questions remain: Is the therapist able to predict danger to self any better than he or she can predict danger to others? If not, at what point does the duty to warn enter? Where does one draw the confidentiality line when the patient is a threat to himself or herself? Here issues of suicide and its active prevention may also ethically relate to the therapist's ideological position. Recently publicized cases of so-called "rational suicide," especially under the psychological and physical specter of terminal illness, along with the call for increased options for dealing with dying, suggest that the psychotherapist may be increasingly faced with the need to respect such choices by patients as part of his or her ethical responsibilities. In each such instance, the therapist and patient alike are obliged to confront and resolve their ethical dilemmas together.

Therapist-Patient Sex and Sexism

The Hippocratic Oath pledges that "with purity and holiness I will practice my art. . . . Into whatever houses I enter I will go into them for the benefit of the sick and will abstain from every voluntary act of mischief and corruption, and further from the seduction of females or males, of freemen and slaves" (53). The *Annotations Especially Applicable to Psychiatry of The Principles of Medical Ethics* (22) less eloquently but no less unequivocally upholds this moral tradition by stating simply, "Sexual activity with a patient is unethical." Indeed, it is the only specific activity deemed unethical between doctor and patient that is presented in so unambiguous a fashion. As part of the requirement that the physician "conduct himself with propriety in his profession and in all the actions of his life" (22), the dictum regarding sexual activity is especially important in the case of the psychiatrist because the patient tends to model his or her behavior after that of the therapist by identification. Further, the intensity of the therapeutic relationship may activate sexual feelings and fantasies on the part of both patient and therapist, while weakening the objectivity required for treatment. Insofar as it has earned a position of such priority, therapist-patient sex may be considered the ultimate expression of the overt misuse and exploitation of the transference relationship.

Nonetheless, sexual activities (including sexual intercourse and various forms of erotic contact between therapist and patient) have been increasingly reported in the literature; they have involved clinicians at all levels of training, from psychiatric resident to training analyst (54–61). Despite appearances, this is hardly a new problem for psychotherapists, who have reported erotic transferences and their vicissitudes since the dawn of psychoanalysis. Mesmer, Breuer, Janet, and Charcot, as well as Freud, have amply described the emergence of strong sexual feelings in treatment and the inevitable problems wrought by their presence. Although affairs between therapist and patient were never sanctioned by Freud or his followers, they did occur. However, therapists were often saved from moral indictment, as they still are, by marriage to the patient (and, of course, the termination of treatment by the spouse-therapist). Such a "shotgun" resolution between therapist and patient may be a rather extreme and limited option for dealing with sexual acting-out deriving from the therapeutic relationship. The question still remains, What are the ethical options if the therapist does not marry the patient?

In a current assessment of the legal and professional alternatives in deterring, disciplining, or punishing sexual activity between therapist and patient, Stone (62) cited four possible avenues of approach: 1) criminal law (e.g., charges of rape by fraud or coercion, 2) civil law (e.g., malpractice suits), 3) medical boards (e.g., revoked licensure), and 4) professional associations (e.g., pressure to limit referrals and threatened career opportunities). Each in its turn has been virtually ineffectual thus far in providing an effective system of control. In the instance of criminal law, rape charges, which were strongly recommended by Masters and Johnson (63), are rarely brought and rarely stick; most cases involve psychological coercion, not physical coercion. Both force and fraud appear to be required, and the prevailing judicial view is that if the patient consents and the therapist never claimed that sexual activity was treatment there has been neither force nor fraud. In the instance of civil law damages or malpractice cases, again no legal course may be available if the therapist has not misidentified the sexual activity as treatment. In one recent publicized incident, two factors were held in the therapist's favor; the patient pressed charges a year and a half after the sexual relationship began, and the patient presumably did not have a normal transference. (Legally the therapist was found "negligent," and he continued to practice without his medical license.) Medical licensing boards are not consistent from state to state and often do not have a close relationship with members who are psychiatrists. Finally, professional associations generally have no subpoena power and little expertise in evidentiary investigation, either to protect the due process rights of the therapist charged or if the therapist sues them. Davidson (34) pointed out that going into treatment may be another way for the seductive psychiatrist to escape censure; treatment thus serves to sabotage efforts at discipline. Given the above failings of sanctions from without, Stone (62) was forced to conclude that in the end "patients must depend on the decent moral character of those entrusted to treat them."

What constitutes "decent moral character," however, may be changing with the times, at least according to the findings of some psychotherapists. We have not only Masters and Johnson's extreme stance on the matter (i.e., therapists who have sex with their patients should be charged criminally with rape, no matter who initiated the seduction) (63) but also attitudes on the other side of the scale. Evidence suggests that the sexual value system of psychiatric clinicians has evolved in the direction of increased sexual permissiveness in terms of what is acceptable for themselves and what is acceptable for others (64). In addition, there is the current overt endorsement of touching and so-called "nonerotic" physical behaviors, especially by advocates of the human potential movement (65, 66). Such activities, far from being regarded as unethical or harmful, are viewed as promoting personal growth and enhancing the therapeutic relationship.

The range of opinions and/or activities on the matter appears to reflect not only individual predilection but also theoretical orientation (65) and major medical specialty (57). Kardener and associates' survey of physicians' erotic and nonerotic physical contact with patients (57) may be relatively heartening in that it found psychiatrists among the lesser offenders in comparison with other medical specialists. Psychiatrists' reported rate of erotic contact — 10% — and sexual intercourse with patients — 5% — were lower than those of general practitioners, surgeons, and obstetrician/gynecologists. Moreover, substantial differences regarding therapist-patient sex were found between psychiatrists with "psychodynamic" and those with other theoretical orientations. For example, although 86% of the therapists with a psychodynamic orientation felt that erotic contact with the therapist would never benefit the opposite-sex patient, this figure was substantially lower for humanistic and behavioral therapists (71% and 61%, respectively). That there is widespread ambivalence on the subject even after the fact is reflected in Taylor and Wagner's review of cases of therapists who had actually had intercourse with their patients (68). Less than half (47%) reported that the experience had had negative effects on either patient or therapist, 32% reported that it had mixed effects, and 21% that it had positive effects. (The authors did not survey the patients.) Butler (58), however, found that 95% of therapists who had sex with their patients reported conflict, fear, and guilt; yet only 40% sought consultation for their problems.

In brief, available evidence suggests that erotic practices with patients do not conform, nor have they ever conformed, to medicine's ethical dictates; neither are any real risks taken by those who engage in them. Those therapists who may not themselves engage in sexual activity with patients have lent subtle support to the practice by protecting their errant colleagues with silence or with treatment (34). Several questions remain: Is such behavior unequivocally unethical regardless of outcome? If erotic contact is decidedly unethical, how ethical is the "nonerotic" kissing, hugging, and touching that more than 50% of a sample of psychiatrists said they engaged in with patients (57)? When, if ever, are these appropriate?

Others raise a more subtle issue: Are sexual relations with a patient (nearly always a female patient) simply the tip of the iceberg of the more pervasive practice of sexism in psychotherapy (69, 70)? The ethics of psychotherapy in relation to patient gender has implications not only for its specific abuses (e.g., sex between the male therapist and the female patient) but for other forms of sexual exploitation and discrimination. They may be manifested in psychotherapy's underlying theory, training practices, and doctor-patient relationship.

Although it may well be difficult (even unethical) to do otherwise because of subtle and pervasive social pressures, therapeutic theories have more often supported than questioned stereotypical assumptions about sex roles. Broverman and associates (71) noted different standards of mental health for women and men, including tacit assumptions that dependency and passivity are normal for women whereas assertiveness and independence are normal for men. Women who are unhappy in their traditional role have often been considered psychopathological (69).

In addition to the unfortunate legacy of an "anti-feminine Freudian position" (69), women may also be harmed by a "blame-the-mother" tradition, especially by therapists positing their potential as "schizophrenogenic" to their children (70). Such sex role biases are then often compounded during the therapist's professional training, in which androcentrism (i.e., male chauvinism) is not likely to be corrected by a male supervisor (70). Indeed, female therapists are much less likely to have had supervisors of their own sex as role models during training; some even have had none (72). By far the most insidious issue of sexism in the practice of psychotherapy has been a function of the predominance of male therapists and the resultant tendency in psychotherapy to replicate within the dyadic relationship the "one-down" position in which women are typically placed. This may encourage the fantasy that an idealized relationship with a powerful other is a more desirable solution to life's problems than taking autonomous action (56, 70). Such a posture, in fact, may set the stage for the kind of sexual exploitation that occurs in instances of therapist-patient sex.

In the final analysis, ethical recommendations for dealing with both sex and sexism in psychotherapy would approximate the constellation of factors found in the new feminist therapies: a greater egalitarianism between therapist and patient in an active attempt to balance the therapist and patient's social power in the therapeutic endeavor and a conscious recognition of the necessity at all times to provide an ethical role model for the patient.

Conclusions

While ethical concerns have no doubt been with the field of psychiatry since its inception, *The Principles of Medical Ethics with Annotations Especially Applicable to Psychiatry* (22) provides a rather modest addendum to suggested standards for the profession. Unfortunately, some therapists feel that, however unprecedented its appearance and despite its noble aspirations, it has serious limitations in assisting them to make ethical decisions in their daily practice. It is understandably disappointing to those who confuse codes with covenants or who expect to magically produce morally scrupulous psychiatrists.

Aside from the merits or failings of a code of ethics itself, Zitrin and Klein (73) insisted that the more pressing problem is not the establishment of guidelines but their enforcement. The sentiment here is that a document can always be revised to better meet the psychiatrist's needs, but there are major problems in self or peer review processes and procedures. These problems include the voluntary nature of complaint investigations, the conflicting roles in which professional committees are required to act (as investigator, prosecutor, judge, and jury), inaccessibility and bureaucratic barriers to the system, inaccurate (and insufficient) case reporting, fear of liability by the professional reviewer, and overconcern with confidentiality, which often takes precedence over other ethical considerations and can be used as a rationalization to resist investigation (74). In actuality, however, it is exceedingly difficult to know what really occurs within the therapeutic relationship. Psychotherapists, like other professionals, are naturally reluctant to judge their colleagues, nor may they feel morally or technically equipped to do so. For example, Sullivan (75) reported that of more than 200 known charges of unethical conduct brought against psychiatrists within a 26-year period (1950–1976), only 8 psychiatrists were more than reprimanded.

The ethics not only of the profession but of peer review is also of concern (75). Here a major criticism is that the patient has been excluded from the design process and has been poorly informed about current procedures. Consequently, a prevailing view suggests that psychiatry at this time is simply unable to police itself (73) and that peer review, as currently constructed, is "bound to fail" (76). Nonetheless, we have made and continue to make positive headway in the peer review process (77).

The expectations held for a code of ethics and for peer review may be over-endowed, especially by practitioners not directly involved in their development and implementation. For example, in his examination of the true roles and functions of a code of ethics, Moore (74) defined two major purposes as "structuring" and "sensitizing." The first has a basically preventive value and aims to hold back impulsive or unethical behavior; the latter has an essentially educative value and aims to raise one's ethical consciousness. However, a code of ethics can be misused by the moralist or therapist with personal motives that are essentially punitive, not educative or preventive. Moore made the point that a code of ethics should not be viewed as a vehicle for revenge, vindication, or private gain. Comparably, Newman and Luft (78) considered the primary purpose of the peer review process to be education, not control.

These authors suggested that an educational peer review system promoting cooperation among professionals would be of greater utility and more acceptable to clinicians than a bureaucratic system of control, which might tend to foster manipulation. Since the question remains as to how much authority should be vested in peer review committees, using such systems involves very powerful and delicate processes. Ultimately the need for continuing and remedial education for the practicing psychotherapist must be addressed, both for the clinician and for the selection, training, and evaluation of reviewers. More active development of codes of ethics as basic guidelines, not disciplinary instruments, can be used to help elucidate ethical conflicts and the part they play in the life of every psychotherapist.

In conclusion, as I have suggested throughout this paper, the problem of ethics in the practice of psychotherapy is not entirely soluble in that there is no single answer to the varied and complex dilemmas psychotherapists face in relation to the patient and to society. Thus at this time we cannot completely rely on codified instruments — nor should we. Ideally, with the guidance of our professional peers, we must seek individual answers to the ethical problems that inevitably arise. I think the following suggestions would maximize the exercise of ethical choices by the psychotherapist:

1. Greater exploration of the philosophical foundations of therapeutic practice and the ethical assumptions on which psychotherapy is predicated.

2. Awareness of one's own self and personal commitments, for example, by constant examination and analysis of attitudes and behaviors within and outside of the therapeutic relationship.

3. Active development within the treatment endeavor of a "therapeutic alliance" or partnership in which there is equal power and participation by both parties toward mutual goals and responsibilities.

4. Greater allegiance to a code of ethics and its development to better sort out one's ethical choices and their implications for both patient and therapist.

5. Greater responsibility by the clinician for the maintenance of professional competence for himself or herself and others of the profession.

6. Openness to consultation with others and receptivity to outside opinions in making the best ethical decisions in treatment.

7. Greater understanding of human nature and morality from which timely and productive ethical alternatives can be derived.

As Bernal y del Rio (79) aptly put it, "By definition, ethical problems remain unresolved. By their unresolved quality, they provoke a continuous anxiety in the practicing psychiatrist and concomitantly a desire to search, to oppose, to think, and to research."

NOTE

1. M. Parloff: Twenty-five years of research in psychiatry. Department of Psychiatry, Albert Einstein College of Medicine, New York, N.Y., Oct. 17, 1975.

REFERENCES

1. Spiegel R: Editorial: on psychoanalysis, values, and ethics. J. Am. Acad. Psychoanal. 6: 271-273, 1978.
2. Osmond H: Psychiatry under siege: the crisis within. Psychiatric Annals 3(11):59-81, 1973.
3. Freedman DX, Gordon RP: Psychiatry under siege: attacks from without, Psychiatric Annals 3(11):10-34, 1973.
4. Michels R: Professional ethics and social values. Int. Rev. Psychoanal. 3:377-384, 1976.
5. Fletcher J: Ethical aspects of genetic control. N. Engl. J. Med. 285:776-783, 1971.
6. Lifton RJ: Advocacy and corruption in the healing professions. Int. Rev. Psychoanal. 3:385-398, 1976.

7. Redlich, F, Mollica R: Overview: ethical issues in contemporary psychiatry. Am. J. Psychiatry 133:125–136, 1976.
8. Jasnow A: The psychotherapist—artist and/or scientist? Psychotherapy: Theory, Research and Practice 15:318–322, 1978.
9. Edelson M: Psychoanalysis as science: its boundary problems, special status, relations to other sciences, and formalization. J. Nerv. Ment. Dis. 165:1–28, 1977.
10. London P: The Modes and Morals of Psychotherapy. New York, Holt, Rinehart and Winston, 1964.
11. Strupp H: Some observations on the fallacy of value-free psychotherapy and the empty organism: comments on a case study. J. Abnorm. Psychol. 83:199–201, 1974.
12. Buckley P, Karasu TB, Charles E, et al.: Theory and practice in psychotherapy: some contradictions in expressed belief and reported practice. J. Nerv. Ment. Dis. 167:218–223, 1979.
13. Erikson E: Psychoanalysis and ethics—avowed or unavowed. Int. Rev. Psychoanal. 3:409–415, 1976.
14. Marcuse H: Eros and Civilization. Boston, Beacon Press, 1955.
15. Szasz T: The Myth of Mental Illness. New York, Hoeber-Harper, 1961.
16. Torrey EF: The Death of Psychiatry. Radnor, Pa., Chilton Book Co., 1974.
17. Hollingshead A, Redlich F: Social Class and Mental Illness: A Community Study, New York, Wiley, 1958.
18. Horney K: New Ways in Psychoanalysis. New York, WW Norton & Co., 1939.
19. Fromm-Reichmann F: Psychoanalysis and Psychotherapy. Chicago, University of Chicago Press, 1959.
20. Freud S: Analysis terminable and interminable (1937–1939), in Complete Psychological Works, vol. 23. Translated and edited by Strachey J. London, Hogarth Press, 1964.
21. American Medical Association: Opinions and Reports of the Judicial Council. Chicago, AMA, 1971.
22. The Principles of Medical Ethics with Annotations Especially Applicable to Psychiatry. Washington, DC, APA, 1968.
23. Fisher S, Greenberg RP: The Scientific Credibility of Freud's Theories and Therapy. New York, Basic Books, 1977.
24. Karasu TB: Psychotherapies: an overview. Am. J. Psychiatry 134:851–863, 1977.
25. Leo J: Danger is found in some remedies: group psychotherapy body urges thorough study. New York Times, Feb. 9, 1969, p. 92.
26. Brill N: Future of psychiatry in a changing world. Psychosomatics 14:19–26, 1973.
27. Kety S: From rationalization to reason. Am. J. Psychiatry 131:957–963, 1974.
28. Yager J: A survival guide for psychiatric residents. Arch. Gen. Psychiatry 30:494–499, 1974.
29. Cerrolaza M: The nebulous scope of current psychiatry. Compr. Psychiatry 14:299–309, 1973.
30. Raskin D: Psychiatric training in the 70s—toward a shift in emphasis. Am. J. Psychiatry 128:119–120, 1972.
31. Vispo R: Psychiatry—paradigm of our times. Psychiatr. Q. 46:208–219, 1972.
32. Szasz T: The Myth of Psychotherapy. New York, Anchor/Doubleday, 1978.
33. Blatte H: Evaluating Psychotherapies. Hastings Center Report, Sept. 1973, pp. 4–6.
34. Davidson V: Psychiatry's problem with no name: therapist-patient sex. Am. J. Psychoanal. 37:43–50, 1977.
35. Garfield S: Values: an issue in psychotherapy. Comments on a case study. J. Abnorm. Psychol. 83:202–203, 1974.
36. Davison GC, Wilson GT: Goals and strategies in behavioral treatment of homosexual pedophilia: comments on a case study. J. Abnorm. Psychol. 83:196–198, 1974.
37. Hadley SW, Strupp HH: Contemporary views of negative effects in psychotherapy: an integrated account. Arch. Gen. Psychiatry 33:1291–1302, 1976.
38. Frank J: Persuasion and Healing: A Comparative Study of Psychotherapy. Baltimore, Johns Hopkins Press, 1961.

39. Greenson R: The Technique and Practice of Psychoanalysis, vol. 1. New York, International Universities Press, 1967.
40. Miller D: The ethics of practice in adolescent psychiatry. Am. J. Psychiatry 134:420-424, 1977.
41. Karasu TB: General principles of psychotherapy, in Specialized Techniques in Individual Psychotherapy, Edited by Karasu TB, Bellak L. New York, Brunner/Mazel, 1980.
42. Goldberg C: Therapeutic Partnership: Ethical Concerns in Psychotherapy. New York, Springer Publishing Co., 1977.
43. Parsons T: The Social System. Glencoe, Ill., Free Press, 1951.
44. Burling T, Lenz EM, Wilson RN: Give and Take in Hospitals: A Study of Human Organization. New York, GP Putnam and Sons, 1956.
45. American Psychiatric Association: Encounter Groups and Psychiatry. Task Force Report 1. Washington, DC, APA, 1970.
46. Goldberg C: Encounter: Group Sensitivity Training Experience. New York, Science House, 1970.
47. Dubey J: Confidentiality as a requirement of the therapist: technical necessities for absolute privilege in psychotherapy. Am. J. Psychiatry 131:1093-1096, 1974.
48. Plaut EA: A perspective on confidentiality. Am. J. Psychiatry 131:1021-1024, 1974.
49. Bloch DA: Family therapy, group therapy. Int. J. Group Psychother. 26:289-299, 1976.
50. Tarasoff v. Regents of the University of California, 118 Calif. Rep. 129, 529 P 2d 553, 1974.
51. Roth LH, Meisel A: Dangerousness, confidentiality, and the duty to warn. Am. J. Psychiatry 134:508-511, 1977.
52. Gurevitz H: *Tarasoff*: protective privilege versus public peril. Am. J. Psychiatry 134:289-292, 1977.
53. Braceland FJ: Historical perspectives of the ethical practice of psychiatry. Am. J. Psychiatry 126:230-237, 1969.
54. Dahlberg C: Sexual contact between patient and therapist. Contemporary Psychoanalysis 6:107-124, 1970.
55. Truax CB, Mitchell KM: Research on certain therapist interpersonal skills in relation to process and outcome, in Handbook of Psychotherapy and Behavior Change: An Empirical Analysis. Edited by Bergin AE, Garfield SL. New York, John Wiley & Sons, 1971.
56. Chesler P: Women and Madness. Garden City, NY, Doubleday, 1972.
57. Kardener S, Fuller M, Mensh I: A survey of physicians' attitudes and practices regarding erotic and nonerotic contact with patients. Am. J. Psychiatry 130:1077-1081, 1973.
58. Butler S: Sexual contact between therapists and patients. Los Angeles, California School of Professional Psychology, 1975 (doctoral dissertation).
59. Robertiello R: Iatrogenic psychiatric illness. Journal of Contemporary Psychotherapy 7:3-8, 1975.
60. Stone M: Management of unethical behavior in a psychiatric hospital staff. Am. J. Psychother. 29:391-401, 1975.
61. Marmor J: Some psychodynamic aspects of the seduction of patients in psychotherapy. Presented at the 129th annual meeting of the American Psychiatric Association, Miami Beach, Fla., May 10-14, 1976.
62. Stone AA: The legal implications of sexual activity between psychiatrist and patient. Am. J. Psychiatry 133:1138-1141, 1976.
63. Masters WH, Johnson VE: Principles of the new sex therapy. Am. J. Psychiatry 133:548-554, 1976.
64. Roman M, Charles E, Karasu TB: The value system of psychotherapists and changing mores. Psychotherapy: Theory, Research and Practice 15:409-415, 1978.
65. Levy RB: I Can Only Touch You Now. Englewood Cliffs, Prentice-Hall, 1973.
66. Pattison JE: Effects of touch on self-exploration and the therapeutic relationship. J. Consult. Clin. Psychol. 40:170-175, 1973.
67. Holroyd JC, Brodsky AM: Psychologists' attitudes and practices regarding erotic and nonerotic physical contact with patients. Am. Psychol. 32:843-849, 1977.

68. Taylor BJ, Wagner NN: Sex between therapists and clients: a review and analysis. Professional Psychology 7:593–601, 1976.
69. Rice JK, Rice DG: Implications of the women's liberation movement for psychotherapy. Am. J. Psychiatry 130:191–196, 1973.
70. Seiden AM: Overview: research on the psychology of women, II, Women in families, work, and psychotherapy. Am. J. Psychiatry 133:1111–1123, 1976.
71. Broverman IK, Broverman DM, Clarkson FE, et al.: sex-role stereotypes and clinical judgments of mental health. J. Consult. Clin. Psychol. 34:1–7, 1970.
72. Seiden A, Benedek E, Wolman C, et al.: Survey of women's status in psychiatric education: report of the APA Task Force on Women. Presented at the 127th annual meeting of the American Psychiatric Association, Detroit, Mich., May 6–10, 1974.
73. Zitrin A, Klein H: Can psychiatry police itself effectively? The experience of one district branch. Am. J. Psychiatry 133:653–656, 1976.
74. Moore RA: Ethics in the practice of psychiatry: origins, functions, models, and enforcement. Am. J. Psychiatry 135:157–163, 1978.
75. Sullivan FW: Peer review and professional ethics. Am. J. Psychiatry 134:186–188, 1977.
76. Klein H: Current peer review system bound to fail. Psychiatric News, July 16, 1975, p. 21.
77. Chodoff P, Santora P: Psychiatric peer review: the DC experience, 1972–1975. Am. J. Psychiatry 134:121–125, 1977.
78. Newman DE, Luft LL: The peer review process: education versus control. Am. J. Psychiatry 131:1363–1366, 1974.
79. Bernal y del Rio V: Psychiatric ethics, in Comprehensive Textbook of Psychiatry, 2nd ed., vol. 2. Edited by Freedman AM, Kaplan HI, Sadock BJ. Baltimore, Williams & Wilkins Co., 1975, p. 2546.

Task Panel on Legal and Ethical Issues

Assuring Patients/Clients of Their Rights: Bills of Rights and Other Mechanisms

Bills of Rights

Recommendation 1.

> *The President's Commission should recommend to the legislatures of the individual States that legislation be enacted providing a "Bill of Rights" for all mentally handicapped persons, both those who are institutionalized and those residing in the community.*

Commentary:

Following the seminal decision by Judge Frank Johnson in *Wyatt v. Stickney*,[1] approximately 14 States have enacted legislation establishing "bills of rights" for psychiatric patients[2] and 12 have promulgated similar legislation for mentally retarded persons.[3] These statutes reflect the specific standards established in *Wyatt* for treatment of mentally handicapped persons[4] and other judicial opinions that, in the words of the *Harvard Law Review*, "have sketched the outlines of a constitutional right to protection of bodily integrity from unwanted State intrusion."[5]

The need for such legislation should be self-evident: The extent of discrimination against mentally handicapped persons needs no lengthy recitation. The pattern of abuse, disenfranchisement and disregard[6] eloquently underscores the need for vigorous, enforceable, prophylactic legislation in each of the States. It should be pointed out that enactment of a "bill of rights" in no way consigns the mentally handicapped to "second class citizen" status. Rather, it is an acknowledgment of the historical fact that such persons have been perceived and treated as second class citizens—or worse—by much of society. Because of this history, prophylactic legislation is necessary.[7]

After analysis of several of the significant State enactments,[8] the Panel has concluded that an adequate bill of rights for mentally handicapped persons should include at least seven basic components:

(a) A statement that all mentally handicapped persons are entitled to the specified rights;

(b) A statement that rights cannot be abridged solely because of a person's handicap or because s/he is being treated (whether voluntarily or involuntarily);

(c) A declaration of the right to treatment, the right to refuse treatment and the regulation of treatment, the right to privacy and dignity, the right to a humane physical and psychological environment and the right to the least restrictive alternative setting for treatment;

(d) A statement of other, enumerated fundamental rights which may not be abridged or limited;

(e) A statement of other specific rights which may be altered or limited only under specific, limited circumstances;

(f) An enforcement provision; and

(g) A statement that handicapped persons retain the right to enforce their rights through *habeas corpus* and all other common law or statutory remedies.

A brief analysis follows.*

(a) The statute should explicitly state that every handicapped person is entitled to all rights set forth in the act and should retain all rights not specifically denied. But for its reference to "patient in treatment" (thus potentially limiting its applicability to institutionalized patients), the New Jersey provision could serve as a model for the draft statute.

> Every patient in treatment shall be entitled to all rights set forth in this act and shall retain all rights not specifically denied him under this Title. A notice of the rights set forth in this act shall be given to every patient within 5 days of his admission to treatment.[9]

(b) The statute should explicitly indicate that the fact that a person is receiving treatment or rehabilitation services cannot by itself justify deprivation of his or her civil rights. This section should specify that there may be no presumption of incompetency because a person has been examined, evaluated, treated or admitted to an institution. It should also specifically ban discrimination because of an individual's status as patient or resident. The kinds of rights to which persons remain entitled regardless of their status as patients include but are not limited to the right to register for and to vote at elections; rights relating to the granting, forfeiture, or denial of a license, permit, privilege, or benefit pursuant to any law; the right to dispose of property, the right to sue or be sued, and the right to obtain housing.[10]

(c) The statute should specify that all persons have a right to treatment in a humane physical and psychological environment, a right to freedom from harm, a right to refuse treatment and a right to the regulation of treatment procedures, a right to basic privacy and dignity, the right to the least restrictive setting for treatment, and the right to be free from discrimination in education, employment, housing and other matters.

(d) The statute should also specify certain treatment rights and conditions of treatment rights which may not be denied under any circumstance — for example, all patients have the absolute rights (1) to be free from unnecessary or excessive medication, (2) not to be subjected to experimental research, shock treatment, psychosurgery, or sterilization, without their express and informed consent after consultation with counsel or an interested party of their choice, (3) to be free from physical restraint and isolation and (4) to be free from corporal punishment.[11] In addition to the above rights, at a minimum patients and residents should have the absolute right to correspond with public officials, attorneys, clergymen and to the appropriate advocacy office[12] and the absolute right to religious freedom.[13]

(e) The statute should also specify other environmental and conditional rights guaranteed to all patients which can only be abridged in specific situations for a limited time and subject to an independent, neutral review mechanism. Thus, the New Jersey law, for example, provides the full panoply of *Wyatt*[14] rights: privacy and dignity, use and wearing of personal possessions and clothes, use of personal money, individual private storage space, daily visitors, reasonable access to telephones, access to letter-writing materials and uncensored correspondence, regular physical exercise, outdoor visitation, interaction with the opposite sex, freedom of religion and adequate medical treatment.[15] Further, the statute should stipulate that patients have the right to control their own assets[16] and the right to compensation for work done.[17]

Many of these rights have already been the subject of discrete court litigation.[18] Nonetheless the Panel feels that they are of such significance that they should be statutorily mandated.

(f) The statute should contain a strong enforcement provision. None of the existing statutes includes such a section; the only step toward such a mechanism is the absolute right to a hearing, built into the New Jersey law, in the case of experimental research and similar treatments in matters involving persons adjudicated incompetent.[19] Optimally, there should be a grievance mechanism comporting with procedural due process, appointment of counsel and an automatic hearing procedure established in the case of denial of any of the rights enumerated in a draft bill.

Regardless of the specific enforcement provision adopted, the Panel feels that a strong, vigorous, independent advocacy system is absolutely mandatory to represent and advise patients at all stages of their institutionalization and on all other matters discussed in this recommendation.[20] It would not be an overstatement to suggest that any "bill of rights" would be meaningless to patients without such an advocacy system.

(g) The statute should include language similar to the following:

Any individual subject to this Title shall be entitled to a writ of habeas corpus upon proper petition by himself, by a relative, or a friend to any court of competent jurisdiction in the county in which he is detained and shall further be entitled to enforce any of the rights herein stated by civil action or other remedies otherwise available by common law or statute.[21]

Although the statutory sections are not complete, they are useful as a model for a bill which can be recommended for endorsement and ultimate enactment. Endorsement of such a bill by the President's Commission on Mental Health would help to ensure "equal access to justice" for mentally handicapped persons.[22] [23]

Recommendation 2.

The President's Commission should recommend to the States that all currently existing laws establishing rights of patients, of persons in treatment and of residents of hospitals, facilities for the retarded or similar institutions should be prominently displayed in all living areas, wards, hallways and other common areas of all such facilities, and should be incorporated into all staff-training and staff-orientation programs as well as in educational programs directed to patients, staff, families and the general public. Explanation of rights to patients should be clearly and simply stated and in a language the patient understands; the explanation should be read to any patient who cannot read.

Commentary:

If there is any expectation that the rights in question will be enforced, it is absolutely necessary that patients and residents be apprised of them and that treatment staff be made aware of them and their significance.[24] This recommendation is a modest first step towards that goal.

It also follows that recognition of rights precedes enforcement and that therefore the education of all citizens as to their rights is imperative. Specifically, persons receiving mental health services and, where appropriate, their guardians, should be informed of the rights they have and of all possible methods of enforcement. Further public information to inform the general population of the rights of mentally handicapped citizens could eliminate some old myths and lead to a better climate in which these rights could be enjoyed.

NOTES

1. 325 *F. Supp.* 781 (M.D. Ala. 1971), 334 *F. Supp.* 1341 (M.D. Ala. 1971), 344 *F. Supp.* 373 (M.D. Ala. 1972), 344 *F. Supp.* 387 (M.D. Ala. 1972), aff'd sub. nom. *Wyatt v. Aderholt,* 503 *F.*2d 1305 (5 Cir. 1974).

2. See "The *Wyatt* Standards: An Influential Force in State and Federal Rules," 28 *Hosp. & Commun. Psych.* 374 (1977).

3. American Bar Association Commission on Mentally Disabled, draft unpublished document pertaining to the rights of institutionalized developmentally disabled persons, in progress. All States surveyed which have enacted a bill of rights for developmentally disabled persons have in place a bill of rights for the mentally ill; but some States which have enacted a bill of rights for the mentally ill have not enacted such a measure for the developmentally disabled.

4. 344 *F. Supp.* at 379–386; 344 *F. Supp.* at 395–407.

5. "Developments—Civil Commitment of the Mentally Ill," 87 *Harv. L. Rev.* 1190, 1345 (1974).

6. In the words of Patricia Wald, the handicapped person is perceived as "someone to whom attention need not be paid," Wald, "Basic Personal and Civil Rights," in Kindred *et al.,* eds., *The Mentally Retarded Citizen and the Law* 3, 18 (1976).

7. The analogy to the passage of the Civil Rights Act of 1964 and 1965 is probably a useful point of comparison in this regard.

8. See, *e.g., N.J.S.A.* 30:4–24.1 *et seq.; Ariz. Rev. Stats.* § 36–504 *et seq.; Minn. Stat.* § 253A.17; *Fla. Stat.* § 394.459 *et seq.; Wis. Stat.* 51.61 *et seq.*

* We note that Federal regulations for Skilled Nursing Facilities and Intermediate Care Facilities, including ICF/MRs, contain a patient bill of rights. The same bill-of-rights context was recently proposed for Federal regulations for general and psychiatric hospitals by Rep. William Cohen (R-Maine), but this amendment to statutorily provide a bill of rights for patients in a Medicare or Medicaid provider facility was withdrawn prior to passage of recent amendments.

9. *N.J.S.A.* 30:4–24.2b.

10. For example, the draft statute might well combine language from the New Jersey and Arizona statutes as well as a portion of the *Wyatt* decision. See *N.J.S.A.* 30:4–24.2a and 24.2c, *Ariz. Rev. Stats.* 36–506, and *Wyatt,* 344 *F. Supp.,* above, at 379.

11. See, for example, *N.J.S.A.* 30:4–24.2d (1) through (4).

12. See *N.Y. Mental Hygiene Law* § 15.05(a); see also, 50 *Penn. Stat.* § 4423(1); *Minn. Stat.* § 253A.17(2).

13. See, *e.g.,* 50 *Penn. Stat.* § 4423(2); *Ariz. Rev. Stats.* § 36–514(4).

14. See *e.g., Wyatt,* 344 *F. Supp.,* above, at 380–381.

15. See *N.J.S.A.* 30:4–24.2e(1) and (3) through (12).

16. See, for example, *Vecchione v. Wohlgemuth,* 377 *F. Supp.* 1361, 1369 (E.D. Pa. 1974), further proceedings 426 *F. Supp.* 1297 (E.D. Pa. 1977), aff'd. 588 *F.*2d 150 (3 Cir. 1977), *cert. den. sub. nom. Beal v. Vecchione,* — U.S. — , 98 S. Ct. 439 (1977); and *Board of Chosen Freeholders of Hudson County v. Connell,* Civ. No. 83870,9 *Clearinghouse Rev.* 585 (N.J. Hudson Cty. Ct. 1975), 9 *Clearinghouse Rev.* 732 (N.J. Hudson Cty. Ct. 1976).

17. See, for example, *Souder v. Brennan,* 367 *F. Supp.* 808 (D.D.C. 1973); *Ariz. Rev. Stats.* § 36–510; *N.Y. Mental Hygiene Law* § 15.09.

18. See, for example, *Schmidt v. Schubert,* 422 *F. Supp.* 57, 58 (E.D. Wis. 1976) (visitation policy); *Brown v. Schubert,* 347 *F. Supp.* 1232, 1234 (E.D. Wis. 1972), supplemented 389 *F. Supp.* 281, 283–284 (E.D. Wis. 1975) (right to send mail); *Gerrard v. Blackmun,* 401 *F. Supp.* 1180, 1193 (N.D. Ill. 1975) (right to private communications with counsel); *Winters v. Miller,* 446 *F.*2d 65, 69–71 (2 Cir. 1971) (freedom of religion); *Carroll v. Cobb,* 139 N.J. Super. 439, 354 A.2d 355 (App. Div. 1976) (right to register to vote).

19. See *N.J.S.A.* 30:4–24. 2d(2).

20. As indicated in the section on "advocacy," above, it is essential that patients and former patients have input into both the advocacy system and suggested draft legislation.

21. N.J.S.A. 30:4-24.2h.

22. Herr, *Advocacy Under the Developmental Disabilities Act* 88 (1976).

23. It has also been suggested that consideration be given to amending Federal law to make future Medicaid/Medicare certification and other third party payment mechanisms contingent upon individual State adoption and implementation of approved "bills of rights."

We note here that the Federal government can play a direct role in fashioning bills of rights, through administrative directive, regulation, or statute, for patients in Veterans' Administration facilities, and we suggest that the Commission give consideration to such a mechanism. The *Wyatt* Standards could, in the absence of a State bill of rights, serve as a guide for minimally adequate standards. Should the State have enacted or should it subsequently enact a bill of rights with standards higher than those in the VA bill of rights, the higher State standards would prevail.

24. See, for example, for a discussion of the lower level of staff comprehension of patients' rights, Laves and Cohen, "A Preliminary Investigation Into the Knowledge and Attitude Toward the Legal Rights of Mental Patients," 1 *J. Psych. & L.* 49 (1973). See also *N.J.S.A.* 30:4-24.2b.

Robert W. Gibson

The Rights of Staff
in the Treatment of the Mentally Ill

The rights of the individual in our society are in danger and must be protected. Perhaps this situation is an inevitable consequence of the increased size, complexity, and power of government, business, and all of our institutions. Whatever the cause, the threat is there. And we can be grateful that dedicated individuals and organizations are trying to counteract it.

The loss of basic personal rights is not a new experience for the mentally ill. Probably no other group has been so consistently persecuted and deprived of basic human rights as those who suffer from psychiatric illness. Many of the problems arise from the dehumanization that comes from the increasing size and complexity of our health care system. Whatever difficulties exist generally are magnified by the underfunding of the facilities and programs for the mentally ill. Added to this are the consequences of suspicion and fear of those whose behavior is seen as deviant.

In an effort to protect the interests of patients generally, the American Hospital Association set forth a Patient's Bill of Rights in 1973. Many of these rights, such as consideration and respect, the right to adequate information, and the right to know the terms and conditions under which care is given, are not unique to health care. Some of the rights do deal with specific treatment issues as, for example, the right to know the risks and medical alternatives, the right to confidentiality, the right to expect continuity of care, and the right to know if human experimentation is to be considered.

The AHA Bill of Rights has received a varied response. Some states have

From *Hospital and Community Psychiatry* 27 (December 1976):855–859. Copyright © 1976 by the American Psychiatric Association. Reprinted by permission of the publisher and the author.

enacted legislation to guarantee those rights. Some hospitals have adopted those rights as policy. The legal counsel to hospitals have generally cautioned that such a bill of rights could be construed as a legal document and be introduced as evidence in court actions. They express concern about the vagueness and open endedness of statements such as "The patient has the right to expect that within its capacity a hospital must make reasonable response to the request of a patient for services." How can the capacity of a hospital to respond be determined? What is a reasonable response? Is there any limitation to the requests that can be made by a patient?

A different concern was expressed by Willard Gaylin, who asserted, "The objection to this well-intended though timid document is that it perpetuates the very paternalism that precipitated the abuses." And, "The hospital has no power to grant these rights. They were vested in the patient to begin with. If the rights have been violated they have been violated by the hospital and its hirelings."[1]

The AHA Patient's Bill of Rights is directed toward the general hospital, and thus does not address many problem areas for the mentally ill. The heavy emphasis on openness of communication and access to medical records overlooks the sensitive nature of much of the material contained within the psychiatric record. The bill of rights was not designed with an awareness of the various defense mechanisms of denial, resistance, and displacement that are inherent in psychiatric treatment.

A bill of rights modified expressly to meet the needs of hospitalized mental patients appeared recently in *Psychiatric Annals,* but even this bill would cause legal counsel considerable concern. Consider the closing statement: "The above rights have been constructed with calculated ambiguity to permit agency personnel to balance patient medical and legal interests appropriately."[2] Ambiguity is undesirable in what may turn out to be a legal document introduced in a malpractice suit.

Hospital staff members who enthusiastically supported the move toward a better deal for their patients have been dismayed to discover they may be the targets of civil actions. They find themselves in seemingly insoluble dilemmas. For example, if a medication is forced upon a patient, it would violate the right to refuse treatment, yet failure to give adequate treatment might be the basis of a charge of neglect.

The efforts to protect the rights of patients are based on good intentions and, on balance, are a positive force. The problem is that at times these efforts have been initiated by individuals who are unfamiliar with the needs of the mentally ill and the potential impact their efforts could have on the treatment process. The adversarial climate gives the impression that the rights of patients are in opposition to the rights of staff; a gain for one is perceived as a loss for the other.

Some suggest, philosophically, that the pendulum, having swung in one direction, will surely swing back and will eventually come to a midpoint. I submit that this is begging the question. The rights of patients must be protected and should not be in opposition to the legitimate interests and concerns of staff.

During the 1960s there evolved in this country a national policy that adequate health care is the right of every individual. If we accept that premise, and if we really mean adequate health care is a right, it follows that the provider, as a basic right, must have the opportunity and the conditions necessary to give adequate health care. Starting from this position there is a commonality of interests, not a conflict. Adequate health care for all is the goal of both patient and provider: the patient has the right to receive it; the provider must have those rights needed to give it.

A Set of Staff Rights

In roughing out a set of staff rights, I have concentrated on those rights that bear directly on the treatment process. Each right supports the common goal of adequate health care for all. I have not addressed issues such as working conditions, right to organize, career ladders, and appeal mechanisms. These also are legitimate concerns. My objective, however, is to begin identifying those staff rights essential to providing adequate treatment of the mentally ill.

The right of staff to have sufficient resources to provide adequate health care. During the past decade the cost of health care has consumed an increasingly greater portion of the gross national product, moving from 5.9 per cent in 1965 to 8.3 per cent in 1975. This increase indicates that more resources (money, personnel, facilities, equipment, and supplies) have been made available for health care. Those resources were needed to meet higher expectations and standards of treatment. The volume of services has increased as unmet needs have been identified. Wages and salaries in the health field have been brought up to a reasonable level. Approximately 8.3 per cent of the GNP is not too much to spend on health care—we probably should spend more; 5.9 per cent was too little.

Whether the increased expenditures for mental health have, in the aggregate, kept up with inflation I am not sure. We hear of hospital facilities in many state systems losing their accreditation. Commissions appointed by state governments, citizen advocate groups, and even the consultation and evaluation services board of the American Psychiatric Association report gross inadequacies in the treatment programs for the mentally ill. Our society does not even come close to providing adequate care for the mentally ill. The assertion that adequate health care is a right will remain a hollow promise unless state and national leaders take steps to ensure equal coverage for the treatment of the mentally ill.

Because there is a limit to the number of dollars, it is unrealistic to expect a blank check. Staff will be challenged to demonstrate that they are using existing resources efficiently and effectively. Nevertheless, staff have a right, and indeed an obligation, to press for all that is needed to provide adequate mental health care.

When staff members seek to expand and improve the quality of treatment programs, they are sometimes accused of acting out of self-interest. Limitations in insurance coverage and benefits of government programs are often portrayed as problems for the provider of care when, in fact, they are problems for those in need of treatment — the consumer. The mentally ill have seldom been articulate spokesmen able to advance their interests. Staff members, individually and collectively through their professional organizations, must serve as advocates seeking coverage for treatment of the mentally ill equal to that of general medical care.

The right of staff to participate in the allocation of resources and the setting of priorities. In the foreseeable future there will not be enough resources available to provide all the treatment programs that are necessary and desirable. The mental health delivery system is going to be under heavy financial pressure. Since it is simply not possible to do everything at once, difficult choices about what to do first will have to be made.

Unfortunately the decision-making process is becoming further and further removed from those providing direct patient care. As the administrative structure has expanded, more and more decisions are made by individuals lacking clinical experience and sometimes even lacking sensitivity to the needs of the mentally ill. The planning and decision-making process must include staff members involved in patient care. Only in this way can treatment programs be developed that are responsive to patient needs.

Even though staff members have the right to participate in the allocation of resources and the setting of priorities, they cannot expect to have the final say; this is a prerogative of top management. To be a part of top management one must have an overview of the total situation. This does not mean that to be heard every clinician must understand all the intricacies of budgeting and personnel management. It does mean, however, that top clinician-administrators must acquire such expertise. Clinical directors of programs, for example, must at least understand fiscal, administrative, and political implications.

The right of staff to be accountable for clinical matters to the highest governing authority. The ultimate responsibility for patient care rests with the governing body, not with the clinical staff. It is true that governing bodies generally look to the staff to develop and to maintain standards of care. But they cannot delegate this responsibility and, therefore, must maintain direct communication with the staff.

There was a time when the director of a major clinical program, the superintendent of a psychiatric hospital, or the director of a state mental health program was always a clinician, usually a physician. As such he was accountable to the highest governing authority, whether it was the board of a private institution, a state legislature, or the chief executive of a state government. As systems have become larger and administrative demands have become greater, there has been an increasing reliance on nonclinical administrators. This change has some merit. Administrative pressures are intense; few clinicians are willing to master a second profession.

In dealing with this issue the Joint Commission on Accreditation of Hospitals, in its standards for governing body and management, indicates: "In any psychiatric hospital in which the chief administrative officer is not a psychiatrist, the ultimate responsibility for the diagnosis and treatment of patients shall rest with a psychiatrist, who is accountable therefore to the governing body."[3] This concept should be applied to any organizational structure so a direct line of communication and accountability is always retained between the clinical staff and the authority with ultimate responsibility.

For clinicians this right carries new responsibilities. The demands and expectations for quality assurance have escalated. The traditional method of clinical conferences and individual supervision is seldom adequate to meet these new expectations. We have just begun to scratch the surface in developing new methodologies for systematic review including utilization review, determinations of medical necessity, medical audit, and medical care evaluation. Clinicians must assume a leadership role in quality assurance by developing the techniques to identify inadequacies in the treatment process and by seeking ways to use such findings systematically to improve the treatment program.

The right of staff to the free and complete exercise of clinical judgment and skill under conditions that will not cause the deterioration of the quality of care. It has long been recognized that clinical practice can be influenced adversely by the particular circumstances or conditions under which it is conducted. Indeed, the American Medical Association code of ethics explicitly forbids physicians from practicing under circumstances that could lead to a deterioration in the quality of care. Obvious abuses such as fee-splitting are forbidden. As the health care system becomes more complex, more subtle problems are being identified. Some of the attempts to control and modify the health care delivery system create new ethical questions.

For example, a concerted effort is being made to shift the locus of care from hospitals to outpatient and day treatment programs within the community. The therapeutic advantages of this approach are so well known that they need no elaboration. Unfortunately the concept of deinstitutionalization has, in some instances, become a political slogan used to empty hospitals for the purpose of saving money rather than promoting the best interests of the patients. This is particularly true when the push to get patients out of the hospital is undertaken without provision of adequate treatment facilities in the community. A staff member can easily be caught in an ethical dilemma if he is directed to discharge patients when he knows that adequate treatment resources are not available.

Of course, the reverse of this problem can occur in an institution that is dependent upon revenues derived from patient care. To maintain the flow of dollars from patient services, staff members could feel pressured to prolong the hospital stay. The point is, staff members must be free to carry out their treatment in accord with their best clinical judgment.

Staff must be wary of still another subtle danger. Numerous studies have shown that staff are more likely to select the attractive, highly verbal patient, presumably because of the greater interest and challenge. Understandably, staff members seek satisfaction from their clinical practice, but in exercising the right to free clinical judgment, they must be scrupulous in keeping the patient's interests in the forefront. The commitment must be to the common goal of staff and patients for adequate health care for all.

The right to have clinical practice reviewed by peers. The clinician, almost as a matter of reflex, perceives the review of treatment practices as an unwarranted intrusion into professional autonomy. Legislation calling for professional standards review organizations evoked violent protest and a spate of lawsuits. At this point, it is no longer a question of whether clinical practice is going to be reviewed, but simply by whom. All federal health programs require such review as a condition of payment, and every national health insurance proposal mandates such review. Private health insurance programs have a less visible but equally potent mechanism in their claims review procedures.

Any attempt to monitor professional services must start with a set of standards and criteria. The American Psychiatric Association has participated vigorously in developing such standards and criteria, and the product of one of these efforts is incorporated into the American Medical Association's *Sample Criteria for Short Stay Hospital Review*. A cursory look at these standards reveals that they are just the beginning; they provide for only the grossest screening to identify those cases that warrant individualized review.[4]

Governmentally mandated systems of PSRO, utilization review, and the like have undoubtedly been stimulated by the desire to contain costs. That causes many professionals to be wary, and with good reason. But cost containment, if properly done, is of considerable merit in that it permits us to use resources with the greatest possible effectiveness. Beyond that, however, the growing attention and support of quality assurance offers clinicians an unparalleled opportunity to get data that will form some rational basis for continuing education, certification and recertification of specialists, and the basic training of mental health professionals.

We must not be turned off by the bureaucratic overtones of federal legislation and regulation. Inherent in all of these systems is the concept of standard-setting, review, and corrective action by professional peers. It is different from what we have known, but it can be used to fulfill traditional responsibilities of professions to maintain standards of practice and the ethical conduct of colleagues.

In my judgment several years of hard work will be required to develop quality assurance systems. Clinicians must provide the leadership in this time-consuming and unfamiliar task. The peer review committees of many APA district branches are demonstrating that it can be done.

The right of staff to practice without excessive and unnecessary regulation. Most of the regulatory efforts are well-intentioned; there have been abuses and less-than-desirable treatment practices. Regulations seem to dig into every aspect of care through utilization review, determinations of medical necessity, standards for medical records, and even control of specific treatment modalities.

Still other controls are aimed at protecting patients' rights, ensuring a safe environment, fixing hospital charges, and eliminating discrimination. Like it or not, the day has passed when we can expect to conduct treatment relatively free from external requirements.

Unfortunately the controls overlap, at times are contradictory, and add directly to the cost of care. Preoccupation with these multiple requirements may distract mental health professionals from their main goal: providing high-quality treatment services appropriate to the patient's needs. In exasperation staff protest that it has become more important to document that some arbitrary requirement has been met than it is to do something that will be really helpful to the patient. The health care industry is not alone. It seems that every aspect of our living is invaded by bureaucratic intrusion. David Mathews, secretary of the Department of Health, Education, and Welfare, has acknowledged that something must be done, but it is not at all clear what that may be.

The most desirable solution would be to effect changes at the source: the regulatory agencies themselves. It would seem that some kind of streamlining and coordination of controls would be possible, but I'm not optimistic they could be carried out. Short of that, we may just have to accept the fact that meeting the regulatory requirements is part of the cost of doing business. Just as we have a financial office to handle fiscal matters and a personnel department to handle the affairs of employees, it may now be time to establish a department to assist in meeting the regulatory demands. For example, the staff of such a department might be involved in each involuntary admission, seeing that all the precise legal requirements are met within the appropriate time frame. Perhaps this sounds drastic, but it may be the only way to prevent external requirements from disrupting the treatment process.

The privilege of staff members to practice their profession. Rapid social changes, new patterns of health care, and technological developments have placed new demands on all of the mental health professions. The increased emphasis on accountability strikes at the core of every profession: self-discipline through standards of training, continuing education, and voluntarily adopted codes of ethics enforced by the professional group itself. The proliferation of formalized regulatory requirements challenge the basic concept that the members of a profession are capable of self-discipline. Have we failed to maintain adequate standards of professional responsibility? Do our systems overlap so much that responsibility must be shared? Have professions lost the public trust?

Instead of looking to the professions, the public is now turning to the courts for answers to questions about voluntary and involuntary admissions, periodic review of confinement, the right to treatment, the right to refuse treatment, civil rights, confidentiality, payment for work, restraints, shock therapy, sterilization, psychosurgery, and legal competence. Some of the court decisions on these matters offer the hope of better treatment services for patients. Some do not. The adversarial climate, the recurrent threat, and the sense of vulnerability push the professional into a defensive position. Forced to direct more attention to the protection of self-interests, the professional is less able to maintain the altruistic goal of service to others.

Many clinicians, particularly physicians, have become so accustomed to society's sanction that they are convinced all aspects of professional practice are prerogatives automatically granted with a degree. This is simply not true. Practice of a profession is not a right. It is a privilege to be earned and repeatedly reaffirmed by responsible actions and behavior.

Thus the rights of patients and the rights of staff are not in conflict; together patients and staff share a common goal — adequate health care for the mentally ill. Staff must have adequate resources and an opportunity to practice their profession under conditions that permit them to use these resources in the best interest of the patients.

The public has a right to expect accountability from the professions. As a consequence, we must strengthen and refine our internal systems of review to keep pace with the advances in mental health care and the increasing complexity of the delivery system. We must press ahead to define more clearly the standards and criteria for quality care. Beyond that we must develop mechanisms to use our findings to improve all elements of professional activity. We must demonstrate that our own voluntary systems of peer review and quality assurance are more effective than the external requirements imposed by government and third-party payers. In short, we must reaffirm our stature as professions worthy of the public trust.

NOTES

1. W. Gaylin, "The Patient's Bill of Rights," *Saturday Review of the Sciences,* Vol. 1, March 1973, p. 22.

2. P. B. Hoffman and R. C. Dunn, "Guaranteeing the Right to Treatment," *Psychiatric Annals,* Vol. 6, June 1976, pp. 258–282.

3. Joint Commission on Accreditation of Hospitals, *Accreditation Manual for Psychiatric Facilities,* Chicago, 1972, p. 22.

4. American Medical Association, Chicago, 1976.

Suggestions for Further Reading

The Therapist-Patient Relationship

Appleton, William S. "The Importance of Psychiatrists' Telling Patients the Truth." *American Journal of Psychiatry* 129 (December 1972):742–745.

Braceland, Frances J. "Historical Perspectives of the Ethical Practice of Psychiatry." *American Journal of Psychiatry* 126 (August 1969):230–237.

Casebook on Ethical Standards of Psychologists. Washington, D.C., American Psychological Association, 1967.

Ethical Standards of Psychologists. Washington, D.C., American Psychological Association, 1977 and 1981.

Foster, H. M. "The Conflict and Reconciliation of the Ethical Interests of Therapist and Patient." *Journal of Psychiatry and Law* 3 (1975):39–48.

Joseph, David I., and Peele, Roger. "Ethical Issues in Community Psychiatry." *Hospital and Community Psychiatry* (May 1975):259–299.

Karasu, Toksoz B. "The Ethics of Psychotherapy." *American Journal of Psychiatry* 37 (1980):1502–1512.

"Mental Health and Human Rights: Report of the Task Panel on Legal and Ethical Issues." *Arizona Law Review* 20 (1978):49–174.

Szasz, Thomas S. *The Ethics of Psychoanalysis.* New York: Basic Books, 1965.

Tancredi, Laurence R., and Slaby, Andrew E. *Ethical Policy in Mental Health Care: The Goals of Psychiatric Intervention.* New York: Prodst/William Heinemann Medical Books, 1977.

Van Hoose, William H., and Kottler, Jeffrey A. *Ethical and Legal Issues in Counseling and Psychotherapy.* San Francisco: Jossey-Bass, 1977.

Veatch, Robert M. "Models for Medicine in a Revolutionary Age." *Hastings Center Report* (June 1972):5–7.

————. "Professional Ethics: New Principles for Physicians?" *Hastings Center Report* (June 1980):16–19.

West, Louis Joylon. "Ethical Psychiatry and Biosocial Humanism." *American Journal of Psychiatry* 126 (August 1969):226–237.

Confidentiality in Psychotherapy

American Psychiatric Association. "Position Statement on the Need for Preserving Confidentiality of Medical Records in Any National Health Care System." *American Journal of Psychiatry* 129 (April 1972):1349.

Annas, George J. "Confidentiality and the Duty to Warn." *Hastings Center Report* 6 (December 1976):6–8.

Appelbaum, Paul S. "Tarasoff: An Update on the Duty to Warn." *Hospital and Community Psychiatry* 32 (January 1981):14–15.

Bennett, Chester C. "Secrets Are for Sharing." *Psychology Today* 2 (February 1969):30ff.

"Confidentiality." In Reich, Warren T., ed. *Encyclopedia of Bioethics.* Vol. I. New York: The Free Press, 1978, pp. 194–200.

Chayet, N. *Confidentiality in Psychiatry.* Los Angeles, Seminar of the University of California's Colloquium on Law and Psychiatry, December 4, 1965.

"The Confidentiality of Health Records." *Psychiatric Opinion* 12 (January 1975).

Curran, William J. "Confidentiality and the Prediction of Dangerousness in Psychiatry." *New England Journal of Medicine* 293 (August 7, 1975):285–286.

Daley, Dennis W. "Tarasoff v. Regents of the University of California and the Psychotherapist's Duty to Warn." *San Diego Law Review* 12 (July 1975): 932–951.

Eger, Charles L. "Psychotherapists' Liability for Extrajudicial Breaches of Confidentiality." *Arizona Law Review* 18 (1976):1061–1094.

Gaylin, Willard, and Callahan, Daniel. "The Psychiatrist as Double Agent." *Hastings Center Report* 4 (February 1974):11–14.

Gurevitz, Howard. "Tarasoff: Protective Privilege Versus Public Peril." *American Journal of Psychiatry* 134 (March 1977):289–292.

"In the Service of the State: The Psychiatrist as Double Agent." Special Supplement, *Hastings Center Report* 8 (1978):1–24.

Klein, Marjorie, et al. "Computers and Psychiatry: Promises to Keep." *Archives of General Psychiatry* 32 (July 1975):837–843.

Kuschner, Harvey, et al. "Case Studies in Bioethics: The Homosexual Husband and Physician Confidentiality." *Hastings Center Report* 7 (April 1977): 15–17.

Laska, Eugene, and Bank, Rheta, eds. *Safeguarding Psychiatric Privacy: Computer Systems and Their Uses.* New York: John Wiley & Sons, 1976.

Menninger, Walter, and English, Joseph T. "Confidentiality and the Request for Psychiatric Information for Nontherapeutic Purposes." *American Journal of Psychology* 122 (1965):638–645.

Noll, John O., and Hanlon, Mark J. "Patient Privacy and Confidentiality at Mental Health Centers." *American Journal of Psychiatry* 133 (November 1976):1286–1289.

Plaut, E. A. "A Perspective on Confidentiality." *American Journal of Psychiatry* 131 (September 1974):1021ff.

Rosen, Catherine E. "Why Clients Relinquish Their Rights to Privacy Under Sign-Away Pressures." *Professional Psychology* (February 1977):17–24.

Roth, L. H., et al. "Dangerousness, Confidentiality, and the Duty to Warn." *American Journal of Psychiatry* 134 (March 1977):508–511.

Rozovsky, Lorne E., and Akhtar, S. N. "Should Psychiatric Communication Be Privileged." *Legal Medical Quarterly* 1 (June 1977):115–118.

Shestack, Jerome J. "Psychiatry and the Dilemmas of Dual Loyalties." In Frank J. Ayd, Jr., ed. *Medical, Moral and Legal Issues in Medical Health Care.* Baltimore: The Williams & Wilkins Co., 1974, Ch. 2.

Sietel, Max. "Privacy, Ethics and Confidentiality." *Professional Psychiatry* 10 (April 1979):249–258.

Slovenko, R. "Psychotherapy and Confidentiality." *Cleveland State Law Review* 24 (1975):375–392.

Smith, Steven. "Constitutional Privacy in Psychotherapy." *The George Washington Law Review* 49 (1980):1–60.

Szasz, Thomas, et al. "Silence Is Golden, Or Is It?" *Mental Hygiene* 57 (Winter 1973):21–27.

Tancredi, Laurence R., et al. *Legal Issues in Psychiatric Care.* New York: Harper & Row, 1975, Ch. 6.

Patient and Staff Rights

Allen, P. "A Bill of Rights for Citizens Using Outpatient Mental Health Services." In Lamb, H. R., ed. *Community Support Systems for the Long-Term Patient.* San Francisco: Jossey-Bass, 1976, pp. 147–170.

Armstrong, Barbara. "A Question of Abuse: Where Staff and Patient Rights Collide." *Hospital and Community Psychiatry,* Vol. 30, May 1979, pp. 348–351.

Bradley, Valerie, and Clarke, Gary, eds. *Paper Victories and Hard Realities: The Implementation of the Legal and Constitutional Rights of the Mentally Disabled.* Washington, D.C.: The Health Policy Center of Georgetown University, 1979.

Collins, Dean T. "The Rights of Mental Health Professionals." *Bulletin of the Menninger Clinic* 44 (May 1980):291–295.

Ennis, Bruce J. *Prisoners of Psychiatry.* New York: Avon Books, 1972.

Ennis, Bruce J., and Emery, Richard D. *The Rights of Mental Patients.* New York: Avon Books, 1978.

Friedman, Paul R. *The Rights of Mentally Retarded Persons.* New York: Avon Books, 1976.

Gibson, Robert W. "The Rights of Staff in the Treatment of the Mentally Ill."

Hospital and Community Psychiatry 27 (December 1976):855–859. See summary in *Esprit* 18 (1977):1–3.

Lamb, H. Richard. "Securing Patients' Rights-Responsibility." *Hospital and Community Psychiatry* 32 (June 1981):393–397.

"Mental Health and Human Rights: Report of the Task Panel on Legal and Ethical Issues." *Arizona Law Review* 20 (1978):49–174.

"Patient Rights." *Consolidated Standards for Child, Adolescent, and Adult Psychiatric Programs, 1981 Edition.* Chicago: Joint Commission on Accreditation of Hospitals, pp. 51–53.

"Rights," in Reich, Warren T., ed. *Encyclopedia of Bioethics,* Vol. IV. New York: The Free Press, 1978, pp. 1507–1516.

The Rights of the Mentally Handicapped. Washington, D.C., The Mental Health Law Project, 1973.

4. Informed Voluntary Consent: Competency to Consent to Treatment and Research

Introduction

The most axiomatic action-guiding principle in contemporary medical and legal ethics is that of informed voluntary consent. The principle is advanced as a morally acceptable way of structuring power relationships within the medical setting. It asserts that diagnostic, therapeutic, and experimental medical procedures should be performed on a competent adult patient only after he or she has knowingly and freely consented. This principle may be reformulated in terms of a doctrine of patient rights and corresponding staff obligations, as follows:

1. Patients have the right to make the final decision about submitting to any medical procedure.
2. Patients have the right to refuse any medical procedure to which they have not given their informed voluntary consent.
3. Medical personnel have a duty to educate and inform their patients with respect to relevant medical procedures and to avoid getting uninformed consent (e.g., by tricking patients into signing consent forms).
4. Medical personnel have a duty to avoid obtaining consent under conditions of coercion (threat or harm) or enticement (undue incentives) which call the voluntariness of the consent into question.

Acceptance of the principle of informed voluntary consent may be grounded in the enlightened commitment to certain fundamental human values. The principle might be accepted on moral grounds because one cherishes rational autonomy as such—or at least the enjoyment thereof—or because one abhors the disvalues (e.g., the distresses) which result when rational autonomy is not respected and affirmed in practice. Violations of rational autonomy involve deception; and they result in a loss of self respect, a sense of no longer being in control, and in alienation and mistrust on the part of patients. There are also self-interested reasons why medical personnel should want to adopt an ethic of informed voluntary consent. The law is usually on the side of the patients in such matters, and medical personnel must obtain their voluntary informed consent in order to avoid civil prosecution for negligence or criminal prosecution for assault and/or battery.

In applying the principle of informed consent, a number of philosophical questions arise. In the first selection by Meisel, Roth, and Lidz, the following questions are explored: What is the meaning of "voluntary," and under what conditions is the voluntariness of consent abrogated? What specific sort of information is relevant, and how much is enough, before a particular consent is considered to be informed? In what does competence consist, and under what conditions should a patient be regarded as incompetent? Who may give consent on behalf of the incompetent patient?

Applying the principle of informed voluntary consent to psychiatric patients is complicated by the fact that, in these cases, the part of the person which controls knowing and willing is the diseased part. This generates the presumption in practice that the patient is not really competent to consent. Such a presumption has doubtless reinforced our resistance to applying this fundamental ethical principle to psychiatric patients themselves. We appeal instead to proxy consent by others on their behalf, a proxy consent often given in the clinical setting by the treating physician, or by family, friends, or guardians. Increasingly, however, we are realizing that to presume the incompetence of an individual is too much like a court's presumption that a defendant is guilty until proven innocent.

Although only an exceptionally alert and sensitive mental hospital staff can and will implement it, the ideal presumption should be that the patient is competent until and unless this presumption is defeated by his or her own behavior. Psychiatric illness is highly episodic, and it is always worthwhile to approach the patient afresh each new day with the presumption of competence. Legally, a formal competency hearing is required when specific areas of competency are at issue; but day to day judgments of the patient's ability to understand and manage must also be made by those who deal with the mentally ill. Most patients have periods of lucidity between psychotic episodes, are able to understand and cope in some areas of life even if they have blocks in others, and can best achieve responsible rational autonomy only if it is constantly being thrust upon them. The most serious difficulty with competence is that a number of different criteria of competence are used. In our second selection by Roth, Meisel, and Lidz, five such criteria and their respective strengths and weaknesses are identified and explored.

Although competency hearings are designed to provide procedural safeguards against exploitation and abuse, there is always the real danger that they will become empty formalities in practice. For example, family members easily deprive mental hospital patients of property by having them declared incompetent to manage their business affairs and obtaining power of attorney over them. This is often done at cursory competency hearings in which the patient is not present, has no legal representation, and is not even informed that court action is taking place. The mere presence of the patient in a mental hospital is taken as sufficient evidence of incompetence at such hearings. Any kind of competency hearing may easily degenerate into such a farce, and procedural safeguards afford real protection only when executed by persons of good will and keen moral and legal sensitivities. Lacking power, status, and money, mental patients often find that even the right of appeal against such legally sanctioned exploitation is just another meaningless procedural safeguard.

The ideal of informed voluntary consent is just as relevant to the research setting as it is to the ordinary therapeutic environment. In our third selection, William T. Blackstone explores the relevance of this ideal to the topic of psychological experimentation on human subjects and attempts to ground the ideal in philosophical theory. In light of the fact that so much research and drug testing has been done on mental hospital patients, often without their knowledge or agreement, it is imperative that the relevance of the principle of informed voluntary consent be applied to their situation, as is done in the final selection drawn from the 1978 report of the President's Task Panel on Legal and Ethical Issues. Both Blackstone and the Task Panel seem to assume the validity of a moral rule such as: If X is incompetent to give informed voluntary consent to risky research, then normally it is morally wrong to perform such research on X. Ask yourself if you accept the validity of this principle where X is (a) a chronic schizophrenic, (b) a profoundly retarded adult, (c) an infant candidate for non-therapeutic research, (d) a fetus, (e) a chimpanzee, (f) a mouse. If you think that the principle is applicable in some of these cases but not in others, where do you draw the line, and why?

Finally, Blackstone's assumption that one must abandon utilitarianism and adopt a deontological ethic in order to attach great significance to human dignity may not be justifiable. If, with Blackstone, we equate human dignity with rational autonomy, and if we regard rational autonomy (or at least the enjoyment thereof) as an immense intrinsic good, there is no incompatibility here with utilitarianism, for utilitarianism is simply the view that we ought to maximize intrinsic goodness.

Alan Meisel, Loren H. Roth, and Charles W. Lidz

Toward a Model of the Legal Doctrine of Informed Consent

There is currently a great deal of debate as to the proper role, if any, of the legal regulation of psychiatry. The recent controversies have focused primarily on the legal safeguards to be afforded people before they may be involuntarily hospitalized and on the rights of patients, especially the right to treatment, after they have been hospitalized (1).

Although both of these focuses trace their origins to similar movements in the last century (2), a third focus has begun to emerge. This involves the sharing of decision-making power within the physician-patient relationship; the vehicle of legal regulation on this issue is the doctrine of informed consent. This doctrine, which had its origin primarily in surgery (3), envisions a physician-patient relationship quite different from the traditional ones described by Szasz and Hollender (4), in which the physician is the predominant agent and the patient is either entirely passive or trusting, cooperative, and submissive. The informed consent doctrine has had the effect of pushing the physician-patient relationship in the direction of Szasz and Hollender's model of mutual participation.

Judicial Sources of Informed Consent

Although the principle of informed consent did not develop into a full-blown doctrine to which courts generally adhere until about 1960, its antecedents

From *The American Journal of Psychiatry* 134 (1977):285–289. Copyright © 1977 by the American Psychiatric Association. Reprinted by permission of the publisher and the author.

date at least as far back as the late-eighteenth-century case of *Slater v. Baker and Stapleton* (5), which is credited with being the first reported case dealing with the problem now addressed under the banner of informed consent.

There do not seem to be any earlier reported cases requiring that a physician obtain the patient's consent before rendering treatment. However, it is clear from *Slater* that it was the professional custom among surgeons not to treat patients without obtaining their consent: "It appears from the evidence of the surgeons that it was improper to disunite the callous without consent; this is the usage and law of surgeons." The court added, "It was ignorance and unskillfulness in that very particular, to do contrary to the rule of the profession, what no surgeon ought to have done." In other words, a deviation from the practice ordinarily adhered to by surgeons — specifically the practice of obtaining consent from the patient before administering treatment — was the ground for imposing liability.

Slater went even further than merely requiring that physicians obtain their patients' consent to treatment. The court also said, "It is reasonable that a patient should be told what is about to be done to him, that he may take courage and put himself in such a situation as to enable him to undergo the operation." Because this case involved the use of an innovative means of treating a fracture, it is possible that the court did not intend to imply that the dual requirements of telling a patient what is to be done and obtaining his or her consent were generally applicable to accepted means of treatment. However, subsequent cases do not seem to support this limited reading of *Slater*.

The ground for imposing liability on the physicians in *Slater* was that they failed to adhere to customary professional standards of practice. However, when the first modern cases involving consent began to appear in the early part of this century they were often based on a different rationale. Justice Cardozo's often quoted dictum in *Schloendorff v. Society of NY Hospital* that "every human being of adult years and sound mind has a right to determine what shall be done with his body" (6) indicates that a basis for imposing liability for unauthorized treatment might also be found in the law of battery.

Cases scattered throughout the first half of the twentieth century (7–11) held physicians liable for failing to disclose information about treatment to the patients before rendering it, but not until the late 1950s did cases of this sort begin to appear with any degree of frequency (12–14). In a three-day period in 1960 the supreme courts of Kansas and Missouri issued opinions that were to revolutionize the law of consent to medical treatment.

Natanson v. Kline (15) was a case in which a woman received radiation therapy after a mastectomy and suffered injuries from the radiation. In *Mitchell v. Robinson* (16) the patient received insulin shock and ECT therapies for the treatment of schizophrenia: the treatment caused the fracture of several vertebrae. In both cases the patients' consent to treatment had been obtained. However, in each case the court held that the patient's consent was insufficient to shield the doctors from liability for untoward results of treatment, even though the physicians may not have been negligent in the performance of the procedures. The consents were judged invalid because the physicians had not "inform[ed the patient] generally of the possibly serious collateral hazards" of the treatments (16).

The doctrine of informed consent both reflects and enforces the ancient concern of Anglo-American law with the individual's right to be free from the conduct of others that affronts bodily integrity, privacy, and individual autonomy. Because "Anglo-American law starts with the premise of thorough-going self determination . . . [it] follows that each man is considered to be master of his own body, and he may, if he be of sound mind, expressly prohibit the performance of, life-saving surgery, or other medical treatment" (15). In addition to protecting these time-honored values, the modern doctrine of informed consent also seeks to promote intelligent decision making by medical patients by assuring that relevant information is available to them (17).

Elements of a Legally Valid Decision

What constitutes a valid decision[1] is an issue with which the courts and commentators have grappled since at least the turn of this century. Although a few commentators have expended a substantial amount of effort in exploring some of the elements of a valid decision (3, 18–22), no comprehensive theoretical model has yet been explicated.

We have drawn together the disparate scholarly and judicial commentaries on consent to treatment in order to develop a comprehensive model of the components in the decison-making process and their interrelationship. The components of a valid decision consist of three main variables (provision of information, competency, and understanding), one precondition (voluntariness), and one consequence of the process (consent or refusal).

Voluntariness

Patients must be so situated as to be able to act voluntarily. They must be free from coercion and from unfair persuasions and inducements (23). There must be social support for their belief in their own freedom, at least to the extent that those responsible for providing medical care have an obligation to make patients aware that they possess the right to make their own decisions regarding treatment.

Provision of Information

Patients must be provided with some quantum of information about treatment before their decision can be considered valid. They must be informed of 1) the risks, discomforts, and side effects of proposed treatments, 2) the anticipated benefits of such treatments, 3) the available alternative treatments and their attendant risks, discomforts, and side effects, and 4) the likely consequences of a failure to be treated at all (3, 15, 16, 20–22, 24–26). The explanation must be made in simple language, but there is no need to provide patients with a medical education (25, 27).

Traditionally, all that was necessary was for patients to be informed that a specified medical procedure was contemplated. A physician could have complied with the law, for example, if he or she told the patient, "I am going to remove your appendix" and the patient acquiesced. A greater quantum of information must now be imparted to patients if their decision is to be considered valid. Patients suffering from appendicitis must still be told that an appendectomy is contemplated, but they must now also be informed of the risks, discomforts, and side effects of treatment, the anticipated benefits of treatment, the probable consequences of foregoing treatment, and any available alternative treatments as well as their risks, discomforts, and side effects.

There are two general exceptions permitting abbreviated disclosure or even nondisclosure. In an emergency, when the patient's decision cannot be obtained (e.g., when the patient is unconscious), treatment may proceed without disclosure or consent (24). If disclosure of certain information — especially the risks of treatment — is likely to upset the patient so seriously that he or she will be unable to make a rational decision, then the physician has the "therapeutic privilege" to withhold such information (28).

There are no rules by which a particular physician may be guided in a particular case as to precisely what information must be disclosed to a patient. Many courts adhere to the general rule that the physician is obligated to disclose that information which physicians practicing in the community are accustomed to disclosing to their patients under similar circumstances (15). However, since 1972 several courts have shifted from a standard of disclosure measured by medical custom to what is referred to as a "reasonable patient" standard. That is, the physician must disclose what an average, reasonable patient would want to know before the patient makes a decision whether to undergo or forego treatment (24–26).

Competency

Patients are presumed to have the capacity to comprehend the information with which they are provided to the extent that a "reasonable" person would understand it. For example, a patient must not be afflicted with any such condition as deafness and blindness, intoxication, or emotional or intellectual deficits that would preclude his or her receiving and/or using the information to the same extent that an average person would. If in fact the patient is not "competent" or of "sound mind," any decision that he or she makes will not be considered valid (23).

Exactly what this requirement means is not clear. Several tests of competency might be applied, e.g., patients may be considered competent if 1) they evidence a choice concerning treatment, 2) this choice is "reasonable," 3) this choice is based on "rational" reasons, 4) the patient has a generalized ability to understand, or 5) the patient actually understands the information that has been disclosed. As we indicate at greater length in our companion paper in this issue of the *Journal* (29), the courts have not settled on any single test of competency; in practice, doctors seem to apply an amalgam of some or all of these tests.

Understanding

The judicial decisions implicitly assume that a free actor who is provided with adequate information and who is competent will in fact understand the information provided and be able to make a reasoned decision concerning the course of his or her medical treatment. So far, the courts have not required that patients actually understand what they are told (30). As long as a reasonable person would have understood the information, it is not clear that the particular patient involved must actually understand in order for the decision to be valid.

Some authorities have suggested that a physician is also obligated to take reasonable steps to ascertain whether or not the patient understands what has been disclosed (22, 31). However, the cases use the words "inform" and "understand" interchangeably without seeming to recognize that the act of informing someone does not assure that one will understand the information that has been imparted (23). It is therefore uncertain what obligation, if any, the physician has to attempt to ascertain the patient's level of understanding.

Decision

The final element is that the patient actually made a decision regarding medical treatment. This decision can be either to accept treatment (consent) or not to accept treatment (refusal). In some cases patients may not articulate a decision, and under certain circumstances patients may be said to imply consent to treatment through their conduct rather than verbally (32).

Summary

It is assumed that information given to a competent, free actor will result in understanding and that understanding will yield a decision. A consent will protect the physician from liability as long as the treatment itself is not negligently rendered; a refusal of treatment will also shield the physician from liability. From the patient's viewpoint, the decision-making process protects bodily integrity, privacy, and the right to make a decision whether to undergo or forego treatment free from coercion and with adequate information so that the decision may be made intelligently.

Alternative Models

Because of the failure of the judicial opinions to confront and discuss squarely the meaning of their requirements of competency and understanding and because of the potential overlap of the two elements depending on how each is defined, we offer two alternative models of a valid consent that take into account these uncertainties. We refer to these models as the objective and the subjective models of valid consent.

Objective Model

The objective model of consent eliminates the element of understanding as an essential part of a valid decision. Rather than making inquiry into whether or not the patient actually understands the information that has been disclosed, this model focuses on the congruence or lack of congruence between the particular patient and a hypothetical reasonable person. What is determinative of the validity of the decision (assuming that the patient is acting voluntarily and that there has been adequate disclosure of information) is not the patient's actual, subjective understanding but his or her generalized ability to function in the world—his or her correspondence to an objectively reasonable person. If patients closely resemble this objective ideal, their decision to accept or refuse treatment is valid and their actual understanding does not affect the validity of the decision.

Subjective Model

The subjective model of consent focuses entirely on the patient's actual understanding of the information the physician has supplied. The fact that the patient may be psychotic, retarded, drugged, or similarly compromised is per se irrelevant to the validity of his or her decision. Rather, the decision is considered to be legally valid if the patient has the requisite degree of subjective understanding of the information or if the physician reasonably believes that the patient has this level of understanding (22). This determination may be extremely difficult to make in practice (29).

Informed Consent and Psychiatry

Three of the elements of the legal model of the decision-making process—voluntariness, competency, and understanding—also play an important role in the treatment of psychiatric disorders. It is arguable that to discuss information with patients in the manner required by the law of informed consent is to compromise the effectiveness of psychiatric treatment. Whether or not this is the case, the law is clear that the presence of mental disorder does not ipso facto eliminate the need for disclosing information to patients about treatment or obtaining their consent. One of the foundation cases of the informed consent doctrine, *Mitchell v. Robinson* (16), involved a psychiatric patient; countless other cases have applied the doctrine to psychiatry.

However, does informed consent apply to psychiatry with the full vigor that it does elsewhere in medicine? It is likely that the psychiatrist may invoke the therapeutic privilege to withhold information more easily than other physicians on the ground that disclosure will seriously upset the patient. The therapeutic privilege is not intended to permit the physician to withhold information that he or she believes will cause the patient to refuse treatment; its purpose is to allow the physician to withhold information that will so upset the patient that rational decision making will be precluded (24). Here, too, no hard and fast rule can be announced that all psychiatric patients will be upset by the disclosure of information to them about the risks of treatment, thus providing the psychiatrist with license to withhold all information. Rather, the applicability of the therapeutic privilege must be dealt with on a case-by-case basis.

To date, relatively few legal cases have raised the issue of informed consent in the context of psychiatric treatment. Of those which have, all have dealt with an organic rather than a psychological therapy. The most famous of these cases is *Kaimowitz v. Michigan Department of Mental Health* (33). However, because this case involved an experimental procedure (amygdalectomy) to be performed on a criminally committed patient as a condition of release, it is an atypical case.

The cases that are likely to be far more common for psychiatry and therefore more problematic than *Kaimowitz* are those involving the applicability of informed consent to involuntarily hospitalized patients who refuse commonly accepted organic therapy, most notably psychoactive medication. Although it has long been assumed that the involuntarily committed patient has been deprived of the right to refuse treatment and that the patient's informed consent is therefore not a prerequisite to treatment, cases challenging this assumption are beginning to come up (34–37). Perhaps even involuntarily committed patients should have the right to accept an alternative form of treatment or to choose confinement without treatment. The patient bears the entire risk of side effects of the treatment (7); some patients may prefer to avoid these side effects even at the cost of a longer and perhaps indefinite period of loss of freedom.

Conclusions

The law of consent to medical care has undergone important changes during the last two decades. For the most part, these changes have been effected through the common-law process, that is, by judicial decisions in particular cases rather than through the legislative promulgation of general rules. As a result, the current status of the law of consent is both incomplete and evolving. What constitutes a valid consent today may not remain so tomorrow; what constitutes a valid consent in one jurisdiction may not be an accurate representation of the law in a neighboring jurisdiction; and what constitutes a valid consent in one branch of medicine may be a less than wholly accurate guide to a valid consent in another branch of medicine. Although the applicability of informed consent to psychiatric practice is still in its incipient stages, it is clear that the doctrine does apply, although some modifications will probably be necessary to reflect some of the fundamental differences between psychiatry and the other medical specialties. The trends are unmistakably clear: the emphasis is on more information, and the consequence may well be an increase in patient participation in decision making.

NOTES

1. Developments in the law—civil commitment of the mentally ill. Harvard Law Review 87: 1190–1406, 1974.
2. Deutsch A: The Mentally Ill in America. New York, Columbia University Press, 1949.
3. Restructuring informed consent: legal therapy for the doctor-patient relationship. Yale Law Journal 79:1533–1576, 1970.
4. Szasz TS, Hollender MH: The basic models of the doctor-patient relationship. Arch. Intern. Med. 97:585–592, 1956.
5. Salter v. Baker and Stapleton, 2 Wils 359, 95 Eng Rep 860 (KB 1767).
6. Schloendorff v. Society of NY Hospital, 211 NY 125, 105 NE 92 (NY 1914).
7. Mohr v. Williams, 95 Minn 261, 104 NW 12 (Minn 1905).
8. Pratt v. Davis, 224 Ill 300, 79 NE 562 (Ill 1906), affirming 118 Ill App 161 (Ill 1905).
9. Hunter v. Burroughs, 123 Va 113, 96 SE 360 (Va 1918).
10. Kenny v. Lockwood [1932] 1 DLR 507 (Ont App 1931).
11. Wall v. Brim, 138 F 2d 478 (5th Cir 1943).
12. Hunt v. Bradshaw, 242 NC 517, 88 SE 2d 762 (NC 1955).
13. Salgo v. Leland Stanford Jr. Univ. Bd. of Trustees, 154 Cal App 2d 560, 317 P 2d 170 (Cal 1957).
14. Bang v. Charles T. Miller Hospital, 251 Minn 427, 88 NW 186 (Minn 1958).
15. Natanson v. Kline, 186 Kan 393, 350 P 2d 1093; rehearing denied, 187 Kan 186, 354 P 2d 670 (Kan 1960).
16. Mitchell v. Robinson, 334 SW 2d 11 (Mo 1960); affirmed after retrial 360 SW 673 (Mo 1962).
17. Katz J, Capron A: Catastrophic Diseases: Who Decides What? New York, Russell Sage Foundation, 1975, pp. 82–90.
18. Goldstein J: For Harold Laswell: some reflections on human dignity, entrapment, informed consent, and the plea bargain. Yale Law Journal 84:683–703, 1975.
19. McCoid AH: A reappraisal of liability for unauthorized medical treatment. Minnesota Law Review 41:381–434, 1957.
20. Plante ML: An analysis of informed consent. Fordham Law Review 36:639–672, 1968.
21. Waltz JE, Scheuneman TW: Informed consent to therapy. Northwestern University Law Review 64:628–650, 1970.
22. Capron AM: Informed consent in catastrophic disease research and treatment. University of Pennsylvania Law Review 123:340–438, 1974.
23. Relf v. Weinberger, 372 F Supp 1196, 1202 (DC 1974).
24. Canterbury v. Spence, 464 F 2d 772 (DC Cir); cert denied 409 US 1064 (1972).
25. Cobbs v. Grant, 8 Cal 3d 229, 104 Cal Rptr 505, 505 P 2d 1 (Cal 1972).
26. Wilkinson v. Vesey, 110 RI606, 295 A 2d 676 (RI 1972).
27. ZeBarth v. Swedish Hospital Medical Center, 81 Wash 2d 12, 499 P 2d 1 (Wash 1972).
28. Informed consent: the illusion of patient choice. Emory Law Journal 25:503–522, 1974.
29. Roth LH, Meisel A, Lidz CW: Tests of competency to consent to treatment. Am. J. Psychiatry 134:279–284, 1977.
30. US Department of Health, Education, and Welfare: Protection of human subjects: proposed policy. Federal Register 39:30647–30657, Aug. 23, 1974.

31. Pennsylvania Department of Public Welfare: Rights of patients and residents in mental health and mental retardation facilities operated by the Department of Public Welfare, Pennsylvania Bulletin 5:2038–2043, 1975.
32. Consent as condition of right to perform surgical operation. American Law Reports 139: 1370–1375, 1942.
33. Kaimowitz v. Michigan Department of Mental Health, Civil Action 73-19434-AW (Wayne County, Mich, Cir Ct 1973).
34. In re Gross, No 16 March term (Pa Supreme Ct 1976, pending).
35. Friedman v. Escalona, 75 C 4414 (ND Ill, filed Dec. 30, 1975).
36. Risley v. Coombs, N-76-234 (D Md, filed Feb. 17, 1976).
37. Scott v. Plante, 532 F 2d 939 (3d Cir 1976).

Loren H. Roth, Alan Meisel, and Charles W. Lidz

Tests of Competency to Consent to Treatment

The concept of competency, like the concept of dangerousness, is social and legal and not merely psychiatric or medical (1). Law and, at times, psychiatry are concerned with an individual's competency to stand trial, to make a will, and to contract (2–5). The test of competency varies from one context to another. In general, to be considered competent an individual must be able to comprehend the nature of the particular conduct in question and to understand its quality and its consequences (3, 6). For example, in *Dusky v. United States* the court held that to be considered competent to stand trial an individual must have "sufficient present ability to consult with his lawyer with a reasonable degree of rational understanding — and . . . a rational as well as a factual understanding of the proceedings against him" (7). A person may be considered competent for some legal purposes and incompetent for others at the same time (3). An individual is not judged incompetent merely because he or she is mentally ill (6).

There is a dearth of legal guidance illuminating the concept of competency to consent to medical treatment (8–11). Nevertheless, competency plays an important role in determining the validity of a patient's decision to undergo or forego treatment. The decision of a person who is incompetent does not validly authorize a physician to perform medical treatment (12). Conversely, a physician who withholds treatment from an incompetent patient who refuses treatment may be held liable to that patient if the physician does not take reasonable steps to obtain some other legally valid authorization for treatment (13).

From *The American Journal of Psychiatry* 134 (1977):279–284. Copyright © 1977 by the American Psychiatric Association. Reprinted by permission of the publisher and the co-authors.

In psychiatry the entire edifice of involuntary treatment is erected on the supposed incompetency of some people to voluntarily seek and consent to needed treatment (14). In addition, the acceptability of behavior modification for the patient who is considered dangerous (15), the resolution of ethical issues in family planning (i.e., sterilization) (16, 17), and the right to refuse psychoactive medications (18) — to cite only a few of the more prominent examples — turn in part on the concept of competency.

As we explain in our companion paper in this issue of the *Journal* (19), competency is theoretically one of the independent variables that is determinative in part of the legal validity of a patient's consent to or refusal of treatment. There is therefore a need to specify how competency can be determined. Related questions include the following: Who raises the question of competency? When is this question raised? and Who makes the determination? Answers to these questions are beyond the scope of this paper.

The objective of the present inquiry is to make sense of various tests of competency, to analyze their applicability to patients' decisions to accept or refuse psychiatric treatment, and to illustrate the problems of applying these tests by clinical case examples from the consultation service of the Law and Psychiatry Program of Western Psychiatric Institute and Clinic.

In a brief presentation it is impossible to provide any serious linguistic analysis of a number of words that are frequently used in discussions of competency — words such as "responsible" (20), "rational" or "irrational" (21, 22), "knowing" (23, 24), "knowingly" (25, p. 99), "understandingly" (24), or "capable" (26). These words are often used interchangeably without sufficient explanation or clear behavioral referents. Only the rare scholarly article attempts to explain with precision what is meant by such terms (11); judicial decisions or statutes generally do not.

In evaluating tests for competency several criteria should be considered. A useful test for competency is one that, first, can be reliably applied; second, is mutually acceptable or at least comprehensible to physicians, lawyers, and judges; and third, is set at a level capable of striking an acceptable balance between preserving individual autonomy and providing needed medical care. Reliability is enhanced to the extent that a competency test depends on manifest and objectively ascertainable patient behavior rather than on inferred and probably unknowable mental status (6).

Tests for Competency

Several tests for competency have been proposed in the literature; others are readily inferable from judicial commentary. Although there is some overlap, they basically fall into five categories: 1) evidencing a choice, 2) "reasonable" outcome of choice, 3) choice based on "rational" reasons, 4) ability to understand, and 5) actual understanding.

Evidencing a Choice

This test for competency is set at a very low level and is the most respectful of the autonomy of patient decision making (10). Under this test the competent patient is one who evidences a preference for or against treatment. This test focuses not on the quality of the patient's decision but on the presence or absence of a decision. This preference may be a yes, a no, or even the desire that the physician make the decision for the patient. Only the patient who does not evidence a preference either verbally or through his or her behavior is considered incompetent. This test of competency encompasses at a minimum the unconscious patient; in psychiatry it encompasses the mute patient who cannot or will not express an opinion.

Even such arch-defenders of individual autonomy as Szasz have agreed that patients who do not formulate and express a preference as to treatment are incompetent. In answer to a question about the right to intervene against a patient's will, Szasz has stated,

> It is quite obvious, and I make this abundantly clear, that I have no objection to medical intervention vis-à-vis persons who are not protesting; . . . [for example,] somebody who is lying in bed catatonic and the mother wants to get him to the hospital and the ambulance shows up and he just lies there. (27)

The following case example illustrates the use of the test of evidencing a choice:

> *Case 1.* A 41-year-old depressed woman was interviewed in the admission unit. She rarely answered yes or no to direct questions. Admission was proposed; she said and did nothing, but looked apprehensive. When asked about admission, she did not sign herself into the hospital, protest, or walk away. She was guided to the inpatient ward by her husband and her doctor after being given the opportunity to walk the other way.

This test may be what one court had in mind when, with respect to sterilization of residents of state schools, it ruled that even legally incompetent and possibly noncomprehending residents may not be sterilized unless they have formed a genuine desire to undergo the procedure (28).

The guidelines proposed by the U.S. Department of Health, Education, and Welfare concerning experimentation with institutionalized mentally ill people also point in this direction by requiring even the legally incompetent person's "assent to such participation . . . when . . . he has sufficient mental capacity to understand what is proposed and to express an opinion as to his or her participation" (29, at 46.504c). Although this low test of competency does not fully assure patients' understanding of the nature of what they consent to or what they refuse, it is behavioral in orientation and therefore more reliable in application; it also guards against excessive paternalism.

"Reasonable" Outcome of Choice

This test of competency entails evaluating the patient's capacity to reach the "reasonable," the "right," or the "responsible" decision (10, 30). The emphasis in this test is on outcome rather than on the mere fact of decision or how it has been reached. The patient who fails to make a decision that is roughly congruent with the decision that a "reasonable" person in like circumstances would make is viewed as incompetent.

This test is probably used more often than might be admitted by both physicians and courts. Judicial decisions to override the desire of patients with certain religious beliefs not to receive blood transfusions may rest in part on the court's view that the patient's decision is not reasonable (31). When life is at stake and a court believes that the patient's decision is unreasonable, the court may focus on even the smallest ambiguity in the patient's thinking to cast doubt on the patient's competency so that it may issue an order that will preserve life or health. For example, one judge issued an order to allow amputation of the leg of an elderly moribund man even though the man had clearly told his daughter before his condition deteriorated not to permit an amputation (32, 33).

Mental health laws that allow for involuntary treatment on the basis of "need for care and treatment" (34) without requiring a formal adjudication of incompetency in effect use an unstated reasonable outcome test in abridging the patient's common-law right not to be treated without giving his or her consent. These laws are premised on the following syllogism: the patient needs treatment; the patient has not obtained treatment on his or her own intiative; therefore, the patient's decision is incorrect, which means that he or she is incompetent, thus justifying the involuntary imposition of treatment.

The benefits and costs of this test are that social goals and individual health are promoted at considerable expense to personal autonomy. The reasonable outcome test is useful in alerting physicians and courts to the fact that the patient's decision-making process may be, but not necessarily is, awry. Ultimately, because the test rests on the congruence between the patient's decision and that of a reasonable person or that of the physician, it is biased in favor of decisions to accept treatment, even when such decisions are made by people who are incapable of weighing the risks and benefits of treatment. In other words, if patients do not decide the "wrong" way, the issue of competency will probably not arise.

Choice Based on "Rational" Reasons

Another test is whether the reasons for the patient's decision are "rational," that is, whether the patient's decision is due to or is a product of mental illness (10, 22). As in the reasonable outcome test, if the patient decides in favor of treatment the issue of the patient's competency (in this case, whether the decision is the product of mental illness) seldom if ever arises because of the medical profession's bias toward consent to treatment and against refusal of treatment.

In this test the quality of the patient's thinking is what counts. The following case example illustrates the use of the test of rational reasons:

> *Case 2.* A 70-year-old widow who was living alone in a condemned dilapidated house with no heat was brought against her will to the hospital. Her thinking was tangential and fragmented. Although she did not appear to be hallucinating, she seemed delusional. She refused blood tests, saying, "You just want my blood to spread it all over Pittsburgh. No, I'm not giving it." Her choice was respected. Later in the day, however, when her blood pressure was found to be dangerously elevated (250 over 135 in both arms), blood was withdrawn against her will.

The test of rational reasons, although it has clinical appeal and is probably much in clinical use, poses considerable conceptual problems; as a legal test it is probably defective (10). The problems include the difficulty of distinguishing rational from irrational reasons and drawing inferences of causation between any irrationality believed present and the valence (yes or no) of the patient's decision. Even if the patient's reasons seem irrational, it is not possible to prove that the patient's actual decision making has been the product of such irrationality. The patient's decision might well be the same even if his or her cognitive processes were less impaired. For example, a delusional patient may refuse ECT not because he or she is delusional but because he or she is afraid of it, which is considered a normal reaction. The emphasis on rational reasons can too easily become a global indictment of the competency of mentally disordered individuals, justifying widespread substitute decision making for this group.

The Ability to Understand

This test—the ability of the patient to understand the risks, benefits, and alternatives to treatment (including no treatment)—is probably the most consistent with the law of informed consent (19). Decision making need not be rational in either process or outcome; unwise choices are permitted. Nevertheless, at a minimum the patient must manifest sufficient ability to understand information about treatment, even if in fact he or she weighs this information differently from the attending physician. What matters in this test is that the patient is able to comprehend the elements that are presumed by law to be a part of treatment decision making. How the patient weighs these elements, values them, or puts them together to reach a decision is not important.

The patient's capacity for understanding may be tested by asking the patient a series of questions concerning risks, benefits, and alternatives to treatment (35). By providing further information or explanation to the patient, the physician may find deficiencies in understanding to be remediable or not (36). The following case examples illustrate the use of the test of the ability to understand:

> *Case 3.* A 28-year-old woman who was unresponsive to medication was approached for consent to ECT. She initially appeared to be unaware of the

examiner. Following an explanation of ECT, she responded to the request to explain its purposes and why it was being recommended in her case with the statement, "Paul McCartney, nothing to zero." She was shown a consent form for ECT that she signed without reading. Further attempts to educate her were unsuccessful. It was decided not to perform the ECT without seeking court approval.

Case 4. A 44-year-old woman who was diagnosed as having chronic schizophrenia refused amputation of her frostbitten toes. She was nonpsychotic. Although her condition was evaluated psychiatrically as manifesting extreme denial, she understood what was proposed and that there was some risk of infection without surgery. Nevertheless, she declined. She stated, "You want to take my toes off; I want to keep them." Her decision was respected. She agreed to return to the hospital if things got worse. A month later she returned, having suffered an auto-amputation of the toes. There was no infection; she was rebandaged and sent home.

Some of the questions raised by this test of competency are, What is to be done if the patient can understand the risks but not the benefits or vice versa? Alternatively, what if the patient views the risks as the benefits? The following case example illustrates this problem:

Case 5. A 49-year-old woman whose understanding of treatment was otherwise intact, when informed that there was a 1 in 3,000 chance of dying from ECT, replied, "I hope I am the one."

Furthermore, how potentially sophisticated must understanding be in order that the patient be viewed as competent? There are considerable barriers, conscious and unconscious and intellectual and emotional (37), to understanding proposed treatments. Presumably the potential understanding required is only that which would be manifested by a reasonable person provided a similar amount of information. A few attempts to rank degrees of understanding have been made (38). However, this matter is highly complex and beyond the scope of the present inquiry. Certainly, at least with respect to nonexperimental treatment, the patient's potential understanding does not have to be perfect or near perfect for him or her to be considered competent, although one court seemed to imply this with respect to experimental psychosurgery (39). A final problem with this test is that its application depends on unobservable and inferential mental processes rather than on concrete and observable elements of behavior.

Actual Understanding

Rather than focusing on competency as a construct or intervening variable in the decision-making process, the test of actual understanding reduces competency to an epiphenomenon of this process (19). The competent patient is by definition one who has provided a knowledgeable consent to treatment. Under this test the physician has an obligation to educate the patient and directly ascertain whether he or she has in fact understood. If not, according to this test the patient may not have provided informed consent (19). Depending on how sophisticated a level of understanding is to be required, this test delineates a potentially high level of competency, one that may be difficult to achieve.

The provisional decision of DHEW to mandate the creation of consent committees to oversee the decisions of experimental subjects (29, at 46.506) implicitly adopts this test, as does the California law requiring the review of patient consent to ECT (40). Controversial as these requirements may be, they require physicians to make reasonable efforts to ascertain that their patients understand what they are told and encourage active patient participation in treatment selection (41).

The practical and conceptual limitations of this test are similar to those of the ability-to-understand test. What constitutes adequate understanding is vague, and deficient understanding may be attributable in whole or in part to physician behavior as well as to the patient's behavior or character. An advantage that this test has over the ability-to-understand test, assuming the necessary level of understanding can be specified a priori, is its greater reliability. Unlike the ability-to-understand test, in which the patient's comprehension of material of a certain complexity is used as the basis for an assumption of comprehension of other material of equivalent complexity (even if this other material is not actually tested), the actual understanding test makes no such assumption. It tests the very issues central to patient decision making about treatment.

Discussion

It has been our experience that competency is presumed as long as the patient modulates his or her behavior, talks in a comprehensible way, remembers what he or she is told, dresses and acts so as to appear to be in meaningful communication with the environment, and has not been declared legally incompetent. In other words, if patients have their wits about them in a layman's sense (19) it is assumed that they will understand what they are told about treatment, including its risks, benefits, and alternatives. This is the equivalent of saying that the legal presumption is one of competency until found otherwise (42). The Pandora's box of the question of whether and to what extent the patient is able to understand or has understood what has been disclosed is therefore never opened.

In effect, the test that is actually applied combines elements of all of the tests described above. However, the circumstances in which competency becomes an issue determine which elements of which tests are stressed and which are underplayed. Although in theory competency is an independent variable that determines whether or not the patient's decision to accept or refuse treatment is to be honored, in practice it seems to be dependent on the interplay of two other variables, the risk/benefit ratio of treatment and the valence of the patient's decision, i.e., whether he or she consents to or refuses treatment.

The phrase "risk/benefit ratio of treatment" is used here in a shorthand way to express the fact that people who determine patient competency make this decision partly on the basis of the risks of the particular treatment being considered and the benefits of that treatment. We do not mean to imply that any formal calculation is made or that any given ratio is determinative of competency. The problems of who decides what is a risk and what is a benefit, the relative weights to be attached to risks and benefits, and who bears the risks and to whom the benefits accrue (e.g., the patient, the clinician, society), are beyond the scope of the present inquiry.

TABLE 1
Factors in Selection of Competency Tests

Patient's Decision	Risk/Benefit Ratio of Treatment	
	Favorable	Unfavorable or Questionable
Consent	Low test of competency (cell A)	High test of competency (cell D)
Refusal	High test of competency (cell B)	Low test of competency (cell C)

Table 1 illustrates the interplay of the valence of the patient's decision and the risk/benefit ratio of treatment. When there is a favorable risk/benefit ratio to the proposed treatment in the opinion of the person determining competency and the patient consents to the treatment, there does not seem to be any reason to stand in the way of administering treatment. To accomplish this, a test employing a low threshold of competency may be applied to find even a marginal patient competent so that his or her decision may be honored (cell A). This is what happens daily when uncomprehending patients are permitted to sign themselves into the hospital. Similarly, when the risk/benefit ratio is favorable and the patient refuses treatment, a test employing a higher threshold of competency may be applied (cell B). Under such a test even a somewhat knowledgeable patient may be found incompetent so that consent may be sought from a substitute decision maker and treatment administered despite the patient's refusal. An example would be the patient withdrawing from alcohol who, although intermittently resistive, is nevertheless administered sedative medication. In both of these cases, in which the risk/benefit ratio is favorable, the bias of physicians, other health professionals, and judges is usually skewed toward providing treatment. Therefore, a test of competency is applied that will permit the treatment to be administered irrespective of the patient's actual or potential understanding.

However, there is a growing reluctance on the part of our society to permit patients to undergo treatments that are extremely risky or for which the benefits are highly speculative. Thus if the risk/benefit ratio is unfavorable or questionable and the patient refuses treatment, a test employing a low threshold of competency may be selected so that the patient will be found competent and his or her refusal honored (cell C). This is what happens in the area of sterilization of mentally retarded people, in which, at least from the perspective of the retarded individual, the risk/benefit ratio is questionable. On the other hand, when the risk/benefit ratio is unfavorable or questionable and the patient consents to treatment, a test using a higher threshold of competency may be applied (cell D), preventing even some fairly knowledgeable patients from undergoing treatment. The judicial opinion in the well-known *Kaimowitz* psychosurgery case delineated a high test of competency to be employed in that experimental setting (39).

Of course, some grossly impaired patients cannot be determined to be competent under any conceivable test, nor can most normally functioning people be found incompetent merely by selective application of a test of competency. However, within limits and when the patient's competency is not absolutely clear-cut, a test of competency that will achieve the desired medical or social end despite the actual condition of the patient may be selected. We do not imply that this is done maliciously either by physicians or by the courts; rather, we believe that it occurs as a consequence of the strong societal bias in favor of treating treatable patients so long as it does not expose them to serious risks.

Conclusions

The search for a single test of competency is a search for a Holy Grail. Unless it is recognized that there is no magical definition of competency to make decisions about treatment, the search for an acceptable test will never end. "Getting the words just right" is only part of the problem. In practice, judgments of competency go beyond semantics or straightforward applications of legal rules; such judgments reflect social considerations and societal biases as much as they reflect matters of law and medicine.

NOTE

This research was supported in part by Alcohol, Drug Abuse, and Mental Health Administration grant MH-27553 from the Center for Studies of Crime and Delinquency, National Institute of Mental Health.

REFERENCES

1. Shah SA: Dangerousness and civil commitment of the mentally ill: some public policy considerations. Am. J. Psychiatry 132:501–505, 1975.

2. Allen RC, Ferster EZ, Weihofen H: Mental Impairment and Legal Incompetency. Englewood Cliffs, NJ, Prentice-Hall, 1968.
3. Hardisty JH: Mental illness: a legal fiction. Washington Law Review 48:735-762, 1973.
4. Alexander GJ, Szasz TS: From contract to status via psychiatry. Santa Clara Lawyer 13: 537-559, 1973.
5. Group for the Advancement of Psychiatry Committee on Psychiatry and Law: Misuse of Psychiatry in the Criminal Courts: Competency to Stand Trial. Report 89. New York, GAP, 1974.
6. Green MD: Judicial tests of mental incompetency. Missouri Law Review 6:141-165, 1941.
7. Dusky v. United States, 362 US 405 (1960) (per curiam).
8. Informed consent and the dying patient. Yale Law Journal 83:1632-1664, 1974.
9. Mental competency of patient to consent to surgical operation or treatment. American Law Reports Annotated, Third Series 25:1439-1443, 1969.
10. Friedman PR: Legal regulation of applied behavior analysis in mental institutions and prisons. Arizona Law Review 17:39-104, 1975.
11. Shapiro MH: Legislating the control of behavior control: autonomy and the coercive use of organic therapies. Southern California Law Review 47:237-356, 1974.
12. Demers v. Gerety, 515 P 2d 645 (NM 1973).
13. Steele v. Woods, 327 SW 2d 187, 198 (Mo 1959).
14. Peszke MA: Is dangerousness an issue for physicians in emergency commitment? Am. J. Psychiatry 132:825-828, 1975.
15. Halleck SL: Legal and ethical aspects of behavior control. Am. J. Psychiatry 131:381-385, 1974.
16. Grunebaum H, Abernethy V: Ethical issues in family planning for hospitalized psychiatric patients. Am. J. Psychiatry 132:236-240, 1975.
17. Relf v. Weinberger, 372 F Supp 1196 (DC 1974).
18. Michels R: The right to refuse psychoactive drugs: case studies in bioethics. Hastings Center Report 3(3):10-11, 1973.
19. Meisel A, Roth LH, Lidz CW: Toward a model of the legal doctrine of informed consent. Am. J. Psychiatry 134:285-289, 1977.
20. A Draft Act Governing Hospitalization of the Mentally Ill, revised. US Public Health Service Publication 51, Washington, DC, US Government Printing Office, 1952, pp. 6, 26, 27.
21. In re Yetter, 62 D&C 2d 619, 624 (CP Northampton County, Pa 1973).
22. Stone AA: Mental Health and Law: A System in Transition. US Department of Health, Education, and Welfare Publication 75-176. Rockville, Md, National Institute of Mental Health, 1975, p. 68.
23. US Department of Health, Education, and Welfare: Protection of human subjects. Federal Register 39:18914-18920, May 30, 1973.
24. Moore v. Webb, 345 SW 2d 239, 23 (Mo 1961).
25. Freidman PR: Legal regulation of applied behavior analysis in mental institutions and prisons. Arizona Law Review 17:39-140, 1975.
26. New York City Health and Hospital Corp v. Stein, 335 NYS 2d 461, 465 (NY 1972).
27. McDonald MC: And things get rough. Psychiatric News, Nov. 5, 1975, pp. 13-14.
28. Wyatt v. Aderholt, 368 F Supp 1383, 1385 (MD Ala 1974).
29. US Department of Health, Education, and Welfare: Protection of human subjects: proposed policy. Federal Register 39:30647-30657, Aug. 23, 1974.
30. United States v. George, 239 F Supp 752 (D Conn 1965).
31. Cantor NL: A patient's decision to decline life-saving medical treatment: bodily integrity versus the preservation of life. Rutgers Law Review 26:228-264, 1973.
32. Judge OKs amputation of south sider's leg. Pittsburgh Press, June 4, 1975, p. 1.
33. Amputate order more human than judicial, Larsen says. Pittsburgh Press, June 8, 1975, p. 1.
34. Developments in the law — civil commitment of the mentally ill. Harvard Law Review 87: 1190-1406, 1974.
35. Miller R, Willner HS: The two-part consent form. N. Engl. J. Med. 290:964-966, 1974.

36. Infelfinger FJ: Informed (but uneducated) consent. N. Engl. J. Med. 287:465–466, 1972.
37. Katz J: Experimentation with Human Beings. New York, Russel Sage Foundation, 1972, pp. 609–673.
38. Olin GB, Olin HS: Informed consent in voluntary mental hospital admissions. Am. J. Psychiatry 132:938–941, 1975.
39. Kaimowitz v. Michigan Department of Mental Health, Civil Action 73-19434-AW (Wayne County, Mich. Cir Ct 1973).
40. California enacts rigid shock therapy controls. Psychiatric News, Feb. 5, 1975, pp. 1, 4–7.
41. Szasz RS, Hollender MH: The basic models of the doctor-patient relationship. Arch. Intern. Med. 97:585–592, 1956.
42. Lotman v. Security Mutual Life Insurance Co., 478 F 2d 868 (3d Cir 1973).

William T. Blackstone

The American Psychological Association Code of Ethics for Research Involving Human Participants: An Appraisal[1]

Introduction

We are all keenly aware of the ethical issues of medical experimentation in which human subjects are used. The Nuremberg Trials seared this on our consciences at the end of World War II.[2] And since then the medical possibilities created by new knowledge, new technology and skill have created complex moral questions, not just in the application and distribution of this new knowledge, but also in the quest for yet additional knowledge and the use of human subjects in furthering that quest. The ethical problems generated by the possibilities of heart transplants (and other vital organs), psychosurgery, and genetic manipulation have had a very wide press. Institutes and Centers have been created whose main purpose is to investigate the ethical issues in medicine and the life sciences.[3] The need for such investigation is more than obvious. Life and death and the quality of human existence hang on principles and practices in these areas. Examples of the blatantly immoral use of human beings in medical experimentation are not difficult to come by. We don't have to go to Nazi Germany. We can go to Tuskegee, Alabama, where U.S. Government doctors withheld penicillin treatment from a control group of several hundred black men in order to study the effects of syphilis in the human body.[4] We can go to New York where cancer cells were injected into elderly and chronically ill individuals who were not informed that malignant cells were being used.[5] Or, to the case where effective penicillin treatment was

From *The Southern Journal of Philosophy* 13 (1975):407–418. Reprinted by permission of the publisher and Mrs. Jean Blackstone.

denied a control group, the result being crippling rheumatic fever for many of the subjects.[6] These and other cases have focused great attention on the ethical issues involved in medical experimentation, quite apart from dramatic cases like having your heart snatched away for another's use before you are quite finished with it.

Less attention has been devoted to the development of an ethic for psychological experimentation. The scene here is generally not one of life or death. Most psychological research is harmless and poses no risk to the subject. But more and more psychological research does involve risk, in some cases considerable risk to the welfare and dignity of the subject. In research projects where drugs are used, privacy is invaded, physical and mental stress is induced in the subject, deception is employed, where subjects are subtly coerced into participation, benefits are withheld from control groups and so on — such research contexts raise fundamental ethical problems. The APA, of course, is well aware of this. It has cited a number of ethically problematic cases in the report of the Ad Hoc Committee on Psychological Research, and it has revised the 1953 Code of Ethics in the 1973 publication, *Ethical Principles in the Conduct of Research with Human Participants*. The procedure used in arriving at this new and tentative code was systematic and well-conceived. The proposed code was widely discussed throughout the profession prior to final adoption. Approximately 200 groups scheduled discussions of the initial draft with many of them feeding back to the Ad Hoc Committee. Efforts were made to examine specific research contexts which generate ethical problems and to seek out the implications of those problems for formulating a set of ethical principles. The procedure was far more empirical and participatory than most philosophers use in formulating normative codes. You may recall that our own Society devoted a symposium to the initial draft at our 1972 meeting.

What I want to do in this paper is to examine briefly the newly published code. A thorough analysis would take us well beyond our limited space, but within my abbreviated analysis, I want to indicate what I consider to be some important limitations and inadequacies of the new code, however much it is an improvement over the old. Also, I will be so bold as to make some suggestions both in terms of the normative base of principles of the code and in terms of devices for the practical implementation of it. These criticisms and suggestions are not intended as some sort of divine moral guidance or moral insight granted me by the Oracle at Delphi. They are made in the same participatory spirit encouraged by the Ad Hoc Committee of the A.P.A. which drafted the code. I am bothered by what the code might permit; also, by some apparent inconsistencies in the code.

Let me begin by granting that the ethical issues involving psychological research are complex. There are a number of competing and conflicting values at stake — prudential, professional, and moral. There is the interest of society in increasing knowledge which bears on psychological health and social stability; and our society is strongly committed to the support of research which increases that knowledge. There is the prudential interest of the investigator himself, whose career is often dramatically affected by the success of his research. There is the interest of the research participant whose welfare and dignity or self-esteem can be damaged by unethical research. All of these interests or values are at stake in decisions to conduct or not conduct research involving human subjects. In contexts where these various interests conflict, how are we to decide? And we must remember that the conflict is often not merely between the prudential interests of the investigator and the welfare of the research participant. Often the conflict is between the welfare of the research participant and the welfare of society as a whole.

The ideal, it goes without saying, is a procedure which realizes the social value of experimentation without any risk or sacrifice to the experimental subjects. But progress in the medical and psychological sciences does require some risk, even when all efforts have been made to minimize it. The question is when or under what circumstances the investigator is justified in proceeding with risk. I would grant that the central control is the conscience of the investigator. He, more than anyone, knows what is going on. But not all consciences, including those of professionals, are fully informed and sensitive to all of the interests at stake. The point of developing ethical guidelines, I take it, is that of assisting in the development of informed and sensitive consciences.

The Cost-Benefit Model

When we turn to the 1973 *Ethical Principles* it is not at all clear what framework emerges as a way of balancing these various interests or values. Seven basic principles are stated and explicated, but the total framework of principles is open to several interpretations. One of these interpretations is that the overall code is a cost-benefit model. Tally the costs of an experiment, including that to research participants. Tally the probable benefits. If the probable benefits outweigh the probable costs, then the experiment is ethically justifiable. Professor John Marshall evinced considerable concern with this possible reading of the APA Code prior to its publication.[8] I have the same fears with the published version. My fear is rooted in the danger of the use of a purely cost-benefit or act-utilitarian model (in which the aggregate good is the sole criterion of ethical evaluation) in any area of human activity and decision, not merely the area of experimentation. The danger is that this model may justify far too much, namely, actions which violate the rights of individuals and fly in the face of our ordinary moral sensitivities.

Let me indicate the basis on which we may infer that the APA endorses this cost-benefit model as an adequate ethic for experimentation with humans. I quote:

> . . . the ethical problems associated with psychological research on human beings cannot be solved by enunciating simple principles that point to absolute rights and wrongs. When ethical questions arise, the situation is usually one of weighing the

advantages and disadvantages of conducting the research as planned. On the one hand there is the contribution that the research may ultimately make to human welfare, on the other, there is the cost to the individual research participant. Put in these stark terms, the essential conflict is between the values to science to benefit all mankind and the values that dictate concern for the research participant.[9]

This model looms large in much of the *Ethical Principles,* It is seen as the "broad framework of competing values" within which there are more specific conflicts (such as that which might occur between the obligation to obtain informed consent and to avoid visiting harm or stress upon a participant).[10] But all conflicts, these passages appear to say, are to be resolved within a cost-benefit model. Though no purely quantitative formula or decision rule is possible, the *Ethical Principles* emphasize, still ". . . an analysis following this approach asks about any procedure, 'Is it worth it, considering what is required of the research participant and other social costs, on the one hand, and the importance of the research, on the other?' Or, 'Do the net gains of doing the research outweigh the net gains of not doing it?' "[11] Exact calculation of consequences is not possible, but it is clearly the ideal espoused. "We need to form a judgment," the *Principles* emphasize, "about the likelihood and seriousness of the costs, the probability and importance of the gains, and the number of people who will be affected."[12] The distinct impression of these passages and the implications of the cost-benefit model is this: If the potential consequential considerations for mankind in carrying out some important research are high enough, then the violation of a research subject's rights—the harm and indignity to the participant—are morally justifiable. Harm to research participants is to be avoided, but not at all costs.

Now the statement of principles properly recognizes that the cost-benefit assessment of any controversial research proposal will be very complex; it also insists that the rights and welfare of research participants must be carefully weighed in that assessment. But let me repeat. On the cost-benefit reading of the basic thrust of those principles, the rights of the research participant as reflected in other parts of the principles (the insistence upon the informed consent of the participant, the right of the participant to withdraw from the experiment and to withdraw his data, *etc.*) can always be overridden if, in the eyes of the investigator and his consultants, the benefits outweigh the costs.

The Deontological Model

Let me now offer another reading of the *Principles,* one which is quite inconsistent with the cost-benefit, act-utilitarian reading. I will call it the deontological model (indicating the position in ethical theory that obligation or duty is not reducible to purely consequential considerations or the aggregate good).

Principle 3 emphasizes the responsibility of the investigator to protect the dignity and welfare of the research participant and Principle 7 reads as follows:

The ethical investigator protects participants from physical and mental discomfort, harm and danger. If the risk of such consequences exists, the investigator is required to inform the participant of that fact, secure consent before proceeding, and take all possible measures to minimize distress. A research procedure may not be used if it is likely to cause serious and lasting harm to participants.[13]

If one combines these two principles with some textual exegesis, what emerges is a strong element of moral absolutism *and* the moral priority of the rights and dignity of the research participant over consequential considerations. I quote again:

. . . in weighing the pros and cons of conducting research involving ethical questions, priority must be given to the research participant's welfare. The nearest that the principles in this document come to an immutable "thou shalt" or "thou shalt not" is in the insistence that the human participants emerge from their research experience unharmed or at least that the risks are minimal, understood by the participants, and accepted as reasonable.[14]

This passage reminds one of John Rawls' lexical ordering of his principles of justice,[15] or of W. D. Ross' ordering of prima facie duties[16] — an ordering of priorities in which a fundamental principle must be fully satisfied before a secondary principle comes into play. What these passages seem to say is that in the ethical assessment of experimental research involving human subjects, priority must always be given to the welfare of the participant. The participant's welfare and dignity take precedence over the import and value of the research. This priority-emphasis on the dignity and welfare of the research participant is completely inconsistent with the cost-benefit, act-utilitarian model.

The same priority emerges late in the *Ethical Principles* in the exegesis of Principle 7. Here is what is said:

Principle 7 summarizes the investigator's responsibilities. It implies that the principles relating to informed consent to participate (Principle 3), to fairness and freedom from exploitation in the research relationship (Principle 6), and to the removal of stressful consequences following completion of the research (Principle 9) must be scrupulously observed with compromise in these principles not to be tolerated insofar as the stress or risk is serious.[17]

If possible stress or risk to the participant is serious, there is to be *no* compromise in the principles. If the physical and mental stress or risk is not very serious and if the research is for a highly important purpose, then the research may be ethically warranted — with the usual stipulations or safeguards for the participant and exploration of alternative procedures. Otherwise risk and the violation of the principles of informed consent and fairness are "not to be tolerated." This, of course, requires an evaluative judgment and different investigators will have different estimates of what is serious risk. But the point I want to stress is that on this reading the ethical framework for decision gives uncompromising priority to the dignity, rights, and welfare of the research participant.

The Consent Requirement

I want to focus briefly now on the consent requirement, which seems to me to be particularly important for the deontological emphasis of a research code. The APA 1973 *Ethical Principles* emphasize the consent of the participant. However, we must recognize two things: (1) If the cost-benefit model is the basic thrust of the code, then the consent requirement can easily be weakened or overridden on utilitarian grounds. (2) Some psychologists plainly do feel that consent, especially informed consent, is a secondary consideration.

Let me cite an example of the denigration of the consent requirement, in this case from a context of discussion on medical experimentation. Dr. Louis Lasagna has said this:

> I want to take issue with (the) notion that consent is the pre-eminent question. Consent is primarily important in the abstract and appeals to those who are interested in civil libertarian problems. The major protection of the patient, however, comes from the review of protocols by peer and non-peer groups, from the competence of the investigator, and all of the ancillary facilities at his disposal, and from monitoring the performance of experiments.[18]

Now I agree that the major protection of the patient, or the subject or participant in the case of psychological experimentation, comes from these kind of factors. Still this does not mean that consent is important simply in the abstract. The consent requirement is a way of emphasizing the intrinsic worth and dignity, and the rights of individuals. Some form of consent seems to me to be an absolutely minimal requirement in most cases of the experimental use of human subjects in medical or psychological research. This device expresses our commitment to a deontological dimension of our value perspective, which is absent in talk about social utility, progress, cost-benefits, and welfare. The consent requirement emphasized by civil libertarians in effect says: we must make the rights of the individual a prime concern in research decisions, for respecting a person's rights is respecting the person. It is far too easy for dedicated researchers to undervalue and overlook the rights and dignity of the research participant, especially when they envisage monumental gains for society as a whole and for future generations. A strong emphasis on consent helps to balance these values.

But consent, like utility, can be overemphasized. Some researchers worry that such overemphasis would impede, perhaps even halt, important research. Much depends on how much is built into the consent requirement. Suppose consent required a fully informed subject, in which "fully informed" includes a complete grasp of research design and objectives. In a number of cases in psychological research, this would defeat the objective of the research itself. But in cases where that is not the case, some willing participants are not capable of fully grasping the research design and objective. Should they be ruled out as acceptable subjects? I think not. Basic information about the experiment should certainly be conveyed in any case, but additional information might justifiably be tailored to the subject's comprehension and interests.

Others insist that the consent requirement must include disinterested motivation of the consenting subject. I am inclined to agree that such strict construal of consent reflects an "excessive ethical fastidiousness," as Louis Jaffe puts it.[19] But the other side of the coin is that we lapse into far too loose a construal of the consent requirement or that we write it off as totally secondary to scientific gains. When either of these happens, the deontological dimension is seriously undercut. Persons are treated as objects, to be used and manipulated according to the researcher's needs. This happens when consent is coerced through economic or academic pressure, when the researcher fails to inform participants on central facts or when he falsifies or lies to the subject.[20]

One must grant that the concept of consent or of informed consent is quite complex. We cannot address those complexities here. But surely there are qualitative degrees of consent and the importance and quality of consent might justifiably vary from one research context to another. Still, in most cases, some minimal fulfillment of the consent requirement is essential. Whatever is required to respect the subject's dignity and his moral and legal rights should be fulfilled. Without this emphasis we are too easily led down the cost-benefit, act-utilitarian line, which can justify most anything in the interest of society's long-range welfare. What I am saying here, and at least in point of emphasis it disagrees with Dr. Lasagna's position (though Lasagna by no means suggests that consent be thrown out as a requirement), is this: review of protocols by peer and non-peer groups, a competent researcher, adequate facilities and careful monitoring of experiments — these criteria do not constitute an adequate framework for ethical assessment. Respect for subjects and their moral rights — the deontological dimension as well as the cost-benefit dimension — must be part and parcel of the perspective of the researcher and of review committees.

This is not to say that consent of the subject is itself sufficient to justify the use of the subject by the investigator. An experiment may be badly designed; it may involve high risks and have no social value. In such cases, the fact of consent by research subjects does not justify the experiment. Also I do not mean to imply that the consent requirement can never be overridden or simply not be required (or be legally renounced). Situations where even a minimal consent requirement can be justifiably overridden or ignored would be very rare. But they are certainly conceivable. Suppose that a horrendous disaster threatened the continued existence of the human race. Such a possibility is at least conceivable in a medical context, though my imagination fails me for a psychological context. But given this supposition, would not our moral framework justify the experimental use of some humans to save the rest of the race, including, of course, an overriding of their interests and rights? It seems to me that it would do so. In extreme circumstances, we waive our ordinary rules and priorities.

But, in formulating an ethic for experimentation, we are *not* concerned with what might be called morally extreme cases or "desert island" situations, where one's basic commitment to individual rights is challenged. We are concerned with ordinary situations where scientific and social progress is at stake but not the future of mankind. In ordinary situations we do not permit individual rights to be overridden. To avert an outright disaster, yes; simply to promote the good of society (longer life or better quality of life), no.

Placed in the context of medical or psychological experimentation, this means that experimentation which required overriding the values of human dignity and respect (embodied in the consent doctrine) might be justified if a case could be made out that it averts some horrendous disaster. This is a high burden of proof. In the case of all medical and psychological experimentation on humans of which I am aware, that proof is not forthcoming. Such experimentation may improve the human condition. It cannot be argued that it averts disaster. Therefore, even for those of us for whom ethical waters are quite muddy—in contrast to the clearcut Cartesians among us—and for whom social utility might override the claims of dignity and consent in some contexts, still the burden of proof for such a state of affairs is so high that it would almost never be justified. For this reason I agree with W. J. Curran and Henry Beecher who holds that "it is unthinkable that we make progress in medicine [and I would add psychology] at the expense of the rights of individuals."[21] (I emphasize the word "progress" here, for I cannot go as far as Curran who says that *no* end of social justification warrants depriving an individual of basic rights.)

A Suggestion About Models

Given the ambivalence, perhaps even the inconsistency, of the APA statement of principles and given the tremendous implications for the conduct of research and the treatment of research subjects which hangs on the choice of a model, it seems to me that the APA Committee on Ethical Standards in Psychological Research should focus on alternative ethical models and their implications for research. I am not suggesting that psychologists try to solve the problems of normative ethical theory or of metaethics, many of which philosophers themselves have left quite unresolved. I am suggesting that they explore more fully the implications of alternative ethical frameworks for psychological research, testing those implications against what might be called our common moral consciousness or prevailing social values and priorities. The intention of the 1973 *Principles* was in part to do this, and to avoid the advocacy of ethical absolutes ("We therefore are concerned with conflict resolution, not the advocacy of ethical absolutes."[22]). The *Principles* properly emphasize the complexity of the ethical issues involved and conflicts of obligation, insisting that "the ethical problems associated with psychological research in human beings cannot be solved by enunciating simple principles that point to absolute rights and wrongs."[23] Furthermore, the exegetical remarks state that the issues are so complex that psychology as a profession is "not yet ready . . . to take a unified stand on the issues . . . ."[24] And yet, what emerges in much of the 1973 statement of principles is a kind of moral absolutism, which comes out as act-utilitarianism in some contexts; as a form of deontologism in others. A more self-conscious exploration of several models for ethical decision-making with special reference to problems generated by the use of research subjects might help to iron out the inconsistencies or at least the appearance of inconsistencies in the *Principles* as presently formulated; also, it might assist in formulating a more adequate set of principles for the research psychologist.

What I have in mind is the clear articulation of the kinds of decisions or results which would be justified or permitted under an act-utilitarian model, and then, an assessment of whether those results square with our considered moral judgments on the matter. The same procedure would be followed with other models, say, a Kantian deontological model; and with a mixed model, one like that of W. D. Ross in which consequential and deontological elements are blended but in which there is a commitment to a hierarchy of *prima facie* duties.[25] An example of priorities in Ross' hierarchical ordering is this: The duty of not doing harm (non-malevolence) is more binding than the duty to do good (beneficence). If accepted, this has particular relevance for an ethic of experimental research.

I believe that the Ross model is more adequate than other models. The problems generated by the Kantian view that duties are unconditional or absolute in all contexts are avoided, and the Ross model offers a way of resolving conflicts of duty without falling into a purely utilitarian framework. It also leaves us with obvious problems. How do we decide which duties are *prima facie*? How do we decide which ones take precedence, generally, over others? How do we determine when there is adequate reason for one *prima facie* duty to override another? We cannot deal with these questions here. But whatever philosophical difficulties confront the Ross model, an exploration and testing of that model and its implications for a research ethic against our considered moral judgments and moral consciousness might be of considerable aid in formulating an adequate ethic of experimental research.[26]

Conclusion

Let me briefly summarize. What emerges from the 1973 APA code of ethics is a mixed bag. In some contexts the cost-benefit model completely dominates. In others, the deontological model, in which the rights and dignity of the research participant have absolute priority over the potential scientific and social progress of the research, dominates. I have suggested that a model similar to that of Ross might be a more adequate and fruitful model for the resolution of ethical issues involving the use of research participants.

Even an adequate model, however, does not assure that ethically proper decisions will be made in research projects using humans. Nothing assures that in any context. What this framework does assure, if given self-conscious attention in research contexts, is that the full range of relevant value considerations are weighed and balanced in the decision-process and that proper priority is given to those values (the dignity and rights of individuals) so essential to any civilized society.

In conclusion, I want to suggest the possible extension of certain procedures which are included in the 1973 *Ethical Principles* but which are not carried out as far as they could be as procedural safeguards for the dignity (and rights) and welfare of research subjects. Let me first indicate what my suggested extensions are extensions to. The 1973 *Principles* insist that the investigator incurs an obligation to consider alternative research approaches and to obtain ethical advice when there is any threat to the research subject (and the higher the risk the greater the obligation). There is no standardized way of getting that advice, but the *Principles* clearly distinguish between a mandatory review of a proposal by an institutional review group and a voluntary, self-initiated consultation process. The former is more of a clearinghouse for funding and an evaluation of the importance and viability of a research project. Except for blatant cases of possible subject mistreatment, it offers little ethical advice. The *Principles* insist on genuine ethical consultation, not simply a mandatory review for funding, and leave open broad alternatives in getting this.

So far, so good. But if genuine and sound ethical assessment and advice is to be had, it is essential that the full range of data bearing on the cost or danger to the participants, including any infringement on their dignity as persons, and the value of the research itself be thoroughly explored. There are several possible ways of assuring such thoroughness. (1) One is to broaden consultative committees so that the full range of opinion on hard cases is heard, and this will require getting committee members from outside of the psychological research complex (and adding to bureaucratic red tape). (2) Secondly, a requirement that the researcher and his institution must compensate all research subjects for harm done and rights violated would assure a more thorough review of research projects. It seems to me that there is little emphasis today on compensatory rights of research participants, nor on compensatory obligations of researchers and research institutions. It may be that the cost of instituting this would be prohibitive. I don't know. Whether it would slow down the pace of important research, I don't know. Hopefully not, since we are talking about hard cases only. I am confident that it would result in a more thorough review, even if only on a cost-benefit model; for when we are forced to assess risks on a monetary basis, our decisions are made in the real world, not in a fabricated or isolated one. (3) My third suggestion builds on a recommendation which Professor Guido Calabresi has made to assure adequate review in the context of medical experimentation on humans. It seems to me to be an important procedure for review of hard cases of psychological experimentation as well. The procedure: publish all of the cases decided by review committees.[27] Such a report could include a description of the research project, its purpose, the potential gains for science, the potential risks to the welfare and dignity of research subjects, the nature of the consent of the subjects, and accounts of the main pro and con arguments of the committee members. Published reports of this type would undoubtedly become objects of close scrutiny by both professional psychologists and non-professionals. Much as with key legal decisions, the pros and cons would be subject to intense analysis and reexamination. Research committee decisions would be critiqued from perspectives representing the full range of social values, not simply from the perspective of the professional complex, and from this open analysis, a more adequate set of guidelines for future decisions would surely emerge.

NOTES

1. This paper is a revised version of the Presidential Address to the Sixty-Seventh Annual Meeting of The Southern Society for Philosophy and Psychology held in New Orleans, La., March 27–29, 1975.

2. See The Nuremberg Code, The Results of Trials of War Criminals Before Nuremberg Military Tribunals Under Control Council Law No. 10 (Oct. 1946–Apr. 1949); in part reprinted in William J. Curran and E. Donald Shapiro, *Law, Medicine, and Forensic Science*, second ed. (Boston, 1970), pp. 887–9.

3. Institute of Society, Ethics, and The Life Sciences, Hastings-on-Hudson, N.Y., and The Kennedy Center, Washington, D.C.

4. See *The Atlanta Constitution,* Saturday, Sept. 14, 1974, p. 8A, for discussion of the legal suit filed against the U.S. Government by the Tuskegee research subjects.

5. Cited by Henry K. Beecher, "Ethics and Clinical Research," *New England Journal of Medicine,* vol. 274 (June 16, 1966), pp. 1354–60; also in Henry K. Beecher, "Medical Research and the Individual," in Daniel Labby, ed., *Life or Death: Ethics and Options* (Seattle: University of Washington Press, 1968), where 12 cases of unethical medical experimentation are discussed. See also M. H. Pappworth, *Human Guinea Pigs: Experimentation on Man* (Boston, 1968).

6. Cited by Beecher, "Medical Research and the Individual," p. 147.

7. Published by the American Psychological Association, Inc., Washington, D.C., 1973, hereafter referred to as *Ethical Principles.*

8. The occasion was the annual meeting of the Southern Society for Philosophy and Psychology, April, 1972. His paper, "Remarks on 'Ethical Standards for Psychological Research Involving Human Subject,'" was part of a symposium designed to critically review the tentative, prepublication statement of principles of the APA on conduct of research with human participants.

9. *Ethical Principles,* p. 10.

10. Ibid.

11. Ibid., p. 11.

12. Ibid., p. 12.

13. Ibid., p. 2.

14. Ibid., p. 11.

15. John Rawls, *A Theory of Justice* (Cambridge, Mass., 1971).

16. W. D. Ross, *The Right and The Good* (Oxford, 1930).

17. *Ethical Principles,* p. 61.

18. Quoted by Louis I. Jaffe, "Law as a System of Control," *Daedalus* 98, no. 2, special issue on "Ethical Aspects of Experimentation With Human Subjects" (Spring, 1969), pp. 420–21.

19. Ibid., p. 424.

20. Hans Jonas' suggestion of a "descending order of permissability" in the use of experimental subjects, in which the use of subjects who are "poorer in knowledge, motivation, and freedom of decision" requires a "more compelling . . . countervailing justification," rings a sound ethical bell. Hans Jonas, "Philosophical Reflections on Experimenting With Human Subjects," *Daedalus* 98, no. 2 (1969), p. 237. This would require stronger justification for the use of children, the insane, and prisoners.

21. Henry K. Beecher, "Medical Research and The Individual," in Daniel Labby, ed. *op. cit.*, p. 118.

22. *Ethical Principles*, p. 11.

23. Ibid., p. 10.

24. Ibid., p. 16.

25. Ross, *op. cit.*

26. I leave the notion of "our considered moral judgments and moral consciousness" unexplicated. I do not mean simply a cultural or national consensus discoverable by statistical survey but something like John Rawls' appeal to "reflective equilibrium" (*A Theory of Justice,* Harvard University Press, 1971), pp. 46–51, or Charles Baylis' appeal to "rational preference" in *Ethics, Principles of Wise Choice* (Henry Holt and Co., 1958), Ch. X. The entire issue of moral knowledge, both its possibility and its foundation, is at stake.

27. Guido Calabresi, "Reflections on Medical Experimentation in Humans," *Daedalus* 98, no. 2 (1969), pp. 400–401.

Task Force on Legal and Ethical Issues

Experimentation With Mentally Handicapped Subjects

Recommendation 1.

An educational campaign must be directed to the general public with regard to individual opportunity and obligation to participate in the advancement of scientific knowledge. A disproportionate share of the risk for the benefit of society as a whole should not be assigned to "convenient"—often institutionalized—populations, including mentally handicapped individuals. Rather, to the extent possible, such persons should bear less risk than those who are more able to make free and uncoerced decisions.

Commentary:

Everyone recognizes the importance of research in advancing our knowledge about the causes, prevention and techniques for curing or ameliorating mental handicaps. But news reports continue to remind us of excesses—sanctioned if not actually devised by governmental authorities—in the area of experimentation with human subjects. The history of abuses in experimentation includes several chapters involving institutionalized mentally disabled persons, such as the infamous Willowbrook (New York) hepatitis experiments (deliberate exposure of retarded children to hepatitis, on the basis of coerced parental consent); a similar but lesser known Willowbrook project using residents to test an ineffective shigella vaccine; the unconsented pneumonia, flu and meningitis experiments on residents of two State institutions in Pennsylvania; and the routine administration of Depo-Provera, an experimental and potentially harmful medication, to the female residents of mental institutions in Tennessee and elsewhere.[1] Such a recitation should also include the experimental psychosurgery, under the auspices of the State of Michigan, which was enjoined by the court in the case of *Kaimowitz* v. *Department of Mental Health.*[2]

On the other hand, such incidents actually represent a small deviation, so far as is known, from the general run of responsible and useful—or at least not harmful—experimentation with mentally disabled and other human subjects.[3] There is no question that some kinds of biomedical and behavioral research are necessary for continued advances in the diagnosis, prevention and treatment of mental and physical disabilities. Moreover, in the absence of a systematic approach, every patient or client becomes an experiment—yet nothing new is learned. Many drugs and procedures in current use are not considered experimental and are assumed to be of value simply because of familiarity or custom; but the only way truly to evaluate the effectiveness of these measures is through controlled clinical research.[4]

The basic issue, then, is the extent to which persons who have been deprived of their personal liberty on the basis of their alleged mental disability, or whose ability to give free and informed consent is otherwise questionable, should bear the burden of scientific progress on behalf of society as a whole. This issue is not just one of ethics. Where the individuals involved are in State institutions or confined pursuant to State law or where the research is conducted, supported or regulated by governmental agencies, it is also one of constitutional right.[5]

Persons confined to mental institutions are not incarcerated for the purpose of providing investigators with a captive population of research subjects, but rather to receive whatever services are necessary to enable them to return to society as quickly as possible.[6] Most institutions in the country, especially the large public institutions, are hard pressed to meet even minimal standards for safety, sanitation, staffing and habilitative and rehabilitative programs, and are hardly in a position to meet the increased demands imposed by the conduct of research projects. Moreover, such projects, if initiated, tend to attract concentrations of the best and most motivated institutional personnel (and the "best" patients or clients as well), to the detriment of patients or clients excluded from research projects as well as those subjected to the experimentation.

Because institutions are by nature removed from direct familial and public scrutiny, the potential for research abuses, intentional or not, cannot be discounted. Finally, patients or clients in institutions may not be able to give truly informed consent to participate in experimentation, both because of their presumably disabled condition and because of the well-recognized coercive effects of institutionalization itself.

Recommendation 2.

(a) Covert experimentation involving risks ought never to be permitted, regardless of the asserted justification, and full disclosure of such matters as research risks, expected benefits and the right to refuse participation must be made to potential subjects and, where appropriate, to their parents, surrogate parents or legal guardians:

(b) Experimentation which is neither directly beneficial to individual subjects nor related to such subjects' mental condition and which poses any degree of risk to such

subjects should not be permitted with institutionalized mentally handicapped individuals.

(c) Research performed for the direct benefit of a mentally handicapped subject after nonexperimental procedures, if any, have been exhausted should be permitted where the risk/benefit ratio is favorable and there are adequate procedures for obtaining the subject's consent or, where appropriate, the consent of the subject's parent, parent surrogate or legal guardian. High-risk experimental procedures such as psychosurgery should be permitted, if at all, only upon the informed consent of the subject himself; some such procedures ought to be prohibited altogether, at least with respect to institutionalized individuals.

Commentary:

Covert experimentation, especially upon mentally handicapped individuals in institutions or the community, has no place in an ethical society. Nor, the Panel feels, dces experimentation with institutionalized mentally handicapped persons which does not benefit them directly or relate to the prevention, diagnosis or treatment of their mental condition. There is no acceptable reason for testing a hepatitis or shigella vaccine, for example, on an institutionalized mentally disabled population when such physical ailments are not peculiar to mentally handicapped individuals and can be identified or induced as readily in experiments with subjects whose capacity and autonomy are not open to question.

On the other hand, research designed to improve an individual mental condition which has not responded to standard techniques ought to be permitted, with proper safeguards, upon mentally handicapped persons. (Ideally, the benefits of such experimentation will extend to others who suffer from a similar or related condition — *i.e.,* there is also an expected gain in general scientific knowledge about that specific condition.) In general, objections to such research by a patient or client should be honored, although the objection of a legally incompetent individual might be overridden (or an experimental procedure might be imposed upon a nonobjecting incompetent subject) where the potential benefit is great and the risk comparatively low. In such cases, appropriate consent should be obtained from parents or legal guardians. Certain procedures, such as psychosurgery, involve such a high degree of risk that they ought never to be employed on the basis of substituted consent, and in some situations should be prohibited altogether. Psychosurgery, even if intended for therapeutic purposes, should be included in any discussion of high-risk experimentation because it is such a drastic and irreversible procedure and because so much uncertainty exists as to its effects and the factors influencing such effects.

Recommendation 3.

At a minimum, research upon mentally handicapped individuals for the purpose of obtaining new scientific or medical information should be conditioned upon the following requirements:

(a) The research protocol must undergo independent review for scientific merit of the research design and for competence of the investigator.

(b) The institution, if any, in which the research is to be conducted must meet recognized standards for medical-care, direct care and other services necessary to meet the increased demands imposed by research activities, in addition to the ordinary requirements of adequate care and treatment.

(c) The proposed research must not reduce the level of habilitative or rehabilitative services available either to research participants or to patients or clients not included in the project.

(d) The experimentation must involve an acceptably low level of risk to the health or well-being of the research subjects;

(e) The proposed research should relate directly to the prevention, diagnosis or treatment of mental disability and should seek only information which cannot be obtained from other types of subjects. Such information should be of high potential significance for the advancement of acknowledged medical or scientific objectives related to mental disability.

(f) Research involving risk may be performed only on patients or clients who are actually competent to consent to participation therein and who have in fact given such consent. Substituted consent to procedures involving risk should not be permitted except in the most unusual and compelling circumstances and never in the face of objections, however expressed, by the patient or client himself. All consent should be subject to review and approval by an independent body, with an opportunity for patients or clients to be advised and represented in this process by an independent advocate (who may be an attorney).

(g) All subjects, and where appropriate their parents or guardians, should be provided with and informed of their right to any follow-up care necessitated by unforeseen harmful consequences of the research project.

Commentary:

The most problematic questions in this area arise with regard to research which does not directly benefit a particular group of subjects but which promises to produce important new knowledge concerning mentally handicapped persons generally. The questions become even more difficult, if not insoluble, when children — by definition incapable of informed consent — are involved as subjects of such experiments.

So long as privacy and confidentiality are respected, the Panel is not particularly concerned with nontherapeutic research which is merely observational in nature or which involves the mere use or sampling of urine, feces or other specimens normally available or obtainable at no risk to the subject. Other, more intrusive types of experimentation, however, should be subject to at least the strictures outlined above. Since there is no anticipated benefit to the individual subject, the objections of patients or clients ought to be binding, whatever the age or legal competence of the person involved, and substituted consent should rarely if ever be permitted. In most instances, affirmative consent—rather than absence of objection—should be a prerequisite for involvement in nontherapeutic research.

In view of the risk inherent in much experimentation and the potential vulnerability of mentally handicapped subjects, particularly in closed institutions, the importance of institutional review boards and other monitoring bodies cannot be overstated. Clearly, such bodies should not be limited to or dominated by peers of the investigating clinicians, but should include attorneys, citizen advocates and mentally handicapped individuals or their representatives.

Recommendation 4.

(a) Whatever schema is eventually put forward by the National Commission for the Protection of Human Subjects of Biomedical and Behavioral Research should be considered as tentative and subject to continuous review.
(b) A permanent National Commission for the Protection of Human Subjects of Biomedical and Behavioral Research, with a membership including mentally handicapped individuals and/or former patients or institutional residents and parents of children with mental handicaps should be established to evaluate and, if necessary, modify the policies resulting from the recommendations of the current Commission and to monitor the performance of institutional review boards and other bodies charged with protection of the rights of research subjects.

Commentary:

In 1973, Congress established the National Commission for the Protection of Human Subjects of Biomedical and Behavioral Research (Public Law 93-348), charged with recommending the standards for the protection of research subjects. Final recommendations on experimentation with the "institutionalized mentally infirm" and on the functions of institutional review boards are anticipated shortly. Final recommendations for research on children have already been submitted.[7] The testimony before and deliberations of the National Commission illustrate the complexity of the issues related to experimentation with human subjects, particularly "special" or "vulnerable" subjects such as some mentally handicapped individuals.

While unequivocal and unambiguous guidelines may be desirable, the area of human experimentation does not lend itself to simplistic answers. Even such basic concepts as "therapeutic" and "nontherapeutic" research, the terms "research" and "experimentation" themselves, "low" or "minimal" risk and "informed consent" need to be defined with new precision. Moreover, the trend toward deinstitutionalization of mentally handicapped individuals raises the questions of the extent to which the protections afforded persons in traditional large institutions can or should be extended to those in other residential settings and to mentally handicapped individuals living in the community, including children enrolled in the public schools.

Because of the difficulty of these questions and the importance of balanced regulation in this area, the Task Panel feels that continued oversight and review is essential. In particular, for the reasons noted above, the functions of institutional review boards and other such monitoring bodies must be a primary focus of the ongoing review process.

NOTES

1. Goldby, S., "Experiments at the Willowbrook State School," 1 *The Lancet* 749 (1971); testimony of Dr. Max Werner, December 12, 1974, *New York State Association for Retarded Children and Parisi v. Carey,* No. 72-C-356/357 (E.D.N.Y.); "Kids Used as Guinea Pigs," *Pittsburgh Post Gazette,* April 14, 1973; hearings, "Quality of Health Care—Human Experimentation, 1973," Subcommittee on Health, Senate Committee on Labor and Public Welfare, February 21–22, 1973.

2. No. 73-19434-AW (Cir. Ct. of Wayne County, Mich., July 10, 1973).

3. See Cardon *et al.* "Injuries to Research Subjects, A Survey of Investigators," 295 *New Eng. Jour. of Med.* 650 (1976).

4. See remarks of Eisenberg, L., in Experiments and Research with Humans: Values in Conflict, at 96 (Washington, D.C. 1975).

5. See *Knecht v. Gillman,* 488 *F.*2d 1136 (8th Cir. 1973); *Mackey v. Procunier,* 477 *F.*2d 877 (9 Cir. 1973); *Kaimowitz v. Department of Mental Health,* No. 73-19434-AW (Cir. Ct. of Wayne County, Mich., July 10, 1973). *Cf. Rochin v. California,* 342 U.S. 165 (1952); Schloendorff v. Society of New York Hospitals, 211 N.Y. 125, 105 N.E. 92 (1914).

6. See *O'Connor v. Donaldson,* 422 U.S. 563 (1975); *Wyatt v. Stickney,* 344 *F. Supp.* 373 and 387 (M.D. Ala. 1972). aff'd sub nom. *Wyatt v. Aderholt,* 503 *F.*2d 1305 (5 Cir. 1974).

7. *Report and Recommendations: Research Involving Children,* The National Commission for the Protection of Human Subjects of Biomedical and Behavioral Research, DHEW Pub. No. (OS) 77-0004 (Washington, D.C.). See also the National Commission's recommendations on research involving prisoners, 42 F.R. 3075 (January 14, 1977), and the rules proposed by the Department of Health, Education, and Welfare, 43 F.R. 1049 (January 5, 1978). The Commission has also made recommendations in the area of psychosurgery. *Report and Recommendations Psychosurgery,* DHEW Pub. No. (OS) 77-0001 (Washington, D.C.).

Suggestions for Further Reading

Abernethy, Virginia, and Lundin, Keith. "Competency and the Right to Refuse Medical Treatment." In Abernethy, Virginia, ed. *Frontiers in Medical Ethics*. Cambridge, Massachusetts: Ballinger Publishing Co., 1980.

Allen, R.C., et al. *Mental Impairment and Legal Incompetency*. Englewood Cliffs: Prentice-Hall, Inc., 1968.

Ayd, Frank J., Jr. *Medical, Moral and Legal Issues in Mental Health Care*. Baltimore: The Williams and Wilkins Co., 1974, Chs. 3 and 4 on psychiatric research.

Blackstone, William T. "The American Psychological Association Code of Ethics for Research Involving Human Participants." *The Southern Journal of Philosophy* 13 (1975):407–417.

Brady, John P., and Brodie, H. Keith, eds. *Controversy in Psychiatry*. Philadelphia: W. B. Saunders Co., 1978, Ch. 24.

Casebook on Ethical Standards of Psychologists. Washington, D.C.: American Psychological Association, 1967.

Chayet, Neil L. "Informed Consent of the Mentally Disabled, A Failing Fiction." *Psychiatric Annals* 6 (June 1976):82ff.

Culver, Charles M., et al. "ECT and Special Problems of Informed Consent." *American Journal of Psychiatry* 137 (May 1980):586–591.

Davidson, Henry A. "Legal and Ethical Aspects of Psychical Research." *American Journal of Psychiatry* 126 (August 1969):237–240.

"Ethical Principles in the Conduct of Research with Human Participants." *American Psychologist* 28 (January 1973):79–80.

Ethical Principles in the Conduct of Research with Human Participants. Washington, D.C.: American Psychological Association, 1973.

Ethical Standards of Psychologists. Washington, D.C.: American Psychological Association, 1977 and 1981.

"Freedom of Inquiry and Subjects." *American Journal of Psychiatry* 134 (August 1977):891–913.

Friedman, Paul R. "Legal Regulation of Applied Behavior Analysis in Mental Institutions and Prisons." *Arizona Law Review* 17 (1975):39–104, especially pp. 75–91.

Garvey, John. "Freedom and Choice in Constitutional Law." *Harvard Law Review* 94 (1981):1756–1794.

Gaylin, Willard. "Who Speaks for the Helpless: The Question of Proxy Consent." *Journal of the American Academy of Child Psychiatry* 18 (Summer 1979): 419–436.

Grisso, Thomas. *Juveniles' Waiver of Rights, Legal and Psychological Competence.* New York: Plenum Publishing Co., 1980.

Guidelines for Psychologists for the Use of Drugs in Research. Washington, D.C.: American Psychological Association, 1971.

Howell, T., and Stack, R. L. "The Ethics of Human Experimentation in Psychiatry: Toward a More Informed Consensus." *Psychiatry* 44 (May 1981):113–132.

"Informed Consent: When Can It Be Withdrawn?" *Hastings Center Review* 2 (1972):10–11. An electroshock case.

Katz, J. "Who's Afraid of Informed Consent?" *Journal of Psychiatry and Law* 4 (1976):315–325.

"Informed Consent in Human Research, Mental Health and Therapeutic Relationship." In Reich, Warren T., ed. *Encyclopedia of Bioethics.* New York: The Free Press, 1978, Vol. II, pp. 751–778.

Kelman, Herbert C. "The Rights of the Subject in Social Research: An Analysis in Terms of Relative Power and Legitimacy." *American Psychologist* 27 (November 1972):989–1016.

Kolata, Gina Bari. "Electroshock Experiment at Albany Violates Ethics Guidelines." *Science* 1988 (October 28, 1977):383–386.

MacKay, Charles R., and Shea, John M. "Ethical Considerations in Research on Huntington's Disease." *Clinical Research* 25 (October 1977):241–247.

Macklin, Ruth. *Man, Mind, and Morality: The Ethics of Behavior Control.* Englewood Cliffs: Prentice-Hall, 1982.

"Medical Experimentation: A Symposium on Behavior Control." *Duquesne Law Review* 24 (1975):375–392.

"Mental Health and Human Rights: Report of the Task Panel on Legal and Ethical Issues." *Arizona Law Review* 20 (1978):111–117.

Milgram, Stanley. *Obedience to Authority.* New York: Harper & Row, 1974.

Murphy, Jeffrie G. "Total Institutions and the Possibility of Consent to Organic Therapies." *Human Rights* (Fall 1975):25–45.

Rada, Richard T. "Informed Consent in the Care of Psychiatric Patients." *National Association of Private Psychiatric Hospitals* 8 (1976):9–12.

"Research, Behavioral." In Reich, Warren T. *Encyclopedia of Bioethics* Vol. IV. New York: The Free Press, 1978, pp. 1470–1481.

Research Involving Psychosurgery — Report and Recommendations — With Appendix

(Bethesda, Maryland: US DHEW, Publication No. (OS) 77-0001 and (OS) 77-0002, March 14, 1977).

Research Involving Those Institutionalized as Mentally Infirm — With Appendix (Bethesda, Maryland: US DHEW, Publication No. (OS) 78-0006 and (OS) 78-0007, February 2, 1978).

Romano, John. "Reflections on Informed Consent." *Archives of General Psychiatry* 30 (January 1974):129–135.

Schlenker, Barry R., and Forsyth, Donelson R. "On the Ethics of Psychological Research." *Journal of Experimental Social Psychology* 13 (1977):369–396.

Shuman, Samuel I. *Psychosurgery and the Medical Control of Violence.* Detroit: Wayne State University Press, 1977, Ch. 7.

Spoonhour, J. M. "Psychosurgery and Informed Consent." *University of Florida Law Review* (Spring 1974):432–452.

Stone, Alan A. "Informed Consent: Special Problems in Psychiatry." *Hospital and Community Psychiatry* 30 (June 1979):407–411.

Tancredi, Laurence, R., et al. *Legal Issues in Psychiatric Care.* New York: Harper & Row, 1975, Chs. 7, 8, and 9.

Turnbull, H. Rutherford, III, ed., *Consent Handbook.* Washington, D.C.: American Association of Mental Deficiency, 1977.

Warwick, Donald P. "Social Scientists Ought to Stop Lying." *Psychology Today* 8 (February 1975):38ff.

Werhofen, Henry, and Usdin, Gene L. "Who Is Competent to Make a Will?" *Mental Hygiene* 54 (January 1970):37–43.

5. Coercion in Commitment Voluntary and Involuntary Hospitalization and Dangerousness

Introduction

There are basically two types of admissions to mental hospitals: voluntary and involuntary. In theory, voluntary patients come of their own accord, whereas involuntary patients are coerced into hospitalization. In our first selection, Peter R. Breggin scrutinizes this contrast and calls attention to the many coercive factors which typically influence even voluntary hospitalization. Most of these commitments are voluntary only in the sense that they are nonjudicial; the presence of coercion remains an open question.

Involuntary hospitalization, which may be on an emergency short-term basis or on a regular long-term basis, is overtly coercive; but there are many subclasses. Patients who are committed through civil and criminal procedures are hospitalized as a consequence of decisions made by others, whether the patients like it or not. Several varieties of criminal commitments will be examined in section 9, and our present focus will be on civil commitment. This actually applies more in theory than practice to persons who have not committed or at least are not being prosecuted for any crimes. As Joseph M. Livermore and his co-authors indicate in our second selection, historically, civil patients have been coerced into hospitalization for an incredible variety of reasons. Among these are the need for treatment or custodial care, being a social nuisance, being an economic burden to others, being incapable of caring for oneself, or being overtly dangerous to self or others. Prior to the relatively recent deinstitutionalization emphasis, our mental hospitals were inundated with unwilling persons unwanted by society and therefore hospitalized (incarcerated?) under such diffuse civil commitment statutes. Civil commitment has been so grossly abused that many critics propose that it be entirely eliminated.

In recent years the trend has been toward tightening up civil commitment laws, instead of eliminating them, limiting coercive noncriminal commitment to persons who are both mentally ill *and* dangerous to others or to self, the latter either overtly or through neglect. Even here there are serious conceptual and empirical difficulties. What is "dangerousness"? It has been construed to mean almost everything from hurting someone's feelings to writing bad checks to threatened or actual homicidal, suicidal, or mutilative behavior (whether to self or others). The better laws define "dangerousness" as applying only to an *imminent* likelihood of *serious physical* harm to self or others, as manifested by actual threats or overtly aggressive acts. At the point of overt aggression, the distinction between civil and criminal commitment tends to collapse. Evidence of dangerousness is constituted by criminal behaviors such as battery, assault, homicide, and attempted suicide. It is simply not true that horrendous injustice is perpetrated against such civil patients because they are incarcerated without having committed a crime (though they have not been tried and convicted for such). The real difference between these individuals and other offenders processed through the criminal justice system is that, somewhere along the way, someone has decided not to take out a warrant or press charges against them, usually for humanitarian reasons. Dangerousness predicated on *threats* of harm is much more troublesome. As predictions of *future* behavior, all pronouncements of dangerousness border on unconstitutional preventive detention; but the problem is especially acute where no overtly aggressive acts have been performed.

Many other difficulties with respect to dangerousness are raised by Livermore et al. as well as by Saleem A. Shah in our third selection. Among these are: Do we predict dangerousness on the basis of our knowledge of the individual person or on the basis of the fact that he or she belongs to a general class of patients with similar diagnoses? Do not mental health professionals grossly over-predict dangerousness far in excess of anything that can be empirically verified to protect themselves against malpractice suits? Are not most predictions of dangerousness horrendously inaccurate anyway; and, if so, has not society placed a heavy responsibility upon psychiatric professionals which they are ill equipped to perform? An 85 percent rate of inaccuracy in predicting dangerousness is very impressive! Why should we preventively detain mental patients for dangerousness when we do not do so for much more dangerous persons such as ex-prison inmates, members of street gangs, or drunken drivers? How can equal protection under the law and due process be assured in civil commitment procedures for persons accused of dangerousness?

There are other important issues as well. Since dangerousness in the absence of mental illness is not a sufficient warrant for involuntary mental hospitalization, what concept of "mental illness" is operative here? This is a critical problem since there is no agreed upon definition of this key general concept in the psychiatric or psychological professions, and since statutory definitions are always incredibly vague or circular. Since dangerous behavior is often regarded as sufficient evidence of mental illness, the requirement of both mental illness and dangerousness often becomes a vacuous tautology.

Finally, what is coercion? The core of this concept consists of the attempt to get someone to do what you want them to do by using force, by threatening them with some harm or actually harming them. But does the concept also include offering them positive inducements as well? Where positive inducements are offered in a setting in which they might be abnormally potent (as for example in dealing with deprived institutionalized persons), it might be best to use some more positive words for the strategies of persuasion involved, such as "enticement," "seduction," "undue incentive," "manipulation," to name a few. All such concepts may refer to morally questionable activities that subvert a person's rational autonomy in some way. "Coercion" also needs to be defined in terms of the intentions of the coercer, not merely in terms of the perceptions of the coercee, as Breggin does in his essay. We should also note that classifying an act as coercive does not thereby render it morally objectionable, though it may typically be so. The threat of legal penalties is always coercive but not always morally wrong, and we do not always object to the coercive punishment of prisoners and children. The problem of how to distinguish between justifiable and unjustifiable coercion still remains. Is there something about mental patients which would justify coercive institutionalization? Once institutionalized, may patients refuse treatment? This final question is so important that the last essay of section 6 will be devoted to it.

Involuntary commitment on the basis of being a danger to oneself becomes an especially acute problem when the issue is suicide prevention. Should we allow suicidal persons to "die with their rights on" without paternalistic intervention, even though at some time a majority of them will greatly appreciate such intervention? Though there probably is such a thing as rational suicide, the most relevant practical rule for dealing with emergency suicidal patients brought to mental hospitals is still "When in doubt, treat." Rational suicides will always find another chance, assuming that they are not incarcerated forever. In the final selection, David F. Greenberg proposes that definite time limits be set for suicidal patients. After all, the severely depressed patients who are the typical suicidal cases are not our paradigms of rational autonomy; so there is a rationale for temporary intervention. But how long is too long? In light of the fact that it often takes three weeks or so for some anti-depressant drugs and other psychotropic medication to become effective, most mental health professionals probably will find Greenberg's twenty-four hour limit to be much too brief; but what about a maximum of from three to five weeks?

Peter R. Breggin

Coercion of Voluntary Patients in an Open Hospital

Author's Note (1982)

"Coercion of Voluntary Patients in an Open Hospital" was written twenty years ago when I was training as an intern in a small psychiatric hospital. The article was a first in the literature — an analysis of the oppression and control of psychiatric patients in an allegedly open, humanistically oriented psychiatric hospital. Unhappily, the article remains a first. I know of no other similar analysis in the official psychiatric literature over the subsequent twenty years.

Psychiatry remains as reluctant as ever to recognize the devastating impact of its treatments upon the minds and brains of its patients. The personal, subjective response of the patient is almost wholly ignored in the psychiatric literature. Meanwhile, in private practice, as well as in clinics and hospitals, the psychiatric patient is subjected to a variety of threats and controls, from the simple authority of the physician to the more concrete menace of *involuntary* drugging, electroshock, and incarceration. Despite many legal attempts to increase the civil liberties of mental patients, it remains true today that even the ostensibly *voluntary* mental patient has almost no protection against assault with the psychiatric armamentorium.

For those psychiatric patients who experience the relatively benign and sometimes helpful experience of psychotherapy in private practice, the threat of psychiatric oppression may seem remote. But should this same patient become "irrational," "self-destructive," "dangerous," "mentally ill," or even "in

From *Archives of General Psychiatry* 10 (1964):173–181. Copyright © 1964 by the American Medical Association. Reprinted by permission of the publisher and the author.

need of hospital treatment" in the opinion of his well-meaning psychiatrist, his civil liberties can be abrogated, and he can be committed to a mental hospital.

Over the years, I have broadened my criticism of institutional psychiatry as a form of political totalitarianism—the use of state power to control the individual.[1-8] Seldom will the liberty and the integrity of an individual be subjected to a greater threat than when he comes under the scrutiny of psychiatric authorities. In the Western world today, psychiatry remains the greatest threat to the civil liberties and the mental integrity of individual citizens. Few people realize the potential danger to which they expose themselves when they ask for help from a psychiatrist or when they voluntarily enter a mental hospital. But at this moment of great need and vulnerability, the mental patient may find himself in a no-win contest with the overwhelming power and authority of psychiatry.

Introduction

The long history of the open hospital, with its goal to limit the coercion of patients, has recently been reviewed.[6,7] The open hospital may also be a field of study for more subtle forms of coercion that might go unnoticed in other hospitals. The absence of outright locked doors tends to draw attention to these more indirect forms of control over the patient. In an environment dedicated to the elimination of coercion, the staff and the patients will then be exquisitely sensitive to any which continues to manifest itself. In addition, the absence of the locked ward means that any coercion must be directed by an individual doctor against an individual patient, making it more painfully obvious to everyone in the hospital.

This ironic situation provides fertile ground for studying coercion. It might also be used by some as evidence for the inadequacy of open hospitals and by others as evidence for the insidiousness of coercion even within ideal circumstances. The topic is so charged with dramatic ethical, legal, and therapeutic considerations that I might best explain my own bias at the start. I am ethically committed to the principle that coercion should be limited as much as possible but believe that the actual extent of this limitation cannot be decided until we know considerably more about the effects of coercion upon the patient.

Definition of Coercion

By coercion is meant any action, or threat of action, which compels the patient to behave in a manner inconsistent with his own wishes. The compelling aspect can be direct physical or chemical restraint, or it can be indirect threatened recriminations or indirect "force of authority" which convinces the patient that no other legal or medical alternative is available to him.

Coercive behavior falls into the general category of manipulative behavior, in which one person feels that his actions are determined by someone else, despite his own wishes. Coercion may be considered the experience of an unusually constraining or intimidating alternative, so that the individual feels his freedom of choice is pre-empted.

This is a practical definition in which the reference point is the patient's feeling of being compelled. It is meant to define a common element in the patient's response to such diverse experiences as enforced confinement to a locked ward; self-imposed restriction to an unlocked ward for fear of certification to another hospital; self-imposed restriction to an unlocked ward after receiving the impression that one has no legal right to leave the ward; or self-imposed restriction because one believes that no other medical alternative is available. The focus must be upon the patient's feeling or response, otherwise the patient is subjected to another imposition whereby he loses even his right to decide what is coercive. Defining coercion from the patient's point of view also takes into account individual variations: some patients may not feel coerced by any of these alternatives, either because they do not fear them or because they do not wish to leave the ward, while other patients will be particularly sensitive to the alternatives either because they strongly wish to leave the ward or greatly fear the threats presented to them.

Definition from the patient's point of view is not without ambiguities. For example, it will often be difficult to distinguish between different levels of response in the patient. The patient may say that he feels coerced, while he behaves as if he is not, or the patient may deny feeling coerced while he acts as if he is. Equally difficult, the patient may perceive coercion in a situation where few others would. These problems cannot be avoided, since coercion is relative to the individual, and to the situation. Life itself exists along a continuum of coercion in which the individual often feels that his behavior is in part determined by direct constraints or threats. The definition cannot do away with the ambiguities and relativity inherent in the situation, but it can draw attention to the patient's response to various constraints, pressures, or threats within the hospital environment.

Description of the Open Hospital

The doors of the hospital and all its wards are all open during the day from 8 AM to 8 PM. Otherwise, the setting is like that of other acute treatment hospitals with active residency training programs. The Syracuse Psychiatric Hospital is part of the New York State Department of Mental Hygiene. It is located in the midst of the city of 250,000, near the Syracuse University Campus, and side-by-side with the State University of New York Upstate Medical Center, from which it draws its staff and residents. The average daily census is 55 patients, and the average stay is 45 days, although some patients stay several months. Each therapist has from six to ten patients most of the time, providing ample time for intense psychotherapy with selected patients. While the bias of the hospital is toward psychotherapy, many patients also receive tranquilizers, and 10% eventually receive electroconvulsive treatment.

The patient population represents a somewhat modified cross-section of the city's more acute psychiatric problems. Some of the city's unusual management problems or recurrently rehospitalized patients may be sent directly to a larger state hospital, but others will be admitted to Syracuse Psychiatric Hospital (S. P. H.) and subsequently sent on to one of the other state hospitals.

Of the several admission forms provided by the laws of New York State, three accounted for all admissions to S. P. H. in 1962. In keeping with the hospital's attitude, 82% of last year's admissions were voluntary. These voluntary patients can be held for 15 days against their will, at which time they may be required to give ten days' notice before leaving the hospital (Chapter 27, Mental Hygiene Law, in the consolidated laws of New York State, available in 1962). As the only appropriate community facility, the hospital does accept a certain number of involuntary admissions. Of these 18%, most are admitted involuntarily by the hospital admitting officer at the request of a responsible member of the community, usually the family physician. The remainder of the involuntary admissions are by a community health officer. The hospital did not admit any court certified patients during the year.

During the past year, 93.2% of the patients admitted were eventually discharged to return to the community. The remaining 6.8% were committed to one of the two larger state hospitals serving the area. This certification is made by the court, after either the family or the Commissioner of Public Welfare has signed the appropriate papers. At least one patient has been certified each month during the past year, so that each patient who stays a month or more witnesses the certification of one or more other patients.

The alternative to admission to S. P. H. is usually admission to one or the larger state hospitals. Few individuals qualify for admission to the Syracuse Veteran's Administration psychiatric wards, the community's one private sanitarium, or the community's one general hospital with a private psychiatric ward. Similarly, the alternative to discharge from S. P. H. is certification to one of these same two large state hospitals. Thus other alternatives at the time of admission and discharge are usually limited to admission or certification to a larger state hospital. The larger state hospitals thereby figure importantly in the patient's attitude to his hospitalization in S. P. H.

The larger state hospital most familiar to the patients and the staff, and symbolic of "The State Hospital," is located about one hour's drive from Syracuse outside a nearby city. The hospital is among the best known and respected within the large and progressive New York State hospital system. The attitudes of the S. P. H. patients and psychotherapists toward this hospital will be described as the topic of coercion is elaborated.

The Physician's Use of Coercion

There are many reasons why the resident therapist may at times feel the need to act against the patient's will, even in the open hospital.

First, he may believe he has an ethical, professional, or religious responsibility to help the patient, even if the patient does not want help. The physician may believe that the patient, like a child, is unable to make the best decision for himself, and therefore must have someone else "take over" for him. The physician knows that patients often resist the initial efforts of their therapists, only to thank them later. He knows that many patients, and society in general, *expect* him to take this responsibility. He may perceive at times that the patient often *wants* him to be coercive. In addition, his medical training has conditioned him to trust his own judgment in determining what will be of benefit to the patient.[9]

Second, the therapist may be motivated to coerce the patient by a sense of responsibility toward the patient's family and toward the society. The therapist may wish to mitigate the patient's hostility, or to restrain the patient from physically or psychologically harming others. He may also wish to rehabilitate the patient into a socially and economically productive human being. He may believe these goals at times transcend the patient's immediate, and perhaps irresponsible, wishes.

Third, the therapist may be concerned about placing himself in legal jeopardy if he does not accept responsibility for his patient and society. For example, he may fear being sued by the family of a patient who harms or kills himself. He may also place his residency appointment in jeopardy if he does not at times coerce his patient. In any contemporary hospital, no matter how "open" its attitude, his superiors will at times hold him responsible for his patient's welfare and the society's welfare. Thus, legal and professional survival add impetus to any other motives which might influence him to coerce his patient.

Fourth, the therapist may be motivated to protect or enhance his own self-image and prestige through the actions of his patient. Thus, he may wish to coerce his patients into avoiding or performing certain acts. A patient who kills someone else, or who kills himself, can deal a severe blow to the resident therapist's self-image and prestige. To a lesser extent, a patient who does not respond in an appropriate fashion to psychotherapy is bound to reflect upon the therapist. An example of this is found in a recent paper which encourages psychiatrists to use the relative number of patients who sign out Against Medical Advice as a reflection of the resident's ineptitude.[4] Such an attitude on the part of supervisors is bound to encourage trainees to coerce their patients into more acceptable forms of behavior. At S. P. H. any such arbitrary "grading system" would be frowned upon. Nonetheless, the residents sometimes feel that the proportion of their patients certified reflects upon them. While few residents, if any, would rationally accept so gross a standard of therapeutic success or failure, most would admit to embarrassment and a sense of failure when one of their patients is certified to a larger state hospital. When it appears that a patient is "in danger of getting certified," a strong impulse then arises to modify the patient's behavior by restricting his liberty, by threat of certification, by electroconvulsive treatment, or by heavy tranquilization.

Fifth, the therapist might coerce the patient for motives entirely inappropriate for the situation. To give an example with infinite variations, one resident became aware that he refused his patient weekend passes in part because he resented her wish to visit home rather than to attend the Saturday therapy session. Many motives to coerce might result from counter-transference of various intensities, many of which the therapist-in-training might not recognize. There is little reason to presume that first or second year residents, or really anyone, would be immune to these motives. Supervision by more highly trained psychiatrists might mitigate some of these motives, if the supervision and the supervisor were oriented in this way. On the other hand, the supervisor usually has his own coercive powers over the trainee, setting an example for one individual to coerce another. In addition, since the supervisor's use of coercion will depend in part upon his evaluation of the trainee's patient, the resident may feel the need to coerce his patient into behavior consistent with the supervisor's expectations.

Finally, the therapist may feel that the existence of the larger state hospitals creates a situation in which, in order to avoid even greater coercion, he must himself act coercively upon the patient. For example, he may anticipate that certain acting out by his patient will eventually lead to certification by the staff. He might then compromise his own antipathy to coercion by using a little "prophylactic coercion," hoping a few restrictions on the patient's liberty, or electroconvulsive therapy, will discourage further acting out. Similarly, if he has a very low opinion of the larger state hospital, he may feel that the "danger of being sent away" is greater than the danger of temporarily coercing his patient. He may feel that separation from the psychotherapy would harm the patient at a crucial time when the patient is acting out. However, even if the therapist has no desire at all to coerce the patient, he may indirectly increase the threat of coercion by communicating his own anxiety about the threat to the patient. For example, the therapist may tell the patient, "I would not want to see you committed, but I feel you should know that your present behavior will lead the hospital administration to advise your commitment."

If the physician decides to use coercion, three basic methods are available to him: restriction of liberty, certification to a larger hospital, or treatment with electroconvulsive therapy and large doses of medication. Each of these can be coercive when used as threats, as direct constraints, or as punishments. In each case, the patient feels compelled to act against his will.

Despite the absence of locked doors, control over the patient's physical liberty remains the most frequent means of coercion. The physician may limit the patient's freedom to move around the hospital, he may refuse weekend passes, or he may insist that the patient remain in the hospital for the full 25 days stipulated in the voluntary admission form. In many instances, nearly every therapeutic hour with a hospitalized patient will revolve around direct or indirect bargaining for increased liberties with improved behavior. For example, the patient may request a pass to leave the ward, and the physician may respond that the patient's behavior still lacks sufficient self-control. No matter what the therapist's attitude, the coerciveness of the implication cannot be avoided—if the patient does not change his behavior, he will not be given more freedom.

From the physician's point of view, coercion through real or threatened physical restriction is often very taxing and very disagreeable. Although most patients will not defy his legal authority, he must on occasion further implement his restrictions to the ward. This is very difficult in an open hospital and places a great deal of strain upon the ward personnel who are directly responsible for watching the patient's movements, and for restraining him, somehow, without the locked door. The use of restrictions on liberty is also frankly contrary to the "open door" attitude, and often extremely repugnant to the physician.

The second means of coercion, threatened or actual certification to a larger state hospital, is so pervasive that it hardly needs to be mentioned by the therapist. This threat is so obvious and overwhelming to many patients, that the physician has little power to increase or ameliorate it. Nearly everyone on the staff is very reluctant to certify anyone, but more than one patient is still certified every month. The effect of this on the remainder of patients will be discussed in the next section.

The third means of coercion is threatened or actual treatment with drugs or electroconvulsive therapy. Many patients will bargain to diminish their drug doses, much as they will bargain to decrease their physical restrictions. Many dislike the associated side effects of phenothiazines, including the dryness of the mouth, chapped lips, blurred vision, stuffy nose, and gastrointestinal symptoms, as well as the more disturbing changes in motor control and affect which almost invariably accompany larger doses. The use of drugs is entirely the prerogative of the physician and is most often a clear method of restraint when the patient is suicidal or homicidal. From the physician's point of view, the drugs have many disadvantages in restraining doses. First, the side-effects often interfere with psychotherapy. Second, it is sometimes difficult to make the patient take the drug. Third, the use of the drug for cercion prejudices the patient against any further use of the drugs.

Electroconvulsive therapy is a more potent means of coercion. In my own experience, most patients have terror of the treatment. Those few who have requested the treatment, still expressed a great fear of it. At S. P. H., the patient and the therapist usually both dislike the use of electroconvulsive therapy. Most patients refuse to sign permission, and the hospital then asks the patients' nearest relatives to sign. The legal implication of the family's consent has never been tested in New York State and is not clearly stated in any law. The device is nonetheless a strong inducement to the patients, who believe it legally binding. This is an example of coercion by implying to the patient that he has no other legal alternative.

In summary, the resident therapist may have many motives to coerce his patient. Some may be characteristic of all human relationships. Some are basic to current legal and social attitudes toward the mentally ill. A number are characteristic of an open hospital which must operate in a fundamentally closed society, represented by the larger state hospitals. If the physician decides to use coercion, he has three basic means: (1) control over the patient's liberty and length of stay in the hospital; (2) certification to a larger state hospital; (3) treatment with drugs or electroconvulsive therapy. Each of these may be used coercively as threats, punishments, or a means of restraint.

The Patient's Response to Coercion

Most patients sign a voluntary admission to the hospital. However, many of these admissions occur as a result of direct or indirect coercion by the patient's family. The patient may be brought to the hospital in a chaotic fashion by his family in the midst of a disintegrating social situation. Usually one or more other members of the family have decided that the patient's admission is the only feasible and immediate solution to the situation.

Often the patient will balk at the last minute when he is told that admission means he can be held for 25 days against his will. At this time, the family may pressure the patient by threats to certify him, or by threats to withdraw support. More rarely, the patient will be accompanied by the police or parole officer who may exert more direct coercion.

On occasion, the resident admitting officer for the day will admit the patient involuntarily at the request of the family and the family physician. More often, the resident is caught up as a passive observer in the family conflict. If he has interviewed the patient through the formal preadmissions clinic, or if he can ascertain quickly that the patient is grossly psychotic, he may also urge the patient to accept a voluntary admission. He may ameliorate the patient's fear of being held 25 days by emphasizing the open doors, and by implying that the patient could not really be held against his will, even though the law permits it.

Very likely more patients would balk at signing the voluntary admission if aware that they could be committed from S. P. H. to a larger state hospital, or that they might feel intimidated to stay considerably longer than the 25 days, or that they might be given electroconvulsive treatment against their will. For this reason, the admitting officer seldom mentions these eventualities at the time of admission. However, soon after admission the patient learns about these possibilities from direct observation of other patients, from discussions with other patients, or through his own experience. This is one of the reasons why the patient often begins to clamor for discharge within ten days or two weeks of hospitalization. He is afraid that the longer he stays the more danger there is that one or more threats will materialize. His fears usually culminate at the time of the official staff meeting which takes place about two weeks after each patient's admission.

Of all the fears, fear of commitment to the large state hospital is by far the most pervasive and intense. From his own prior knowledge and from hospital scuttlebutt, the patient learns that the larger state hospital (1) carries a greater social stigma; (2) has much tighter controls on personal freedom, including locked doors; (3) is more isolated from friends and family, with more limited visiting hours; (4) places more emphasis on chemical and electroconvulsive therapy; and (5) tends to hold patients for longer periods.

Beyond these specific fears about the larger hospital, there is an indefinable awe. In part, it stems from the not-too-distant past when most large state hospitals were "snakepits." In part, it stems from a fear of being mentally ill. Commitment to the larger hospital implies a degree of mental illness far greater than implied in the original voluntary admission to S. P. H. Similarly, the patient may feel that commitment implies incurability. On top of all this, the patient often looks upon commitment as an outright rejection by his physicians and family.

Fear of commitment to the larger state hospital can be reinforced by some commitments of other patients which he is likely to witness in the small hospital. Often the other patients will display overwhelming anxiety concerning their commitment. They may be given large doses of drugs, or transferred to the third floor for closer observation just prior to commitment. Then they are whisked off to the other hospital, leaving behind a wake of spreading fear throughout the hospital.

For many patients, the fear of commitment to the larger state hospital becomes a major motive during the hospital stay. Thus the smaller hospital, despite its open doors, becomes in some ways an annex or way station to the other hospital. For some patients, the threat becomes as real as if the smaller hospital were no more than a ward attached to the larger hospital.

The patient who lives under the threat of commitment, as well as the threat of a prolonged hospitalization, greater restrictions, or electroconvulsive therapy, soon develops ideas about what kind of behavior is likely to cause these threats to materialize. These ideas are often thrashed out in patient bull sessions in preparation for staff meetings. They include the following: (1) failure to respond satisfactorily to therapy, or failure to show an interest in therapy; (2) unmanageable or destructive behavior; (3) suicidal attempts or repeated suicidal threats; (4) immoral acts; (5) behavior disturbing to other patients; (6) repeated attempts to run away from the hospital; (7) any behavior which antagonizes hospital doctors, nurses or personnel; and (8) any behavior which antagonizes the patient's family.

The fear that running away will lead to eventual commitment to the larger hospital is especially important, for it most directly modifies the hospital's "open door policy." It effectively "locks the door." The patient may realize that he would rarely be forcibly returned to the hospital after running away, but he may feel that the hospital would thereafter deny him readmission. This would limit his future alternatives to the larger hospitals. Indirectly, then, the fear of the larger hospital might compel him to stay on in the ward.

In summary, the patient learns, soon after admission, that his voluntary status leaves him vulnerable to certain eventualities, the most disturbing being involuntary electroconvulsive therapy and certification to a larger state hospital. He also tries to find out what kind of behavior will cause these threats to materialize, so that he can modify his behavior accordingly.

Illustration of Cases

The following cases are illustrations of how coercion may effect different patients and their physicians.

The first patient is a 20-year-old girl who became suicidal, stuporous, and mute during her first few months at college. She was diagnosed schizophrenic and was voluntarily hospitalized three times in rapid succession during the next several months. She felt that each hospitalization brought her closer to being "sent away," yet she herself recognized the need for each hospitalization, and may have unconsciously wished for commitment and more prolonged treatment at the larger hospital. Prior to her third voluntary admission, her out-patient therapist had to reassure her that she would again be discharged if she showed some improvement. After a few weeks, her new hospital therapist felt she was making progress, but the hospital administration felt it was time to commit her for long-term treatment. Her new therapist told the patient he himself was against her commitment. The patient confided she imagined the larger hospital as a kind of Hell, and she threatened to run away. However, when the commitment papers were finally signed, she did a turnabout, and tearfully thanked everyone for committing her. She asked for tranquilizers to make her transition to the new hospital easier.

The second patient is a 26-year-old man who had developed paranoid schizophrenia during his first year of college. At that time he had been admitted voluntarily and then given electroconvulsive therapy against his wishes. He bitterly remembered these treatments and partly for this reason refused voluntary admission a second time. He was brought in involuntarily. After several weeks of psychotherapy his paranoid ideation ceased to function overtly in the patient-physician relationship. When his period of involuntary hospitalization drew to a close, he reluctantly agreed to sign a voluntary admission for continued hospitalization. In retrospect, he probably did this out of fear that he would otherwise be committed. When the therapist subsequently had to leave the hospital prior to the completion of therapy, the therapist decided to commit the patient for further treatment at a larger hospital. The patient again became acutely paranoid. At first he denounced his therapist but then tried to mollify him. He was finally placed on large doses of chlorpromazine to prevent his fleeing the hospital prior to commitment.

The first patient was always reluctant to be admitted voluntarily, for fear of eventual certification, and when certification did occur, she threatened to run away. Eventually, her basically passive-dependent orientation led her to "accept what's best." In the second case, the patient resisted admission at the start, but accepted voluntary status later on during his hospitalization. Very possibly, he thought that he would be certified if he refused voluntary status, as he would have been. When he was eventually certified, his basically paranoid orientation led him to reincorporate the therapist into his paranoid system. However, when he realized that the display of paranoid ideation and hostility would only further insure his certification, he attempted to mollify his therapist.

Often, the threat of commitment is itself potent enough to obviate the need for commitment. The third case, an addict to meperidine (Demerol), was admitted involuntarily at night when the doors are locked. In the morning, after several hours of unmanageable behavior, he fled past the attendant. The police were called to pick up the patient, who was thought dangerous to his wife. They were instructed to return him to jail in preparation for more speedy commitment to the larger state hospital. However, the policeman turned out to be an old high school chum of the patient. He warned the patient about the danger of commitment and returned him to the hospital. Despite the apprehension of the doctors, the patient was docile after this.

The vast majority of patients would not yield such clear-cut illustrations of coercion. One example, from an unusual follow-up opportunity, demonstrates that responses to coercion may be concealed from the therapist. The patient is a 35-year-old mother of four children who came in voluntarily after several months of bitter struggle between herself and her husband. In the last days before admission the patient had become agitated, threatened suicide, and finally became mute and stuporous. Rapport seemed to develop quickly between the patient and the therapist, and the patient made a remarkable symptomatic improvement after ventilating her rage and receiving support for her self-esteem. She appeared as the victim of an extremely sadomasochistic relationship. After the patient's discharge in two weeks, she somewhat reluctantly entered into a weekly family therapy project with the same therapist. During the first session, one daughter told how the patient's husband had threatened her with commitment to a larger state hospital just prior to her voluntary admission. During the second session, another daughter made a slip of the tongue which uncovered that the patient had always included the therapist among those hostile male figures whom she had to resist passively. She had put up a front of rapport during her hospitalization to insure her speedy discharge and to guard against the threat of commitment to the larger state hospital. To what extent some kernel of rapport did exist could not be ascertained against the background of motivation to deceive.

Comment

The proportion of patients actually affected by direct and threatened coercion, and the degree to which these patients accordingly modify their behavior, require some quantification. Many psychiatrists have already stated the opinion that so long as the threat of coercion exists, most or all patients will respond to it.[1,3,5,8,10,11] I have the impression that nearly every patient is affected by the threat of coercion but that only the more intact patients are able to modify their behavior in response. Thus the case illustrations present two schizophrenic patients who were unable to disguise their symptoms despite the threat of coercion, and a drug addict and a neurotic patient who were able to modify their behavior and, in the latter case, to disguise the response to the coercion. Beyond this kind of impression, it is not at present possible to quantify the degree of response, since every patient, voluntary or involuntary, is subjected to the same threats. Under these conditions, there are no control groups upon which to base a study of the effect of coercion. *

Because the effects of coercion are not fully understood, it is not easy to decide if we should, or could, do away with all coercion in mental hospitals. However, there are some cogent reasons to do away with the pretense about coercion and to recognize, as some have already done,[1] that the voluntary mental hospital experience is thoroughly permeated with coercion. If we gloss over the implications of coercion, we put the patient into a dangerous double bind. On the one hand, we tell him he is voluntary and encourage him to establish a relationship of mutual confidence. On the other hand, we use actual restraint, certification, and undesired treatments to control or intimidate him. On top of this, we then close our eyes to the problem and thus indirectly warn against too much concern about the realistic ambiguities of the situation. As one patient confided, "Is it true, Doctor, that you get committed if you look too eager to go home?" Naturally, openness and frankness about the pervasiveness of coercion is likely to help the physician as well as the voluntary patient, for it encourages a feeling of greater self-respect on the part of the physician and removes a taboo from important areas of the patient-physician relationship.

A concrete step can be taken to increase frankness and honesty in this regard. A requirement could be made that the patient be informed prior to admission about the possibilities of involuntary treatment, restrictions on liberty, and certification. In New York State this would be little more time-consuming or difficult than the current requirement that the patient be told prior to admission that he can be held for 15 days against his will at the discretion of the staff, and that he may then be required to give ten days' notice before leaving.

After being given this information, some patients might choose not to sign a voluntary admission. This occasionally happens now, when the patient is told that he can be held against his will. In keeping with the spirit of the voluntary admission, this should be the patient's prerogative. If the patient eventually does need involuntary hospitalization, the community then has means for obtaining this more directly through the various forms of mental hospital commitment. In New York State, for example, there is no lack of these forms and therefore little reason for physicians to fear for the future of patients who might refuse voluntary admission.

Frank recognition of the implications of voluntary admission would seem justified on ethical grounds, as well as on therapeutic grounds. Hopefully, frank recognition might also lead to codification of more real legal distinctions between voluntary and involuntary admissions in our state laws pertaining to the mentally ill. This would further the goal of a more frank and unambiguous patient-physician relationship. It would also make possible comparative studies of the effects of voluntary and involuntary hospitalization, studies now hampered by the absence of truly voluntary admissions.

Summary

An open hospital environment provides the opportunity for observing the more covert and indirect means of coercion found in most mental hospitals. Coercion is viewed from the patient's point of view as any action, or threat of action, which makes the patient feel compelled to behave in a manner contrary to his own wishes. Special attention is given to restriction of liberty around the hospital, certification to a larger and more remote state hospital, and involuntary treatment with drugs or electroconvulsions. Each of these can function coercively as a direct means of constraint, as a threat, or as a punishment. Case illustrations are given. The therapist's wish to coerce the patient is also presented.

A suggestion is made to inform voluntary patients prior to admission about the eventualities of coercion in the hospital. This would establish a more frank patient-physician relationship at the start and encourage future definitive legal distinctions between voluntary and involuntary patients.

REFERENCES TO AUTHOR'S NOTE

1. Breggin, Peter R.: "Psychotherapy as Applied Ethics." *Psychiatry* 34:59–75, 1971.

2. Breggin, Peter R.: *The Crazy from the Sane* (a novel). Lyle Stuart Publisher, New York, 1971.

3. Breggin, Peter R.: *After the Good War* (a novel). Stein and Day Publisher, New York, 1972.

4. Breggin, Peter R.: "Therapy as Applied Utopian Politics." *Mental Health and Society* 1:129–146, 1974.

5. Breggin, Peter R.: "Psychiatry and Psychotherapy as Political Processes." *American Journal of Psychotherapy* 29:369–382, 1975.

6. Breggin, Peter R.: "Needed: Voluntaristic Psychiatry," *Reason*, September, 1975.

7. Breggin, Peter R.: *The Psychology of Freedom*, Prometheus Books, Buffalo, 1980.

8. Breggin, Peter R.: "A Libertarian Critique of Psychiatry and Psychology," *Psychiatric Quarterly*, in press.

REFERENCES

1. Bickford, J. A. F.: Shadow and Substance: Some Changes in the Mental Hospital, Lancet 1:423–424, 1958.

2. Cameron, D. E.: An Open Psychiatric Hospital, Mod. Hosp. 74:84–88, 1950.

3. Freedom in Mental Hospitals: The End and the Means, Lancet 2:964–966, 1954.

4. Greenwald, A. F., and Bartemeier, L. H.: Psychiatric Discharges Against Medical Advice, Arch. Gen. Psychiat. 8:117–119, 1963.

5. Hunt, R. C.: "Ingredients of a Rehabilitation Program," in An Approach to the Prevention of Disability from Chronic Psychoses: The Open Mental Hospital Within the Community, New York, Milbank Memorial Fund, 1958, pp. 9–28, cited in Rubin and Goldberg.[7]

6. Knoff, W. F.: Modern Treatment of the "Insane": An Historical View of Nonrestraint, NY J. Med. 60:2236–2243, 1960.

7. Rubin, B., and Goldberg, A.: An Investigation of Openness in the Psychiatric Hospital, Arch. Gen. Psychiat. 8:269–276, 1963.

8. Szasz, T.: Discussions at the State University of New York, Upstate Medical Center, Department of Psychiatry.

9. Szasz, T., and Hollender, M. H.: A Contribution to the Philosophy of Medicine: The Basic Modes of the Doctor-Patient Relationship, AMA Arch. Intern. Med. 97:585, 1956.

10. The Unlocked Door, Lancet 2:953–954, 1954.

11. Winston, F.: Beyond the Open Door, Ment. Hyg. 46:11–19, 1962.

Joseph M. Livermore, Carl P. Malmquist, and Paul E. Meehl

On the Justifications
for Civil Commitment

Involuntary confinement is the most serious deprivation of individual liberty
that a society may impose. The philosophical justifications for such a deprivation by means of the criminal process have been thoroughly explored. No such
intellectual effort has been directed at providing justifications for societal use
of civil commitment procedures.[1]

When certain acts are forbidden by the criminal law, we are relatively
comfortable in imprisoning those who have engaged in such acts. We say that
the imprisonment of the offender will serve as an example to others and thus
deter them from violating the law. If we even stop to consider the morality of
depriving one man of his liberty in order to serve other social ends, we usually
are able to allay anxiety by referring to the need to incarcerate to protect society from further criminal acts or the need to reform the criminal. When
driven to it, at last, we admit that our willingness to permit such confinement
rests on the notion that the criminal has justified it by his crime. Eligibility for
social tinkering based on guilt, retributive though it may be, has so far
satisfied our moral sensibilities.[2]

It is, we believe, reasonably clear that the system could not be justified
were the concept of guilt not part of our moral equipment. Would we be comfortable with a system in which any man could go to jail if by so doing he
would serve an overriding social purpose? The normal aversion to punishment
by example, with its affront to the principle of equality, suggests that we would
not. Conversely, could we abide a rule that only those men would be punished

From *University of Pennsylvania Law Review* 117 (1968):75–96. Copyright © 1968. Reprinted by permission of the publisher and the co-authors.

whose imprisonment would further important social ends? Again, the thought of vastly different treatment for those equally culpable would make us uneasy.[3]

Similarly, if we chose to justify incarceration as a means of isolating a group quite likely to engage in acts dangerous to others, we would, without the justification of guilt, have difficulty explaining why other groups, equally or more dangerous in terms of actuarial data, are left free. By combining background environmental data, we can identify categories of persons in which we can say that fifty to eighty per cent will engage in criminal activity within a short period of time.[4] If social protection is a sufficient justification for incarceration, this group should be confined as are those criminals who are likely to sin again.[5]

The same argument applies when rehabilitative considerations are taken into account. Most, if not all of us could probably benefit from some understanding psychological rewiring. Even on the assumption that confinement should be required only in those cases where antisocial acts may thereby be averted, it is not at all clear that criminals are the most eligible for such treatment. In addition, most people would bridle at the proposition that the state could tamper with their minds whenever it seemed actuarially sound to do so.

Fortunately, we can by reason of his guilt distinguish the criminal from others whom we are loathe to confine. He voluntarily flouted society's commands with an awareness of the consequences. Consequently, he may serve utilitarian purposes without causing his imprisoners any moral twinge.

This same sort of analysis is not available once we move beyond the arena of the criminal law. When people are confined by civil process, we cannot point to their guilt as a basis for differentiating them from others. What can we point to?

The common distinguishing factor in civil commitment is aberrance. Before we commit a person we demand either that he act or think differently than we believe he should. Whether our label be inebriate,[6] addict,[7] psychopath,[8] delinquent,[9] or mentally diseased,[10] the core concept is deviation from norms.[11] Our frequently expressed value of individual autonomy, however, renders us unable to express those norms, however deeply they may be felt, in criminal proscriptions. We could not bring ourselves to outlaw senility, or manic behavior, or strange desires. Not only would this violate the common feeling that one is not a criminal if he is powerless to avoid the crime, but it might also reach conduct that most of us feel we have a right to engage in. When a man squanders his savings in a hypomanic episode, we may say, because of our own beliefs, that he is "crazy," but we will not say that only reasonable purchases are allowed on pain of criminal punishment. We are not yet willing to legislate directly the Calvinist ideal.

What we are not willing to legislate, however, we have been willing to practice through the commitment process. That process has been used to reach two classes of persons, those who are mentally ill and dangerous to themselves or others[12] and those who are mentally ill and in need of care, custody or treatment.[13] While those terms seem reasonably clear, on analysis that clarity evaporates.

Mental Illness

One need only glance at the diagnostic manual of the American Psychiatric Association[14] to learn what an elastic concept mental illness is. It ranges from massive functional inhibition characteristic of one form of catatonic schizophrenia[15] to those seemingly slight aberrancies associated with an emotionally unstable personality,[16] but which are so close to conduct in which we all engage as to define the entire continuum involved. Obviously, the definition of mental illness is left largely to the user and is dependent upon the norms of adjustment that he employs. Usually the use of the phrase "mental illness" effectively masks the actual norms being applied.[17] And, because of the unavoidably ambiguous generalities in which the American Psychiatric Association describes its diagnostic categories, the diagnostician has the ability to shoehorn into the mentally diseased class almost any person he wishes, for whatever reason,[18] to put there.

All this suggests that the concept of mental illness must be limited in the field of civil commitment to a necessary rather than a sufficient condition for commitment. While the term has its uses, it is devoid of that purposive content that a touchstone in the law ought to have. Its breadth of meaning makes for such difficulty of analysis that it answers no question that the law might wish to ask.[19]

Dangerousness to Others

The element of dangerousness to others has, at least in practice, been similarly illusive. As Professors Goldstein and Katz have observed, such a test, at a minimum, calls for a determination both of what acts are dangerous and how probable it is that such acts will occur.[20] The first question suggests to a criminal lawyer the answer: crimes involving a serious risk of physical or psychical harm to another. Murder, arson and rape are the obvious examples. Even in criminal law, however, the notion of dangerousness can be much broader. If one believes that acts that have adverse effects on social interests are dangerous, and if one accepts as a generality that the criminal law is devoted to such acts, any crime can be considered dangerous. For example, speeding in a motor vehicle, although traditionally regarded as a minor crime, bears great risk to life and property, and thus may be viewed as a dangerous act. Dangerousness can bear an even more extensive definition as well. An act may be considered dangerous if it is offensive or disquieting to others. Thus, the man who walks the street repeating, in a loud monotone, "fuck, fuck, fuck," is going to wound many sensibilities even if he does not violate the criminal law. Other examples would be the man, found in most cities, striding about town lecturing at the top of his lungs, or the similar character in San Francisco who spends his time shadow boxing in public. If such people are dangerous, it is not because they threaten physical harm but because we are made uncomfortable when we see aberrancies. And, of course, if dangerousness is so defined, it is at least as broad a concept as mental illness. The cases are unfortunately silent about what meaning the concept of danger bears in the commitment process.[21]

Assuming that dangerousness can be defined, the problem of predictability still remains. For the man who can find sexual release only in setting fires, one may confidently predict that dangerous acts will occur. For the typically mentally aberrant individual, though, the matter of prediction is not susceptible of answer. However nervous a full-blown paranoiac may make us, there are no actuarial data indicating that he is more likely to commit a crime than any normal person. Should he engage in criminal activity, his paranoia would almost certainly be part of the etiology. But on a predictive basis we have, as yet, nothing substantial to rely on.[22]

Even if such information were available, it is improbable that it would indicate that the likelihood of crime within a group of individuals with any particular psychosis would be any greater than that to be expected in a normal community cross-section.[23] Surely the degree of probability would not be as high as that in certain classes of convicted criminals after their release from prison or that in certain classes of persons having particular sociological or psychological characteristics.

Dangerousness to Self

The concept of "dangerousness to self" raises similar problems. The initial thought suggested by the phrase is the risk of suicide. But again it can be broadened to include physical or mental harm from an inability to take care of one's self, loss of assets from foolish expenditures, or even loss of social standing or reputation from behaving peculiarly in the presence of others.[24] Again, if read very broadly this concept becomes synonymous with that of mental illness. And, of course, reliable prediction is equally impossible.

In Need of Care, Custody, or Treatment

The notion of necessity of care or treatment provides no additional limitation beyond those imposed by the concepts already discussed. One who is diagnosably mentally ill is, almost by definition, in need of care or treatment.[25] Surely the diagnostician reaching the first conclusion would reach the second as well. And, if a man is dangerous, then presumably he is in need of custody. The problem, of course, lies with the word "need." If it is defined strictly as, for example, "cannot live without," then a real limitation on involuntary commitment is created. In normal usage, however, it is usually equated with "desirable," and the only boundary on loss of freedom is the value stricture of the expert witness.

It is difficult to identify the reasons that lie behind incarceration of the mentally ill. Three seem to be paramount:

(1) It is thought desirable to restrain those people who may be dangerous;

(2) It is thought desirable to banish those who are a nuisance to others;

(3) It is thought humanitarian to attempt to restore to normality and productivity those who are not now normal and productive.

Each of these goals has social appeal, but each also creates analytic difficulty.

As already mentioned, in order to understand the concept of danger one must determine what acts are dangerous and how likely is it that they will occur. There is a ready inclination to believe that experts in the behavioral sciences will be able to identify those members of society who will kill, rape, or burn. The fact is, however, that such identification cannot presently be accomplished. First, our growing insistence on privacy will, in all but a few cases, deny the expert access to the data necessary to the task of finding potential killers. Second, and of much greater importance, even if the data were available it is unlikely that a test could be devised that would be precise enough to identify only those individuals who are dangerous. Since serious criminal conduct has a low incidence in society, and since any test must be applied to a very large group of people, the necessary result is that in order to isolated those who will kill it is also necessary to incarcerate many who will not. Assume that one person out of a thousand will kill. Assume also that an exceptionally accurate test is created which differentiates with ninety-five per cent effectiveness those who will kill from those who will not. If 100,000 people were tested, out of the 100 who would kill 95 would be isolated. Unfortunately, out of the 99,900 who would not kill, 4,995 people would also be isolated as potential killers.[26] In these circumstances, it is clear that we would not justify incarerating all 5,090 people. If, in the criminal law, it is better that ten guilty men go free than that one innocent man suffer, how can we say in the civil commitment area that it is better that fifty-four harmless people be incarcerated lest one dangerous man be free?

The fact is that without any attempt at justification we have been willing to do just this to one disadvantaged class, the mentally ill. This practice must rest on the common supposition that mental illness makes a man more likely to commit a crime. While there may be some truth in this, there is much more error. Any phrase that encompasses as many diverse concepts as does the term "mental illness" is necessarily imprecise. While the fact of paranoid personality might be of significance in determining a heightened probability of killing, the fact of hebephrenic schizophrenia probably would not. Yet both fit under the umbrella of mental illness.

Even worse, we have been making assessments of potential danger on the basis of nothing as precise as the psychometric test hypothesized. Were we to ignore the fact that no definition of dangerous acts has been agreed upon, our standards of prediction have still been horribly imprecise. On the armchair assumption that paranoids are dangerous, we have tended to play safe and incarcerate them all. Assume that the incidence of killing among paranoids is five times as great as among the normal population. If we use paranoia as a basis for incarceration we would commit 199 non-killers in order to protect ourselves from one killer.[27] It is simply impossible to justify any commitment scheme so premised. And the fact that assessments of dangerousness are often made clinically by a psychiatrist, rather than psychometrically and statistically, adds little if anything to their accuracy.[28]

We do not mean to suggest that dangerousness is not a proper matter of legal concern. We do suggest, however, that limiting its application to the mentally ill is both factually and philosophically unjustifiable. As we have tried to demonstrate, the presence of mental illness is of limited use in determining potentially dangerous individuals. Even when it is of evidentiary value, it serves to isolate too many harmless people.[29] What is of greatest concern, however, is that the tools of prediction are used with only an isolated class of people. We have alluded before to the fact that it is possible to identify, on the basis of sociological data, groups of people wherein it is possible to predict that fifty to eighty per cent will engage in criminal or delinquent conduct. And, it is probable that more such classes could be identified if we were willing to subject the whole population to the various tests and clinical examinations that we now impose only on those asserted to be mentally ill. Since it is perfectly obvious that society would not consent to a wholesale invasion of privacy of this sort and would not act on the data if they were available, we can conceive of no satisfactory justification for this treatment of the mentally ill.

One possible argument for different treatment can be made in terms of the concept of responsibility.[30] We demonstrate our belief in individual responsibility by refusing to incarcerate save for failure to make a responsible decision. Thus, we do not incarcerate a group, eighty per cent of whom will engage in criminal conduct, until those eighty per cent have demonstrated their lack of responsibility—and even then, the rest of the group remains free. The mentally diseased, so the argument would run, may be viewed prospectively rather than retrospectively because for them responsibility is an illusory concept. We do not promote responsibility by allowing the dangerous act to occur since, when it does, we will not treat the actor as responsible. One way of responding to this is to observe that criminal responsibility and mental illness are not synonymous, and that if incarceration is to be justified on the basis of irresponsibility, only those mentally ill who will probably, as a matter of prediction, commit a crime for which they will not be held responsible should be committed.[31] A more fundamental response is to inquire whether susceptibility to criminal punishment is reasonably related to any social purpose. Granted that there is a gain in social awareness of individual responsibility by not incarcerating the responsible in advance of their crime, it does not necessarily follow that it is sufficiently great to warrant the markedly different treatment of the responsible and the irresponsible.

The other possible justification for the existing differential is that the mentally diseased are amenable to treatment. We shall explore the ramifications of this at a later point. It is sufficient now to observe that there is no reason to believe that the mentally well, but statistically dangerous, individual is any less amenable to treatment, though that treatment would undoubtedly take a different form.

Another basis probably underlying our commitment laws is the notion that it is necessary to segregate the unduly burdensome and the social nuisance. Two cases typify this situation. The first is the senile patient whose family asserts inability to provide suitable care. At this juncture, assuming that the family could put the person on the street where he would be unable to fend for himself, society must act to avoid the unpleasantness associated with public disregard of helplessness. This caretaking function cannot be avoided. Its performance, however, is a demonstration of the psychological truth that we can bear that which is kept from our attention. Most of us profess to believe that there is an individual moral duty to take care of a senile parent, a paranoid wife, or a disturbed child. Most of us also resent the bother such care creates. By allowing society to perform this duty, masked in medical terminology, but frequently amounting in fact to what one court has described as "warehousing,"[32] we can avoid facing painful issues.

The second case is the one in which the mentally ill individual is simply a nuisance, as when he insists on sharing his paranoid delusions or hallucinations with us. For reasons that are unclear, most of us are extremely uncomfortable in the presence of an aberrant individual, whether or not we owe him any duty, and whether or not he is in fact a danger to us in any defensible use of that concept. Our comfort, in short, depends on his banishment, and yet that comfort is equally dependent on a repression of any consciousness of the reason for his banishment. It is possible, of course, to put this in utilitarian terms. Given our disquietude, is not the utility of confinement greater than the utility of liberty? Perhaps so, but the assertions either that we will act most reasonably if we repress thinking about why we are acting or, worse yet, that our legislators will bear this knowledge for us in order to preserve our psychic ease makes us even more uncomfortable than the thought that we may have to look mental aberrance in the eye.

Again, we do not wish to suggest that either burden or bother is an inappropriate consideration in the commitment process. What we do want to make clear is that when it is a consideration it ought to be advertently so. Only in that way can intelligent decisions about care, custody, and treatment be made.

The final probable basis for civil commitment has both humanitarian and utilitarian overtones. When faced with an obviously aberrant person, we know, or we think we know, that he would be "happier" if he were as we are. We believe that no one would want to be a misfit in society. From the very best of motives, then, we wish to fix him. It is difficult to deal with this feeling since it rests on the unverifiable assumption that the aberrant person, if he saw himself as we see him, would choose to be different than he is. But since he cannot be as we, and we cannot be as he, there is simply no way to judge the predicate for the assertion.

Our libertarian views usually lead us to assert that treatment cannot be forced on anyone unless the alternative is very great social harm. Thus while we will require smallpox vaccinations[33] and the segregation of contagious tuberculars, we will not ordinarily require bed rest for the common cold, or a coronary, or even require a pregnant woman to eat in accordance with a medically approved diet. Requiring treatment whenever it seemed medically sound to do so would have utilitarian virtues. Presumably, if death or serious incapacitation could thereby be avoided society would have less worry about unsupported families, motherless children, or individuals no longer able to support themselves. Similarly, if the reasoning were pursued, we could insure that the exceptionally able, such as concert violinists, distinguished scholars, and inspiring leaders would continue to benefit society. Nonetheless, only rarely does society require such treatment.[34] Not only does it offend common notions of bodily integrity and individual autonomy, but it also raises those issues of value judgment which, if not insoluble, are at least discomforting. For example, is the treatment and cure of the mentally ill individual of more benefit to society than the liberty of which he is deprived and the principle (lost, or tarnished) that no one should assert the right to control another's beliefs and responses absent compelling social danger?

The reason traditionally assigned for forcing treatment on the mentally ill while making it voluntary for other afflicted persons is that the mentally ill are incapable of making a rational judgment whether they need or desire such help.[35] As with every similar statement, this depends on what kind of mental illness is present. It is likely that a pederast understands that society views him as sick, that certain kinds of psychiatric treatment may "cure" him, and that such treatment is available in certain mental institutions. It is also not unlikely that he will, in these circumstances, decide to forego treatment, at least if such treatment requires incarceration. To say that the pederast lacks insight into his condition and therefore is unable to intelligently decide whether or not to seek treatment is to hide our real judgment that he ought to be fixed, like it or not.[36] It is true that some mentally ill people may be unable to comprehend a diagnosis and, in these instances, forced treatment may be more appropriate. But this group is a small proportion of the total committable population. Most understand what the clinician is saying though they often disagree[37] with his view.

We have tried to show that the common justifications for the commitment process rest on premises that are either false or too broad to support present practices. This obviously raises the question of alternatives. Professor Ehrenzweig has suggested in another context that the definition of mental illness ought to be tailored to the specific social purpose to be furthered in the context in question.[38] That is what we propose here.

Returning to the first of our considerations supporting commitment, we suggest that before a man can be committed as dangerous it must be shown that the probabilities are very great that he will commit a dangerous act. Just how great the probabilities need be will depend on two things: how serious the probable dangerous act is and how likely it is that the mental condition can be changed by treatment. A series of hypotheticals will indicate how we believe this calculus ought to be applied.

Case 1: A man with classic paranoia exhibits in clinical interview a fixed belief that his wife is attempting to poison him. He calmly states that on release he will be forced to kill her in self defense. The experts agree that his condition is untreatable. Assume that statistical data indicate an eighty per cent probability that homicide will occur. If society will accept as a general rule of commitment, whether or not mental illness is present, that an eighty per cent probability of homicide is sufficient to incarcerate, then this man may be incarcerated. In order to do this, of course, we must be willing to lock up twenty people out of 100 who will not commit homicide.

Case 2: Assume the same condition with only a forty per cent probability of homicide.[39] We do not know whether, if the condition is untreatable, commitment is justified in these circumstances. If lifetime commitment is required because the probabilities are constant, we doubt that the justification would exist. Our own value structure would not allow us to permanently incarcerate sixty harmless individuals in order to prevent forty homicides. On the other hand, if incarceration for a year would reduce the probability to ten per cent, then perhaps it is justified. Similarly, if treatment over the course of two or three years would substantially reduce the probability, then commitment might be thought proper.

Case 3: A man who compulsively engages in acts of indecent exposure has been diagnosed as having a sociopathic personality disturbance. The probability is eighty per cent that he will again expose himself. Even if this condition is untreatable, we would be disinclined to commit.[40] In our view, this conduct is not sufficiently serious to warrant extended confinement. For that reason, we would allow confinement only if "cure" were relatively quick and certain.

The last case probably is more properly one of nuisance than of danger. The effects of such conduct are offensive and irritating but it is unlikely that they include long-term physical or psychical harm. That does not mean, however, that society has no interest in protecting its members from such upset. Again, the question is one of alternatives. Much nuisance behavior is subject to the control of the criminal law or of less formal social restraints. In mental institutions patients learn that certain behavior or the recounting of delusions or hallucinations will be met with disapproval.[41] Accordingly, they refrain from such behavior or conversation. There is no reason to believe that societal disapproval in the form of criminal proscriptions or of less formal sanctions will be less effective as a deterrent.[42] And, from our standpoint, the liberty of many mentally ill individuals is worth far more than the avoidance of minor nuisances in society.

Case 4: A person afflicted with schizophrenia walks about town making wild gestures and talking incessantly. Those who view him are uncomfortable but not endangered. We doubt that commitment is appropriate even though it would promote the psychic ease of many people. Arguably we would all be happier if our favorite bogey man, whether James Hoffa, Rap Brown, Mario Savio, or some other, were incarcerated. Most of us would be outraged if any of these men were committed on such a theory. If we cannot justify such a commitment in these cases, we doubt that it is any more justifiable when social anxiety is a consequence of seeing mentally ill individuals. While it might be proper to commit if speedy cure were possible, such cures are, as a matter of fact, unavailable. Moreover we have some difficulty distinguishing the prevention of psychic upset based on cure of the mentally ill and prevention based on neutralizing other upsetting behavior.[43]

The next justification of commitment is more solid, though it too presents the question of the necessity of utilizing less burdensome alternatives. This is the rationale of care for the person who is unable to care for himself and who has no one else to provide care for him. As we suggested earlier, such care must be provided if we are unwilling to allow people to die in the streets.

Case 5: An elderly woman with cerebro-vascular disease and accompanying cerebral impairment has the tendency to leave her home, to become lost, and then to wander helplessly about until someone aids her.[44] At other times she is perfectly able to go shopping or visit friends. She has no relatives who will care for her in the sense that they will prevent her from wandering or will find her when she has become lost. In some ways, this is another case of public nuisance and it may well be that it is impossible to find a justification for incarcerating this woman. On the other hand, to allow this woman to die from exposure on one of her forays is as disquieting as the loss of her freedom. Since her condition is untreatable, provision of treatment offers no justification for confinement. It might be justifiable to exercise some supervision over her, but surely that justification will not support total incarceration. In these circumstances, we believe that if the state wishes to intervene it must do so in some way that does not result in a total loss of freedom.[45] The desire to help ought not to take the form of simple jailing.

Case 6: A schizophrenic woman is causing such an upset in her family that her husband petitions for commitment. It is clear that the presence of this woman in the family is having an adverse effect on the children. Her husband is simply unwilling to allow the situation to continue. The alternatives here are all unpleasant to contemplate. If the husband gets a divorce and custody, he may accomplish his end. But the social opprobrium attaching to that solution makes it unlikely. The question, then, is whether the state should provide a socially acceptable alternative. If that alternative is her loss of freedom, we find it hard to justify. Assuming that the condition is untreatable, that the woman is not dangerous, and that her real sin is her capacity to disrupt, it is almost incomprehensible that she should be subject to a substantial period of incarceration. Yet that is what it has meant. Presumably, in order to isolate the woman from her family, it is necessary to transport her to a location where she will no longer bother her family. Then, if she is able to support herself she could have complete freedom. If she is not able, the state will have to provide care. That care, of course, need not involve a total deprivation of freedom.[46]

The final justification for commitment — the need to treat — is in many ways the most difficult to deal with. As we have said before, society has not traditionally required treatment of treatable diseases even though most people would agree that it was "crazy" for the diseased person not to seek treatment.[47] The problem has been complicated by the fact that religious beliefs against certain forms of treatment often are present[48] and by the fact that most cases of stubborn refusal to accept treatment never come into public view.[49] There is, however, a competing analogy that suggests that mandatory treatment may sometimes be appropriate.

Without going into unnecessary detail, we think it can be said that one of the reasons society requires compulsory education is that it believes a certain minimum amount of socialization is necessary for everyone lest they be an economic burden or a personal nuisance.[50] That principle can also be used to support mandatory psychiatric rewiring if the individual to be refurbished is in fact a burden or nuisance and can be fixed. The difficulty, of course, lies in the extent to which the principle can be carried. To take a mild example outside the field of mental disease, assume an unemployable individual who is unable to support his large and growing family. Could society incarcerate him until he had satisfactorily acquired an employable skill?[51] In the context of mental disease, then, can society demand that an individual obtain an employable psyche?

Case 7: An individual has been suffering from paranoid schizophrenia for several years without remission and has lost his job because of his behavior. He is divorced, but he is able to support himself from prior savings. He is not dangerous, and if he is committed it is unlikely that he will be cured since the recovery rates from such long-term schizophrenia are very low.[52] In addition, the availability of treatment in a state mental institution is problematic.[53] We doubt that he can justifiably be committed. If treatment is an adequate basis for confinement, it surely ceases to be so either when the illness is untreatable or when treatment is in fact not given or given in grossly insufficient amounts. No other basis for commitment being present, it is unjustifiable.

Case 8: A distinguished law school professor, known for a series of brilliant articles, is suffering from an involutional depression. His scholarship has dried up, and, while he is still able to teach, the spark is gone and his classes have become extremely depressing. There is a chance, though probably not more than twenty-five per cent,[54] that he will commit suicide. He has been told that he would recover his old élan if he were subjected to a series of electro-shock treatments but this he has refused to do. In fact, in years past when he was teaching a course in law and psychology, he stated that if he ever became depressed he wanted it known that before the onset of depression he explicitly rejected such treatment.

Should he be compelled to undergo treatment? The arguments of social utility would suggest that he should. Yet we are unable to dislodge the notion that potential added productivity is not a license for tampering.

Case 9: A woman suffers from a severe psychotic depression resulting in an ability to do little more than weep. Again shock treatment is recommended with a reasonable prospect of a rapid recovery. The woman rejects the suggestion saying that nothing can make her a worthy member of society. She is, she claims, beyond help or salvation. It is possible to distinguish this from the preceding case on the ground that her delusional thought processes prevent her from recognizing the desirability of treatment. But any distinction based on a proposed patient's insight into her condition will probably be administered on the assumption that any time desirable treatment is refused, insight is necessarily lacking. And that, of course, would destroy the distinction.

These cases suggest that the power to compel treatment is one that rarely ought to be exercised. We are unable to construct a rationale that will not as well justify remolding too many people to match predominant ideas of the shape of the ideal psyche. We recognize, of course, that we are exhibiting a parade of horrors. In this instance, however, we believe such reference justified. The ease with which one can be classified as less than mentally healthy, and the difficulty in distinguishing degrees of sickness, make us doubt the ability of anyone to judge when the line between minimum socialization and aesthetically pleasing acculturation has been passed. Regardless of our views, however, it seems clear that if society chooses to continue to exercise the power to compel treatment, it ought to do so with constant awareness of the threat to autonomy thus posed.

Different considerations are present when commitment is not based on the need to treat. If one is committed as dangerous, or as a nuisance, or as unable to care for oneself, and treatment can cure this condition, then it is easier to strike the balance between deprivation of liberty and the right to refuse treatment in favor of compulsory treatment. If told that this is the price of freedom, the patient may accede; if he prefers confinement to treatment, perhaps the state ought not to override his wishes. But at least in this situation the question is ethically a close one.

The difficulty with present commitment procedures is that they tend to justify all commitments in terms that are appropriate only to some, and to prescribe forms of treatment that are necessary in only some cases. Thus, while danger stemming from mental illness may be a proper basis for commitment, it does not follow that all mentally ill are dangerous, or that the standards of danger should be markedly less rigid in cases of mental illness. Similarly, because mentally ill people may be a nuisance and some means of preventing such nuisance must be found, it does not follow that nuisance commitments ought to involve the same restraints as commitments based upon potential danger. Finally, because treatment is humanitarian when applied to those confined for danger, nuisance, or care, does not in itself suggest that treatment can be applied whenever administrators believe it proper or humane to do so.

We recognize that many people will not agree with the manner in which we have drawn the balance in individual cases. We hope that few will disagree that the balance must be drawn. We suggest, therefore, that in each case of proposed commitment, the following questions be asked:

I. What social purpose will be served by commitment?

    A. If protection from potential danger, what dangerous acts are threatened? How likely are they to occur? How long will the individual have to be confined before time or treatment will eliminate or reduce the danger so that he may be released?[55]

    B. If protection from nuisance, how onerous is the nuisance in fact? Ought that to justify loss of freedom? If it should, how long will confinement last before time or treatment will eliminate or reduce the risk of nuisance so that release may occur?

    C. If the need for care, is care in fact necessary? If so, how long will confinement last before time or treatment will eliminate the need for care so that release may occur?

II. Can the social interest be served by means less restrictive than the total confinement?

III. Whatever standard is applied, is it one that can comfortably be applied to all members of society, mentally ill or healthy?[56]

IV. If confinement is justified only because it is believed that it will be of short term for treatment, is the illness in fact treatable? If it is, will appropriate treatment in fact be given?

If these questions are asked — and we view it as the duty of the attorney for the potential patient to insure that they are — then more intelligent commitment practices may follow.[57]

NOTES

Our reflections on the justifications for civil commitment were greatly aided and in part actuated by the excellent collection of material in J. KATZ, J. GOLDSTEIN & A. DERSHOWITZ, PSYCHOANALYSIS, PSYCHIATRY AND LAW (1967). *See also* T. SZASZ, LAW, LIBERTY AND PSYCHIATRY (1963); Dershowitz, *Psychiatry in the Legal Process: A Knife That Cuts Both Ways,* 4 TRIAL, Feb./Mar. 1968, at 29. The latter article is particularly perceptive.

    1. *But see* Ross, *Commitment of the Mentally Ill: Problems of Law and Policy,* 57 MICH. L. REV. 945,

954–964, (1959). It will become obvious that we share the point of view of C. S. Lewis and Francis Allen that confinement is confinement regardless of the name under which it parades.

> To be taken without consent from my home and friends; to lose my liberty; to undergo all those assaults on my personality which modern psychotherapy knows how to deliver; to be re-made after some pattern of "normality" hatched in a Viennese laboratory to which I never professed allegiance; to know that this process will never end until either my captors have succeeded or I have grown wise enough to cheat them with apparent success—who cares whether this is called Punishment or not?

Lewis, *The Humanitarian Theory of Punishment,* 6 RES JUDICATAE 224, 227 (1953).

> Measures which subject individuals to the substantial and involuntary deprivation of their liberty contain an inescapable punitive element, and this reality is not altered by the fact that the motivations that prompt incarceration are to provide therapy or otherwise contribute to the person's well-being or reform. As such, these measures must be closely scrutinized to insure that power is being applied consistently with those values of the community that justify interference with liberty for only the most clear and compelling reasons.

F. ALLEN, THE BORDERLAND OF CRIMINAL JUSTICE 37 (1964).

2. *See generally* H. L. A. HART, PUNISHMENT AND RESPONSIBILITY (1968); H. M. Hart, *The Aims of the Criminal Law,* 23 LAW & CONTEMP. PROB. 401 (1958).

3. Of course, arbitrary punishment would lose its utility if its nature were widely known, but even if it were useful it would generally be viewed as morally wrong. *See* H. L. A. HART, PUNISHMENT AND RESPONSIBILITY 77–80 (1968). Perhaps the reason that inequality in application can exist in the civil commitment area is that, like secret, arbitrary punishment, it does not make us conscious of any threat to our own liberty.

4. *See* Briggs, Wirt & Johnson, *An Application of Prediction Tables to the Study of Delinquency,* 25 J. CONSULTING PSYCHOLOGY 46 (1961); Craig & Glick, *A Manual of Procedure for Application of the Glueck Prediction Table,* in J. KATZ, J. GOLDSTEIN & A. DERSHOWITZ, PSYCHOANALYSIS, PSYCHIATRY AND LAW 394–99 (1967); Thompson, *A Validation of the Glueck Social Prediction Scale for Proneness to Delinquency,* 43 J. CRIM. L.C. & P.S. 451 (1952). *But see* S. HATHAWAY & E. MONACHESI, ADOLESCENT PERSONALITY AND BEHAVIOR: MMPI PATTERNS OF NORMAL, DELINQUENT, DROPOUT, AND OTHER OUTCOMES (1963); S. HATHAWAY & E. MONACHESI, AN ATLAS OF JUVENILE MMPI PROFILES (1961); S. HATHAWAY & E. MONACHESI, ANALYZING AND PREDICTING JUVENILE DELINQUENCY WITH THE MMPI (1951); Wirt & Briggs, *The Efficacy of Ten of the Glueck's Predictors,* 50 J. CRIM. L.C. & P.S. 478 (1960). *See generally* Briggs & Wirt, *Prediction,* in JUVENILE DELINQUENCY, RESEARCH AND THEORY 170 (H. Quay ed. 1965).

In addition to the legal, ethical, and social policy issues upon which we focus in this paper, there is a difficult problem concerning the application of actuarial results to the disposition of the individual case. In the text we have simply referred to the betting odds, the "chances per hundred" that behavior of a stated kind will subsequently occur, without examining such questions as how such numerical estimates are best arrived at, or what should be their precise interpretation when applied to an individual. To go into the logical, epistemological and mathematical issues involved therein (*e.g.,* the very technical controversy over the several alleged meanings of the word "probability") is beyond the scope of this paper. The leading treatment of the so-called "clinical-statistical" issue in the behavioral sciences is P. MEEHL, CLINICAL VERSUS STATISTICAL PREDICTION (1954). *See also* G. KIMBLE & N. GARMEZY, PRINCIPLES OF GENERAL PSYCHOLOGY 589 (3d ed. 1968); B. KLEINMUNTZ, PERSONALITY MEASUREMENT 344 (1967); P. MARKS & W. SEEMAN, THE ACTUARIAL DESCRIPTION OF ABNORMAL PERSONALITY (1963); RESEARCH IN CLINICAL ASSESSMENT (E. Megargee ed. 1966); W. MISCHEL, PERSONALITY AND ASSESSMENT 128 (1968); N. SUNDBERG & L. TYLER, CLINICAL PSYCHOLOGY: AN INTRODUCTION TO RESEARCH AND PRACTICE 197–224 (1962); Gough, *Clinical Versus Statistical Prediction in Psychology,* in PSYCHOLOGY IN THE MAKING 526 (L. Postman ed. 1962); Kleinmuntz, *The Processing of Clinical Information by Men and Machine,* in FORMAL REPRESENTATION OF HUMAN JUDGMENT 149 (B. Kleinmuntz ed. 1968); Meehl, *What Can the Clinician Do Well?* in PROBLEMS IN HUMAN ASSESSMENT 594 (D. Jackson

& S. Messick eds. 1967); Meehl, *When Shall We Use Our Heads Instead of the Formula?* 4 J. COUNSEL-ING PSYCHOLOGY 268 (1957). Without digressing into the merits of that controversy, we cannot avoid at least entering two caveats for the benefit of our law-trained readers who will, in general, be unfamiliar with the relevant research literature, by now very considerable in scope. First, one should not simply assume as somehow obvious that "individual prediction" is fundamentally different from "actuarial prediction," a quick-and-easy distinction very commonly presupposed in many quarters. Second, one should not simply assume that "intensive, clinical, psychological understanding of the individual" leads generally to more trustworthy forecast of behavior than a more behavioristic-actuarial approach to the predictive task. This second assumption seems still to be taken blithely for granted by almost all psychiatrists and—surprisingly, given the research evidence—by many clinical psychologists. The comparative efficacy of different methods of predicting behavior is, of course, a factual question; and in spite of the armchair plausibility of the above mentioned assumptions (to be sceptical of "understanding the individual" is rather like being against motherhood), there exists a very sizable body of empirical evidence to the contrary. The latest published summary of factual evidence is Sawyer, *Measurement and Prediction, Clinical and Statistical,* 66 PSYCHOLOGICAL BULL. 178 (1966), which also presents a very sophisticated and fair-minded methodological reformulation. Of some five dozen published and unpublished research studies known to us, there is only a single study showing, given an acceptable research design, a clearcut superiority of clinical judgment over actuarial prediction. *See* Lindzey, *Seer Versus Sign,* 1 J. EXPERIMENTAL RESEARCH IN PERSONALITY 17 (1965); Meehl, *Seer Over Sign: The First Good Example,* 1 J. EXPERIMENTAL RESEARCH IN PERSONALITY 27 (1965). *But see* Goldberg, *Seer Over Sign: The First "Good" Example?* 3 J. EXPERIMENTAL RESEARCH IN PERSONALITY — (1968). It would be difficult to mention any other domain of social science research in which the trend of the data is so uniformly in the same direction, so that any psychiatrist or psychologist who disfavors the objective, actuarial approach in a practical, decision-making context should be challenged to show his familiarity with this research literature and invited to rebut the theoretical argument and empirical evidence found therein.

5. The habitual criminal statutes may be thought of as one instance where incarceration is based on a judgment that the person incarcerated is dangerous. But such statutes also serve a deterrent function by a Bethamite increase in punishment for those who are viewed as especially likely to commit a crime.

6. *See, e.g.,* CONN. GEN. STAT. REV. § 17–155e (Supp. 1965).

7. *E.g.,* ALA. CODE tit. 22, §§ 249–50 (1958); *see In re* Spadafora, 54 Misc. 2d 123, 281 N.Y.S.2d 923 (Sup. Ct. 1967).

8. *E.g,* Boutilier v. Immigration & Naturalization Service, 387 U.S. 118 (1967); MINN. STAT. ANN. § 526.09 (1947). *See* Minnesota *ex rel.* Pearson v. Probate Court, 309 U.S. 270 (1940).

9. *E.g.,* MD. CODE ANN. art. 31B, § 5 (1967); *see* Sas v. Maryland, 334 F.2d 506 (4th Cir. 1963); Director of Patuxent Institution v. Daniels, 243 Md. 16, 221 A.2d 397 (1966), *cert. denied,* 385 U.S. 940 (1966).

10. *E.g.,* MASS. ANN. LAWS ch. 123, § 1 (1965):

"Mentally ill" person, for the purpose of involuntary commitment to a mental hospital or school under the provisions of this chapter, shall mean a person subject to a disease, psychosis, psychoneurosis or character disorder which renders him so deficient in judgment or emotional control that he is in danger of causing physical harm to himself or to others, or the wanton destruction of valuable property, or is likely to conduct himself in a manner which clearly violates the established laws, or ordinances, conventions or morals of the community.

11. The concept "abnormal" or "aberrant" is sorely in need of more thorough logical analysis than it has, to our knowledge, as yet received. It seems fairly clear that several components—perhaps even utterly distinct kinds of meaning—can be discerned in the current usage of medicine and social science. The most objective meaning is the purely statistical one, in which "abnormal" designates deviation from the (statistical) "norm" of a specified biological or social population of organisms. Whether an individual specimen, or bit of behavior, is abnormal in this sense is readily ascertained by adequate sampling methods plus a more or less arbitrary choice of

cutting score (*e.g.*, found in less than 1 in 100 cases). But for legal purposes this purely statistical criterion does not suffice, because the *kind* and *direction* of statistical deviation from population norms, as well as the *amount* of deviation which threatens a protected social interest sufficiently to justify legal coercion, are questions not answerable by statistics alone. Thus, anyone who has an IQ of 180, or possesses absolute pitch, or is color-blind, is statistically abnormal but hardly rendered thereby a candidate for incarceration, mandatory treatment, or deprivation of the usual rights and powers of a "normal" individual. A second component in the concept of normality relies upon our (usually inchoate or implicit) notions of biological health, of a kind of proper functioning of the organism conceived as a teleological system of organs and capacities. From a biological viewpoint, it is not inconsistent to assert that a sizable proportion — conceivably a majority — of persons in a given population are abnormal or aberrant. Thus, if an epidemiologist found that 60% of the persons in a society were afflicted with plague or avitaminosis, he would (quite correctly) reject an argument that "Since most of them have it, they are okay, *i.e.*, not pathological and not in need of treatment." It is admittedly easier to defend this non-statistical, biological-fitness approach in the domain of physical disease, but its application in the domain of behavior is fraught with difficulties. *See* W. Schofield, Psychotherapy: The Purchase of Friendship 12 (1964). Yet even here there is surely something to be said for it in extreme cases, as, for example, the statistically "normal" frigidity of middle-class Victorian women, which any modern sexologist would confidently consider a biological maladaptation in need of repair, induced by "unhealthy" social learnings. A third component invokes some sort of subjective norm, such as an aesthetic, religious, ethical, or political ideal or rule. Finally, whether an a priori concept of "optimal psychological adjustment" should be considered as yet a fourth meaning of normality, or instead subsumed under one or more of the preceding, is a difficult question. In any event, it is important to keep alert to hidden fallacies in legal and policy arguments that rely upon the notion of abnormality or aberration, such as subtle transitions from one of these criteria to another. It is especially tempting to the psychiatrist or clinical psychologist, given his usual clinical orientation, to slip unconsciously from the idea of "sickness," where treatment of a so-called "patient" is the model, to an application that justifies at most a statistical or ideological or psychological-adjustment usage of the word "norm." Probably the most pernicious error is committed by those who classify as "sick" behavior that is aberrant in *neither* a statistical sense *nor* in terms of any defensible biological or medical criterion, but solely on the basis of the clinician's personal ideology of mental health and interpersonal relationships. Examples might be the current psychiatric stereotype of what a good mother or a healthy family must be like, or the rejection as "perverse" of forms of sexual behavior that are not biologically harmful, are found in many infra-human mammals and in diverse human cultures, and have a high statistical frequency in our own society. *See generally* F. Beach, Sexual Behavior in Animals and Men (1950); H. Ellis, Studies in the Psychology of Sex (1936); C. Ford & F. Beach, Patterns of Sexual Behavior (1951); A. Kinsey, W. Pomeroy & C. Martin, Sexual Behavior in the Human Male (1948); A. Kinsey, W. Pomeroy, C. Martin & P. Gebhard, Sexual Behavior in the Human Female (1953); W. Masters & W. Johnson, Human Sexual Response (1966); Ellis, *What is "Normal" Sexual Behavior,* 28 Sexology 364 (1962); S. Freud, *Three Essays on the Theory of Sexuality,* in 7 Complete Psychological Works 123 (J. Strachey ed. 1962).

12. *E.g.,* Tenn. Code Ann. § 33–604(d) (1967).

13. *Id.* For a discussion of standards applied in the various states, see American Bar Foundation, The Mentally Disabled and the Law 17, 44–51 (1961).

14. Diagnostic & Statistical Manual of Mental Disorders (2d ed. 1968) [hereinafter cited as DSM-II]. The first edition of this manual, published in 1952, will be referred to as DSM-I.

15. DSM-II, 295.24, at 33.

16. In such cases the individual reacts with excitability and ineffectiveness when confronted with minor stress. His judgment may be undependable under stress, and his relationship to other people is continuously fraught with fluctuating emotional attitudes, because of strong and poorly controlled hostility, guilt, and anxiety. DSM-I, 000-x51, at 36. In DSM-II, this disorder is characterized as hysterical personality. DSM-II, 301.5, at 43.

17. "Normal and abnormal, one sometimes suspects, are terms which a particular author

employs with reference to his own position on that curve." A. KINSEY, W. POMEROY & C. MARTIN, SEXUAL BEHAVIOR IN THE HUMAN MALE 199 (1948). *See also* Boutilier v. Immigration & Naturalization Service, 387 U.S. 118, 125 (1967) (Douglas, J., dissenting); W. SCHOFIELD, PSYCHOTHERAPY: THE PURCHASE OF FRIENDSHIP 12–13 (1964); Weihofen, *The Definition of Mental Illness,* 21 OHIO ST. L.J. 1 (1960).

18. The usual reason for variance in diagnosis is a variance in the theoretical orientation of the diagnosticians.

19. We are not saying that mental illness does not exist or that the disease concept should not be used in the field of "functional" behavior disorders. *Compare* T. SZASZ, THE MYTH OF MENTAL ILLNESS (1961); Albee, *Models, Myths, and Manpower,* 52 MENTAL HYGIENE 168 (1968); Szasz, THE MYTH OF MENTAL ILLNESS, 14 AM. PSYCHOLOGIST 113 (1960), *with* Ausubel, *Personality Disorder is Disease,* 16 AM. PSYCHOLOGIST 69 (1961); Meehl, *Schizotaxia, Schizotypy, Schizophrenia,* 17 AM. PSYCHOLOGIST 827 (1962); Meehl, *Some Ruminations on the Validation of Clinical Procedures,* 13 CAN. J. PSYCHOLOGY 102 (1959). The most objective and sophisticated methodological analysis known to us of the general problem of taxonomy, types, and disease entities in the domain of "nonorganic" behavior disorders is Dahlstrom, *Types and Personality Systematics,* in HANDBOOK OF MODERN PERSONALITY THEORIES (R. Cattell ed. [in press]). *See also* R. CATTELL, PERSONALITY AND MOTIVATION, STRUCTURE AND MEASUREMENT 382 (1957); M. LORR, C. KLETT & D. McNAIR, SYNDROMES OF PSYCHOSIS (1963); W. MAYER-GROSS, E. SLATER & M. ROTH, CLINICAL PSYCHIATRY 6 (2d ed. 1960); W. SARGANT & E. SLATER, AN INTRODUCTION TO PHYSICAL METHODS OF TREATMENT IN PSYCHIATRY 4, 14, 305 (4th ed. 1963); Cattell, *Taxonomic Principles for Locating and Using Types,* in FORMAL REPRESENTATION OF HUMAN JUDGMENT 99 (B. Kleinmuntz ed. 1968); Foulds, *Psychotic Depression and Age,* 106 J. MENTAL SCIENCE 1394 (1960); Kiloh & Garside, *The Independence of Neurotic Depression and Endogenous Depression,* 109 BR. J. PSYCHIATRY 451 (1963); McQuitty, *Pattern Analysis Illustrated in Classifying Patients and Normals,* 14 EDUCATIONAL & PSYCHOLOGICAL MEASUREMENT 598 (1954); McQuitty, *Typal Analysis,* 21 EDUCATIONAL & PSYCHOLOGICAL MEASUREMENT 677 (1961); Meehl, *Detecting Latent Clinical Taxa by Fallible Quantitative Indicators Lacking an Accepted Criterion,* REP. PR-65-2, RESEARCH LABORATORIES, DEP'T OF PSYCHIATRY, UNIV. OF MINN. (1965); Meehl, *Detecting Latent Clinical Taxa II: A Simplified Procedure, Some Additional Hitmax Cut Locators, a Single-Indicator Method, and Miscellaneous Theorems,* REP. PR-68-4, RESEARCH LABORATORIES, DEP'T OF PSYCHIATRY, UNIV. OF MINN. (1968); Rao & Slater, *Multivariate Analysis Applied to Differences Between Neurotic Groups,* 2 BR. J. PSYCHOLOGY (STATISTICAL SECT.) 17 (1949); Wender, *On Necessary and Sufficient Conditions in Psychiatric Explanation,* 16 ARCH. GEN. PSYCHIATRY 41 (1967); Wittenborn, *Symptom Patterns in a Group of Mental Hospital Patients,* 15 J. CONSULTING PSYCHOLOGY 290 (1951). *See generally* EXPLORATIONS IN TYPING PSYCHOTICS (M. Lorr ed. 1966) with its extensive bibliography. For a beautiful methodological analysis of the relation between specific etiology and other quantitative contributors—still very much worth reading in spite of the author's later repudiation of his substantive thesis—see S. FREUD, *On the Grounds for Detaching a Particular Syndrome from Neurasthenia Under the Description "Anxiety Neurosis,"* and *A Reply to Criticisms of My Paper on Anxiety Neurosis,* in 3 COMPLETE PSYCHOLOGICAL WORKS 90, 123 (J. Strachey ed. 1962).

Even a nodding acquaintance with these works should suffice to convince any scholar that the complexities are enormous, and that writers who find easy solutions to the disease-entity problem (*e.g.,* with a few clichés about "pigeonholing" and "the unique individual") are not even beginning to grapple with it. A fair statement of the present situation in psychiatry and clinical psychology with regard to "disease entities" would be that nobody knows whether or not such entities exist outside the domain of the "organic" psychoses associated with demonstrable damage to the brain by trauma, toxins, infections, vascular disorder, senile changes, etc. The conceptual and statistical problems involved are difficult, recondite, and highly technical. We can only caution our law-trained readers against being "taken in" by plausible, quick and easy verbal resolutions of the issue, which are all too common among psychologists and psychiatrists. The most difficult class is the major functional disorders (*e.g.,* schizophrenia, manic-depression) where hereditary factors appear to play an important causal role, but where the concept "disease" does not have quite its usual medical meaning. We do not think that the moral, policy and legal questions before us hinge upon the resolution of these empirical issues. The clinical status of a psychologically aberrated individual (*e.g.,* "Can he think rationally about his condition?"), his prognosis (with and without hospitalization and treatment), and his probability of socially dangerous or intolerable conduct if left in the community are the relevant considerations. Given a particular quantitative balance among these three behavioral factors, what does it matter whether the behavior-syndrome is truly "taxonomic," and whether the aberration, taxonomic or not, is mainly attributable to germs, genes, toxins, or social learning experiences? It is, we submit, a mistake to rest the cases for and against civil commitment upon the slippery semantics of the term "disease," or upon the unsettled empirical questions concerning the etiology of mental disorder, as does Szasz.

20. Goldstein & Katz, *Dangerousness and Mental Illness: Some Observations on the Decision to Release Persons Acquitted by Reason of Insanity,* 70 YALE L. J. 225, 235 (1960). *See* Note, *The Nascent Right to Treatment,* 53 U. VA. L. REV. 1134, 1141–43 (1967).

21. *But see* United States v. Charnizon, 232 A.2d 586 (D.C. Ct. App. 1967), where the probability of the issuance of checks drawn on insufficient funds was found to render the defendant "dangerous."

22. While there is an inclination to equate mental illness and dangerousness, "the fact is that the great majority of hospitalized mental patients are too passive, too silent, too fearful, too withdrawn" to be dangerous. Statement of Albert Deutsch, *Hearings on Constitutional Rights of the Mentally Ill Before the Subcomm. on Constitutional Rights of the Senate Comm. on the Judiciary,* 87th Cong., 1st Sess. 43 (1961) [hereinafter cited as *1961 Hearings*]. *See also* THE CLINICAL EVALUATION OF THE DANGEROUSNESS OF THE MENTALLY ILL (J. Rappeport ed. 1967); Statement of Thomas Szasz, *1961 Hearings* 270; Dershowitz, *Psychiatry in the Legal Process: A Knife that Cuts Both Ways,* 4 TRIAL, Feb./Mar. 1968 at 29; Giovannoni & Gurel, *Socially Disruptive Behavior of Ex-Mental Patients,* 17 ARCH. GEN. PSYCHIATRY 146 (1967); Rappeport & Lassen, *The Dangerousness of Female Patients: A Comparison of the Arrest Rate of Discharged Psychiatric Patients and the General Population,* 123 AM. J. PSYCHIATRY 413 (1966); Weihofen, *Institutional Treatment of Persons Acquitted by Reason of Insanity,* 38 TEX. L. REV. 849, 855–7 (1960).

23. Of course, the probability of dangerous conduct would increase if the computation was made on the basis of a subclass comprised only of mentally ill individuals who had engaged in dangerous behavior before. Even here, though, we have no solid data upon which to rely.

24. *E.g.,* Statement of Hugh J. McGee, *1961 Hearings* 56. Another example of danger to self can be found in a woman enmeshed in a masochistic marriage. Not only may she suffer physical harm at the hands of her sadistic husband but her need for such sadism and her consequent willingness to endure it may lead to more serious psychical deterioration. *See* Snell, Rosenwald & Robey, *The Wife Beater's Wife—A Study of Family Interaction,* 11 ARCH. GEN. PSYCHIATRY 107 (1964).

25. That one needs treatment does not answer two other crucial questions: whether there is any known effective treatment for the affliction and whether treatment will be made available.

26. *See* Meehl & Rosen, *Antecedent Probability and the Efficiency of Psychometric Signs, Patterns, or Cutting Scores,* 52 PSYCHOLOGICAL BULL. 194 (1955); Rosen, *Detection of Suicidal Patients: An Example of Some Limitations in the Prediction of Infrequent Events,* 18 J. CONSULTING PSYCHOLOGY 397 (1954).

27. Even if we applied the psychometric test earlier hypothesized to a group of paranoids, we would still isolate ten harmless individuals for every dangerous one.

28. *See* note 4 *supra.*

29. This is compounded by the natural inclination of institutional psychiatrists and committing courts to protect themselves against possible censure by retaining patients until any possibility of danger has passed. *See, e.g.,* Ragsdale v. Overholser, 281 F.2d 943 (D.C. Cir. 1960). This conclusion is reinforced by a study to which Dr. Guttmacher alluded, *1961 Hearings* 152, when he said that "people who were released against hospital advice made about as good an adjustment rate as the people who were released by the hospital." *See also* Lewin, *Disposition of the Irresponsible: Protection Following Commitment,* 66 MICH. L. REV. 721 (1968).

30. *See* Note, *Civil Commitment of the Mentally Ill: Theories and Procedures,* 79 HARV. L. REV. 1288, (1966); Project, *Civil Commitment of the Mentally Ill,* 14 U.C.L.A. L. REV. 827 (1967).

31. It would be even more difficult to predict irresponsibility than it is to predict dangerous

conduct. In addition, it is unlikely that the irresponsible will represent a high percentage of the mentally ill. *See* Livermore & Meehl, *The Virtues of M'Naghten*, 51 MINN. L. REV. (1967).

32. Sas v. Maryland, 334 F.2d 506, 516 (4th Cir. 1963).

33. Jacobson v. Massachusetts, 197 U.S. 11, 27 (1905): "Upon the principle of self-defense, of paramount necessity, a community has the right to protect itself against an epidemic of disease which threatens the safety of its members."

34. *See generally,* Note, *Compulsory Medical Treatment,* 51 MINN. L. REV. 293 (1966).

35. *See generally* Slovenko, *The Psychiatric Patient, Liberty and the Law,* 13 KAN. L. REV. 59 (1964); Note, *Civil Commitment of Narcotics Addicts,* 76 YALE L. J. 1160, 1168–1174 (1967); Note, *Civil Commitment of the Mentally Ill: Theories and Procedures,* 79 HARV. L. REV. 1288, 1295–98 (1966).

36. The circularity of argument is obvious when the refusal to accept treatment is used as evidence of incompetence to decide, which in turn justifies compulsion. It is also present, however, in more refined formulations suggesting that mental illness diminishes liberty and that "mental health treatment should be required when the increase in liberty resulting from treatment outweighs the limitations necessary for the therapeutic process." Comment, *Liberty and Required Mental Health Treatment,* 114 U. PA. L. REV. 1067 (1966). The circularity is buried even deeper when incompetence to decide is premised on a psychiatric judgment that while the proposed patient cognitively appreciates the nature of the decision, his emotional response or affect is inappropriate.

37. *See, e.g.,* M. TWAIN, THE MYSTERIOUS STRANGER *passim* (1916).

38. Ehrenzweig, *A Psychoanalysis of the Insanity Plea — Clues to the Problems of Criminal Responsibility and Insanity in the Death Cell,* 73 YALE L.J. 425 (1964).

39. THE CASE BECOMES EVEN MORE INTERESTING WHEN THE CONDITION IS USUALLY COMPENSATED, THUS MAKING THE INDIVIDUAL A FUNCTIONING MEMBER OF SOCIETY, BUT CAN ON RARE OCCASIONS BECOME BRIEFLY DECOMPENSATED WITH POSSIBLY DISASTROUS RESULTS. CONSIDER THE CASE OF THE MAN WHO OVER A PERIOD OF 15 YEARS HAD TWO EPISODES OF CATATONIC EXCITEMENT IN WHICH HE BECAME VIOLENTLY ASSAULTIVE. EACH OCCURRENCE CAME WITHOUT WARNING.

40. IT SHOULD BE POINTED OUT, HOWEVER, THAT SUCH CONDUCT WOULD MOST PROBABLY VIOLATE THE CRIMINAL LAW, SO THAT CRIMINAL PROSECUTION AND INCARCERATION MIGHT BE IN ORDER, EVEN THOUGH CIVIL COMMITMENT WOULD BE IMPROPER.

41. *See* E. GOFFMAN, ASYLUMS (1961).

42. For example, a bus driver in Minneapolis began to annoy passengers by inflicting his paranoid ideas on them in conversation. He was advised by his employer that if he continued to do this, he would lose his employment. The offensive conduct stopped and the driver continued to work for many more years.

43. The most famous case of incarceration to relieve psychic anxiety is the segregation of the Japanese in World War II. *See* Ex parte Endo, 323 U.S. 283 (1944); Korematsu v. United States, 323 U.S. 214 (1944). This episode, however, has never been cited as one that had favorable precedential value. *See* Rostow, *The Japanese American Cases — A Disaster,* 54 YALE L.J. 489 (1945).

A STATUTE IN THE DISTRICT OF COLUMBIA, D.C. CODE § 24–301(d) (1961), providing for mandatory commitment after acquittal by reason of insanity was passed in part to add to "the public's peace of mind." Lynch v. Overholser, 369 U.S. 705, 717 (1962), *quoting* S. REP. No. 1170, 84th Cong., 1st Sess. 13 (1955); H.R. REP. No. 892, 84th Cong., 1st Sess. 13 (1955). In the case of Bolton v. Harris, 395 F.2d 642 (D.C. Cir. 1968), the mandatory commitment provision was attacked as failing to provide equal protection of the laws. Judge Bazelon agreed, but instead of holding the entire provision invalid, the court merely read the procedural safeguards of the civil commitment statute into subsection (d). *See* Comment, *Commitment Following Acquittal by Reason of Insanity and the Equal Protection of the Laws,* 116 U. PA. L. REV. 924 (1968). *See also* MODEL PENAL CODE § 4.08, Comment (Tent. Draft No. 4, 1955).

44. *See* Lake v. Cameron, 364 F.2d 657 (D.C. Cir. 1966).

45. *Id. See also* ASSOCIATION OF THE BAR OF THE CITY OF NEW YORK, MENTAL ILLNESS AND DUE PROCESS 43 (1962).

46. If nothing short of total confinement can keep the woman away from her family, we may have to temporarily deprive her of all freedom. If this occurs frequently enough, deterrence may

be effected. If that, too, fails, then long term confinement may be necessary, barbaric as that may seem. Obviously, the disruption ought to be very great before this last alternative is embraced.

47. *See* note 34 *supra* and accompanying text.

48. *E.g.,* Jehovah's Witnesses v. King County Hosp., 278 F. Supp. 488 (W.D. Wash. 1967).

49. *See In Memory of Mr. Justice Jackson,* 349 U.S. xxvii, xxix (1955).

50. "A primary purpose of the educational system is to train school children in good citizenship, patriotism and loyalty to the state and the nation as a means of protecting the public welfare." *In re* Shinn, 195 Cal. App. 2d 683, 686, 16 Cal. Rptr. 165, 168 (Dist. Ct. App. 1961). *See also* State v. Superior Court, 55 Wash. 2d 177, 346 P.2d 999 (1959), *cert. denied,* 363 U.S. 814 (1960).

51. Consider the comment of the Minnesota court in Leavitt v. City of Morris, 105 Minn. 170, 175, 117 N.W. 393, 395 (1908): "The state has the power to reclaim submerged lands, which are a menace to the public health, and make them fruitful. Has it not, also, the power to reclaim submerged men overthrown by strong drink, and help them to regain self-control?" *But see* Golding, *Ethical Issues in Biological Engineering,* 15 U.C.L.A. L. Rev. 443 (1968).

52. *See, e.g.,* Dragsow, *A Criterion for Chronicity in Schizophrenia,* 31 Psychiatric Q. 454 (1957).

53. That a certain form of treatment is useful in one type of case, of course, does not mean it is uniformly efficacious or even helpful with respect to all mental illnesses. Thus, while milieu therapy, the provision of a structured environment, may be a positive benefit to a psyche that must be removed from existing pressures or stresses, it may be useless or even harmful in other cases requiring other forms of treatment. We applaud the humanitarian concern of the Court of Appeals for the District of Columbia in recognizing a right to treatment in Rouse v. Cameron, 373 F.2d 451 (D.C. Cir. 1966), but we view that effort as misconceived. It suggests that if a patient is receiving any treatment, the state may continue his commitment. This can only be so if the provision of treatment is itself a basis of commitment, a proposition that we find horrifying in its implications. It also tends to direct attention to the limited question of provision of treatment rather than to the more fundamental question whether the state may incarcerate. Finally, by necessity it requires assessment of adequacy of treatment, an issue that because the treating professionals are in disagreement, the courts are ill-equipped to judge. *See generally* Commonwealth v. Page, 339 Mass. 313, 159 N.E.2d 82 (1959); *Position Statement on the Adequacy of Treatment,* 123 Am. J. Psychiatry 1458 (1967); Note, *Civil Restraint, Mental Illness, and the Right to Treatment,* 77 Yale L.J. 87 (1967); Note, *Due Process for All — Constitutional Standards for Involuntary Civil Commitment and Release,* 34 U. Chi. L. Rev. 633 (1967); Note, *The Nascent Right to Treatment,* 53 U. Va. L. Rev. 1134 (1967).

54. 1 American Handbook of Psychiatry 543 (S. Arieti ed. 1959).

55. *See generally* Dession, *Deviation and Community Sanctions,* in Psychiatry and the Law 1, 11 (P. Hoch & J. Zubin eds. 1955).

56. *See* Morris, Impediments to Penal Reform, 33 U. Chi. L. Rev. 627, 640 (1966).

57. The proposed statutory formulation that most nearly approaches ours is contained in Royal Commission on the Law Relating to Mental Illness and Mental Deficiency, 1954–1957, Report, Cmd. No. 169, at 111 (1957):

> We consider that the use of special compulsory powers on grounds of the patient's mental disorder is justifiable when: —
>
> (a) there is reasonable certainty that the patient is suffering from a pathological mental disorder and requires hospital or community care; and
>
> (b) suitable care cannot be provided without the use of compulsory powers; and
>
> (c) if the patient himself is unwilling to receive the form of care which is considered necessary, there is at least a strong likelihood that his unwillingness is due to a lack of appreciation of his own condition deriving from the mental disorder itself; and
>
> (d) there is also either
>
>   (i) good prospect of benefit to the patient from the treatment proposed—

an expectation that it will either cure or alleviate his mental disorder or strengthen his ability to regulate his social behaviour in spite of the underlying disorder, or bring him substantial benefit in the form of protection from neglect or exploitation by others; or

(ii) a strong need to protect others from anti-social behaviour by the patient.

Saleem A. Shah

Dangerousness and Civil Commitment of the Mentally Ill: Some Public Policy Considerations

Concern about the alleged dangerousness of an individual is raised in a variety of contexts, e.g., involuntary civil commitment of the mentally ill, sexual psychopathy, confinement and release of persons acquitted of criminal responsibility by reason of insanity, and sentencing and release of "dangerous" offenders. The issues and problems pertaining to dangerousness have been the subject of much discussion. Often, however, these issues might best be viewed in reference to a specific area of psychiatric and legal decision making. This presentation will focus on the use of the concept of dangerousness to others in the involuntary civil commitment of the mentally ill. Commitment criteria phrased in terms of dangerousness to self, grave disablement, or the need for care and treatment will not be addressed.

At present, there are 15 jurisdictions in the United States that authorize commitment *only* if the individual is mentally ill and dangerous to himself and others or is unable to care for his physical needs. Fourteen other states provide for such commitment of the mentally ill person if the individual is dangerous or is in need of care or treatment. Various other jurisdictions require that commitment be necessary to protect the welfare of the individual or the welfare of others; still other states permit involuntary commitment when the individual is in need of care and treatment or in need of hospitalization because of mental illness (1, 2).

From *The American Journal of Psychiatry* 132 (1975):501–505. Copyright © 1975 by the American Psychiatric Association. Reprinted by permission of the publisher and the author.

Defining Dangerousness: Public Policy and Sociopolitical Factors

Since involuntary civil commitment represents an exercise of state power that may deprive an individual of his liberty and may also compel him to undergo psychiatric treatment, it raises public policy and legal questions regarding the circumstances which justify such coercive state action (1). According to a basic principle in common law, restraint of insane persons without the usual legal process is justified when the use of such restraint is limited to situations involving imminent danger to persons or property (2). This inherent power to protect the safety and welfare of the public is referred to as the police power of the state. Thus involuntary civil commitments that are justified by reference to a broad societal interest rather than to protection of the interests of the mentally ill person constitute an exercise of police power. There are various restrictions, including Constitutional provisions, that govern and regulate the proper exercise of this power.

Historically, the sovereign, as father of the country, was also responsible for the care and custody of persons who were incompetent to care for themselves. This parens patriae function may be viewed in its current use as a power that citizens have granted to the state for their personal protection. Even though they are less closely regulated or restricted than police power actions, the benevolent intentions and actions of the state have to conform to a number of Constitutional restrictions, e.g., that such actions are reasonably related to a valid state goal (1).

The initial and fundamental question that must be asked when the state wants to use its power and authority to involuntarily confine an individual is, What potential harms to society or to the individual are sufficiently serious to justify resorting to coercive confinement (3)?

Clearly, this question involves public policy, sociopolitical, and legal considerations. It is *not* in this context a medical, psychiatric, psychological, or mental health question. However, determination of dangerousness is often left to representatives of these professions, who may testify as expert witnesses, as a function of the vague statutory language that typifies civil commitment and related laws and of the failure of courts to make explicit judicial determinations and findings of fact (4, 5). This situation leads to a confounding of public policy and legal issues with psychiatric and mental health concerns (6).

Thus two interacting questions are involved in the issue of dangerousness. The first asks, What kinds of behavior are sufficiently threatening to society to be officially defined as dangerous? This is fundamentally a public policy question. The second question is, With what degree of certainty can one say that an individual will in the future engage in dangerous behavior and, if so, over what period of time? This question is essentially empirical and poses a most difficult challenge to the predictive and prognostic skills of mental health professionals.

Some Official Definitions and Criteria

Despite the frequent use of the concept of dangerousness, there are few specific and clear official definitions as to the precise behaviors it encompasses. The vague statutory language referring to "danger to self and others" barely addresses this need. However, even a quick review of some of the relevant case law during recent years, especially that which has developed in the United States Court of Appeals for the District of Columbia, indicates that the courts have tended to move away from their earlier and very global notions of dangerousness and toward narrower definitions.

In the case of *Overholser v. Russell* (7), for example, it was stated that competent evidence that the individual may commit any criminal act was sufficient to indicate the likelihood of dangerousness to the community. In this particular case, the criminal charge for which the individual had received an insanity acquittal was writing a check against insufficient funds. Similarly, in the case of *United States v. Charnizon* (8), a defendant who had been involuntarily confined to a mental hospital following an insanity acquittal (on two counts of false pretenses) was denied release from the hospital because he was judged to be likely to pose a danger to himself or to others "in the sense of writing bad checks."

However, in *Millard v. Cameron* (9), a case involving the District of Columbia sexual psychopath law, the court ruled that the statute required that "dangerous conduct be not merely repulsive or repugnant but must have serious effect on the viewer." Later, in *Millard v. Harris* (10), a court stated that the possible harm from the patient's exhibitionism to "very seclusive, withdrawn, shy, sensitive" women was insufficient in regard to the "limits on the extent to which the law can sweep the streets clear of all possible sources of occasional distress to such women." Similarly, in *Cross v. Harris* (11), the court pointed out that "a mere possibility of injury is not enough; the statute requires that harm be *likely*." The court also emphasized that decisions pertaining to the dangerousness of an individual must consider both the likelihood of harm and the magnitude of the anticipated harm.

The quest by the courts for more limited and carefully defined uses of the dangerousness criterion points to the need for mental health professionals to begin to seriously reexamine their uses of this concept and criterion. In the past, there has been a tendency on the part of many physicians and psychiatrists to behave as though there were no particular difficulties in assessing dangerousness. Regrettably, fairly brief, conclusory statements about a patient's mental illness and potential dangerousness—based on equally brief examinations—have often typified involuntary civil commitment proceedings in many jurisdictions (12, 13).

The Conceptualization of Behavior

A major problem in efforts to assess, predict, prevent, and treat dangerous and deviant behavior pertains to the way behavior is conceptualized. Behavior—

be it socially defined as dangerous, peaceful, social, or antisocial—is often viewed as stemming largely (if not entirely) from within the individual, i.e., as deriving from his personality. From this perspective, behavior tends to be viewed as a fairly enduring and consistent characteristic of the individual. Moreover, a specific behavioral act may not only be assessed and labeled as dangerous, but the assumption may be made that such samples of behavior are fairly representative of the individual. Hence, through a conceptual shortcut, certain aspects of the individual's behavior are defined as dangerous and then the individual himself comes to be viewed and labeled as dangerous. This, of course, may be misleading and unnecessarily stigmatizing, since violent and dangerous behaviors are often not representative of the individual's typical behavioral repertoire (5).

It is most important that behavior be understood in reference to its social, situational, and environmental context. In other words, behavior should be viewed as involving an interaction between an individual and a particular physical and social environment. This environment may exert major influence on the form, frequency, and range of possible behaviors. Some situational and environmental factors may tend to elicit, facilitate, and even provoke certain behaviors; other factors may tend to have an inhibiting and suppressive effect (14, 15).

Why the Link Between Illness and Dangerousness?

The behavioral characteristic of dangerousness often tends to be linked with mental illness not only in reference to civil commitment statutes but also in regard to issues of exculpatory insanity, sexual psychopathy, and even the sentencing of so-called dangerous offenders (16). Typically, an individual cannot be involuntarily confined to a mental institution simply because of his/her anticipated—or even demonstrated—dangerousness. There has to be a finding first of mental disorder and then of an associated propensity or predicted likelihood for engaging in dangerous behavior.

It is somewhat difficult to discern how this link between mental illness and dangerous behavior came about and why it continues to be maintained with such enduring zeal with regard to the entire group of persons officially defined as mentally ill. As noted earlier, to protect the community against dangerous individuals, the state typically uses its police powers. However, the criminal process is invoked *after* the individual has engaged in some harmful act, i.e., is alleged to have committed a criminal act. The Constitution has generally been interpreted as prohibiting the use of preventive detention against persons who are expected or presumed to be dangerous but have not yet engaged in a criminal act. How far this interpretation carries is illustrated by a case which involved a 39-year-old man who had a criminal history that included successive convictions for manslaughter, shooting with intent to kill, assault with intent to kill, assault with a pistol, assault and robbery, assault and battery, and attempted robbery (17). On the expectation that the man would again resort to a violent crime, steps were taken to involuntarily commit him to a mental institution on the ground of his being potentially dangerous to others.

In upholding a writ of habeas corpus that freed the man from the hospital, the Court of Appeals stated,

> However commendable was the court's purpose to protect the public from the release to society of a man "potentially dangerous to others," there is no District of Columbia statute or inherent equity power permitting commitment to any institution upon that showing alone. Many persons who are released to society upon completing the services of sentences in criminal cases are just as surely potential menaces to society as is this petitioner, having a similar pattern of antisocial behavior, lack of occupational adjustment, and absence of remorse and anxiety; *yet the courts have no legal basis of ordering their continued confinement on mere apprehension of future unlawful acts,* and must await until another crime against society is committed or they are found insane in proper mental health proceedings before confinement may again be ordered. (18. p. 876, emphasis added)

The reader is invited to ponder the implications of this comment. The court ruled that dangerousness alone, without the commission of some new criminal act or a finding of mental illness, was not sufficient ground for the involuntary confinement of an individual with a clear—even blatant—history of violent and dangerous acts. If, on the other hand, a finding of mental illness had been forthcoming, indeterminate and involuntary hospitalization could have been effected. It would appear, therefore, that (at least in part) the linking of dangerousness with mental illness enabled society to utilize preventive detention against certain groups of individuals, a practice which would otherwise run afoul of the Constitution.

How Dangerous Are the Mentally Ill?

As Nunnally (19) found several years ago, there are fairly stereotyped public impressions of the mentally ill as "relatively dangerous, dirty, unpredictable, and worthless." Mental patients appear to have taken the place of lepers as the targets of public dislike and rejection (20).

Mental health professionals, particularly those who testify in courts as expert witnesses, have a clear obligation to inform themselves, the courts, and lawyers, as well as the general public, on the extent to which the behavioral characteristic of dangerousness is associated with mental illness. There have been several studies on this subject that have examined arrest records of patients released from mental institutions. These studies, although not free from methodological problems, do not support the public stereotype of the mentally ill as highly dangerous and unpredictable.

Several of the earlier studies found that discharged mental patients had lower arrest rates than the general population (21–23). More recent studies, however, have tempered this picture somewhat. For example, Rappeport and Lassen (24, 25) found higher rates of arrest for robbery and rape among male ex-patients and for aggravated assault among female ex-patients than among the general population. Their studies also found that patients with alcohol problems were most heavily represented in both pre- and posthospitalization arrests.

Giovannoni and Gurel (26) obtained results that were rather similar to those of Rappeport and Lassen in a follow-up of 1,142 Veteran's Administration patients, all of whom were functionally psychotic men. These investigators used several indices of "socially disruptive behavior" (namely, time spent in jail or other penal detention, arrests by police, and all instances of socially disruptive behavior, including criminal activity that may not have come to the attention of the police). They found that arrest and detention rates for patients were higher for certain crimes against persons but lower for crimes against property than among the general population.

Alcohol abuse was a serious problem among these VA patients, 65.8 percent of whom had had some type of alcohol-related problem. Of these, 20.6 percent had an arrest only for drunkenness and 45.2 percent had an offense other than drunkenness and were rated as having trouble with alcohol. It is important to note that alcoholism was not the primary diagnosis for any of these patients; they had all been admitted into the study as functionally psychotic, with 95 percent diagnosed as schizophrenic.

It would seem likely, therefore, that ex-mental patients (i.e., those who have been hospitalized) are not necessarily less dangerous, as a group, then the general population. However, it also seems necessary to consider factors such as the high prevalence of alcohol problems and the probability that psychotic patients would be more likely than other offenders to attract attention to their behavior. Moreover, as Giovannoni and Gurel (26) pointed out, it is quite likely that arrest rates among released hospital patients differ considerably as a function of differing admission, retention, and discharge policies and practices of various jurisdictions and mental hospitals. They pointed out that "none of the data cited [in our study] would suggest any accuracy in the distorted view of the average mental patient as an unusually and predominantly dangerous person."

Thus even though persons diagnosed as suffering from serious mental illness (i.e., those likely to be hospitalized) may not be any less dangerous than persons not so diagnosed, the available evidence points strongly to the conclusion that the mentally ill do not constitute one of the most dangerous groups in our society. Indeed, compared to groups of criminal offenders, ex-felons, or even persons convicted of drunken driving, it seems very probable that the mentally ill would not constitute the most dangerous group.

Prediction of Dangerous Behavior

Given the numerous court proceedings in which the dangerousness of a mentally ill person is at issue and the very serious decisions affecting life and liberty that must be made, one might assume that some reasonably accurate means of predicting dangerous behavior are available. This assumption would be false. No instrument has yet been developed that can predict violent and other dangerous behavior in a reasonably accurate and satisfactory manner. Indeed, as Megargee (27) noted, no psychological test has been developed that can adequately identify such behavior retrospectively—let alone predict it.

Despite the absence of an adequate prediction instrument, one might still assume that psychiatrists and other mental health professionals who typically make assessments and predictions of dangerousness would have some demonstrated skills in this regard. Once again, the assumption would be false. The available studies indicate quite clearly and consistently that psychiatrists and other professionals overpredict dangerousness to an extraordinary degree. In other words, the overwhelming majority of mentally ill persons who are committed to mental institutions or are denied release from such facilities because of their presumed dangerousness do not engage in dangerous behavior following release (4, 28–31).

It should, however, come as no surprise that very high rates of error are often associated with efforts to predict infrequent events (i.e., events with very low base rates). Nearly two decades ago, Rosen (32) explained on statistical grounds why attempts to predict behaviors with low base rates are invariably associated with very high rates of false positives (in this case, persons who are identified as likely to be dangerous but who in fact do not display such behaviors). Using suicide among psychiatric in-patients as his example, Rosen demonstrated that there would be between 50 and 99 false positives for every 1 correct prediction.

Moreover, given the particular kinds of social and political consequences that attend the two types of error possible in predictions of an individual's dangerous behavior, it is quite understandable that the error to be avoided is the one which would incur undesirable publicity when a released mental patient later displayed violent behavior in the community. Thus the number of false positives would tend to be further increased in efforts to avoid such societal responses.

Psychiatrists and other mental health professionals are thus presented with some very perplexing decisional problems as well as related public policy questions in the assessment and prediction of dangerousness. These basically difficult problems become more complicated when differing—or conflicting—decision rules enter the picture (6, 33). For example, in the criminal process, rather elaborate safeguards have been instituted to ensure due process for the accused. In addition, in criminal trials a decision rule is used that requires proof of guilt beyond a reasonable doubt—to ensure that any error will be consistent with the values of our society, i.e., will result in erroneous acquittals—not erroneous convictions. Medical decision rules, which obviously are concerned with very different types of consequences, appear to be quite different. The cautious physician operates on the rule "When in doubt, suspect illness." Certainly, the social values and consequences to be avoided are quite different from those in criminal trials.

However, in view of the fact that involuntary civil commitment of the mentally ill pertains, fundamentally, to public policy and legal questions and involves the state in coercive intervention in the lives of individuals, legal rather than medical decision rules would seem to be clearly indicated. Stated differently, when the individual faces involuntary confinement in a situation that involves legal and judicial decisions, as contrasted with the typical physician-patient relationship, mental health professionals need to be very cautious about their decisions. There are already rather clear indications that the relatively weaker decision rules of various civil proceedings (e.g., preponderance of the evidence) are moving toward stricter burden of proof requirements (34–36).

Some Public Policy Implications

Issues of dangerousness and the involuntary commitment of the mentally ill exemplify rather strikingly the manner in which public policy and legal questions have been translated into psychiatric and mental health terms. Stated differently, what would appear essentially to be issues relevant to the state's use of its police powers seem to have been rephrased and shifted to the exercise of parens patriae functions. It is almost as though the recitation and announcement of benevolent societal intentions is necessary for the justification (rationalization?) of practices that suggest social control rather than therapeutic concerns.

By blurring and obscuring the fundamentally moral and public policy issues intrinsically imbedded in the balancing of competing societal interests and values and turning them into mental health questions, it has been possible to justify societal practices that infringe grievously upon the rights and liberties of the mentally ill.

It is not surprising, therefore, that some of the most predictably and demonstrably dangerous persons are *not* preventively detained (as in the case discussed earlier) or handled with greater concern for public safety. For example, numerous studies have provided rather consistent evidence that about 50 percent of all fatal accidents involve drunken drivers. It also appears that less than 10 percent of the driving population (namely, those with serious drinking problems) account for almost two-thirds of all alcohol-related traffic fatalities (37, 38). However, our society demonstrates a truly astonishing tolerance for this group of demonstrably dangerous persons. It is likely that more persons are killed and seriously injured by drunken drivers during the course of a single week than by all combined categories of psychotic individuals over an entire year — perhaps even several years.

In view of the very vague definitions of "dangerousness," the very low predictive accuracy and the glaring overpredictions of such behavior, and the involuntary and indeterminate loss of liberty that follows civil commitments, the labeling of the mentally ill as dangerous could in itself be regarded as a rather dangerous activity. One might well wonder whether, in the various civil and parens patriae proceedings in which psychiatric concepts are invoked and mental health professionals are involved, the societal practices seem to be more concerned with using these professionals as agents of social control rather than as individuals functioning in their usual and traditional therapeutic roles (29). In the final analysis, we must assume greater responsibility for the ways in which our services are used—or misused.

REFERENCES

1. Note: Developments in the law: civil commitment of the mentally ill. Harvard Law Review 87:1190–1406, 1974.
2. Brakel SJ, Rock RS: The Mentally Disabled and the Law, revised ed. Chicago, University of Chicago Press, 1971.
3. Livermore JM, Malmquist CP, Meehl PE: On the justifications for civil commitment. University of Pennsylvania Law Review 117:75–96, 1968.
4. Dershowitz AM: The psychiatrist's power in civil commitment. Psychology Today, Feb 1969, pp. 43–47.
5. Shah SA: Some interactions of law and mental health in the handling of social deviance. Catholic University Law Review 23:674–719, 1974.
6. Shah SA: Crime and mental illness: some problems in defining and labeling deviant behavior. Mental Hygiene 53:21–33, 1969.
7. Overholser v. Russell, 283 F 2d 195 (1960).
8. United States v. Charnizon, 232 A 2d 586, 588 (1967).
9. Millard v. Cameron, 373 F 2d 468, 471 (1966).
10. Millard v. Harris, 406 F 2d 964, 978 (1968).
11. Cross v. Harris, 418 F 2d 1095, 1100 (1969).
12. Maisel R: Decision-making in a commitment court. Psychiatry 33:352–361, 1970.
13. Wexler DB, Scoville SE: The administration of psychiatric justice: theory and practice in Arizona. Arizona Law Review 13:1–259, 1971.
14. Mischel W: Personality and Assessment. New York, John Wiley & Sons, 1968.
15. Moos RH: Conceptualizations of human environments. Am. Psychol. 28:652–665, 1973.
16. National Council on Crime and Delinquency, Council of Judges: Model sentencing act—second edition. Crime and Delinquency 18:335–370, 1972.
17. Williams v. United States, 250 F 2d 19 (1957).
18. In re Williams, 157 F suppl. 871 (1958).
19. Nunnally JC: Population Conceptions of Mental Health. New York, Holt, Rinehart and Winston, 1961.
20. Rabkin JG: Opinions about mental illness: a review of the literature. Psychol. Bull. 77:153–171, 1972.
21. Pollack HM: Is the paroled patient a menace to the community? Psychiatr. Q. 12:236–244, 1938.
22. Cohen LH, Freeman H: How dangerous to the community are state hospital patients? Connecticut State Medical Journal 9:697–699, 1945.
23. Brill H, Malzberg B: Statistical Report on the Arrest Record of Male Ex-Patients, Age 16 or Over, Released from New York State Mental Hospitals During the Period 1946–48. Mental Hospital Service Supplemental Report 153. Washington, DC, American Psychiatric Association, 1962.
24. Rappeport JR, Lassen G: Dangerousness—arrest rate comparisons of discharged mental patients and the general population. Am. J. Psychiatry 121:776–783, 1965.

25. Rappeport, JR, Lassen G: The dangerousness of female patients: a comparison of the arrest rate of discharged psychiatric patients and the general population. Am. J. Psychiatry 123: 413–419, 1966.

26. Giovannoni JF, Gurel L: Socially disruptive behavior of ex-mental patients. Arch. Gen. Psychiatry 17:146–153, 1967.

27. Megargee EI: The prediction of violence with psychological tests, in Current Topics in Clinical and Community Psychology, vol. 2. Edited by Spielberger CD. New York, Academic Press, 1970, pp. 97–156.

28. Hunt R, Wiley E: Operation Baxstrom after one year. Am. J. Psychiatry 124:974–978, 1968.

29. Steadman HJ: The psychiatrist as a conservative agent of social control. Social Problems 20: 263–271, 1972.

30. Steadman HJ, Keveles G: The community adjustment and criminal activity of the Baxstrom patients: 1966–1970. Am. J. Psychiatry 129:304–310, 1972.

31. Wenk EA, Robison JO, Smith GW: Can violence be predicted? Crime and Delinquency 18: 393–402, 1972.

32. Rosen A: Detection of suicidal patients: an example of some limitations in the prediction of infrequent events. Journal of Consulting Psychology 18:397–403, 1954.

33. Scheff TJ: Decision rules, types of error and their consequences in medical diagnosis. Behav. Sci. 8:97–107, 1963.

34. In re Winship, 397 US 358 (1970).

35. Tippett v. Maryland, 436 F 2d 1153 (4th Cir 1971]).

36. Lessard v. Schmidt, 349 F suppl. 1078 (ED Wis [1972]).

37. Alcohol and Highway Safety: A Report to the Congress from the Secretary of Transportation. Washington, DC. US Department of Transportation, Aug. 1968.

38. Voas RB: Alcohol as an underlying factor in behavior leading to fatal highway crashes, in Research on Alcoholism: Clinical Problems and Special Populations. Proceedings of the First Annual Alcoholism Conference of the National Institute on Alcohol Abuse and Alcoholism, US Department of Health, Education, and Welfare Publication 74-670. Edited by Chafetz ME, Washington, DC, US Government Printing Office, 1973, pp. 324–331.

David F. Greenberg

Involuntary Psychiatric Commitments to Prevent Suicide

I. Introduction

This article will evaluate the civil sanctions presently used by the state to prevent people from committing suicide. In particular, we will examine involuntary civil commitments to psychiatric hospitals, as well as lesser degrees of preventive restraint. Although suicides and suicide attempts are illegal and can be punished under the criminal law in a few states,[1] the use of such statutes is infrequent and enjoys no substantial advocacy, probably because the more serious suicide attempter is seen as more sinned against than sinner, more to be pitied than blamed.[2] By contrast, civil commitment procedures for persons believed to be suicidal enjoy wide support, particularly, but not exclusively, within the psychiatric profession.[3]

The emphasis of this study will be conceptual; although it will draw heavily on published social scientific research concerning suicide, it will not be primarily concerned with documenting existing abuses in commitment practices or with portraying deplorable conditions in mental institutions. There are two reasons for this choice of emphasis. First, one's attitude toward abuses may depend on the outcome of a conceptual inquiry, for if it can be established that some practice is, at least in principle, a good idea, then one might look for ways to remedy abuses; but if the practice is objectionable in principle, one may wish to aim at the different target of abolishing it altogether.

The second reason for our emphasis is that very little empirical information

From *New York University Law Review* 49 (1974):227–245. Reprinted by permission of the publisher and the author.

about the use of specific coercive measures to prevent suicide is available. The observation of the United States Supreme Court that, considering the number of people affected, it was surprising how little litigation there had been concerning the substantive constitutional limits to civil commitment proceedings[4] is especially applicable to commitments justified on grounds of suicide prevention. Consequently, the empirical research that might have been stimulated by litigation has not been done. Nor has research with other motivation filled the gap. We do not know how many persons are committed each year under this justification, how long they stay in mental institutions,[5] or, in any detail, what happens to them while they are there.

The conceptual framework for considering such commitments has remained equally undeveloped. Neither the legal nor the medical profession has explored the issues involved in any depth. The careful consideration of issues found in discussions of preventive confinement of persons considered dangerous to others[6] is simply absent when the preventive confinement involves persons considered dangerous to themselves.[7] Hopefully this preliminary effort will stimulate further analysis and encourage empirical research.

II. Rationales for Legal Coercion to Prevent Suicide

Both long-term commitments (hospitalization or institutionalization) and emergency detention to prevent suicide are made possible by state mental health legislation authorizing such measures for persons who are considered mentally ill, dangerous to themselves or in need of care or treatment. The wording of the relevant statutes varies: some states require the establishment of both dangerousness and mental illness; others require only one or the other.[8] One state includes in its definition of mentally ill persons any person "who is of such mental condition that he is dangerous to himself."[9] The existence of these statutes and their sometimes erratic operation in practice[10] pose the question of whether the prevention of suicide is a goal so weighty as to justify infringing cherished values of liberty and autonomy. Our consideration of this question requires a discussion of the various rationales advanced for legal coercion to prevent suicide.

Early rationales for such coercion rested on religious or political grounds: to commit suicide was to reject God's gift of life or to deprive the state of its property.[11] These are no longer persuasive in a secular and democratic age. Contemporary discussions of suicide prevention, on the few occasions when they trouble to discuss the justifications for coercive prevention, emphasize one or more of the following themes: the prevention of harm to survivors, the prevention of harm to the suicide attempter and suicide as the product of mental illness. We shall consider each in turn.

A. Prevention of Harm to Others

A suicide can be devastating in its impact. Intimate survivors may feel guilty, blaming themselves for having caused the suicide or for having failed to prevent it.[12] Alternatively, they may be blamed by others.[13] These responses may, of course, take place independently of the wishes of the deceased. In some instances, however, the person suiciding may attempt to elicit guilt or blame through a suicide note.[14]

While such posthumous accusations may be injurious to a survivor's reputation or peace of mind, and may be difficult to rebut, we have no reason to assume that they are necessarily undeserved or so serious in their consequences as to justify coercive state intervention.

Other kinds of harm to survivors of suicide include financial loss to surviving dependents, which, in extreme cases, may seriously affect their life chances, and lives made more difficult for reasons other than financial.[15] Sometimes a suicide will induce intimate survivors to commit suicide.[16] Someone who suicides may also leave behind unfulfilled legal commitments (*e.g.,* contractual obligations).

In addition to the harm to intimate survivors there may also, in some cases, be harm to society. When the suicide possesses some rare talent, all of us may be diminished by what appears to be a premature death.

Yet, even where an injury to others can clearly be identified, state intervention may not be justified, at least if the intervention is coercive. There are many areas of social life for which we provide no legal channels by which one person can seek redress for harm occasioned by another's actions. In some cases, this is because fault would be difficult to assign. In others, official enforcement would require extreme invasion of privacy and strangling regulation of our private lives. Indeed, since state intervention tends to be crude and mechanical, it is often more likely to make matters worse than better.

Significantly, much of the harm to others occasioned by a suicide involves aspects of life that seem ill-suited to legal regulation. Such harm, when it arises from other causes, does not ordinarily provide the basis for a legally recognized claim (*e.g.,* sparing someone from experiencing grief). Often it is unclear why we should prefer the claims of the survivors who seek protection from distress to those of the potential suicide attempter, who may experience considerable unhappiness if forced to continue living.

In other cases, a basis for a legal claim may be more solidly founded. Just as a parent may be jailed for failure to make child support payments, so the child of a suicide attempter may be legally entitled to support. The difficulty here is that the cost to the person kept alive — the psychic distress of the person who wishes to die — may far exceed the harm prevented, especially when preservation of life requires long-term confinement to a mental institution. Thus, it seems clearly preferable to permit the suicide and use welfare payments to survivors to alleviate financial hardship.

The case for coercion to prevent injury to others from a suicide clearly is weak, and should not ordinarily constitute grounds for state interference with a suicide attempter. Exceptions might be made only in the very rare case when a suicide would result in extremely serious injury to others. For example, if the potential suicide is the only witness to an alibi for a defendant on trial for a serious crime, the latter might reasonably argue that his right to be absolved is sufficiently important to justify the temporary prevention of suicide until after the witness testifies.

B. Prevention of Harm to Self

Upon reflection, the claim that suicide is necessarily harmful must be rejected. We know nothing of the fate of those who kill themselves; conceivably, their souls are transported to an especially favored spot on the Isle of the Blessed. More to the point, however, it is hardly difficult to imagine circumstances where suicide, if not a positive good, would readily be recognizable as the lesser of evils. One obvious case would be the victim who suicides to escape the pain of an excruciating terminal illness.[17] Many other possibilities can be imagined, or discovered in case histories in the suicide literature: to prevent the enemy from obtaining secrets through torture, to end a life that has become lonely and tedious, to preserve honor or reputation in the face of threatened scandal, to call attention to a political injustice or to control one's final "scene" in the theatre of life.

In other instances, however, suicide may seem clearly disproportionate to the precipitating cause. For example, suicide attempts have been attributed to feelings of intense guilt over matters that may seem to many others to be venial or totally inconsequential (*e.g.*, sexual experiences). Yet distress is subjective. The anguish of the person who finds continued life intolerable is not mitigated by another's opinion that the occasion for distress is minor. That most others might not commit suicide in a given situation indicates only that the suicidal person has experienced the situation differently. To prevent suicide in this case is to permit someone else to decide that the potential attempter is better off alive and suffering than dead and to impose that decision on the attempter. This violates the right to die when one wishes, which would seem to be a necessary part of the right to live with dignity and privacy, a right to be denied only if there were some other, overriding interest to be served by the denial. This right would mean little if it could be exercised only when consistent with others' views of what is reasonable or appropriate. While it may seem anomalous to speak of "a right to die," the infringement of this right seriously jeopardizes the right to live one's life as one wishes, and not to live it when it is no longer possible to do so as one wishes.

C. Suicide as the Product of Mental Illness

The case for benevolent coercion to prevent suicide has not rested entirely on the prevention of self-injury. Most commitment statutes specify not only that the defendant must be thought likely to be dangerous to himself if permitted to remain at liberty, but also that he be mentally ill. Sometimes it is specified that the dangerousness must be a *consequence* of the mental illness. The reason for requiring that mental illness be present presumably is that while libertarian principles might allow a sane person to engage in activity others considered self-injurious, a person who is not sane—whose mental processes are so disordered by illness as to preclude a rational choice—forfeits no valued prerogative when prevented from committing suicide, because such a person cannot meaningfully be said to have chosen to die.[18]

There are several problems with this claim. First, the diagnosis of mental illness is far from an exact science. The boundary between behavior that is merely eccentric and behavior that arises from malfunctioning of the faculties of the mind may be extremely difficult, some would say conceptually impossible, to draw.[19] This may be one cause of the wide variation in estimates of the incidence of mental illness among suicide populations.[20] The requirement that mental illness not only be present but in addition be the *cause* of the dangerousness only compounds the difficulty, since the causal element may be difficult to establish even when it is possible to achieve consensus as to the *presence* of "mental illness."

It is safe to assume that these fine points are ignored in present commitment practice. Questions of mental illness are now often decided either by lay notions of mental health or by physicians using psychiatric classifications or, perhaps, their own moral judgments concerning defendants' lifestyles.[21] In the absence of vigorous legal representation (and sometimes in the absence of the defendant as well—not all states require notification or the presence of the defendant at the commitment hearing), delicate questions of causation are likely to be brushed aside, and the working assumption made that dangerousness and mental illness imply one another.

The second problem concerns the empirical relationship between mental illness and suicide. The popular stereotype linking suicide and mental illness[22] is reflected in the emphasis in psychiatric research on suicide on the determination of suicide rates among patients with various psychiatric diagnoses. Possible links between suicide and depression have been particularly stressed. It has been estimated that anywhere between 10 and 40 percent of all suicides suffer from depression.[23] Yet, as Kobler and Stotland point out, a distinction must be made between the presence of *symptoms* of depression and the presence of a depressive psychosis. As an unusual degree of unhappiness is a symptom of depression, investigators may mistakenly infer the presence of depressive illness from evidence that someone who committed suicide had been unhappy.[24]

Other investigators have examined such matters as purposefulness and reality orientation among suicide attempters. One study of schizophrenics who committed suicide found:

> There was surprising (and fairly strong) evidence . . . that suicide did not occur in schizophrenics in response to impulsive delusional thoughts or hallucinations but rather that self-destruction occurred in a somewhat planned and organized attempt at extrication from intolerably stressful life situations. . . .[25]

In fact, a study of suicide attempts among depressive patients found the attempt rate to be quite a bit lower among depressed persons who had persistent obsessions than among those whose obsessions were transient or who had no obsessions at all. Apparently, patients with obsessions were kept so preoccupied thinking about their obsessions that they were unable to think about other matters, such as killing themselves.[26] To plan and carry through a suicide attempt may require more ability to think coherently and to act in a realistic, organized fashion than a patient with delusions or obsessions possesses. Among both schizophrenics and depressives (that is, patients labeled as such; we leave aside the question of correspondence between label and inner psychological state) it has been observed that suicide tends to occur not in the acute phase (in response to hallucinations, delusions or panic) but rather when the patient is improving and unable to cope with problems.[27]

Thus, the mere fact of a suicide attempt or the presence of a threat or a desire to commit suicide cannot by any means be taken as conclusory evidence for the presence of mental illness, especially if by mental illness one means an inability to perceive reality accurately, to reason logically and to make plans and carry them out in an organized fashion.

Quite apart from this empirical question, it is not so obvious that to prevent someone who is mentally ill from committing suicide is necessarily to bestow a blessing. The woman who, despite medical evidence to the contrary, is convinced she has cancer may be mistaken, but, if her delusion persists, she may nevertheless find death preferable to a protracted life of fear and anxiety. Though her beliefs may be in error, her emotions may be just as acute and distressing as if they had been well-founded in physiological reality.

III. Reformulating the Suicide Debate

We have considered the traditional benefits advocated for suicide prevention policies. Our analysis suggested that preventing injury to others or to self rarely would constitute adequate grounds for prevention of suicide through coercive means. That analysis, however, accepted hidden premises that require further examination. In fact, it has not thus far been noticed that much of the discussion of involuntary commitment has tended to rest on premises that may not be valid. The advocate of intervention typically assumes that the individual under consideration *is* suicidal, not someone mistakenly thought to be suicidal or maliciously and wrongfully accused of being suicidal.[28] Consequently, he may pay insufficient attention to the problem of screening. In addition, he is likely to assume that intervention motivated by the goal of preventing suicides will, at least some of the time, attain its goal. Yet this need not be the case. The effectiveness of any given measure in preventing suicides is an empirical question the answer to which may not simply be assumed.[29] The libertarian, on the other hand, assumes, perhaps with no greater justification, that suicide attempters want to die, so that abstaining from interference conforms to their wishes. This assumption, too, may be wide of the mark. These hidden assumptions require careful examination before an objective look at the suicide prevention debate may be had.

A. Do Suicide Attempters Want to Die?

Unlike early research on suicide,[30] recent studies have considered the conscious, self-perceived motivations of suicide attempters to be worthy of study, and have attempted to situate these motivations in the life experiences and circumstances of the attempters. Researchers are in agreement that most attempters do not unequivocally want to die. For example, sociologist Jack Douglas concludes:

> In the vast majority of cases, . . . individuals committing dangerous acts against themselves do have what they themselves see as some degree of intention to die. . . . But there is also every indication that in the great majority of cases where there is such an intention to die, there is also an intention to use suicide, through the construction of certain meanings for others involved, so that they can live better either in this world or the next. Suicide, then, is generally a highly ambivalent action. Even those individuals with very serious intentions of dying by suicide rarely give up hope of living. After taking pills, they call for help or move toward others; when cutting their throats they make "hesitation" cuts; and most individuals who attempt or commit suicide have given their friends and relations serious warnings of their intentions to kill themselves.[31]

In accord with the foregoing observations is the report of a team of psychiatrists: "[W]e have come to regard attempted suicide not as an effort to die but rather as a communication to others in an effort to improve one's life."[32] Although a suicide attempt may seem like a peculiar way to improve one's life, we should not assume without further investigation that a suicide attempt is irrational or foolish. For adults, at least, a suicide attempt frequently is successful in bringing about an improved relationship with significant others. According to one psychiatrist, "[t]he suicidal act . . . usually arouses sufficient sympathy to bring about some change in the circumstances surrounding the person who makes the attempt."[33] Similarly, the authors of another study made the following observation: "We regard these 34 attempts as successful in the sense that desired changes in the life situation of the patient occurred as a consequence of the attempt."[34]

The foregoing research findings as to the motivation of suicide attempts and the responses which these attempts often elicit suggest the relevance of a game theory perspective. From this angle the suicide attempter is a player in a game, so desperate as to be willing to risk a highly unfavorable outcome (death) in order to obtain a favorable outcome (survival and transformed relationships with others, or solved problems).[35] It becomes easier, then, to understand the efforts of so many attempters to bring about life-saving intervention[36] as well as the high survival rate among attempters. It is estimated that only about one of every eight or ten suicide attempts result in death.[37]

Studies of the subsequent mortality rate among survivors of suicide attempts tend to confirm the view of attempters as persons who, for the most part, are not intent on dying. Only about 1% of all surviving attempters kill themselves within a year of the attempt.[38] This is still quite a bit higher than the suicide rate in the general population, but far lower than would be anticipated if most attempters unambivalently wanted to die.

The long-range suicide rate among surviving attempters is somewhat higher. Follow-up studies lasting as long as 15 years suggest that eventually somewhere between five and 15 percent of surviving attempters will kill themselves.[39] Not surprisingly, subsequent suicide may depend on the response to the initial attempt. Thus, the authors of one study "found consistently that recovery requires a major change in the life situation."[40] This, of course, is just what we would expect if most attempters prefer to live, and, at least in part, have used the suicide attempt in order to manipulate a relationship to better advantage.[41] Those who are successful in doing this, and they seem to be the majority, do not attempt suicide again.[42] Others, discovering after a period of time has elapsed that their lives have not improved or have deteriorated, may well attempt suicide again, perhaps with greater definiteness of purpose in bringing about death.

B. Suicide Prevention Behind the Veil of Ignorance

If most suicide attempters either do not want to die or change their minds within a very short time after an attempt, a posited "right to commit suicide" may be a weak basis for defending a policy of non-interference with suicide attempts. Were there no other pertinent considerations, the saving of lives of the high proportion of attempters who, having been restrained, would then want to live and who would be grateful for having been saved[43] would seem to constitute adequate grounds for authorizing interference.[44] As is often the case, there are other considerations, such as our desire to remain free from erroneous or unnecessary interference. The attempt, then, must be to find a suicide prevention policy that will reconcile our goal of saving lives with the preservation of values we consider it important not to jeopardize.

Let us imagine that we are asked to agree upon a suicide prevention policy, given what is known about suicide but prevented by a "veil of ignorance"[45] from knowing who among us will attempt or commit suicide, who may mistakenly be identified or vindictively accused of being suicidal, who will have easy access to top-quality legal representation, and so on. We insist upon the presence of the veil to prevent persons from demanding conditions or provisions tailored in advance to meet their own individual contingencies. Thus, a man who is fairly certain that he never would be falsely identified as suicidal and therefore wrongly threatened with deprivation of liberty might be willing to sacrifice the interest of others in not being misidentified. Such a person, therefore, should not be allowed to formulate a policy taking that knowledge into account.

It seems clear that behind the veil of ignorance we would be willing to tolerate some degree of interference with suicide attempts. We would want to save the lives of those among us who would attempt suicide, but who research indicated did not desire the outcome of death, and who later would be grateful for having been rescued. Moreover, there often are times when we decide to do something on the spur of the moment that we later regret. When the consequences of impulsive action are as extreme as they are in the case of suicide, we might well want some form of intervention to compel us to reflect on whether we really want the choice we have made. Here the motivation for intervention is not that the attempter does not at the moment of the attempt want to die, but that after some consideration he may not want to do so. This later, more considered judgment is preferred over the impulsive one, perhaps because we think it more accurately represents his "true" wishes.

We might also reasonably want to be restrained against committing suicide when our judgment is clouded or distorted, as it might be through chemical processes affecting the functioning of the brain (toxic psychosis) or when a highly upsetting event (such as a death in the family) occurs.

While rationally we would be willing to authorize some measure of interference to prevent us from committing suicide under circumstances such as those mentioned above, we also would insist that a number of limitations on the extent and methods of interference with suicidal individuals be imposed, lest other values be jeopardized. Central among these would be the retention of the ultimate right to commit suicide for those who found the pain or distress of living intolerable, and for whom the desire to end life represented something more than momentary dejection or discouragement. This ultimate control over the decision whether to continue living is something we would be extremely loath to give up, lest we be forced to live in misery for a long time. Moreover, since we would recognize that distress is subjective, we would be reluctant, in making provision for the right to die, to permit others to pass on the rationality of our decision to end life.

As a further requirement, we unquestionably would insist on procedural and substantive safeguards designed to protect non-suicidal individuals from wrongful intervention, mistaken or deliberate.[46] The more extensive the intervention, the more safeguards we would require. When the intervention is so drastic as to entail loss of liberty for an extended period, loss of some civil rights, loss of earnings, separation from family and friends and serious stigmatization, we would want to be careful indeed that only those who were actually suicidal should be the subjects of intervention.

A third concern would be that the intervention not be excessively painful, unpleasant or protracted, for, if it were, the human costs of prevention might well be thought to exceed its benefits.

This analysis suggests that the ideal suicide prevention policy is one that would: (1) save, through methods entailing minimal unpleasantness, the lives of as many as possible of those who do not wish to die; (2) interfere as little as possible with those who after some chance for consideration persist in wanting to die; and (3) afford maximum protection against interference with the liberty of those who pose no threat of suicide. This suggested policy goes very far toward respecting individual choice, but, on the basis of a principle of retrospective gratitude,[47] departs from the most extreme libertarian position to allow very limited paternalistic intervention.

IV. Interference with a Suicide Attempt

The first of the suicide prevention policies we consider is the "minimal" policy of interfering with a suicide attempt in progress or about to begin and providing medical assistance, where needed, to the attempter. The degree of interference here is quite minor; it might include, for example, removing a person from a building ledge from which he was about to leap, giving artificial respiration to a person found unconscious from gas inhalation, or lavaging the stomach of someone who has taken sleeping pills. Where necessary, because of medical considerations or for purposes of restraint, transportation to a hospital emergency room or detention facility would be authorized. The duration of intervention, however, would be limited; the time span required for the kind of intervention we have in mind would not exceed 24 hours, and might frequently be less.[48]

At the end of this brief period, restraint would no longer be authorized; persons wishing to go about their business would be free to do so. In particular, they would be free to resume their suicidal behavior. To prevent the minimal policy from escalating into more protracted restraint, it would be necessary to require a waiting period before intervention could be repeated.

The foregoing policy confers benefits and also entails costs. The major benefit is that it would save the lives of almost all suicide attempters. There is abundant testimony from psychiatrists experienced in the treatment of suicide attempters that survivors of an attempt rarely pose a danger of immediate suicide, even when opportunities for further attempts are not lacking.[49] For this reason, the stringent time limit on intervention would entail a sacrifice of very few lives. This feature makes the policy especially attractive. Moreover, even the small number of subsequent suicides that will continue to occur need not necessarily be considered failures of the policy, since those persons will at least have been provided a chance for reconsideration.[50]

There are several disadvantages to this policy. Some small number of individuals will die who would have changed their minds had they been held for a longer period. Others, firmly committed to suicide, will be detained for a period of some hours. This may be annoying, perhaps extremely distressing. Nevertheless, there are reasons for not being too concerned with this small number of individuals. First, their distress will come to an end in a few hours; secondly, those concerned with avoiding this delay could simply choose a time, place and method unlikely to attract attention.[51]

To reduce some of this imposition, the state might even accommodate determined attempters by granting immunity from any interference to those who register their intention to commit suicide in advance, or by providing resources for painless suicide following a short waiting period so as to be confident that only those who wish to die kill themselves.[52] Despite these provisions, however, some genuinely suicidal persons are likely to be subjected to distress, embarrassment and inconvenience because, contrary to plans, their suicide attempt has been interrupted.

A third class of individuals who may suffer from the minimal policy consists of those who are falsely identified as having been engaged in a suicide attempt or whose attempt would have had no serious consequences and who would not have gone on to a more serious attempt in the absence of intervention. These persons may incur inconvenience and some degree of stigmatization as the result of having been considered suicidal.

Nevertheless, the negative consequences of mistaken identification do not seem serious enough to constitute fatal objections to this proposal. An analogy to arrests for criminal law violations is instructive. Under the "probable cause" standard some innocent persons undoubtedly are wrongly arrested and charged. Though regrettable, the undeserved inconvenience and stigmatization are thought to be unavoidable consequences of law enforcement practices believed to be necessary to the public welfare. Our desire to minimize the unavoidable evil might, for example, lead to protection of the confidentiality of arrest records, but not to outright elimination of the power to arrest, absent an alternative procedure to handle the charging of individuals with crimes and the production of them at trial. The judgment is made that our interest in safety from crime is sufficient to warrant risking some interference with our activities through wrongful arrest.[53] On the other side of the coin, a person suspected of criminal activity cannot lawfully be taken into custody unless there is at least "probable cause" to believe that he committed the crime. Relaxation of this restriction might result in the taking into custody of some criminals who at present are free to continue preying on innocent victims, but we forfeit this potential benefit in order to remain free from arrest based on mere suspicion of involvement in criminal activity.

It is doubtful that coercive suicide prevention is as justifiable as coercive crime prevention; the social consequences of unpunished serious crime probably are much greater than those of unprevented suicide. Failing to attach legal sanctions to acts seriously harmful to the life of another, for example, may lead to vigilantism. Nevertheless, the considerable benefits to be obtained from minimal restraint of suicide attempters seem to us sufficient to justify the limited degree of interference proposed here, notwithstanding its costs for "truly" suicidal persons and for those who are not suicidal at all.

NOTES

The author's views on suicide prevention policy were largely crystallized during his tenure with the Committee for the Study of Incarceration. Some of the material presented here appeared previously in an unpublished staff memorandum of the Committee for the Study of Incarceration, co-authored with Andrew von Hirsch. Comments and discussions with the Committee's Executive Director, Andrew von Hirsch, and with its members, notably Dr. Willard Gaylin and Professor Alan Dershowitz, are gratefully acknowledged. Neither the Committee for the Study of Incarceration nor the aforementioned individuals are responsible for the views expressed here. This essay is dedicated to Caleb Foote.

1. For a brief history of the criminal prohibition of suicide and a list of states in which suicides or attempted suicides are illegal, see Schulman, *Suicide and Suicide Prevention: A Legal Analysis,* 54 A.B.A.J. 855 (1968). A list of states where the criminal law prohibits committing, aiding, assisting, encouraging or abetting suicide is contained in Litman, *Police Aspects of Suicide,* in THE PSYCHOLOGY OF SUICIDE 519, 520 (E. Shneidman, N. Farberow & R. Litman eds. 1960) [hereinafter THE PSYCHOLOGY OF SUICIDE].

2. This has been the supposition. A recent study, however, found evidence of virtually unanimous negative attitudes toward suicide attempters on the part of the general public as well as specific occupational groups dealing with attempters. Psychiatric residents had negative attitudes more often and more intensely than other groups. Ansel & McGee, *Attitudes Toward Suicide Attempters,* 8 BULL. OF SUICIDOLOGY 22, 27 (1971).

3. *See* text accompanying notes 54–56 *infra.*

4. Jackson v. Indiana, 406 U.S. 715, 737 (1972).

5. Limited information about the length of hospitalization of 138 suicidal patients admitted to a British psychiatric ward in 1946 is presented in E. STENGEL, SUICIDE AND ATTEMPTED SUICIDE 80–82, 89–91 (1964) [hereinafter STENGEL, SUICIDE]. Generalization to another country a quarter of a century later would obviously be unwarranted.

6. *E.g.,* Dershowitz, *The Law of Dangerousness: Some Fictions About Predictions,* 23 J. LEGAL ED. 24 (1970); Dershowitz, *Psychiatry in the Legal Process: A Knife that Cuts Both Ways,* 4 TRIAL, Feb./Mar. 1968, at 29; Ervin, *Foreword: Preventive Detention—A Step Backward for Criminal Justice,* 6 HARV. CIV. RIGHTS—CIV. LIB. L. REV. 291 (1971); Foote, *The Coming Constitutional Crisis in Bail,* 113 U. PA. L. REV. 959 (1965); Tribe, *An Ounce of Detention: Preventive Justice in the World of John Mitchell,* 56 VA. L. REV. 371 (1970); von Hirsch, *Prediction of Criminal Conduct and Preventive Confinement of Convicted Persons,* 21 BUFFALO L. REV. 717 (1972). The conceptual framework of this essay on preventive confinement to stop suicide is deeply indebted to von Hirsch's work on the preventive confinement of persons considered dangerous to others.

7. Some of the issues involved in preventive confinement to prevent danger to self were raised in Siegel, *The Justifications for Medical Commitment—Real or Illusory,* 6 WAKE FOREST INTRA. L. REV. 21 (1969). It is testimony to the legal profession's neglect of civil commitments that the issues Siegel raised in this article have not been explored in greater depth in the several years since it appeared.

8. Three convenient tabulations of psychiatric commitment statutes and procedures have appeared recently: S. BRAKEL & R. ROCK, THE MENTALLY DISABLED AND THE LAW (rev. ed. 1971); B. ENNIS & L. SIEGEL, THE RIGHTS OF MENTAL PATIENTS app. A (1973); Roth, Dayley & Lerner, *Into the Abyss: Psychiatric Reliability and Emergency Commitment Statutes,* 13 SANTA CLARA LAW. 400, 412–15 (1973).

9. IDAHO CODE § 66-317(b) (1973).

10. A recent empirical study of civil commitments in Arizona, Wexler & Scoville, *The Administration of Psychiatric Justice: Theory and Practice in Arizona,* 13 ARIZ. L. REV. (1971), illustrates the discrepancy between the provisions of a commitment statute and actual commitment procedure. The project investigators found that although the legal criteria for civil commitment required a showing of dangerousness, in some counties testifying psychiatrists did not even bother expressing an opinion as to the issue of dangerousness. At least one judge openly admitted to blatantly illegal commitments for the "benefit" of the defendant, *id.* at 3–4, and the project team suggests generally that the wording of the statute has little bearing on decision outcomes, since the law can be and is interpreted, twisted or ignored to accomplish the commitment. *Id.* at 113–17. In a few states is the wording of the relevant statute sufficiently precise as to make this at all difficult. This use of psychiatric commitment statutes suggests that they are not so much an expression of *norms,*

but *resources* to be used in accomplishing the goals of those who seek commitments. For a general discussion of this way of looking at formal rules, see Johnson, *The Practical Uses of Rules,* in THEORETICAL PERSPECTIVES ON DEVIANCE 215 (R. Scott & J. Douglas eds. 1972).

Statutory differences among states in *procedure* for commitments are discussed in BRAKEL & ROCK, *supra* note 8, and in R. ROCK, M. JACOBSON & R. JANOPAUL, HOSPITALIZATION AND DISCHARGE OF THE MENTALLY ILL (1968).

11. A. ALVAREZ, THE SAVAGE GOD 50, 69 (Bantam ed. 1973); 4 W. BLACKSTONE, COMMENTARIES ⅓ 189.

12. Henslin, *Guilt and Guilt Neutralization; Response and Adjustment to Suicide,* in DEVIANCE AND RESPECTABILITY: THE SOCIAL CONSTRUCTION OF MORAL MEANINGS 192, 200–01 (J. Douglas ed. 1970) [hereinafter DEVIANCE AND RESPECTABILITY]. *But see* S. WALLACE, AFTER SUICIDE 268 (1973), a recent study of adjustment to suicide among widows of Boston-area men who committed suicide, which found that some widows experienced relief, rather than grief, at their husbands' deaths. *See also* Breed, *Suicide and Loss in Social Interaction,* in ESSAYS IN SELF-DESTRUCTION 188 (E. Shneidman ed. 1967) [hereinafter ESSAYS].

13. Henslin, *supra* note 12, at 204–205.

14. Tuckman, Kleiner & Lavell, *Emotional Content of Suicide Notes,* 116 AM. J. PSYCHIATRY 59, 60 (1959).

15. *See* Cain & Fast, *Children's Disturbed Reactions to Parent Suicide,* 56 AM. J. ORTHOPSYCHIATRY 873 (1966); Cain & Fast, *The Legacy of Suicide: Observations on the Pathogenic Impact of Suicide upon Marital Partners,* 29 PSYCHIATRY 406 (1966) [hereinafter Cain & Fast, *Legacy*].

16. *See* Cain & Fast, *Legacy, supra* note 15, at 410. One commentator has observed that "suicidal efforts seem not infrequently to follow the patterns of suicidal attempts by father, mother, older brother, or older sister." Kubie, *Multiple Determinants of Suicide,* in ESSAYS, *supra note 12,* at 455, 458; *accord,* Teicher & Jacobs, *Adolescents Who Attempt Suicide: Preliminary Findings,* 122 AM. J. PSYCHIATRY 1248, 1257 (1966).

17. A study of suicides in King County, Washington (Seattle), found that 70% of suicides had active physical illness; illness was considered to have contributed to 51% of the suicides. Dorpat, Anderson & Ripley, *The Relationship of Physical Illness to Suicide,* in SUICIDAL BEHAVIOR: DIAGNOSIS AND MANAGEMENT 209, 210–11 (H. Resnik ed. 1968) [hereinafter Resnik].

18. For a typical expression of this viewpoint, see Ringel, *Suicide Prevention as a Contribution to the Re-evaluation of Human Life,* 7 LEX ET SCIENTIA 11, 14–15 (1970).

19. *See* T. SZASZ, LAW, LIBERTY AND PSYCHIATRY 11–36 (1963); M. Pollner, "The Very Coinage of Your Brain": The Resolution of Reality Disjunctures (May 1973) (copy on file at offices of *New York University Law Review*); Blum, *The Sociology of Mental Illness,* in DEVIANCE AND RESPECTABILITY, *supra* note 12, at 31; Sarbin, *The Scientific Status of the Mental Illness Metaphor,* in CHANGING PERSPECTIVES IN MENTAL ILLNESS 9 (S. Plog & R. Edgerton eds. 1969); Rosenhan, *On Being Sane in Insane Places,* 179 SCIENCE 250 (1973).

20. Figures given [for the percentage of suicides who are mentally ill] rest largely on the definition of mental illness, however, and therefore run the gamut from as low as 20 per cent to as high as 90 to 100 per cent. Such a wide variation reflects the difficulty of defining and categorizing mental illness in the first place and the relative independence of suicide and present day psychiatric nosology. . . .

C. LEONARD, UNDERSTANDING AND PREVENTING SUICIDE 273 (1967). *See also* M. KRAMER, E. POLLACK, R. REDICK & B. LOCKE, MENTAL DISORDERS SUICIDE 286 (1972).

21. *See* D. MECHANIC, MENTAL HEALTH AND SOCIAL POLICY 129–31 (1969); T. SCHEFF, BECOMING MENTALLY ILL ch. 5 (1969); Kutner, *The Illusion of Due Process in Commitment Proceedings,* 57 Nw. U.L. REV. 383 (1962).

22. Thus, Erwin Ringel states:

Any man who has given serious and scientific thought to the problem of suicide knows that death — that state of not being — is for the most part chosen under pathological circumstances or under the influence of diseased feelings, and even then I put it to you that the word choice is wrong because an overwhelming imperative compulsion renders any free choice null and void.

Ringel, *supra* note 18, at 15. According to Ilza Veith, "the act [of suicide] clearly represents an illness." *Quoted* in Szasz, *The Ethics of Suicide,* 31 ANTIOCH REV. 7, 8 (1971).

23. Pokorny, *Myths About Suicide,* in Resnik, *supra* note 17, at 57, 62 [hereinafter Pokorny, *Myths*].

24. A. KOBLER & E. STOTLAND, THE END OF HOPE 3-4 (1964). The issue of mistaken attribution of depressive psychosis has also been raised in a recent study of adolescent suicides, Jacobs & Teicher, *Broken Homes and Social Isolation in Attempted Suicides of Adolescents,* 13 INT'L J. SOCIAL PSYCHIATRY 139 (1967). The authors criticize psychiatrically oriented diagnosticians for failure to investigate the experiences that might lead to a suicide attempt, an omission they attribute to a self-confirming assumption that suicide must be the consequence of mental pathology. *Id.* at 147-48. Their own efforts to obtain life histories for the attempters they studied suggest that, at least for adolescents, symptoms of depression may be a perfectly understandable response to their experiences.

25. Farberow, Shneidman & Leonard, *Suicide among Schizophrenic Mental Hospital Patients,* in THE CRY FOR HELP 78, 91 (N. Farberow & E. Shneidman eds. 1965) [hereinafter THE CRY FOR HELP]. Similarly, Jacob Tuckman, Robert J. Kleiner and Martha Lavell comment:

> In this study the writers were impressed with the possibility that in a number of cases the suicide could have resulted from a conscious, "rational" decision reached by weighing the pros and cons of continuing to live, although to a lesser extent unconscious factors may have been operating.

Tuckman, Kleiner & Lavell, *supra* note 14, at 62. Jerry Jacobs and Joseph D. Teicher are likewise impressed with "the matter-of-fact presentation found in suicide notes." Jacobs & Teicher, *supra* note 24, at 148.

26. Gittleson, *The Relationship between Obsessions and Suicidal Attempts in Depressive Psychoses,* 112 BRIT. J. PSYCHIATRY 889 (1966). This is consistent with Norman Farberow's finding that suicide attempters appear less psychologically abnormal or disturbed than suicide threateners or non-suicidal mental patients. Farberow, *Personality Patterns of Suicidal Mental Hospital Patients,* 42 GENETIC PSYCHOLOGY MONOGRAPHS 3, 67 (1950) [hereinafter Farberow, *Personality Patterns*].

27. Pokorny, *Myths, supra* note 23, at 64. Consequently, treatment of mental illness may lead to suicide rather than prevent it:

> If psychosis is . . . an escape from intolerable stresses of reality, perhaps the partial easing of the psychotic state through medication or tranquilizing drugs brings these patients to a state of painful insight before they are able to cope with new insights.

Farberow, Shneidman & Leonard, *supra* note 25, at 91. The process is illustrated in the following tragi-comic story:

> One resident whom I supervised spent a year and a half working to establish a relationship with a regressed hebephrenic woman who lived largely in a hallucinatory world of self-fulfilling fantasies in which she was a socially active debutante. Gradually she gave up these delusions as her ingenious therapist made headway. When after 18 months of painstaking work she surfaced in the world of reality, she discovered that she was fat, forty, and friendless, and made a drastic suicide attempt.

Stone, *Suicide Precipitated by Psychotherapy,* 25 AM. J. PSYCHOTHERAPY, 18, 22 (1971).

28. The problem of prediction in commitments to prevent suicide is discussed in text accompanying notes 107-22 *infra.*

29. The effectiveness of suicide prevention measures is discussed in text accompanying notes 91-106 *infra.*

30. *E.g.,* E. DURKHEIM, LE SUICIDE: ETUDE DE SOCIOLOGIE (1897); H. MORSELLI, SUICIDE: AN ESSAY ON COMPARATIVE MORAL STATISTICS (1882).

31. Douglas, *The Absurd in Suicide,* in ON THE NATURE OF SUICIDE 111, 117-18 (E. Shneidman ed. 1969).

32. Rubinstein, Moses & Lidz, *On Attempted Suicide,* 79 A.M.A. ARCHIVES OF NEUROLOGY & PSYCHIATRY 103, 111 (1958). Characteristically, the authors of this study found:

> The patient was involved in a struggle with the persons important to him and sought a modification of their attitudes or a specific change in his relationships with them. After a

crisis was reached in this struggle, the patient sought to effect these changes through a suicide attempt. . . . Patients sometimes told of seeking such changes prior to their suicide attempt, of seeking them through the attempt, and by still other means afterward. . . . *Id.* at 109. A similar conclusion was reached in a study of suicidal behavior on the part of Irish women. Lukianowicz, *Suicidal Behavior: An Attempt to Modify the Environment,* 6 PSYCHIATRICA CLINICA 171, 185 (1973). *See also* Sacks, *The Search for Help: No One to Turn To,* in ESSAYS, *supra note* 12, at 203, 211.

33. Weiss, *The Suicidal Patient,* in AMERICAN HANDBOOK OF PSYCHIATRY 115, 121 (S. Arieto ed. 1966 [hereinafter Weiss, *The Suicidal Patient*].

34. Rubinstein, Moses & Lidz, *supra* note 32, at 105. Similar conclusions are reported in E. STENGEL & N. COOK, ATTEMPTED SUICIDE: ITS SOCIAL SIGNIFICANCE AND EFFECTS 119–29 (1958) [hereinafter STENGEL & COOK, ATTEMPTED SUICIDE], and in STENGEL, SUICIDE, *supra* note 5, at 95–99.

Adolescents seem less successful than adults at turning a suicide attempt to their advantage. *See* Teicher & Jacobs, *supra* note 16, at 1249.

35. *See* Firth, *Suicide and Risk-Taking in Tikopia Society,* 24 PSYCHIATRY 2 (1961); Weiss, *The Gamble with Death in Attempted Suicide,* 20 PSYCHIATRY 17 (1957). Edwin Lemert discusses the relevance of risk-taking to deviance theory generally in E. LEMERT, HUMAN DEVIANCE, SOCIAL PROBLEMS, AND SOCIAL CONTROL 11–12 (1967).

36. Many suicide attempters give at least one, sometimes more than one, clear warning of an impending suicide during the days and weeks prior to an attempt. Delong & Robins, *The Communication of Suicidal Intent Prior to Psychiatric Hospitalization: A Study of 87 Patients,* 117 AM. J. PSYCHIATRY 695, 699–700 (1961); Dorpat & Ripley, *A Study of Suicide in the Seattle Area,* 1 COMPREHENSIVE PSYCHIATRY 349, 355 (1960); Pokorny, *Characteristics of Forty-Four Patients Who Subsequently Committed Suicide,* 2 ARCHIVES OF GEN. PSYCHIATRY 314, 315–16 (1960); Robins, Gasser, Kayes, Wilkinson & Murphy, *The Communication of Suicidal Intent: A Study of 134 Consecutive Cases of Successful (Completed) Suicide,* 115 AM. J. PSYCHIATRY 724, 733 (1959); Wilson, *Suicide in Psychiatric Patients Who Have Received Hospital Treatment,* 125 AM. J. PSYCHIATRY 752, 753 (1968); Yessler, Gibbs & Becker, *On the Communication of Suicidal Ideas,* 3 ARCHIVES OF GEN. PSYCHIATRY 612, 613 (1960). A problem generally encountered in such studies is that of retrospective interpretation of the sometimes ambiguously worded "warning."

37. Pokorny, *Myths, supra* note 23, at 60.

38. Tuckman & Youngman, *Assessment of Suicide Risk in Attempted Suicide,* in Resnik, *supra* note 17, at 190, 192–93; Gardner, Bahn & Mack, *Suicide and Psychiatric Care in the Aging,* 10 ARCHIVES OF GEN. PSYCHIATRY 547, 550 (1964); Rosen, *The Serious Suicide Attempt: Epidemiological and Follow-Up Study of 886 Patients,* 127 AM. J. PSYCHIATRY 764, 766, (1970) [hereinafter Rosen, *Serious Attempt*]; Tuckman & Youngman, *Identifying Suicide Risk Groups Among Persons Attempting Suicide,* 78 PUB. HEALTH REP. 585 (1963) [hereinafter Tuckman & Youngman, *Identifying Suicide Risk Groups*].

39. N. RETTERSTOL, LONG-TERM PROGNOSIS AFTER ATTEMPTED SUICIDE 95 (1970); STENGEL, SUICIDE, *supra* note 5, at 81–84; STENGEL & COOK, ATTEMPTED SUICIDE, *supra* note 34, at 116; Oltman & Friedman, *Life Cycles in Patients with Manic-Depressive Psychoses,* 119 AM. J. PSYCHIATRY 174, 175 (1962); Pitts & Winokur, *Affective Disorder: Diagnostic Correlates and Incidence of Suicide,* 139 J. NERVOUS & MENTAL DISEASE 176, 179 (1964); Pokorny, *A Follow-Up Study of 618 Suicidal Patients,* 122 AM. J. PSYCHIATRY 1109, 1111 (1966) [hereinafter Pokorny, *Follow-Up Study*]; Stengel, *Recent Research into Suicide and Attempted Suicide,* 118 AM. J. PSYCHIATRY 725 (1962).

40. Moss & Hamilton, *Psychotherapy of the Suicidal Patient,* in CLUES TO SUICIDE 99, 107 (E. Shneidman & N. Farberow eds. 1957) [hereinafter CLUES TO SUICIDE].

41. Even when manipulation is not the purpose of an attempt, the attempt may nevertheless have the consequence of improving the attempter's social environment sufficiently to allay further attempts. Some psychoanalytic theorizing on suicide has emphasized aggressive elements, *e.g.,* hostility toward others redirected inward. S. FREUD, *Mourning and Melancholia,* in 14 THE STANDARD EDITION OF THE COMPLETE PSYCHOLOGICAL WORKS OF SIGMUND FREUD 252 (J. Strachey ed. 1957) [hereinafter COMPLETE PSYCHOLOGICAL WORKS]; K. MENNINGER, MAN AGAINST HIMSELF (1938).

If newly evoked sympathy and attention reduced the intensity of such feelings we might expect a low repeat rate even though there was no conscious or unconscious "appeal" element to the original attempt. Indeed, Ronald Akers has suggested that, from a social learning perspective, the increased attention a suicide attempt elicits may reinforce suicidal behavior, so that, if the attention does not resolve the crisis which precipitated the original attempt, the attempter will be likely to repeat the reinforced behavior. R. AKERS, DEVIANT BEHAVIOR: A SOCIAL LEARNING APPROACH 251 (1973).

42. KOBLER & STOTLAND, *supra* note 24, at 10.

43. J. CHORON, SUICIDE 50 (1972), cites several studies from different countries in which 90% to 100% of rescued suicide attempters reported they were glad they had been saved. *Accord,* RETTERSTOL, *supra* note 39, at 96.

44. Alan Dershowitz has called this line of reasoning the "Thank you, doctor" doctrine (private conversation with the author). The concept also is employed under the label "future-oriented consent" in Wexler, *Therapeutic Justice,* 57 MINN. L. REV. 289, 330–32 (1972). We shall refer to the concept in this article as the principle of retrospective gratitude.

45. J. RAWLS, A THEORY OF JUSTICE 136–42 (1971).

46. Thus, in Litman & Farberow, *Emergency Evaluation of Suicidal Potential,* in THE PSYCHOLOGY OF SUICIDE, *supra* note 1, at 259, 268, an example is given of a woman who claimed that her husband was living "in a dream world" and wanted him committed on grounds that he was likely to kill himself. Upon investigation it turned out that he frequently lost much of his wages gambling. The woman wanted him committed so that she could use his money to straighten out their financial affairs. Sympathetic as we might be with her plight, we would want to provide protection against the use of suicide prevention commitment proceedings to advance goals having nothing to do with suicide prevention. Even where there is no deliberate attempt to deceive or misuse statutory provisions, we still would need to be on guard against family members who are sincere but mistaken in their belief that a suicide attempt may be imminent.

47. *See* text accompanying notes 43–44 *supra.*

48. As defined here, then, minimal interference includes simple restraint at the scene, arrest and removal from the scene and very short-term detainment. Although we consider these together as "minimal," it ultimately might prove useful to distinguish among them and perhaps permit only the least restrictive. These distinctions need not be discussed here.

49. Stengel & Cook, *Recent Research into Suicide and Attempted Suicide,* 1 J. FORENSIC MEDICINE 252 (1954); Shneidman, *Some Reflections on Suicide Theory and Prevention,* in PROCEEDINGS OF A SECOND TECHNICAL ASSISTANCE PROJECT CONFERENCE ON SUICIDE AND DEPRESSION 35 (1967); Weiss, *The Suicidal Patient, supra* note 33, at 121.

50. This need not mean that we should be complacent about suicides, only that this particular coercive policy cannot be made to shoulder the burden of suicide prevention.

51. Ordinarily this should not be too difficult. A major exception might be individuals incarcerated in total institutions where suicide, though certainly not impossible, can be made much more difficult by intensive surveillance and deprivation of materials from which weapons can be constructed. I am indebted to Andrew von Hirsch for this observation.

52. This procedure was employed in the Greek colonies at Marseilles and Ceos. ALVAREZ, *supra* note 11, at 59.

53. On the other hand, we become much more alarmed at more extended pretrial detention, as its disruptive effects mount rapidly when its duration begins to exceed 24 hours. It is clear that, behind the veil of ignorance, we would never accept the class bias built into current pretrial release procedures.

Suggestions for Further Reading

The Concept of Coercion

Bayles, Michael D. "Coercive Offers and Public Benefits." *The Personalist* 55 (Spring 1974):139–144.

Benditt, Theodore. "Threats and Offers." *The Personalist* 58 (October 1977): 382–384.

Beran, Harry. "The Relation Between Coercion and Threat of Force." *Journal of Critical Analysis* 6 (July 1976):77–82.

Chrzanowski, Gerard. "Psychotherapy with Schizophrenics: Parameters of Freedom and Coercion." *American Journal of Psychoanalysis* 36 (September 1976):181–183.

Dworkin, Gerald. "Compulsion and Moral Concepts." *Ethics* (April 1968): 227–233.

Gaylin, Willard. "On the Borders of Persuasion: A Psychoanalytic Look at Coercion." *Psychiatry* 37 (February 1974):1–9.

Halleck, Seymore L. "Legal and Ethical Aspects of Behavior Control." *The American Journal of Psychiatry* 131 (1974):381–385.

Lyons, Daniel. "Welcome Threats and Coercive Offers." *Philosophy* 50 (October 1975):425–436.

McCloskey, H. J. "Coercion: Its Nature and Significance." *The Southern Journal of Philosophy* XVIII (Fall, 1980):335–351.

Nozick, Robert. "Coercion." In Morgenbesser, Sidney; Suppes, Patrict; and White, Morton, eds. *Philosophy, Science, and Method: Essays in Honor of Ernest Nagel.* New York: St. Martin's Press, 1969, pp. 440–472.

Pennock, J. Roland, and Chapman, John W. *Coercion.* Chicago: Aldine,

Atherton, Inc., 1972, especially definitional essays by Pennock, Michael D. Bayles, Bernard Gert and Virginia Held.

Rudinow, Joel. "Manipulation." *Ethics* 88 (July 1978):338–347.

Shapiro, Michael H. "Legislating the Control of Behavior Control: Autonomy and the Coercive Use of Organic Therapies." *Southern California Law Review* 47 (February 1974):237–257.

Van De Veer, Don. "Coercion, Seduction, and Rights." *The Personalist* 58 (October 1977):374–381.

Voluntary and Involuntary Commitments and Dangerousness

Bradley, Valerie, and Clarke, Garry, ed. *Paper Victories and Hard Realities: The Implementation of the Legal and Constitutional Rights of the Mentally Disabled.* Washington, D.C.: The Health Policy Center at Georgetown University, 1976.

Brady, John P., and Brodie, H. Keith, ed. *Controversy in Psychiatry.* Philadelphia: W. B. Saunders Co., 1978, Ch. 23.

Brody, Baruch A., and Engelhardt, H. Tristram, Jr. *Mental Illness: Law and Public Policy.* Boston: D. Reidel, 1980.

Chodoff, Paul. "The Case for Involuntary Hospitalization of the Mentally Ill." *American Journal of Psychiatry* 133 (May 1976):496–501.

Columbia University Task Force on Behavior Modification. "The Case of Jose." *Man and Medicine* 4 (1979):1–21.

Dershowitz, A. "Psychiatrist's Power in Civil Commitment." *Psychology Today* 2 (February 1969):43–47.

Ennis, Bruce J., and Emery, Richard D. *The Rights of Mental Patients.* New York: Avon Books, 1978, Chs. II, III and IV.

Friedman, Julian, and Daley, Robert W. "Civil Commitment and the Doctrine of Balance: A Critical Analysis." *Santa Clara Lawyer* 13 (Spring 1973): 503–517.

Gove, Walter R. "A Comparison of Voluntary and Committed Psychiatric Patients." *Archives of General Psychiatry* 34 (1977):669–676.

Greenberg, David F. "Involuntary Psychiatric Commitments to Prevent Suicide." *New York University Law Review* 49 (May–June 1974):227–269.

Halleck, Seymour L. *The Politics of Therapy.* New York: Harper and Row, 1971.

Kaplan, L. "As You Like It: The Civil Commitment of God." *Boston Law Review* 49 (1969):14–45.

"The Dangerous Patient." Special Issue of *Psychiatric Quarterly* 52 (Summer 1980).

Katz, J. "Dangerousness: A Theoretical Reconstruction of the Criminal Law." *Buffalo Law Review* 19 (Spring 1970):1–32.

Kittrie, Nicholas N. *The Right To Be Different.* Baltimore: The Johns Hopkins Press, 1971, Chs. 1 and 2.

Kozol, H. R., Boucher, R., and Garofalo, R. "The Diagnosis and Treatment of Dangerousness." *Crime and Delinquency* 8 (October 1972):371–392.

Kumasaka, Y. et al. "Criteria for Involuntary Hospitalization." *Archives of General Psychiatry* 26 (May 1972):399–404.

"Legal Issues in State Mental Health Care: Proposals for Change—Civil Commitment." *Mental Disability Law Reporter* 2 (July–August 1977):75–159.

"Mental Health and Human Rights: Report of the Task Panel on Legal and Ethical Issues." *Arizona Law Review* 20 (1978):117–125.

Miller, Kent S. *Managing Madness: The Case Against Civil Commitment.* New York: The Free Press, 1976.

Norton, Alan. "The Concept of Dangerousness." *Journal of Medical Ethics* 2 (December 1977):160–162.

Offir, Carole Wade. "Civil Rights and the Mentally Ill: Revolution in Bedlam." *Psychology Today* 8 (October 1974):60ff.

Olin, Grace B., and Olin, Harry S. "Informed Consent in Voluntary Mental Hospital Admission." *American Journal of Psychiatry* 132 (September 1975): 938–941.

"Overt Dangerous Behavior as a Constitutional Requirement for Involuntary Commitment of the Mentally Ill." *University of Chicago Law Review* 44 (Spring 1977).

Peszke, Michael A. *Involuntary Treatment of the Mentally Ill: The Problem of Autonomy.* Springfield, Illinois: Charles C. Thomas, 1975.

Pfohl, Stephen J. *Predicting Dangerousness.* Lexington, Massachusetts: Lexington Books, 1978.

Rofman, Ethan S., et al. "The Prediction of Dangerous Behavior in Emergency Civil Commitment." *American Journal of Psychiatry* 37 (September 1980): 1061–1064.

Roth, Loren H. "A Commitment Law for Patients, Doctors, and Lawyers." *American Journal of Psychiatry* 136 (September 1979):1121–1127.

Shah, Saleem A. "Dangerousness and Civil Commitment of the Mentally Ill: Some Public Policy Considerations." *American Journal of Psychiatry* 132 (May 1975):501–505.

Szasz, Thomas S. "The Crime of Commitment." *Psychology Today* 2 (March 1969):55–57.

Tooley, Kay. "Ethical Considerations in the 'Involuntary Commitment' of Children and in Psychological Testing as a Part of Legal Procedure." *Mental Hygiene* 54 (October 1970):484–489.

Wexler, David B. *Mental Health Law: Major Issues.* New York: Plenum Publishing Co., 1980.

Suicide

Alvarez, A. *The Savage God: A Study of Suicide.* New York: Random House, 1972.

Battin, M. P., and Mayo, D. J., eds. *Suicide: The Philosophical Issues.* New York: St. Martin's Press, 1980.

Beauchamp, Tom L., and Childress, James F. *Principles of Biomedical Ethics.* New York: Oxford University Press, 1979, pp. 85–94.

Beck, Aaron T., et al. "Classification of Suicidal Behaviors: II. Dimensions of Suicidal Intent." *Archives of General Psychiatry* 33 (July 1976):835–837.

Choron, Jacques. *Suicide.* New York: Charles Scribner's Sons, 1972.

Farberow, Norman L. "Suicide Prevention in the Hospital." *Hospital and Community Psychiatry* 32 (February 1981):99–104.

Glover, Jonathan. *Causing Death and Saving Lives.* New York: Penguin Books, 1977, Ch. 13.

Greenberg, David F. "Involuntary Psychiatric Commitments to Prevent Suicide." *New York University Law Review* 49 (May–June 1974):227–269.

Hankoff, L. D. "Categories of Attempted Suicide: A Longitudinal Study." *American Journal of Public Health* 66 (June 1976):558–563.

Hook, Sidney. "The Ethics of Suicide." *International Journal of Ethics* 37 (1927): 173–189.

Jellinek, Michael, Brandt, Richard B., and Litman, Robert E. "A Suicide Attempt & Emergency Room Ethics." *Hastings Center Report* (August 1979): 12–13.

Kieu, A. *The Suicidal Patient: Recognition and Management.* Chicago: Nelson Hall, 1977.

Litman, R. E., and Farberow, N. L. "The Hospital's Obligation Toward Suicide-prone Patients." *Hospitals* 40 (1966).

Murphy, G. E. "Suicide and the Right to Die." *American Journal of Psychiatry* 130 (1973):472–473.

Olin, Harry S. "Psychotherapy of the Chronically Suicidal Patient." *American Journal of Psychotherapy* 321 (October 1976):570–575.

Osmond, H., and Hoffer, A. "Schizophrenia and Suicide." *Journal of Schizophrenia* 1 (1967):54–64.

Pearson, Linnea, et al. *Separate Paths: Why People End Their Lives.* New York: Harper & Row, 1977.

Perlin, Seymore. *A Handbook for the Study of Suicide.* New York: Oxford University Press, 1975.

Portwood, Doris. *Common Sense Suicide: The Final Right.* New York: Dodd, Meade & Co., 1978.

Portwood, Doris. "A Right to Suicide?" *Psychology Today* 11 (January 1978): 66ff.

Pretzel, P. W. "Philosophical and Ethical Considerations of Suicide Prevention." *Bulletin of Suicidology* (July 1968):30–38.

Reynolds, David K., and Farberow, Norman L. *Suicide Inside and Out.* Berkeley: University of California Press, 1976.

Rosen, David H. "The Serious Suicide Attempt: Five-Year Follow-Up Study of 886 Patients." *Journal of the American Medical Association* 235 (May 10, 1976):1205–1209.

Shein, Harvey M. "Suicidal Care: Obstacles in the Education of Psychiatric Residents." *Omega* 7 (1976):75–81.

Slater, Eliot. "Assisted Suicide: Some Ethical Considerations." *International Journal of Health Services* 6 (1976):321–30.

Sletten, Ivan W., and Barton, John L. "Suicidal Patients in the Emergency Room: A Guide for Evaluation and Disposition." *Hospital and Community Psychiatry* 30 (June 1979):407–411.

Solomon, P. "The Burden of Responsibility in Suicide and Homicide." *Journal of The American Medical Association* 199 (1967):99–102.

Szasz, Thomas S. "The Ethics of Suicide." *The Antioch Review* 31 (Spring 1971): 7–17.

Treffert, Darold A. "Dying with Their Rights On." *American Journal of Psychiatry* 130 (1973):1041.

Wallace, Samuel E., and Eiser, Albin, eds. *Suicide and Euthanasia: The Rights of Personhood.* Knoxville, The University of Tennessee Press, 1981.

Weissman, M., et al. "Hostility and Depression Associated with Suicide Attempts." *American Journal of Psychiatry* 130 (1973):450–455.

Abuses of Institutionalization and Therapy

Arnold, William. *Shadowland.* New York: McGraw-Hill Book Co., 1979. (A biography of Frances Farmer.)

Beers, Clifford. *A Mind That Found Itself.* Garden City, New Jersey: Doubleday, 1953.

Blatt, Burton. *Exodus From Pandemonium.* Boston: Allyn and Bacon, Inc., 1970.

Block, Sidney, and Reddaway, Peter. *Psychiatric Terror: How Psychiatry Is Used to Suppress Dissent.* New York: Basic Books, 1977. On Soviet suppression.

Donaldson, Kenneth. *Insanity Inside Out.* New York: Crown Publishers, 1976.

Ennis, Bruce. *Prisoners of Psychiatry: Mental Patients, Psychiatrists, and the Law.* New York: Avon Books, 1974.

Gross, Martin. *The Psychological Society.* New York: Random House, 1978.

Halleck, Seymour L. *The Politics of Therapy.* New York: Jason Aronson, 1971.

Kesey, Ken. *One Flew Over the Cuckoo's Nest.* New York: Viking Press, 1962.

Robitscher, Jonas. *The Powers of Psychiatry.* Boston: Houghton Mifflin Co., 1980.

Rosenham, David L. "On Being Sane in Insane Places." *Science* 179 (January 1973):250–258. See replies in *Science* 180 (1973):356–369. See also replies by R. L. Spitzer in *Archives of General Psychiatry* 33 (1976):459–470 and in *Journal of Abnormal Psychology* 84 (1975):442–452.

Sheehan, Susan. "Reporter at Large—Creedmore." *The New Yorker* (May 25, 1981):49ff. Continued in later issues.

Spitzer, Therese. *Psychobattery: A Chronicle of Psychotherapeutic Abuse.* Clifton, New Jersey: The Humana Press, 1980.

Steir, Charles, ed. *Blue Jolts: True Stories From the Cuckoo's Nest.* Washington: New Republic Books, 1978.

Szasz, Thomas. *Sex by Prescription.* New York: Penguin Books, 1982.

Torrey, E. Fuller. "The Serbsky Treatment." *Psychology Today,* Vol. 11, June 1977, pp. 38–44. (On Russian mental hospitals as political prisons.)

6. Coercion in Therapy Paternalism and the Rights to Choose and Refuse Treatment

Introduction

In the first selection, Jonas Robitscher explains that since Morton Birnbaum introduced the concept of a "right to treatment" for mental hospital patients in 1960, its scope of application has been much narrower than the phrase itself might suggest. Recent discussions of this proposed right have had a restricted legal focus instead of a broad, moral one. It is not being suggested that voluntary patients have a right to treatment, since *in theory* they are free to leave the hospital at any time. The right applies only to involuntary patients. Its logic is disjunctive because it is in effect a right *either* to be released in the absence of effective treatment *or* to be provided with necessary conditions for adequate treatment in exchange for involuntary loss of liberty. The goal of such treatment should not be absolute cure but rather a restoration to minimal functioning sufficient for the earliest possible return to constitutionally guaranteed liberty. In response to this right, many states have chosen to release the majority of their incarcerated psychiatric patients rather than go to the trouble and expense of providing treatment, even though they are required to supply only *minimal* conditions for treatment, as Robitscher explains. The necessity for providing the minimal humane living conditions essential for a therapeutic environment, which a recognition of this right generates, has been a powerful impetus for deinstitutionalization.

One peril involved in the recognition of a right to treatment is that it might easily degenerate into another rationale for forcing treatment upon unwilling patients. To be compatible with a right to refuse treatment, the right to treatment should be interpreted as a right to *choose* (or refuse) treatment, to which there is a corresponding duty of the institution to *make it available* to those who would choose it, without forcing it upon them.

Involuntary commitment to residence in a mental hospital is not the same thing as a complete suspension of the right to refuse treatment, which non-mental patients enjoy and exercise without serious challenge, given the moral and legal principles recognized in our democratic society. Even if involuntary commitment is for purposes of treatment, this still leaves the question of involuntary therapy partially unresolved, for it is certainly not a license allowing hospital employees to do anything whatsoever to mental patients in the name of therapy. Nevertheless, *some* kinds of paternalistic, coercive treatment of *some* patients may be perfectly justifiable. In the selection by Loren Roth, the possibilities are explored that involuntary treatment is appropriate if the patient is either imminently dangerous to self or others while still competent to choose or refuse therapy, or incompetent to either choose or refuse. Procedural safeguards for protecting the rights of refusal by competent and nondangerous patients are developed.

Legally, some courts have recognized the right of mental patients to refuse psychosurgery; and as Ruth Macklin points out, recent court decisions (in Massachusetts and New Jersey) have given involuntary patients the right to refuse drug therapy. The courts have yet to explore very deeply the application of this right to insulin and electroshock therapies, aversion therapies, denial-of-privileges therapies, and recreational and occupational therapies, among others. Ruth Macklin develops philosophical grounds for paternalistic denials of the right to refuse treatment to dangerous and/or incompetent patients.

Jonas Robitscher

Courts, State Hospitals, and the Right to Treatment

During the 1960s, when community psychiatry was being developed and emphasized, the state hospital patient continued to suffer from neglect. In the 1970s a remarkable series of legal decisions has created a surge of interest in the state hospital patient by enunciating a doctrine of judicial responsibility for the maintenance of state hospital standards.

Although most fair-minded people would applaud the long overdue recognition of the need for a more therapeutic approach to the state hospital patient, court intervention into the state hospital scene raises questions as to the appropriateness of judicial supervision of psychiatric institutions. It marks a new era in psychiatry when psychiatrists must do their institutional reforming and their state hospital housecleaning in public, under the scrutiny of the court, and when they must conform their practices to court-approved standards.

The cases revolve around the concept of the right to treatment. As legal concepts go, this is a novel concept. It dates back only to 1960, when the term was used for the first time in connection with mental hospital patients in an article that appeared in the *American Bar Association Journal* (1). The concept has been often misunderstood because the right to treatment is a shorthand expression for much more than a statement about health care delivery; it means the right of involuntarily hospitalized mental patients to receive adequate therapy as an exchange for their being deprived of their liberty.

Morton Birnbaum, the physician-lawyer who originated the concept, was not advocating psychiatric treatment as a right for all. He addressed himself

From *The American Journal of Psychiatry* 129 (1972):298–304. Copyright © 1972 by the American Psychiatric Association. Reprinted by permission of the publisher and Mrs. Jean Robitscher.

solely to the plight of the involuntarily hospitalized state hospital patient who was not receiving the same quality or quantity of care that was available to private psychiatric patients and who presumably therefore was being held for a longer period than those patients.

Birnbaum's proposal originally suffered from neglect; then it was applied to cases that fell outside the scope of his argument; now it is being applied, among other examples, by a federal judge to the Alabama state hospital system. But in the process the court is becoming involved in the internal administration affairs of state hospitals in a more all-encompassing way than Birnbaum proposed.

Legal and Political Aspects

Birnbaum's concept was both legal and political in nature. Involuntary mental hospitalization is a deprivation of liberty. The Fifth Amendment prohibits the deprivation of liberty without due process of law. The benefit that accrues to patients who get adequate psychiatric treatment enables them to regain their liberty at the earliest possible time and so gives legal legitimacy to the hospitalization. But if the hospitalization is only a "warehousing" operation and does not provide the care that would promote recovery, the due process standard is not met and the patient should be released even if he represents a potential danger to himself or to others. Birnbaum is not a Szaszian who denies the propriety of all involuntary hospitalization. The main thrust of his campaign is to equalize the treatment programs of private hospitals, which he sees as designed to restore the patient to freedom at the earliest possible time, and the state hospital, which has traditionally held on to patients.

The concept that not even dangerousness should be the excuse for deprivation of liberty, which has been elaborated upon by eminent legal authorities such as Alan Dershowitz (2), a professor at Harvard Law School, has both civil libertarian and political implications. Freeing inadequately treated patients would represent justice to the patient; it is also designed to put pressure on state legislatures to appropriate funds for proper treatment programs in order that dangerous patients will not have to be freed. Birnbaum has cited variations in commitment rates (a high of 657 per 100,000 in the District of Columbia and a low of 61 per 100,000 in Utah) and in acts of violence (the jurisdictions with low commitment rates are not high in homicide and suicide rates) as "proof" that mental hospitalization cannot be justified on the grounds of protection of the individual or of society (3).

The heart of Birnbaum's proposal is to use very simple yardsticks; the one he originally relied on most was the ratio of personnel to patients to gauge adequacy of treatment. Even though Birnbaum is a lawyer and although he is not a psychiatrist, he is a physician and identifies with the therapist; he has always emphasized that courts are not the suitable agent to consider details of a treatment plan or to determine appropriateness of therapy.

The enforcement of the right to treatment under the Birnbaum proposal would be by a habeas corpus proceeding. By demonstrating that hospitals were staffed below a minimum ratio or that consultations were spaced farther than minimal periods of time the patients would be entitled to release. Recently, expanding his pragmatic standards for proof of adequacy of treatment, Birnbaum spelled out a more complete list of desirable institution-wide standards (4) that must be met for an inmate to be retained: 1) accreditation by the Joint Commission on Accreditation of Hospitals; 2) qualification for Medicare and Medicaid funds through Social Security Administration certification (many state hospitals forfeit such funds because of their failure to meet certification standards); 3) physical standards that meet minimums set by the American Psychiatric Association; 4) personnel-patient ratios that meet the standards for private hospitals that were set by APA and were used until 1969, when patient-personnel ratios were discarded as "meaningless as a general standard" (5); 5) state licensing of all professional hospital personnel; 6) regularly recorded progress notes reflecting patient-physician consultation; and 7) presence of halfway houses and other intermediate facilities.

The cooperation of state legislatures, which have control over finances, is needed in order to have effective treatment. Some courts may not go as far as Birnbaum might wish in enunciating this right. The legal process is time-consuming. For some or all of these reasons, Birnbaum has also advocated a second approach to the right of treatment, by state legislative action. A bill to specify this right has been introduced into the state legislature of Pennsylvania every year since 1967 (6); a version of this bill is currently under consideration.

Important Court Decisions

The first reaction to Birnbaum's proposal in 1960 was a prompt and enthusiastic endorsement in an editorial in the *American Bar Association Journal*: "A precedent which held that the patient in a public mental institution has a right to reasonable medical and psychiatric attention might work wonders" (7). But little more was heard of the idea until it was seized upon by Judge David Bazelon six years later in a District of Columbia case that involved an offender who had pled not guilty by reason of insanity when charged with a minor offense and had been held in St. Elizabeths Hospital for a period far in excess of the maximum criminal penalty (8).

The position of the offender who is diverted from the criminal process and committed to a mental hospital raises interesting constitutional questions, but this is not the type of situation with which Birnbaum had been concerned. On the one hand, the criminal offender is in a better position than the average mental hospital patient to claim an abridgment of freedom when he is held for an indeterminate period; he often does not meet the criteria of mental illness (the appellant in Judge Bazelon's case was diagnosed as a "sociopath") and he can argue that criminal justice procedural safeguards are not being met. The argument can also be advanced that there is no recognized psychiatric treatment for sociopathy and that hospitalization until the person is "cured" can represent a life term. In contrast, the average involuntary state hospital patient can be seen as being deprived of his liberty without having infringed any law; he has no recourse to a strict system of procedural safeguards — like the criminal law system of safeguards — to guarantee that the deprivation of liberty will be appropriate, effective, and for no longer than a minimum period. This is the patient for whom Birnbaum devised his legal remedy.

The Rouse case (8), in which the right to treatment was first judicially noted, applied the Birnbaum concept only to a class of patients being held for purposes other than merely restoration of mental competency; it did not deal with the average committed patient not under criminal charges. The case further disappointed Birnbaum because it failed to adopt the idea of rough yardsticks that would automatically determine if appropriate treatment were available.

Instead of trying to enunciate such a yardstick as patient-personnel ratios, the court sent the case back to the lower court for a full hearing on the adequacy of treatment. This was the Pandora's box which Birnbaum had said should not be opened; courts do not have the time or the competence to decide in individual cases if patients should have one type of treatment in preference to another. The Rouse rehearing, which is transcribed in a record of more than 500 pages, required the attention of the whole court for varying parts of four different days: it required the time of a United States District Judge, three lawyers for Rouse, two lawyers for St. Elizabeths, the director of the hospital, a staff psychiatrist, a staff clinical psychologist, two ward attendants, a psychiatrist on the staff of the District of Columbia Commission on Mental Health, and two psychiatrists to serve as expert witnesses for Rouse (3, p. 46).

Although the Rouse case clearly said there was a right to treatment, the basis for this right again a disappointment to Birnbaum, was said to be a District of Columbia statute; the question of the applicability of a constitutional Fifth Amendment right based on deprivation of liberty without due process of law went unanswered.

Additional cases in the District of Columbia and Massachusetts affirmed the concept of the right to treatment, but until the recent case of *Wyatt v. Stickney* (9) no case clearly affirmed this as a constitutional right and as a right for all (not merely quasi-criminal) patients. In one Pennsylvania case, the court expressly declined to consider the right to treatment when this was demanded for the inmates of the state hospital for the criminally insane because then the court "quite possibly would have to supervise the therapy of several hundred persons."

> If . . . we were to hold Section 404 unconstitutional either on its face or in its application to the plaintiffs and to others of their class, we quite possibly would have to supervise the therapy of several hundred persons. Could we compel the staff of Farview and other Pennsylvania mental institutions to perform the tasks the prayers of the complaint would have performed by them and determine the

status of each individual? These questions, since several hundred individuals are involved, could present a lengthy, if not almost interminable, process and might perhaps be unmanageable (10).

(The court in a related case later did find the commitment procedure, by medical certification, unconstitutional; the plaintiffs were thus granted substantial relief and the court did not have to delve into the treatment question [11].)

Two recent Bazelon decisions have defined further how far the courts will involve themselves with the appropriateness of the treatment of quasi-criminals confined to mental institutions. Conscious of the quagmire that judicial review of hospital administration could enter, Bazelon apparently is narrowing the role of the court. In *Tribby v. Cameron* (12) it is stated that it is not the function of the court to substitute its own judgment for the judgment of the hospital administrators but it *is* a function of the court to see that the administrators have made permissible decisions. A permissible decision is one that demonstrably takes account of the relevant information which was available or should have been available to the decision-maker. *Covington v. Cameron* (13) further defined the limited judicial review that Bazelon favors; the court must assure itself that the decision-makers "have: 1) reached a reasoned and not unreasonable decision, 2) by employing the proper criteria, and 3) without overlooking anything of substantial relevance." Said Bazelon: "More than this the courts do not pretend to do. To do less would abandon the interests affected to the absolute power of administrative officials" (13).

Such decisions by the courts, in which they show a willingness to exert some control over the internal management of psychiatric hospitals, is part of a general movement that became obvious in the late 60s of court concern in areas where the person operates at a disadvantage because of the power of the system, such as the administration of corrections, the juvenile justice system, and public welfare law.

In two important decisions, courts have meticulously examined the internal affairs of mental hospitals, found much that is wanting, and ordered the hospital to remedy conditions. One of these cases does not take us too far from the Rouse case; like most of the cases in this area, it dealt with a quasi-criminal and the imposition of an indeterminate hospital commitment in place of a jail sentence. *McCray v. Maryland* (14) involved the Patuxent Institution, which is an intermediate institution with features of both a hospital and a prison. The court has issued 35 pages of rules and regulations covering all phases of the internal administration of the institution, down to the details of the personal possessions the inmate can have in his cell (not more than three undershirts and three undershorts) and the edibles he can possess (including three rolls of Tums). The main body of the decision, 46 pages long, considers the treatment available at Patuxent. The court found that sections of the institution used for solitary confinement and disciplinary confinement were not treatment facilities (although the psychiatric staff had stated that these were used as "negative reinforcers" as part of a therapy program). The court found that the program's aim of a total approach to rehabilitation was not being met by the institution's program. Declared the court: "Treatment in the Patuxent Institution should be immediately accelerated without regard to strict budgetary limitations imposed by the state. The institution must perform its responsibilities to the patients to comply with constitutional guarantees" (14).

The Alabama Case

The one case that clearly embraces Birnbaum's right to treatment theory by applying it to all involuntary patients (not merely those who because of law violations might be given extra criminal law procedural safeguards) and by asserting that this is indeed a Fifth Amendment right is *Wyatt v. Stickney* (9), a 1971 Federal Court decision concerning patients at Alabama's Bryce Hospital. The Wyatt case decision ordered the institution, its superintendent, and the Commission of Mental Health for the state to mount an effective treatment plan; it specifically retained jurisdiction over the case so the court could see that this was done. "Indeed," said a commentary in the *Alabama Law Review*, "the court seemed prepared to commit Bryce Hospital to judicial 'receivership' if necessary to ensure proper treatment for the patients there confined" (15). The two other Alabama state hospitals, Searcy and Partlow School for the Retarded, were included in later aspects of the case.[1]

The court found that "the purpose of involuntary hospitalization for treatment purposes is *treatment* and not mere custodial care or punishment. This is the only justification, from a constitutional standpoint, that allows civil commitments to mental institutions . . ." (9, p. 784). (Original emphasis.)

In an order six months later, on December 10, 1971, Judge Johnson specified the three fundamental conditions that his court would examine to ascertain if adequate and effective treatment was available. These were: 1) a humane psychological and physical environment; 2) qualified staff in numbers sufficient to administer adequate treatment; and 3) individualized treatment plans. We can note that the court was aware of the quagmire it would be involved in if it considered the appropriateness of treatment plans; it stated it would require only that there be individual plans.

The court noted that the dormitories were barn-like structures with no privacy for the patients; for most patients there was not even a space provided that a person could think of as his own. The toilets in the rest rooms seldom had partitions between them; the wearing apparel was shoddy; and the work assigned to patients was nontherapeutic ("mostly compulsory, uncompensated housekeeping chores"). Only 50 cents per patient per day was spent for food. (It can be pointed out that in another state, Maryland, some patients in state mental hospitals have been diagnosed as having pellagra and that in addition to being deficient in niacin, diets in the state's six facilities for the mentally ill and mentally retarded have also been found to have been deficient in protein, iron, and calcium [16].)

Concerning a qualified and numerically sufficient staff, the Alabama court stated that "more psychiatrists, Doctor of Philosophy level psychologists, and qualified Medical Doctors are not only a medical but are also a constitutional necessity in this public institution."

Responding to Judge Johnson's order, the State of Alabama's Department of Mental Health has submitted a budget more than double that of previous years. It would provide for a patient-staff ratio of better than one-to-one, a per diem per patient expenditure of more than $25 (in contrast to the expenditure at Bryce in 1971 of $6.86), and an increase in hospital pay scales to match those of the Veterans Administration (17).

Standard Setting by the Court

The court has not only decreed that psychiatrists, psychologists, and social workers — whom it calls "qualified mental health professionals" — must meet the same licensing and certification requirements as are met by persons of the same profession in private practice but has also set a schedule of minimum staffing for every 250 patients: one unit director, two psychiatrists, four physicians, 12 registered nurses, six licensed practical nurses, 92 aides and ten orderlies, one Ph.D. psychologist, one M.A. psychologist, two B.S. psychologists, two M.S.W. social workers, and five B.A. social workers. Requirements for other health personnel, clerks, typists, and even a chaplain (one-half chaplain for every 250 patients) bring the total to 207.5 personnel for 250 patients, a 1 to 1.25 ratio (18). The requirement of two psychiatrists for every 250 patients will mean that a state system that employed only four psychiatrists will now have to employ 42 (19).

By insisting that qualified mental health professionals meet private practice standards, the court has adopted the idea of Dr. F. Lewis Bartlett, a psychiatrist on the staff of Pennsylvania's Haverford State Hospital and an associate of Birnbaum's in a crusade for improved state hospital standards (20), that exceptions for foreign-trained physicians should not be made (21). The court has also accepted another of Bartlett's ideas that may be even more costly than the improved patient-staff ratios; patient labor will have to be compensated for in accordance with minimum wage laws of the Fair Labor Standards Act if patient labor is to help operate and maintain the hospital (22).

The Alabama case has set a train of other cases in motion. In Georgia the American Civil Liberties Union has filed a suit alleging patients in that state receive inadequate diagnosis, care, and treatment (23). *The New York Times* (24) has noted that institutions for the retarded in New York and Massachusetts are the objects of pending suits and that several national mental health organizations and legal associations have said they plan to file similar suits in many other states. According to the *Times*: "The suits are expected by their sponsors to have little difficulty in winning favorable decisions, many people in the field conceding that elimination of injustices done toward the mentally disabled is long overdue" (24).

The Wyatt case ruling goes very far in creating a legal right to the kind of mental hospital treatment that meets court-determined standards of care. This agrees with the policy of a number of groups that have supported the court proposals in "friend of the court" briefs; these have included the American Psychological Association, the National Legal Aid and Defenders Association, the American Orthopsychiatric Association, the American Civil Liberties Union, and the Center for the Law and Social Policy. The last three of these groups have formed a National Council on the Rights of the Mentally Impaired to bring similar suits in other states (24).

The case raises many questions, including the important matter of logistics: Will well-qualified mental health personnel be found to fill the jobs that the court has ordered created, or will the discrepancy between the incomes of public and private practitioners and the differences in working conditions continue to shunt less well-qualified practitioners into the state hospital system?

Another question concerns the relationship of therapists to other personnel, especially administrative and custodial. The 250 patients will be required to have the services of 207.5 personnel (including the half a chaplain), but only two of these will be psychiatrists. Would a different kind of personnel structure, emphasizing therapy by psychiatrists and giving less emphasis to other medical personnel as well as to custodial and ancillary personnel, give the institution a different kind of atmosphere?

This leads to a further question: Should large sums of money be spent now to rebuild existing institutions, or should the money be spent to find alternatives to the state hospital system? Perhaps the two approaches are not mutually exclusive. An American Civil Liberties Union attorney, Bruce Ennis, has said that states affected by similar rulings in the future will probably find it less expensive to provide alternate facilities for mental patients and that the effect of the ruling will be to release many patients to facilities such as halfway houses (18). Such alternate facilities would eventually have to face court scrutiny to determine if they were providing adequate care, but since they would be caring for voluntary patients this would be a legally less compelling but not necessarily a socially less important issue.

A Suggested New Approach

In a more detailed consideration of the right to treatment (25), I have outlined a program that would recognize the right to treatment but would see treatment not as an automatic consequence of improved patient-staff ratios or greater per patient expenditures but as a result of a changed attitude of psychiatry toward the state hospital system. The changed attitude would have to include a greater interest by the "private sector" of psychiatry university programs and private practitioners in the state system; it would have to lead eventually to the phasing out of the dual system of patient care with different standards for public and private hospitals; it would require greater responsibility by psychiatrists for the determination of objective standards of patient care so that the quality of the product delivered by psychiatry can be measured.

As difficult as the measurement of good psychiatric care may be (and it is even more difficult than the measurement of good medical care), some objective standards will have to be set by psychiatry so that patients, third party payees, state legislatures, and courts can compare hospital A and hospital B, treatment A and treatment B, psychiatrist A and psychiatrist B. The myth that all psychiatric care is equivalent to all other psychiatric care must be abandoned, and realistic methods of appraisal of care must be substituted. The measurement of psychiatric effectiveness is belatedly receiving attention; in a recent article Linn (26) pointed out the difficulties but also the necessity of evaluating what is done for patients during their hospitalization.

Innovative approaches to hospitalization including the abandonment of many present institutions and practices will be needed before patients receive adequate treatment. Only an approach far more comprehensive and far more sophisticated than the Wyatt case approach will succeed in upgrading the state hospital system.

We can debate whether the Wyatt case is progressive or regressive. It provides justice for patients who have been denied justice, but it also brings the courts into the mental health movement in a way that may turn out to be harmful for both courts and hospitals.

Psychiatrists at this time must deal with the problem of the camel whose snout is in our tent. We can recognize that there is a right to treatment. We can also insist that courts use simple yardsticks which psychiatry will have to develop quickly to keep the legal determination of treatment adequacy from usurping psychiatric authority and determining hospital policy.

NOTES

1. A motion to amend the complaint was granted August 12, 1971.

REFERENCES

1. Birnbaum M: The right to treatment. American Bar Association Journal 46:499–505, 1960.
2. Dershowitz AM: The psychiatrist's power in civil commitment: a knife that cuts both ways. Psychology Today 2(9):42–47, 1969.
3. Birnbaum M: A rationale on the "Right to Treatment" and some comments on the potentiality of this right for abuse. Read at the 120th annual meeting of the American Psychiatric Association, Detroit, Mich., May 8–12, 1967.
4. Birnbaum M: Some remarks on the "Right to Treatment." Alabama Law Review 23:623–639.
5. De Marneffe F: The new APA standards for psychiatric facilities. Amer. J. Psychiat. 126:879–880, 1969.
6. Halpern CR: A practicing lawyer views the right to treatment. Georgetown Law Journal 57:782–817, 1969, p. 811 (Appendix: Senate Bill 1274 and House Bill 2118, General Assembly of Pennsylvania, 1968).

7. A new right. American Bar Association Journal 46:499–505, 1960.
8. Rouse v. Cameron 373 F 2d 451 (DC Cir 1966).
9. Wyatt v. Stickney 325 F Supp 781 (MD Ala 1971).
10. Dixon v. Commonwealth 313 F Supp 653 (MD Pa 1970).
11. Dixon v. Commonwealth 325 F Supp 966 (MD Pa 1971).
12. Tribby v. Cameron 379 F 2d 104 (DC Cir 1967).
13. Covington v. Cameron 419 F 2d 617 (DC Cir 1969).
14. McCray v. Maryland mise pet 4363 et seq. Cir Ct for Montgomery County, Md., opinion and order, Nov. 11, 1971.
15. Commentary, Alabama Law Review 23:642–656, 1971.
16. Pellagra found in Md state hospitals. Psychiatric News, May 5, 1971, p. 18.
17. Sharp RG: Alabama MH system faces court-engineered upgrading. Psychiatric News, Mar. 1, 1972, pp. 1, 10.
18. Alabama judge sets rigid mental health standards; wide impact on state mental hospitals foreseen. Mental Health Scope, Apr. 26, 1972, p. 1.
19. Court sets guide for mental care. New York Times, Apr. 14, 1972, p. 67.
20. Robitscher J: Controversial crusaders (the mentally ill and psychiatric reform). Medical Opinion & Review 4(9):54–67, 1968.
21. Bartlett FL: Present-day requirements for state hospitals joining the community. New Eng. J. Med. 276:90–94, 1967.
22. Bartlett FL: Institutional peonage. Atlantic 214(1):116–119, 1964.
23. Suit attacks state mental hospitals. Atlanta Constitution, Mar. 30, 1972, p. 2B.
24. Impending ruling by federal judge promises hope for neglected in mental institutions around country. New York Times, Mar. 26, 1972, p. 35.
25. Robitscher J: The right to treatment: a social-legal approach to the plight of the state hospital patient. Villanova Law Review (to be published).
26. Linn LS: Measuring the effectiveness of mental hospitals. Hosp. Community Psychiat. 21: 381–386, 1970.

Loren H. Roth

A Commitment Law for Patients, Doctors, and Lawyers

Man cares because it is his nature to care.
Man survives because he cares and is cared for.
(1, p. 13)

Recent clashes among the parties to mental health commitment have been inevitable and heuristic. Not unlike Greta Garbo, many mental patients want to be alone (2). Their point of view should be respected. In the absence of incompetency to consent to or refuse treatment, or absent an emergency, mental patients should not be treated involuntarily (3).

Next come the mental health lawyers, who are keen to advocate for clients (and to protect civil rights for all persons) and who are reluctant to recognize the legitimate role of paternalism in a caring society. However, no caring society can ignore the health needs of persons demonstrably unable to care for themselves. As Marcus noted, "You can degrade people by taking care of them and you can degrade people by not taking care of them and I see no simple answer to such questions" (quoted in reference 4).

Finally come the physicians, who understandably want to treat severely mentally ill individuals who can benefit from treatment and are frustrated by the new laws emphasizing patient dangerousness as a prerequisite for involuntary treatment (3, 5). However, physicians at times also fail to acknowledge the bankruptcy of past commitment approaches that sanctioned hospitalization of the mentally ill solely on the basis of their need for care and treatment.

From *The American Journal of Psychiatry* 136 (1979):1121–1127. Copyright © 1979 by the American Psychiatric Association.. Reprinted by permission of the publisher and the author.

As a consequence of the failed dialogue among these parties, the stakes have escalated. Recent trends in mental health law, for example, point in a paradoxical direction. The judicially committed mental patient may soon be permitted to refuse customary psychiatric treatments that are likely to reverse or stabilize his or her condition (6). The risk is that the mental hospital will again become custodial, which would ensure the patient's civil rights while failing to restore health. Such a scenario seems all the more paradoxical when one considers that the severely mentally ill are more treatable now than ever before (7).

It is the thesis of this article that a new synthesis for the law of commitment is possible. The following approach to the law of commitment is one which respects persons and gives credence to both medical and legal values. I believe it may be acceptable to all parties concerned, except the most vocal groups of disaffected ex-mental patients and the abolitionists, who would do away with commitment altogether.

Parens Patriae Commitment: Safeguarded Paternalism

The *parens patriae* approach to mental health commitment described herein modifies and tightens considerably an approach previously suggested by Stone (5). Brief periods of mental health commitment are permitted based on the principle of *parens patriae,* the interest of the state in caring for persons unable to care for themselves. As envisioned here, commitment under the *parens patriae* power explicitly sanctions the formerly implicit: commitment is based on the specific legal incompetency of the patient to consent to or refuse treatment. It is an acknowledged period of temporary guardianship in the patient's best interest. Procedural protections are afforded the *parens patriae* patient. The aim is to reconcile mental health commitment with other state laws, which have always permitted substitute permission for treatment of medical patients who are demonstrated incompetent to consent to or refuse medical treatment. This is the medical model for mental health commitment. It ensures that mental patients would be treated similarly to other medical patients, namely, in the absence of their incompetency to consent or refuse, or absent an emergency, patients may not be treated against their will (3).

Proposed Procedures for Parens Patriae Commitment

If the person suffers from a severe and reliably diagnosed mental illness (e.g., psychosis), and 1) absent treatment the immediate prognosis is for major distress of the person, 2) treatment is available, 3) the diagnosed illness substantially impairs the person's ability to understand or to communicate about the possibility of treatment, and 4) the risk/benefit ratio of treatment is such that "a reasonable man would consent to it" then a brief trial of treatment in the patient's best interest is both ethically proper and legally sanctioned (modified from reference 5).

Most state commitment hearings do not at present adjudicate specific legal incompetency to consent or refuse. They are therefore defective, although some might dispute this assertion. In the past the "hidden competency" addressed by most commitment statutes has concerned the patient's ability to judge his own need for treatment. Rather than a more elemental approach to competency (compatible with informed consent doctrine and evaluating whether or not the patient understands the consequences of treatment) a "judgment about treatment" standard was applied. If the person's judgment was so defective that he or she did not voluntarily seek or willingly accept psychiatric treatment, then the patient was committed and involuntarily treated. In operation this standard (and its legal meaning) is vague and imprecise. This approach is heavily susceptible to value judgments, so that unlike other medical patients, the mentally ill patient may be treated simply because he needs such treatment, whether he wants it or not or is capable of deciding for himself. The ethical, legal, and practical problems in implementing this approach have accounted for its rejection by civil libertarians and for a return to dangerousness to self or others as the only acceptable standard for civil commitment. Inspection of the wording of the 1966 Pennsylvania Mental Health statute (now repealed) illustrates this problem. Persons were committed and involuntarily treated upon a finding that mental disability "lessen(ed) the capacity of the person to use his customary self control, judgment, and discretion in the conduct of his affairs and social relations" so as to render the person in "need of care or treatment by reason of such mental disability" (8). The approach to competency to consent proposed here attempts instead to clarify the standard for determination of competency, bringing the determination for psychiatry more into line with that of general medicine and making this determination more viable.

The approach proposed here acknowledges that absent a specific adjudication of incompetency, even those patients properly judicially committed have the right to refuse subsequent treatment. The proposed *parens patriae* system would therefore alter future commitment hearings to address, at the time of commitment, the patient's specific competency to consent to or refuse treatment. Absent patient incompetency to consent or to refuse, no patient may be committed under the *parens patriae* power because a requisite step in the logic of involuntary medical treatment is missing (9).

Recent developments in the law commend such an approach. The report of the National Commission for the Protection of Human Subjects of Biomedical and Behavioral Research advocates that greater reliance be placed on the concept of limited incompetency in adjudicating the rights of the mentally ill (10). The Commission cites with favor the statute of Washington State, which includes the following wording:

(T)he court shall impose . . . only specific limitation and disabilities on a disabled person to be placed under a limited guardianship as the court finds necessary for such person's protection and assistance. (cited in reference 10, p. 80)

It is proposed that such limited incompetency be adjudicated at commitment. The patient remains "generally competent." He or she therefore loses no other civil rights as a consequence of commitment but the right to refuse customary treatment, which is the only civil right that should be abridged by commitment.

There are today no universally accepted criteria for adjudicating a patient's competency to consent to or refuse treatment (11). The following criteria are proposed for trial application. The three-pronged standard for competency to consent or refuse is as follows:

1. Does the patient understand the generally agreed upon consequences (the potential benefits and the potential risks) both of being treated and of not being treated?

2. Does the patient understand why a particular form of treatment, e.g., psychotropic medication, is being considered or recommended in his case?

3. Does the patient express a choice for or against treatment?

Patients who fail on one, two, or three of the three competency criteria may, at the discretion of a legal decision maker, be adjudicated incompetent to consent to or refuse treatment.

A major purpose of the commitment hearing is to adjudicate the patient's competency or incompetency to consent to or refuse treatment, but the legal decision maker, in sanctioning commitment for the patient, attends to other requisite elements in the logic of commitment (e.g., see Stone's 5 criteria above). This approach is practical. Based on outpatient or inpatient evaluation (e.g., following three to five days of emergency psychiatric treatment) professional opinion is usually clear as to whether or not a patient requires treatment with, for example, psychotropic medications. Such plans are part of the patient's general treatment plan. While the professional may later recommend either increases or decreases in medication (or even a change of medication) the general purpose of receiving psychotropic medication is explored with the patient before the commitment hearing. The patient's capacity or incapacity to use this information is then presented to the judge or other legal decision maker in order to adjudicate the patient's competency.

The court does not order that treatment be given. Whether or not the patient is subsequently treated is a matter for further in-hospital deliberation between the patient's physicians, the appointed substitute decision makers (the temporary guardians), and the patient. The court appoints others to act as a limited guardian for the patient for the duration of the commitment order. The patient's relatives, the patient's friends, two or more physicians, a treatment evaluator (12), an interdisciplinary institutional treatment committee, or a human rights committee might each, under differing circumstances or jurisdictions, be appropriate as substitute decision makers (temporary limited guardians) for the patient (13).

The physician solicits an informed permission to treat the patient from the substitute decision maker. The substitute decision maker is empowered to elect or to reject treatment for the patient that is objectively in the patient's "best interest" or under a more subjective approach (14), to make the decision that the patient would have made were he or she competent to consent. While ethical considerations and the demand of good clinical practice dictate that the physician continue attempts to secure an informed consent for treatment from the patient (and to explore variations in the patient's treatment plan that may be more acceptable to the patient) ultimately it is the physician's prerogative, assuming substitute informed permission is obtained, to treat the patient nonconsensually. In-hospital advocacy service is provided for the patient, but the deliberations of the substitute decision maker are fact-finding and information-gathering rather than adversary in nature.

Commitment under the *parens patriae* power is for brief periods of time, e.g., 6 weeks. The court order is renewable for an additional 6 weeks only if it is shown to the court, or an equivalent legal decision maker (e.g., a court-appointed Master) that the patient is benefiting or is likely to benefit from continuing treatment.

At the conclusion of a 12-week period of treatment under the *parens patriae* power, the court order for commitment and for specific incompetency to consent to or refuse treatment is automatically terminated. If the patient has not by this time agreed to voluntary treatment, it is unlikely he will do so. Subsequent periods of hospitalization are permitted only if it is shown that the patient constitutes a clear and continuing danger to others or to self.

The purpose of *parens patriae* treatment is to restore the patient to functioning (competency) over a relatively brief period of time, using common and accepted methods of therapy. Once this is accomplished, the person is in a position to evaluate whether or not he or she has been helped by the interventions that were made over his or her initial objection. This type of help should not be forced again and again in the name of a person's best interest or because of incompetency to consent. The patient should in fact, and not only in theory, say "thank you" (5). If the patient recovers, he or she should be allowed to declare, when no longer a patient, that no such treatment is desired in the future. There should be a "living will" for involuntary treatment delivered under *parens patriae* power. There are complex philosophical problems here concerning the definition and duration of personhood along the life arc. In logic (assuming that repetitive treatment is required for efficacy and that the newly restored person is not yet in a good position to understand what should or would be his future choice were he to become ill again) *parens patriae* might justify involuntary treatment on more than one occasion. However, this has the potential for a "shell game" and should not be permitted to go on indefinitely.

The initial *parens patriae* court hearing is a full legal hearing with the usual due process protections afforded the patient. The patient is afforded counsel, the right to an independent mental health examination, the right to question his doctors as to their rationale for treatment, etc. (15). *Parens patriae* hearings may occur at two times: after a period of outpatient examination or, alternatively, 3 to 5 days after a period of emergency control for the patient under the police power of the state.

Comment

As here proposed, a *parens patriae* commitment makes explicit and legally sanctioned what is now implicit and only questionably legally sanctioned under the law of commitment. The purpose of involuntary commitment is to provide those patients with demonstrated functional incapacity the treatment they need. A *parens patriae* commitment would be a proper medical approach to the involuntary treatment of some patients who are acutely psychotic or schizophrenic, severely and/or delusionally depressed, manic, or have confusional or other organic syndromes that compromise orientation and understanding. Failing a trial of treatment that benefits the patient and absent the patient's consent to continue treatment, involuntary commitment is subsequently permitted only under the "dangerousness to others or self" rationales.

Emergency Commitment

Under emergency circumstances, and before a formal court adjudication of specific competency, involuntary treatment with medication is permitted only to the extent necessary to control the emergency. The purpose of emergency treatment, similar to all medical treatment under the emergency exception to informed consent law (the patient's consent is implied) (16), is to preserve the patient's health and/or to protect others until the court is able to rule on the suitability of a *parens patriae* or a "dangerousness" type commitment.

Police Power Commitments

Is commitment justified for mentally ill patients who are a danger to others? While some psychiatrists have understandably discounted the appropriateness of this approach for the mental health system (5), few legislatures are willing to ground involuntary commitment solely on the basis of *parens patriae*. There remains the question of how to handle mentally ill persons who do not profit from brief treatment and who at the time of expiration of a *parens patriae* commitment may still constitute a danger to others. While it has been argued that a single system of social control for deviant behavior should be sufficient for our society (17) (e.g., the criminal justice system with mental health treatment offered opportunistically), this point of view has not been accepted. A second rationale for commitment, with a differing procedural approach, is therefore proposed.

A major problem with commitment under the dangerousness to others approach is that such patients, many of whom manifest character type problems, are not incompetent to consent or to refuse treatment. It is therefore both legally and ethically unclear whether such mentally ill but competent persons may be treated against their will with, for example, psychotropic medications.

Police power commitments . . . are based on potential dangerousness but do not necessarily require a level of mental disability amounting to incompetency. Police power patients, therefore, may be in a position to refuse intrusive treatment, although . . . their continuing confinement while dangerous may, for public protection purposes, be constitutionally affirmed. (18, p. 15)

The physician's identity as a helping person is both distorted and degraded when he treats competent objecting patients at the behest of society. Furthermore, the patient's rights are violated. It is thus no surprise that recent and ongoing law suits have questioned this point, asserting that in the absence of a clear-cut emergency (imminent danger) involuntary treatment with medication, even for patients committed under the dangerousness to others rationale, is not constitutionally permitted (19). The problem here is one of imminent danger versus "dangerousness" over the long-term, or the proclivity for dangerous behavior. Under the police power there is no doubt as to society's right to restrain dangerous persons and to prevent the continuation of violent behavior. However, it is not clear that preventive treatment may continue once the emergency is controlled. This leaves in limbo the treatment of mentally ill persons who have been assaultive, who are judicially committed, but who are not assaultive in the hospital. Unfortunately, this type of person rather than the person who can profit from treatment is the paradigm of commitment under the "dangerousness to others" approach, honestly applied.

While treatment is presumably part of the purpose for commitment, it is argued that such patients cannot be treated against their will without additionally being adjudicated incompetent to consent or refuse (6, 19).

Roth (3) and Meisel have previously described a "segregation model" for the commitment of dangerous, competent, and mentally ill persons. Under this model the purposes of commitment are served by segregating such persons so as to decrease the risks for others. Treatment is offered but cannot be compelled. The mentally ill, competent, dangerous person may choose to refuse treatment at the risk of continuing confinement. The patient, not the doctor, balances the risk for the patient of continuing confinement as opposed to unwanted treatment. Under the proposed commitment law described below this approach (which I believe is both legally and ethically compelled for dangerous competent persons) is given formal recognition.

Proposed Approach to Commitment of Dangerous, Competent Patients

Dangerousness is adjudicated by a court only when it has been shown that the patient has perpetrated a recent act of violence, either a threat or (preferably for purposes of reliable ascertainment) an attempted or an accomplished act. Future dangerousness is difficult to predict. Courts will no doubt continue to rely on past dangerousness in establishing the likelihood of future dangerousness (for purposes of equity if no other).

The due process protections of the criminal justice system are afforded the patient at the court hearing. Dangerousness must be proved beyond a reasonable doubt.

Commitment is for a 90-day period. The commitment is renewed only after another court hearing establishes the reoccurrence of dangerous behavior during the previous 90 days. Elaboration of this rule is necessary for the treatment of mentally abnormal offenders (e.g., persons found not guilty by reason of insanity). Discussion of this point is beyond the scope of this paper.

If competency is not adjudicated at the time of commitment (as is the present approach in most state laws) the dangerous, competent, committed patient has the right to refuse all treatment save that treatment necessary to control an ongoing emergency (i.e., imminent danger to others or self) in the hospital. Forced treatment of the patient for purposes of making treatment more definitive requires an additional finding of incompetency. To treat nonconsensually the dangerous committed patient, physicians would need to return to court (or to present their recommendations to some other not yet identified legal decision maker) for a second due process competency hearing. This scenario is no pipe dream. It is an approach analogous to that recently proposed by most of the members of the Task Force on Legal and Ethical Issues of the President's Commission on Mental Health (15) and may be constitutionally required depending on the outcome of ongoing legal actions (19).

The dangerousness to others approach might be modified to include adjudication of competency at the time of the commitment hearing, but clinical experience suggests the proposed standard for competency (honestly applied) would adjudicate most patients who are dangerous to others as competent to consent or to refuse. Under a combined approach (dangerousness plus incompetency) many patients who are dangerous to others would not be committed. Alternatively, if found competent but nevertheless committed, the dangerous patient has the right to refuse treatment. The willingness of physicians to provide treatment and to work in mental institutions under these circumstances is problematic (3), and there is the additional problem of ensuring that dangerous patients do not harm other patients. The dangerousness to others approach may well force the creation of a new type of quasi-penal setting for the long-term detention of the dangerous mentally ill patient who refuses treatment.

Combined Commitments: Dangerousness to Self

Commitment under the "dangerousness to self" rationale combines elements of both *parens patriae* and police power. Most patients dangerous to self (e.g., the suicidal and delusionally depressed patient or the patient with an acute confusional psychosis) would be treated under the *parens patriae* approach as above. Persons who are gravely disabled due to mental illness and therefore pose a danger to themselves over the long run may instead be committed under the dangerousness to self system. Such cases, which clinically include some patients with chronic schizophrenia and functional impairment or with organic brain syndromes (e.g., alcoholic dementia, senile dementia with psychosis) resemble more nearly "care" than treatment type cases. In such cases, a 90-day renewable court commitment is permitted contingent on a finding in court that the patient is or continues to be a danger to self.

Commitment under the dangerousness to self rationale is permitted only when the following criteria are satisfied.

1. The person's preference for no care or treatment whatsoever is respected unless it is likely that serious harm to the person's physical health will ensue without care and treatment.

2. Although the person may not be fully treatable, treatment will be attempted.

3. The diagnosed illness impairs the person's ability to understand or to communicate about the possibilities of care and treatment, i.e., the patient is incompetent to consent to or to refuse care and treatment.

4. The quality of care and treatment available (and subsequently delivered) is clearly superior to that care and treatment the person would otherwise receive were he or she not committed.

5. The locus of care is that environment least restrictive of the person's freedom, that which is medically and socially advisable, and which is consistent with the person's needs. A person's preference of environments where care is to be received is given great weight.

The patient who is dangerous to self, since he or she must also be found incompetent to consent to or refuse care and treatment, is not permitted to refuse subsequent care or treatment necessary to maintain health and to stabilize his or her condition. A system for substitute decision making similar to that previously discussed under *parens patriae* commitments is put into place for patients who are dangerous to self. The dangerousness to self approach to commitment is a system of protective services for chronically disabled patients. Much of the care and treatment delivered under this system might be community rather than institutionally based.

Discussion

I cannot review in depth here the philosophical arguments that justify an approach of safeguarded paternalism (15, 20) in the treatment of mental patients. It is clear that some alternative to the dangerousness approach is required, however, if the helping potential of the mental health system is to be realized and if treatment is to be afforded severely mentally ill persons who can profit from treatment and who may be unable, because of their illness, to understand their need for treatment. Unless specific incompetency to consent or to refuse is adjudicated at the time of commitment, the custodial and social control functions of the mental hospital are elevated at the expense of its treatment functions. Allowing commitment without permission to treat is essentially the abolitionist position in disguise.

Complementing the *parens patriae* approach is a back-up system for patients dangerous to self or to others over the long run. A finding of dangerousness (and not solely treatability and incapacity) is required if persons are to be deprived of freedom for long periods of time. The patient must have committed or be likely to commit a criminal act; alternatively, his or her physical as well as mental health must be in obvious jeopardy. Dangerousness, which is a political and not a medical concept, is the sole justification for long-term commitment.

Standards and procedures concerning mental health commitment must be assessed in terms of their pragmatic impact as well as through a consideration of attendant societal values. Over the last few years there have been some studies pointing to the value of brief involuntary treatment for the psychiatric patient. Most patients are helped, not victimized, by involuntary treatment (21–23). A substantial proportion of patients continue to participate in treatment voluntarily following a period of involuntary treatment (24, 25). Furthermore, the course of involuntary treatment is usually fairly brief. In one recent study, 67% of involuntary patients were discharged within 38 days (21). Follow-up interviews with the patients suggested "that although the committed patients were generally hospitalized against their will, with the advantage of hindsight they tended to have a positive attitude toward their hospitalization" (21). Another study found that 63% of the involuntary patients were discharged in less than 3 months (26). While more and better controlled research is needed (not all studies have been so encouraging; see, for example, reference 27), these are the type of findings that I believe help justify brief trials of involuntary treatment for mentally ill patients who are genuinely incompetent to consent to or to refuse it, where such treatment is available. The paradigm case for evaluating the law of commitment is not the harmless eccentric who receives indefinite segregation and overtranquilization in a medieval institution, but the previously functioning person, with an acute or subacute mental decompensation, where the possibility of improvement with treatment can be assessed readily.

The proposed *parens patriae* system treats the psychiatric patient similarly to any other medical patient. In the absence of a formal court adjudication of incompetency to consent or refuse (or absent an emergency) the adult, competent mental patient has the right to refuse treatment. For the incompetent patient, procedural protections are provided and durational limits are defined (15).

Patients who are both dangerous to others and competent to consent to or refuse treatment are committed for detention so that they may be offered an opportunity for treatment and in order to decrease societal risk. The types of acts required to establish dangerousness to others under the dangerousness system are also violations of the criminal law. Such patients in fairness may and, arguably, should be handled in the criminal justice system and not the mental health system.

A final virtue of the proposed system is that it would facilitate research and evaluation of the commitment process. From the outset, all commitment cases are clearly defined and labeled as either of the *parens patriae* type or of the dangerousness type (either to self or to others). Absent this type of approach, precisely targeted evaluation studies of the commitment process have been difficult to perform. The type of law proposed above would be modified subsequently on the basis of empirical data.

If the mental health bar were to accept the approach I have proposed, it would be necessary to concede that the reliability of psychiatric diagnosis is improving (5, 28), that customary treatment should be made available for patients who are incompetent to consent to or to refuse it, and that the principle of beneficence (10) (not misplaced authority) underlies the desires of mental health professionals to provide trials of treatment for persons who are severely mentally ill and functionally impaired. We do no less for kith and kin.

The traditional mental commitment approach, wherein two physicians declare that the patient is ill and that he will be treated at the doctor's discretion (doctor knows best), must also give way. Substitute decision makers, and not solely doctors, must give informed permission for the patient to be treated. Physicians must be willing to participate in formal court hearings that adjudicate patient competency and to subject themselves to cross examination about their opinions. Perhaps most importantly, physicians must recognize that while it is one thing to want to help the impaired patient, if there is evidence that help is not forthcoming it is time to quit.

REFERENCES

1. Gaylin W: Caring. New York, Alfred A Knopf, 1976.
2. Chamberlin J: On Our Own: Patient-Controlled Alternatives to the Mental Health System. New York, Hawthorn Books, 1978.
3. Roth LH: Involuntary civil commitment: the right to treatment and the right to refuse treatment, in Psychiatrists and the Legal Process: Diagnosis and Debate. Edited by Bonnie RJ. New York, Insight Communications, 1977.
4. Shenker I: Milk of kindness sours, experts find. New York Times, March 8, 1976, p. 22.
5. Stone AA: Mental Health and Law: A System in Transition. DHEW Publication ADM 75-176. Washington, DC, US Government Printing Office, 1975.
6. Plotkin R: Limiting the therapeutic orgy: mental patients' right to refuse treatment. Northwestern University Law Review 72:461-525, 1977.
7. Klein DF, Gittelman-Klein R (eds): Progress in Psychiatric Drug Treatment. New York, Brunner/Mazel, 1975.
8. Meisel A: Pennsylvania civil commitment procedures—a practical guide. Pennsylvania Medicine 77:47-50, 1974.
9. Developments in the law—civil commitment of the mentally ill. Harvard Law Review 87:1190-1406, 1974.
10. National Commission for the Protection of Human Subjects of Biomedical and Behavioral Research: Report and Recommendations, Research Involving Those Institutionalized as Mentally Infirm. DHEW Publication OS 78-0006. Washington, DC, DHEW, 1978.
11. Roth LH, Meisel A, Lidz CW: Tests of competency to consent to treatment. Am. J. Psychiatry 134:279-284, 1977.
12. Hoffman PB, Dunn RC: Guaranteeing the right to treatment, in Psychiatrists and the Legal Process: Diagnosis and Debate, Edited by Bonnie RJ. New York, Insight Communications, 1977.

13. Position statement on the right to adequate care and treatment for the mentally ill and mentally retarded (off acts). Am. J. Psychiatry 134:354–355, 1977.
14. Superintendent of Belchertown State School v. Saikewicz, 370 NE 2d 417 (Sup. Jud. Ct., Mass., 1977).
15. Report of the Task Panel on Legal and Ethical Issues: Task Panel Reports submitted to the President's Commission on Mental Health, vol 4, Appendix. Washington, DC, US Government Printing Office, 1978.
16. Prosser WL: Law of Torts, 4th ed. St. Paul, Minn. West Publishing Co., 1971.
17. Monahan J: The psychiatrization of criminal behavior: a reply. Hosp. Community Psychiatry 24:105–108, 1973.
18. Wexler, DB: Criminal Commitments and Dangerous Mental Patients: Legal Issues of Confinement, Treatment, and Release. DHEW Publication ADM 76-331. Washington, DC, US Government Printing Office, 1976.
19. Brief from Amici Curiae, The Mental Health Association, The Civil Liberties Union of Massachusetts, The Mental Patients Liberation Front, in Okin v. Rogers. Mental Disability Law Reporter 2:43–50, 1978.
20. Murphy JG: Incompetence and paternalism. Archiv. Für Rechts-Und Sozialphilosophie 60: 465–485, 1974.
21. Gove WR, Fain T: A comparison of voluntary and committed psychiatric patients. Arch. Gen. Psychiatry 34:669–676, 1977.
22. Sata LS, Goldenberg EE: A study of involuntary patients in Seattle, Hosp. Community Psychiatry 28:834–837, 1977.
23. Ginzburg HM, Rappeport JR, Paskewitz D: A followup study of involuntary commitments. Paper presented at the 130th annual meeting of the American Psychiatric Association, Toronto, Ont., Canada, May 11–15, 1977.
24. Spensley J, Barter JT, Werme PH, et al.: Involuntary hospitalization: what for and how long? Am. J. Psychiatry 131:219–222, 1974.
25. Peele R, Chodoff P, Taub N: Involuntary hospitalization & treatability: observations from the District of Columbia experience. Catholic University of America Law Review 23:744–753, 1974.
26. Tomelleri CJ, Lakshminarayanan N, Herjanic M: Who are the "committed"? J. Nerv. Ment. Dis. 165:288–293, 1977.
27. Zwerling I, Karasu T, Plutchik R, et al.: A comparison of voluntary and involuntary patients in a state hospital. Am. J. Orthopsychiatry 45:81–87, 1975.
28. Helzer JE, Clayton PH, Pambakian R, et al.: Reliability of psychiatric diagnosis. II. The test/retest reliability of diagnostic classification. Arch. Gen. Psychiatry 34:136–141, 1977.

Ruth Macklin

Refusal of Psychiatric Treatment
Autonomy, Competence, and Paternalism

I.

Let me begin by quoting from a short news article that appeared in the *New York Times* on November 1, 1979. Entitled "Judge Curbs Forced Medication in Treatment of Mental Patients," the article raises a number of central issues that receive a detailed analysis below:

> Federal District Judge Joseph L. Tauro has ruled that a mental patient has the right to refuse tranquilizing medication unless he is likely to become violent. The judge called such forced medication "an affront" to human dignity.
>
> Judge Tauro ruled Monday in favor of former patients at Boston State Hospital who had filed a class action suit seeking restrictions on the use of mind-altering drugs and on seclusion at the facility.
>
> "Given a nonemergency, it is an unreasonable invasion of privacy and an affront to basic concepts of human dignity to permit forced injection of a mind-altering drug," Judge Tauro ruled . . . .
>
> "The desire to help the patient is a laudable if not noble goal," he said. "But a basic premise of the right to privacy is the freedom to decide whether we want to be helped or whether we want to be left alone."
>
> He rejected a contention by attorneys for the hospital that a patient, whether voluntarily or involuntarily admitted, was incompetent to decide whether to accept treatment.

An earlier version of this essay appeared in *Man, Mind and Morality* (Prentice-Hall, 1981), Chapter 3. Copyright © 1981 by Prentice-Hall. Reprinted by permission of the publisher and the author.

"The weight of the evidence persuades this Court that, although committed mental patients do suffer at least some impairment of their relationship to reality, most are able to appreciate the benefits, risks and discomfort that may reasonably be expected from receiving psychotropic medication," he said.

Forced injection of mind-altering drugs also violates the provisions of the freedom of speech guarantees of the First Amendment, he added.

"The First Amendment protects the communication of ideas," the judge said. "That protected right of communication presupposes a capacity to produce ideas. As a practical matter, therefore, the power to produce ideas is fundamental to our cherished right to communicate and is entitled to comparable constitutional protection.

"Whatever the powers the Constitution has granted our Government, involuntary mind control is not one of them, absent extraordinary circumstances."

Although this recent ruling reported in the newspaper addresses the issues from a legal standpoint, rather than from the perspective of moral philosophy, the concepts and principles involved are virtually identical.

Before turning to the specific issues raised by the judge's ruling—including issues that arise from the way he chose to formulate his decision—I want to lay down several premises on which my later arguments will be based. First of all, it is too narrow an approach to look at the question of refusal of psychiatric treatment as if the only value at stake were the freedom or liberty of the psychiatric patient. Decisions involving refusal of treatment are often couched in terms of the patient's "right to decide." Although I think this *is* the central issue in cases in which the patient is competent, other considerations enter into the picture when the patient is either clearly incompetent or when there is uncertainty surrounding the patient's competency. In fact, it is just this question of competency that Judge Tauro's decision glosses over much too quickly— a question to which I shall return. My first premise, then, is to acknowledge that freedom is a fundamental value—one that should be respected and promoted in medical (psychiatric) settings, as well as elsewhere in personal and social life.

Following quickly upon this first premise is a second: though freedom is a value of fundamental importance, it is not the only value that needs to be preserved, promoted, or respected in medical practice. To name just a few other salient values, we have justice, equity, equality, self-respect, self-esteem, autonomy, preservation of life itself, improving the quality of life, benevolence, and humaneness. Some of these values are more typical in medical contexts than others and, as we are all too often reminded, these cherished values often come into conflict with one another, making it impossible to satisfy more than one simultaneously.

My third premise is this. Freedom to choose is a *hollow* value if the individual facing a choice lacks the capacity or the opportunity for rational deliberation, adequate understanding, or reasonable assessment of the consequences of the options being offered. The discerning reader will, of course, recognize all the baggage I have packed into this third premise. What constitutes the *capacity* for rational deliberation? Or *adequate* understanding? Or *reasonable* assessment of consequences? What do we mean by "rational," "reasonable," and "adequate"? I do not intend to dodge these hard questions entirely and will come back to them shortly. But however difficult it may be to arrive at a precise formulation of the meanings of these problematic notions, and however hard it may be to devise criteria for their correct application in practice, these difficulties should not lead us to dismiss the premise entirely. Sometimes hard questions are just that — hard. They are not resolved by pretending that conflicting values do not exist, or that people are less complex than they really are. Now I realize that it is not very illuminating to point out that an incompetent patient is one who lacks the capacity for rational deliberation, adequate understanding, or reasonable assessment of the consequences of the options that are available. But neither is it helpful to deny that the distinction between the competent and the incompetent patient is relevant to the question of the patient's right to refuse psychiatric treatment.

What values are central to debates surrounding the right to refuse psychiatric treatment? I have already mentioned individual liberty or freedom. The term now widely used to denote *limitations* on liberty, justified by appeal to a person's own good, well-being, happiness, or interests, is "paternalism." Paternalism has enjoyed an especially bad press in recent years, particularly in areas related to medical treatment, the doctor-patient relationship, the actions of the FDA and other government agencies that regulate the actions of citizens, presumably for their own good. But are all paternalistic acts and practices unjustified? I shall argue shortly that although many are unreasonable, there still remains a class of justifiable paternalistic acts. These are ones in which the person or persons being coerced are incompetent. But before mounting that argument, let me introduce another key concept I will need for developing my further remarks about refusal of psychiatric treatment. The third major concept to be invoked in what follows is that of *autonomy.* To be autonomous is to have a "self-legislating will," in Kantian terms. It is to be author of one's own beliefs, desires, and actions. The autonomous agent is one who is self-directed, rather than one who obeys the commands of others. These various senses of autonomy presuppose an idea of an authentic self, a self that can be distinguished from the reigning influences of other persons and, more importantly for our present topic, a self that has a continuity of traits over time. I will argue below that if individual autonomy is a value that should be protected, promoted, and preserved, libertarians should recognize that autonomy may be lost by a patient's refusal of psychiatric treatment — treatment that might have prevented deterioration, humiliation, or decline. But that is a conclusion, rather than a premise of my argument, so let me turn next to some philosophical considerations — conceptual as well as moral.

II.

It is clear that coercion for paternalistic reasons limits people's freedom.

Even if arguments in favor of controlling the behavior of rational adults for their own good remain unconvincing, there is still a question about those who are less than fully competent.

The principle of liberty, as urged by John Stuart Mill and others, appears to prohibit paternalistic interferences with anyone's liberty of actions for reasons other than that of protecting innocent people from harm. It seems to rule out intervention into the behavior of suicide attempters, electric shock treatments for mental patients who are opposed to them, and involuntary commitment of those who are judged mentally ill and in need of care, custody, or treatment. But is this the proper way to interpret Mill's writings?

The word "paternalism" derives its meaning from the notion of treating others in what the dictionary describes as a "fatherly" manner. The clearest cases of paternalistic acts are found in the behavior of responsible parents or caretakers toward young children. Not only do we think we should interfere with the liberty of action of children in order to protect them from harm, we believe it is our duty to coerce or limit small children in many ways. There is usually no quarrel, in principle, with this view. Debates and quibbles begin over the particular age at which intervention ceases to be warranted or about just which forms of coercion are allowable, and in what areas of a child's life. But it is generally held to be fully justifiable to limit children's liberty of action both in order to prevent them from destroying themselves and also to foster their growth and thriving. At least in the case of very young children, and probably even up to adolescence, paternalistic reasons for controlling behavior appear sound.

The clearest cases of unjustifiable paternalistic acts are those in which obviously rational adults, who know what they are doing, are coerced against their wishes presumably for their own good. This is surely the group Mill had in mind when he asserted his libertarian principle, as a closer look at his position reveals. Mill would no doubt support a justification for involuntary commitment where a high probability exists that a person judged dangerous to others will commit an act of violence or other harm. It hardly seems as though Mill could support involuntary commitment on the grounds that someone is "dangerous to self," for that would be paternalistic. But would it be an unjustifiable form of paternalism? Caution is needed to avoid treating every paternalistic act as wrongful interference, even on a view that appears at first glance as strongly anti-paternalistic as Mill's. In applying his principle, we need to ask: does the prohibition against interfering with another's liberty apply to *everyone's* liberty? Does Mill himself recognize any exceptions to the prohibition against paternalistic acts? Mill's answer is explicit, but not wholly clear:

It is, perhaps, hardly necessary to say that this doctrine is meant to apply only to human beings in the maturity of their faculties. We are not speaking of children, or of young persons below the age which the law may fix as that of manhood or womanhood. Those who are still in a state to require being taken care of by others, must be protected against their own actions as well as against external injury. For the same reason, we may leave out of consideration those backward states of society in which the race itself may be considered as in its nonage. . . . Despotism is a legitimate form of government in dealing with barbarians, provided the end be their improvement, and the means justified by actually effecting that end. Liberty, as a principle, has no application to any state of things anterior to the time when mankind have become capable of being improved by free and equal discussion.[1]

Even though Mill's focus lay on the laws and actions of government, rather than on acts or practices of psychiatrists, the issues in both contexts are largely the same. The major task is to produce adequate criteria for judging when individuals are "in a state to require being taken care of by others" or when they are not (yet) "capable of being improved by free and equal discussion." In spite of his stalwart defense of the libertarian principle, Mill might well be prepared to accept a wide range of paternalistic interventions—precisely those directed at human beings who have not attained "the maturity of their faculties." He offers no clear or practically workable criterion for distinguishing between those who have attained such maturity and those who have not; but he nonetheless countenances a class of cases of justified paternalism. Not only does Mill approve of the imposition of paternalism in the case of children— those who are "still in a state to require being taken care of by others." He actually urges a paternalistic line of conduct. He is quite explicit in holding children and "those backward states of society in which the race itself may be considered as in its nonage" exempt from his injunctions against paternalism. Notice also that Mill does not need a notion of "mental illness," or even that of competency, to refer to the condition he describes here.

But what about other individuals who are "child-like" in a number of ways, especially in their inability to be "improved by free and equal discussion"? Among these are a majority of those correctly labeled mentally retarded, many who suffer some form of mental illness, emotional disturbance or behavior disorder, and the senile. Members of all these groups manifest the lack of full-scale rationality as a permanent or relatively enduring trait. Injunctions against paternalism seem not to apply in cases where people satisfy Mill's rather vaguely worded conditions—"being in a state to require being taken care of by others" and "incapable of being improved by free and equal discussion." Recall that Mill, in applying his own principle, claims that "despotism is a legitimate mode of government in dealing with barbarians, provided the end be their own improvement." This brand of paternalism is morally and politically unacceptable in today's world climate of anticolonialism. Yet it is consistent with this view to hold that coercion of people who are clearly nonrational or incompetent to manage their own affairs is a legitimate mode of treatment provided the end be their own improvement. Mill says his doctrine is meant to apply only to human beings "in the maturity of their faculties." On one plausible reading of this condition, retarded persons, the senile, and those afflicted with what psychiatrists call "thought disorders" are not in the maturity of their faculties in any but the chronological sense of "maturity." The relevant sense of "maturity" here is having "fully developed" mental capacities, where the lack of full development may be a result of chronological immaturity (children), decline of mental faculties (the senile), disease (mental patients), or unexplained developmental failures (many mentally retarded persons). The law now recognizes an intermediate category termed "diminished capacity"—a category used to mitigate criminal responsibility for some persons who have committed offenses.

So even an attack on paternalistic interference as strong as Mill's leaves room for a measure of justifiable paternalism in controlling, modifying, or improving the behavior of less than fully rational individuals. For those judged rational (in some appropriate sense of that complex and slippery notion), paternalistic intervention would not be justified. Since the profoundly retarded and the severely depressed have many of the same characteristics as helpless children, the same moral principle of humaneness applies: do not let harm befall those who, if left alone, would probably perish. In the case of parents and children this moral precept is strengthened by the role parents occupy and the special duties and obligations that flow from that role. The borderline cases pose the most difficulty, since the arguments could go either way depending on how close to the paradigm the analogous cases are drawn. If the notion of being inhumane has any moral force at all, it applies to situations where those who are clearly psychologically incapable of caring for their own needs are simply left to fend for themselves or perish.

A major problem lies in the fact that disagreement exists over where to draw the line conceptually between competence and incompetence. Part of the reason for this disagreement is that competence and incompetence are not discrete, separable states. One shades into the other, and people may be highly competent in some respects yet wholly incompetent in others. Failure to recognize this can result in mistreatment of those who are classed as incompetent according to specific criteria recognized by the law. For example, those judged incompetent to manage their own finances or to make a will may still be sufficiently rational to grant or to refuse consent for treatment using some medical procedure—say, electroconvulsive therapy. To be incompetent in some ways is not necessarily to be incompetent in all ways. Some mental patients suffer primarily from mood disorders, yet their cognitive capacities remain basically intact. The mildly retarded are slow to grasp concepts and may be incapable of abstract reasoning, yet they may understand, when it is carefully explained, what is involved in sterilization. All this suggests the need for a notion of variable competence, which would allow for a cluster of criteria to be used when determinations of competency must be made. This would result in appropriately specific judgments of competence rather than the kind of global assessment that is either too sweeping or turns out to be false. In the end, however, disagreement may remain over the question of whether people ought to assume responsibility for others (aside from children and maybe adult relatives) who cannot care for themselves.

III.

The problem now shifts to the search for appropriate criteria for making judgments of rationality or competence. It is usually easier to get clear about things by looking at paradigms, or clear cases, than by offering definitions or criteria, however. Normal adults are presumed to be rational or competent, and so are allowed to go about their business without interference. Five-year olds are generally presumed incompetent in many respects, and so are watched carefully and their behavior interfered with, when the need arises, by caretaking adults. With the retarded and the mentally ill, it is simply unclear where the general presumption ought to lie. We seek to avoid erring in either of two opposite directions: being too paternalistic, and therefore unjustifiably coercive; or too permissive, thereby opening the door to self-destructive or other irresponsible acts. The one evil consists of violating the cherished value of individual freedom; the other, allowing harm, destruction, or even death to befall an innocent, helpless human.

It is dismaying but not too surprising to discover that the grounds on which judgments of competency are made—usually by psychiatrists, in courts of law—are neither wholly objective nor generally agreed upon by experts in the mental health field. There just is no generally accepted, overall *theory* in psychology or psychiatry on which to base judgments about an individual's rationality, competence, or sanity. Instead, there exist a variety of subtheories and isolated criteria, a small number of which psychiatrists adhere to when they are legally authorized to testify in court.

Yet even in the absence of a solid theoretical foundation for making legal judgments about competence—judgments that may have direct consequences for licensing psychiatric treatment—wide areas remain in which people's competence needs to be assessed. The one that concerns us here is the need to gain informed consent from patients for treatments of various sorts. There is not a great deal of helpful written material on the meaning of "competency" in this context, but a recent article in a psychiatric journal advances the discussion considerably. In an article entitled "Tests of Competency to Consent to Treatment,"[2] the authors describe the various tests of competency used today. They cite (1) evidencing a choice; (2) "reasonable" outcome of choice; (3) choice based on "rational" reasons; (4) ability to understand; and (5) actual understanding, as the five basic categories proposed in the literature or readily inferable from judicial commentary. The authors note further that a useful test for competency is one that can be reliably applied; is mutually acceptable or at least comprehensible to physicians, lawyers, and judges; and finally, is capable of striking an acceptable balance between preserving individual autonomy and providing needed medical care.[3] Thus, although a firm theoretical basis for making judgments of competency may still be lacking, efforts are underway to develop sound, practical criteria that psychiatrists can apply objectively.

If there are, as I would urge, justifiable as well as unjustifiable instances of paternalism, then it is a mistake to deplore all paternalistic interventions as unethical because they interfere with an individual's freedom. Individual liberty can only be exercised when a person is in a reasonable state of health (mental or physical) and has reached an adequate age or degree of competence. Unless we hold—as some people do—that liberty is more important than life itself, limitations on freedom are justified in the interest of preserving life, health, and even autonomy.

The general issue of paternalism and its possible justifications should, moreover, be considered in connection with who serves as the intervening agent: outside authorities, such as the state; parents or relatives; or caretakers from private or voluntary groups. Some responsibilities and authorities derive from specific roles, such as those of teacher, physician, or employer. In some cases, the right to intervene in various ways is contractually determined. In other cases, authority to act is an implicit yet integral feature of an established relationship. The need to make these distinctions becomes evident upon the realization that not all paternalistic interventions should be seen as unjustifiable simply because they involve a measure of coercion. The problem is compounded by the fact that invasive procedures and forcible means can be used to attain highly desirable ends.

Take, for example, compulsory drug treatment or electrical brain stimulation performed on those who engage in acts of self-mutilation; or behavior modification using aversive conditioning on the mentally retarded or on autistic children; or medication to subdue those suffering from what psychiatrists call "manic flight." Some patients after treatment are more self-reliant, function more independently, and enjoy a heightened sense of well-being. These qualities are, by general agreement, judged to be desirable or positive ones, and should therefore be considered objective criteria for the purpose of determining what "really is" in a person's best interest. In these situations, the subjects' *dignity* is enhanced—the quality Judge Tauro invoked in his decision; they are enabled to function more autonomously; their self-satisfaction is increased; they are helped to thrive, rather than merely to subsist. These are reasonably clear cases. But what about paternalistically justified modes of behavior control used in prisons and social control of deviants as practiced in mental institutions? Are these actions so obviously for the subjects' own benefit? They are surely practices that those in control, given their commitment to predominant social values and institutional norms, deem to be for the good of those controlled. If the subjects of control disagree about what is in their best interest, their failure to concur may be taken by those in power as evidence that they are less than fully rational and so may justifiably be coerced for their own good.

Consider now how a range of facts about the special populations on whom paternalistic regulation is practiced aid in drawing moral conclusions. The use of powerful behavior control techniques with severely retarded or disturbed persons can often result in their functioning more independently or with greater self-reliance, thus enhancing their own well-being as well as making them less dependent on others. Using the same powerful technologies on prisoners may, in contrast, reduce their autonomy, render them more passive and, perhaps, more submissive to the will of others. It is hard to arrive at a fully satisfactory, objective account of which characteristics constitute "changes for the better" as a result of psychiatric treatment. In accordance with the Kantian precept that dictates respect for the dignity of human beings, it is incumbent on theorists and practitioners of behavior control to promote the welfare of all persons, even those who are functionally incapacitated or deemed socially undesirable. In the absence of universally agreed upon criteria for determining what really is in the best interests of the subject, paternalistically justified modes of behavior control directed at rational or even incompetent persons should be employed only with great caution.

In the case of the mentally retarded, their level of competency can actually increase as a result of special education, vocational training, behavior modification, or simply undergoing life's experiences. Nevertheless, their retardation will almost surely remain an enduring trait rather than a temporary condition. So the issue of paternalistic intervention may continue to arise throughout their lives, with little likelihood of their attaining a full state of normalcy.

The situation is somewhat more complicated with the mentally ill, however, since there is greater likelihood that their condition is a temporary one. Consider, for example, a mental patient who has intermittent lapses and remissions and who begs—while lucid—not to have electric shock treatment administered. Is ECT, aimed at improving the patient's condition, justified during lapses when he or she may correctly be held incompetent or irrational? Or should the wishes of such patients be honored on the grounds that their desires were expressed at a time when they were rational agents—persons who deserve not to be treated paternalistically?

Perhaps the hardest cases are those of so-called "manic flights." These persons appear rational by virtue of their verbal coherence and occasional bursts of artistic and other creativity. What's more, people who undergo these episodes often refuse even to see a psychiatrist, much less submit to treatment. At least part of the reason is that they enjoy the hypermanic experience.

So why is intervention of any sort felt to be necessary or even desirable? A colleague of mine who is a psychiatrist described some cases to me. In some instances, those who underwent manic episodes engaged in public behavior that threatened their careers, their reputation, their family's well-being, and perhaps even their own self-respect. Sexual exhibitionism, giving away all their money and property, soliciting twelve-year-old boys, often leads such persons to suicide attempts or other self-destructive acts. In most cases, those who were victims of hypermania expressed overwhelming gratitude—once they returned to "normalcy"—to psychiatrists, family members, and others who had intervened, even over their protests. In all cases, those who exhibit such behavior act uncharacteristically. It is not simply that they act differently from other people—that they are "deviant," in the usual sense. They are deviant in the additional sense that they depart from their *own* established character. They are not their *true selves,* they lack continuity with their typical or normal or characteristic personality. Such people could be said to be wholly lacking in autonomy when in those states. If they are offered psychiatric treatment and refuse it, if they are cajoled or manipulated or even coerced into therapy of some sort, is their autonomy being violated? I think something more like the opposite is true. All evidence points to a lack of genuine autonomy in those who behave out of character in hypermanic, self-destructive ways.

I have tried to avoid as much as possible using terms like "mental illness," "emotional or psychiatric disorder," "sanity and insanity, and other concepts that have aroused so much debate in scholarly and now popular literature. This is because I think none of the issues I have raised or the arguments I have examined require that we settle those debates or even that we come down on one side or the other. Nothing whatever hangs on whether mental illness is a myth, whether personality disorders are diseases, whether there should be a legal insanity defense, and so on. I have been talking only about the concepts of competence, paternalism, and autonomy and their applications in the context of refusal of psychiatric treatment. I surely have not given an adequate analysis of those concepts here, nor have I been very thorough in describing or analyzing the examples I chose to illustrate them. Yet there remain solid moral principles—principles of humaneness, of benevolence, of concern for the interests and well-being of others who demonstrably are not competent to act in their own interests. *Autonomous* agents who act in ways that others believe are against their own interest have the right to be let alone. The truly incompetent lack full autonomy, and so that quality cannot be violated by imposing treatment. If there is a reasonable likelihood that their autonomy can be preserved or restored by medication, then forced treatment of such patients is warranted. I am, however, opposed to more invasive treatments being imposed involuntarily, such as psychosurgery or ECT, for purely *behavioral* symptoms.

There will probably always remain some degree of conceptual uncertainty surrounding the notions of freedom, competence, and autonomy. And there will surely never be agreement on which moral principles, or which values ought to prevail when they come into conflict. Yet a careful, systematic approach will yield solutions that are morally superior to those arrived at by a dogmatic adherence to a stance that either rules out paternalism in principle, or else accepts its legitimacy uncritically.

NOTES

1. John Stuart Mill, *On Liberty,* in Max Lerner (ed.), *Essential Works of John Stuart Mill* (New York: Bantam Books, 1961), pp. 263–64.

2. Loren H. Roth, Alan Meisel, and Charles W. Lidz, "Tests of Competency to Consent to Treatment," *American Journal of Psychiatry* 134:3 (March 1977).

3. *Ibid.,* p. 280.

Suggestions for Further Reading

The Rights to Choose and to Refuse Treatment

Annas, George J. "Refusing Medication in Mental Hospitals." *Hastings Center Report* 10 (February 1980):21–22.

Bazelon, J. D. L. "Implementing the Right to Treatment." *University of Chicago Law Review* 36 (1969):742ff.

Birnbaum, Morton. "Rationale for the Right." *Georgetown Law Journal* 57 (1968):752–781.

———. "The Right to Treatment." *American Bar Association Journal* 46 (1960): 499–505.

———. "The Right to Treatment: Some Concepts on Its Development." In Ayd, Frank J., Jr. *Medical, Moral and Legal Issues in Mental Health Care.* Baltimore: The Williams and Wilkins Co., 1974, pp. 97–141.

Bradley, Valerie, and Clarke, Gary, eds. *Paper Victories and Hard Realities: The Implementation of the Legal and Constitutional Rights of the Mentally Disabled.* Washington, D.C.: The Health Policy Center of Georgetown University, 1976.

Bulletin of the American Academy of Psychiatry and the Law 5 (Nov. 1, 1977):1–19. (Several articles on the right to refuse treatment.)

Burris, Donald S., ed. *The Right to Treatment.* New York: Springer Publishing Co., 1969.

Ennis, Bruce J., and Emery, Richard D. *The Rights of Mental Patients.* New York: Avon Books, 1978, Ch. VI.

Golan, Stuart, and Fremouw, William, eds. *The Right to Treatment for Mental Patients.* New York: Irvington Publishers, 1973.

Hentoff, Nat. "Justice in the Cuckoo's Nest." *Inquiry* (Published by the Cato Institute, San Francisco), January 7 and 21, 1980.

Himmelstein, Jack, and Michels, Robert. "Case Studies in Bioethics: The Right to Refuse Psychoactive Drugs." *Hastings Center Report* 6 (1973):8–11.

Johnston, Robert, and Frasier, Margaret. "Right to Treatment." *Mental Hygiene* 56 (1972):*13*-19.

Katz, Jay. "The Right to Treatment—An Enchanting Legal Fiction?" *University of Chicago Law Review* 36 (Summer 1969):755-783.

Kaufman, Edward. "The Right to Treatment Suit as an Agent of Change." *American Journal of Psychiatry* 136 (November 1979):1428-1432.

Kittrie, Nicholas N. *The Right to Be Different.* Baltimore: The Johns Hopkins Press, 1971, Ch. 9.

"Life, Liberty, and the Pursuit of Madness—The Right to Refuse Treatment." Special section in *American Journal of Psychiatry* 137 (March 1980):327-358.

Maham, Shirley, et al. "A Mechanism for Enforcing the Right to Treatment: The Human Rights Committee." *Law and Psychology Review* 1 (1975):131-149.

"Mental Health and Human Rights: Report of the Task Panel on Legal and Ethical Issues." *Arizona Law Review* 20 (1978):98-111.

Michels, Robert. "The Right to Refuse Treatment: Ethical Issues." *Hospital and Community Psychiatry* 32 (April 1981):251-255.

Perlin, Michael L., and Zusman, Jack. "The Right to Refuse Treatment." *Advocacy Now: The Journal of Patient Rights and Mental Health Advocacy* 1 (1979):8-18.

Putten, Theodore Van. "Drug Refusal in Schizophrenia: Causes and Prescribing Hints." *Hospital and Community Psychiatry* 29 (1978):111.

"Right to Refuse Medical Care." In Reich, Warren T., ed. *Encyclopedia of Bioethics* Vol. IV. New York: The Free Press, 1978, pp. 1498-1507.

Robitscher, Jonas. "Courts, State Hospitals, and the Right to Treatment." *American Journal of Psychiatry* 129 (1972):298-304.

———. "The Right to Psychiatric Treatment: A Social-Legal Approach to the Plight of the State Hospital Patient." *Villanova Law Review* 18 (November 1972):11-36.

Roth, Loren H. "A Commitment Law for Patients, Doctors, and Lawyers." *American Journal of Psychiatry* 136 (September 1979):1121-1127.

Sadoff, Robert L. "On Refusing Treatment: Rights and Remedies." *Advocacy Now: The Journal of Patient Rights and Mental Health Advocacy* 1 (1979):57-60.

Schwitzgebel, Ralph K. "Implementing a Right to Effective Treatment." *Law and Psychology Review* 1 (1975):117-130.

Shapiro, Michael H., and Spece, Roy G., Jr. *Bioethics and Law.* St. Paul, Minnesota: West Publishing Co., 1981, Part II.

Shuman, Samuel I. *Psychosurgery and the Medical Control of Violence.* Detroit: Wayne State University Press, 1977, Ch. 9.

Spece, Roy G. "Preserving the Right to Treatment." *Arizona Law Review* 20 (1978):1-47.

Steinbock, Elizabeth A., et al. "Civil Rights of the Mentally Retarded: An Overview." *Law and Psychology Review* 1 (1975):151-178.

Stone, Alan. "Overview: The Right to Treatment—Comments on the Law and Its Impact." *American Journal of Psychiatry* 132 (November 1975):1125-1134.

Stone, Alan. "The Right to Refuse Treatment." *Archives of General Psychiatry* 38 (March 1981):358–362.

Szasz, Thomas S. "The Ethics of Therapy." *National Forum* 58 (Spring 1978): 25–29.

Tancredi, Laurence R., et al. *Legal Issues in Psychiatric Care.* New York: Harper & Row, 1975.

The Right to Treatment in Mental Health Law. Raleigh, North Carolina: Committee on the Office of Attorney General, 1976.

The Rights of the Mentally Handicapped. Washington, D.C.: The Mental Health Law Project, 1973, especially Chs. I and III.

Torrey, E. Fuller. "Refusing to Take Your Medicine." *Psychology Today* 14 (September 1980):12ff. A negative view.

Veatch, Robert M. *Death, Dying, and the Biological Revolution.* New Haven, Connecticut: Yale University Press, 1976, Ch. 4 on "The Right to Refuse Treatment."

Paternalism

Beauchamp, Tom L. "Paternalism and Biobehavioral Control." *The Monist* 60 (January 1977):62–80.

Beauchamp, Tom L., and Childress, James F. *Principles of Biomedical Ethics.* New York: Oxford University Press, 1979, pp. 153–164.

Bok, Sissela. *Lying, Moral Choice in Public and Private Life.* New York: Vintage Books, 1979, Chs. 14 and 15.

Buchanan, Allen. "Medical Paternalism." *Philosophy and Public Affairs* 7 (June 1973):5–10.

Childress, James. "Liberty, Paternalism and Health Care." *Social Responsibility: Journalism, Law, Medicine* Vol. 4, Louis W. Hodges, ed. Lexington, Virginia: Washington and Lee University, 1978.

Dworkin, Gerald. "Paternalism." *The Monist* 56 (1972):64–84.

Feinberg, Joel. "Legal Paternalism." *The Canadian Journal of Philosophy* 1 (1971): 105–124.

Fotion, N. "Paternalism." *Ethics* 89 (January 1979):191–198.

Gert, Bernard, and Culver, Charles. "Paternalistic Behavior." *Philosophy and Public Affairs* 6 (Fall 1976):45–57.

———. "The Justification of Paternalism." *Ethics* 89 (January 1979):199–210.

Graber, Glenn. "On Paternalism and Health Care." In Davis, John W., et al., eds. *Contemporary Issues in Biomedical Ethics.* Clifton, New Jersey: Humanities Press, 1978.

Marsh, Frank H. "An Ethical Approach to Paternalism in the Physician-Patient Relationship." *Ethics in Science and Medicine* 4 (1977):135–138.

May, Larry. "Paternalism and Self-Interest." *Journal of Value Inquiry* 14 (Fall and Winter 1980):195–216.

Morawetz, Thomas. *The Philosophy of Law.* New York: Macmillan, 1980, Ch. 3.

Wikler, Daniel. "Paternalism and the Mildly Retarded." *Philosophy and Public Affairs* 8 (Summer 1979):377–392.

Zembaty, Jane S. "A Limited Defense of Paternalism in Medicine." *Proceedings of the 13th Conference on Value Inquiry: The Life Sciences and Human Values.* Geneseo, New York: State University of New York, 1979, pp. 145–158.

7. Controversial Behavior Control Therapies Psychosurgery, Electroshock, and Electrostimulation

Introduction

Whether we realize and admit it or not, we are all in the business of controlling behavior, either that of ourselves or of other people. What are the most morally acceptable forms of behavior control? From the point of view of any ethic that attaches a great deal of significance to rational autonomy, the most acceptable method for controlling our behavior will be the sort of *direct* self control involved in properly informed volition, will power, freewill, choice, or whatever we wish to call it. Most of us also accept certain *indirect* techniques for modifying our own behavior, those that help us to bring about desirable changes as a result of having performed some previous act. We can modify our own behavior indirectly by voluntarily using certain drugs such as coffee, tea, cola drinks, tobacco, alcohol, street drugs, and physician prescribed psychotropic drugs. Voluntary submission to techniques such as rational persuasion, psychotherapy, psychosurgery, or electroshock also may be used to influence our own behavior; but a need becomes apparent immediately for criteria to distinguish between acceptable and unacceptable forms of the many artificial techniques of indirect self-modification currently available.

What are morally acceptable forms of controlling or influencing the behavior of others? All of these techniques are in some sense indirect, and again we need criteria for distinguishing between the morally acceptable and unacceptable. Both inside and outside of mental hospitals, many indirect forms of behavior modification are used including: parental discipline, public opinion, advertising, religious training, emotionalistic revivals, economic restraints and incentives, education, moral teaching, indoctrination, governmental regulations, laws, courts, prisons, and jails. In addition, many techniques have special uses in psychotherapy, and the readings that follow in this section

347

continue our exploration of some of the more prominent of these. Though the list is not exhaustive, one or more of the following criteria may be used in distinguishing between acceptable and unacceptable forms of indirect behavior control, whether applied to ourselves or to others. A technique may be judged to be acceptable to the degree that:

1. It is used with voluntary informed consent on competent adults.
2. Its use does not infringe on basic legal and/or moral rights.
3. There is a high probability of a favorable cost/benefit ratio, using some ideal of intrinsic good and evil.
4. It enhances or at least does not diminish, a person's capacity for rational autonomy.
5. It involves no physical intrusion into a person's body.
6. It does not have irreversible bad effects. (Irreversible good effects are acceptable if we are confident that we can identify them.)
7. No less objectionable and less restrictive forms of behavior control are readily available.
8. Its monetary costs are not prohibitive.

Judged by such criteria, let us evaluate the techniques of behavior control commonly used on mental patients.

Psychosurgery, the modification or destruction of brain tissue for the purpose of altering mental functions like thinking, feeling, and willing, thus modifying the corresponding behaviors, is probably the most controversial of all the therapies used on mental patients. Peter R. Breggin documents the astonishing extent of its present and former uses, both here and abroad. Many problems of value arise in connection with its use. First, most of it was and still is being done in violation of the informed consent of patients; more often than not it is performed on women, children, the aged, the institutionalized, and other disadvantaged minorities. The notorious obscurity of the concept of "mental illness" is well illustrated by the fact that psychosurgery has been performed to correct such undesirable disorders as neurotic anxieties, hyperactivity, restlessness, warm heartedness, conscientiousness, perfectionism, thoughtfulness, homosexuality, frigidity, promiscuity, strong emotions, gambling, alcoholism, drug addiction, depression, violence, and childhood misbehavior, among others. Equally ambiguous, value-laden concepts such as "cure" or therapeutic "success" are exemplified by the fact that the primary criteria of success are passivity or manageability, along with the cessation of the aforementioned undesirable deviancies, even at the price of terminating practically all conscious functions and activities that are distinctively human. In addition, very serious quality of life problems arise when we realize that psychosurgery eliminates more than just undesirable behavior; other very desirable human functions are also destroyed. Typically, the price paid is an irreversible and severe blunting of numerous capacities including those for thought, memory, motivation, emotion, spontaneity, creativity, moral sensitivity, love, empathy, enjoyment, self-knowledge, and self-control. The resulting emptiness of consciousness is something that only a Zen Buddhist would envy! Newer psychosurgical techniques attempt to avoid some of these unwanted side effects, however.

Vernon Mark, one of the most prominent and outspoken practitioners of psychosurgery, defends this procedure against certain standard objections. He also wishes to circumscribe its use to cases involving "recognized disease," and then only as a last resort. The Breggin article makes it clear that in fact the procedure is not being used by psychosurgeons throughout the world only where all other treatments and helping professions have failed. The response to Mark by Stephan Chorover explores the diffuse nature of Mark's concept of "recognized disease" as well as his questionable criteria of success and methods for obtaining consent. Chorover proposes even stricter limits on the uses of psychosurgery.

Although William B. Scoville (in the Breggin article) and Vernon Mark suggest that the effects of electroshock are often as intrusive, devastating, and permanent as those of psychosurgery, David Avery defends this procedure for use in cases of extreme depression where all else has failed. In the final selection, Elliot S. Valenstein replies to José M. R. Delgado and others who defend the uses of electrostimulation. Valenstein insists that such fantasies of brain control are not readily available to give would be oppressors immense and precise control over the behavior of those deviants of whom society disapproves. In anticipation of the topic of drug therapy to be covered in our next section, Valenstein makes extremely pertinent remarks on the topic of brain chemistry toward the conclusion of his article.

Peter R. Breggin

The Return of Lobotomy
and Psychosurgery

Author's Note (1982)

In 1971, I discovered that a substantial group of psychosurgeons had again become active, and were planning an international resurgence of lobotomy and other forms of psychosurgery. "The Return of Lobotomy and Psycho-surgery" was written to alert the media and the general public to this potential menace. When no one could be found to publish this controversial document, I had it inserted into the Congressional Record by Congressman Gallagher. Gallagher's assistant, Charles "Chip" Witter, had encouraged the congressman to be critical of government-sponsored behavior control projects.

Following the publication of the Record, I contacted the Associated Press and was pleasantly surprised when they showed a willingness to put the story on the AP wire. That wire story kicked off what would become an inter-national campaign to prevent the resurgence of lobotomy and psychosurgery. The campaign had been largely successful. Through a combination of public pressure, law suits, and legislation, many American psychosurgeons have been forced to give up performing the operations. The "second wave of psychosurgery" which they were touting in 1972 has not developed, and today the number of operations has declined to 200–300 per year in the United States. No doubt, however, the psychosurgeons will attempt to resurrect their surgery as soon as public criticism abates. H. T. Ballentine in particular remains very vocal in support of his surgery.[6]

Originally published in the *Congressional Record* (February 24, 1972). Copyright © 1972 by Peter R. Breggin, M.D. Reprinted by the kind permission of the author.

Although the Congressional Record was not intended as a scientific document, its scientific observations have held up over the years.[1-7] My major error was in naively accepting the reports on electrical stimulation of the brain which described the capacity to control specific kinds of behavior. All forms of psychosurgery remain relatively crude and grossly destructive. The individual's behavior and mental activity can be levelled or impaired, but more specific effects cannot be achieved with any regularity.[2,6]

Since writing "The Return of Lobotomy and Psychosurgery" I have gone on to develop the brain-disabling hypothesis which states that *all* the major psychiatric interventions—the major tranquilizers, lithium, the antidepressants, electroshock, and psychosurgery—achieve their primary clinical effect by impairing brain function.[3-7] This impairment produces either euphoria (a false impression of happiness) or apathy (an enforced docility). I have given the name. *iatrogenic helplessness*[5-7] to these common effects of all the major somatic treatments in psychiatry.

The political issues surrounding psychosurgery became more clearly defined as the campaign against psychosurgery grew. I discovered, among other things, that the National Institute of Mental Health and the Justice Department were sponsoring a joint project involving psychosurgery for the control of violence.[2] Neurosurgeon Vernon Mark, psychiatrist Frank Ervin, and their associate, neurosurgeon William Street, had been advocating psychosurgery for the control of the black urban uprisings which were threatening America in the late 1960s and early 1970s. With the documentation of these seemingly unbelievable disclosures, the anti-psychosurgery movement gained considerable momentum. The federal project was terminated, and Mark, Ervin, and Sweet felt compelled to modify their original statements about the potential efficacy of psychosurgery in the political arena.[2]

I have changed some of my own political views with further experience. My efforts led directly to the formation of a National Commission on Psychosurgery; but I learned the bitter lesson that government sponsored commissions support the establishment, not the critics of the establishment. This practical consideration has discouraged me from pushing for federal regulation of various activities, including psychiatric "treatments." More important, I have come to the conclusion that no one, *including me,* has the right to impose his views about therapy upon other consenting adults.[3,7] I have therefore changed the position which I advocate in this paper, and now believe that no form of treatment should be banned by legislation. Voluntary patients should be allowed to choose any therapy they wish for themselves, even if it is brain-damaging. However, patients have the right to be fully informed about the controversial nature of the treatments and about their damaging effects. If they have not given informed consent for the treatment, they should be encouraged to sue for damages. I continue to favor outlawing brain-disabling treatments for children, involuntary mental patients, prisoners, and persons adjudicated incompetent.[3]

Following the publication of "The Return of Lobotomy and Psychosurgery," the Center for the Study of Psychiatry was formed to educate the public concerning the threat of psychiatric technology to political freedom and individual well-being. The Center eventually distributed 10,000 copies of the Congressional Record article, and tens of thousands of additional copies were reprinted and distributed around the world by patient rights organizations. It became an underground bestseller in the movement to curtail psychiatric oppression. Nowadays my views no longer seem so radical, and my more scientifically oriented critiques of psychiatric technology are even finding their way into the professional literature. It's hard to believe that it was ten years ago when I turned to the Congressional Record as a "last resort" for the publication of "The Return of Lobotomy and Psychosurgery." I want to thank Prometheus Books and Rem B. Edwards for at last making it available in book form to the reading public.

(By Hon. Cornelius E. Gallagher, of New Jersey, in the House of Representatives)

Mr. GALLAGHER. Mr. Speaker, I rise today to insert into the Congressional Record one of the most shocking documents I have ever seen. "The Return of Lobotomy and Psychosurgery," by Dr. Peter R. Breggin has not been previously published and represents the first critical review of the current resurgence of this mutilating operation on a wide scale. Dr. Breggin covers the world scene in the first section, concentrates on its use in the United States in the next two sections and concludes with a sensible program for prompt action. His bibliography is extensive and indicates the depth of his research.

Psychosurgery is now being used to control so-called "hyperactive" children and it is even used on children as young as 5 years old. Dr. Breggin describes the frightening use of this surgery on individuals who suffer from "anxiety" and "tension" and other forms of behavior which might be classified as neuroses, and he documents an increasing tendency to select women, older people and now children as targets. He cites dozens of on-going projects.

While there was a strong negative response to the original wave of psychosurgery which claimed up to 50,000 victims in the United States alone, this human revulsion was not widely expressed in the medical literature. I have been informed that the decline of lobotomy in America during the late 1950's was because of the increasing use of electroshock and drugs, not because of any public or professional outcry. This current wave of lobotomy and psychosurgery of all forms should be met with a prompt public interest and, in no case, should it be allowed to spread without informed scrutiny. Dr. Breggin performs a distinct public service by bringing forward an immense amount of information which has hitherto been buried in somewhat arcane journals.

*   *   *

Mr. Speaker, I have used the words "shocking and "frightening" to describe what Dr. Breggin has disclosed. I am especially upset to discover that irreversible brain mutilation is being used on hyperactive children. When my privacy inquiry held a hearing on the use of behavior modification drugs on grammar schoolchildren in September 1970, we learned that there was nothing wrong with these children in the medical sense. It was behavior and behavior alone that created the diagnosis of minimal brain dysfunction and perhaps the only proper definition of that term was presented by Dr. Francis Crinella: "one of our most fashionable forms of consensual ignorance." At least 250,000 children, in all parts of the country, are now receiving drugs to mask the effects of MBD, but the drug therapy can be stopped. Nothing can undo brain mutilation, according to Dr. Breggin, and I am convinced that public debate must take place over the use of such irrevocable destruction of the creative personality.

Mr. Speaker, "shocking" and "frightening" are too mild to describe my reaction to this material. The following article, "The Return of Lobotomy and Psychosurgery," is copyrighted by Dr. Peter R. Breggin in 1972 and I think many Americans will be grateful to Dr. Breggin for allowing its publication in the RECORD. As a man who has been concerned about the erosion of human values for some 7 years and who has taken effective steps in the past to guarantee our citizens the right to pursue happiness in their own way, let me say that I am personally grateful to Dr. Breggin for his courage, scholarship, and humanity. I am proud to insert his copyrighted article in the RECORD at this point:

Introduction

The purpose of this report is to alert the American public to the details of a current resurgence of lobotomy and psychosurgery in America and around the world.

In lobotomy and psychosurgery parts of the brain that show no demonstrable disease are nonetheless mutilated or cut out in order to affect the individual's emotions and personal conduct. In each of the studies presented here, the expressed purpose will be the control of some form of behavior—most often aggressive behavior—or the blunting of an emotion, usually "tension" or "anxiety."

The surgical methods vary widely both here and around the world, including the old-fashioned "modified" pre-frontal lobotomy, essentially a mutilating operation in which the surgeon cuts a narrow slice through the midline base of the frontal lobes, partially incapacitating the highest and most refined functions of the human brain and the human being. These frontal lobes, the highest evolutionary organ in the human being, are also being attacked with ultrasound, electrical coagulations and implanted radium seeds.

Newer operations also attack the amygdala of the temporal lobe of the brain, the cingulum which lies beneath the frontal lobes between the hemispheres, the thalamus, hypothalamus and related structures. As you will see in this survey, the great body of evidence supports the notion that all these operations accomplish the same thing—a "blunting" effect upon the human's emotional responsiveness. They are partial lobotomies.

The first wave of lobotomy and psychosurgery, which claimed 50,000 persons in the United States alone, was primarily aimed at state hospital patients with chronic disabilities. The current wave is aimed at an entirely different group—individuals who are relatively well-functioning, the large majority of them with the diagnosis of "neurosis," many of them individuals who are still living at home and performing on the job.

Women constitute the majority of the patients, with old people and children as other large groups. In Japan, Thailand, and India, children have been large target populations for some time; but now in America, for the first time in many years, numbers of children are again being submitted to psychosurgery, particularly at the University of Mississippi, where O. J. Andy is operating on "hyperactive"children as young as age five.

The current rate of psychosurgery in the United States is difficult to ascertain, but you will be able to make your own estimates from the mass of material presented here, including about 1,000 cases since 1965 which have come to my personal attention during my informal survey and review of the literature. Three American psychosurgeons have accounted for more than 500 among themselves in recent years, and I have counted at least 40 individuals currently involved in psychosurgical projects. In addition, several psychosurgeons who will be quoted have estimated a current rate of 400–600 cases per year, and most important, every psychosurgeon agrees that we are just beginning to witness a massive increase in psychosurgery to rival the wave of 50,000 two decades ago.

There are a number of signals indicating the start of a major resurgence. A new International Association for Psychosurgery has been formed with an American, William Scoville, as its head. Many promotional statements are again appearing in print in widely circulated magazines such as *Newsweek, Medical World News* and *Psychiatric News*. Current textbooks in psychiatry and current year books of treatment will be found reviving psychosurgery, and major publications such as the *Journal of the American Medical Association* and the *American Journal of Psychiatry* have been offering pro-lobotomy articles based upon inadequate scientific studies.

Current scientific studies will be found as wanting as those which originally led the prestigious Group for the Advance of Psychiatry to condemn the entire body of lobotomy literature as promotional and marred by exaggerations of success and denials of grossly mutilating effects upon the personality. Those few follow-up studies with matched controls (56, 73, 93) will describe a disastrous first wave which leaves little optimism for the future.

The material will be prescribed in three parts:

I. Current Psychosurgery Around the World. II. Current Psychosurgery in the United States, and III. Newest Advances in Mind Control. It is useful to start with the material around the world because it more clearly documents the menace of psychosurgery.

The bibliography is by far the most extensive published on psychosurgery since 1965. The great majority of articles describe current psychosurgery, while a few are retrospective evaluations, and most refer to the United States (1, 2, 10, 18, 22, 23, 26, 28, 29, 30, 37, 38, 39, 40, 42, 43, 44, 50, 51, 54, 58, 61, 65, 66, 71, 72, 77, 78, 79, 81, 85, 86, 87, 95, 96, 98), England (3, 12, 20, 21, 24, 42, 46, 47, 48, 53, 55, 57, 58, 70, 76, 78, 79, 82, 83, 84, 88, 89, 90), and Canada (4, 5, 7, 18, 52, 56, 59, 60, 88, 89, 90, 91, 99).

Finally, I am grateful to Congressman Cornelius Gallagher for the opportunity to present the body of my research to the general public.

I. Current Psychosurgery Around the World

Psychosurgery is currently being done in Canada, Australia, France, Spain, Italy, West Germany, Norway, Sweden, Denmark, Finland, Switzerland, Thailand, India, and the world's leaders, Japan, England and the United States, nearly all of whom were represented among the one hundred psychosurgeons gathered in Denmark for the Second International Conference on Psychosurgery in the summer of 1970 (79–80). Russia outlawed lobotomy and psychosurgery in 1951, and Khachaturian published a lengthy polemic explaining why.

My survey is based upon material which was presented at the International Conference, published in the literature or sent to me by the psychosurgeons with whom I have been in contact here in the United States. It is bound to be selective, since only the better work tends to get published or reported, while the less satisfactory work is discarded or kept out of sight. This will be particularly true in regard to a procedure like psychosurgery that has received considerable negative publicity.

Similarly, the published work and reported cases in any field of medicine are likely to reflect only a small portion of what is going on, and in the field of psychosurgery, the effects of the current promotion may not show up for some time.

Now for a review of psychosurgery around the world.

Some of the most candid reports come from Madras, India, one of the leading medical centers in that part of the world, where several high ranking medical and psychiatric authorities are deeply involved in the psychosurgery of children. The chief investigator is Dr. Balasubramaniam, Honorary Neurosurgeon, Government General Hospital and Government Mental Hospital, Madras. He is well-known among western psychosurgeons, delivered a paper at the Second International and publishes in English language journals.

He headlines his basic theoretical paper "Sedative Neurosurgery" and then opens with one of the most forthright and simplistic descriptions in the psychosurgery literature: "Sedative neurosurgery is the term applied to that aspect of neurosurgery where a patient is made quiet and manageable by an operation." P. 377.

Classical prefrontal lobotomy, the operation done on so many tens of thousands, is one variant of sedative surgery, he says. His own up-to-date amygdalotomy and more occasional hypothalotomy are newer variants. His work heavily involves children who are hospitalized, and he tells us: "The patient who requires this operation may manifest with one of the various behavioral disorders listed below. The commonest is restlessness." B. 377.

You will see that this is not a practice limited to India, and that both Japan and the United States are doing psychosurgery on hyperactive children.

Writing in July, 1970 in the American Journal, *International Surgery*, Balasubramaniam summarizes his results with 115 patients, three of them *under age five* and another 36 *under age eleven*. Using diathermy or injections of foreign matter, such as olive oil, to destroy areas of these childrens' brains, he produces this result: "The improvement that occurs has been remarkable. In one case a patient had been assaulting his colleagues and the ward doctors; after the operation he became a helpful addition to the ward staff and looked after other patients. In one case the patient became quiet, bashful and was a model of good behavior." P. 21.

Balasubramaniam sums up in his concluding sentence: "This operation has proved to be useful in the management of patients who previously could not be managed by any other means." P. 22.

If this turns out to be true, as I believe it will, then amygdalotomy surgery will be the ultimate "therapeutic weapon" for any state hospital superintendent or prison warden.

A bizarre report comes out of Thailand, where Chitanondh is also performing amygdalotomies on brain damaged patients, psychotics, neurotics, epileptics and behavior problems under the psychiatrically absurd rubric of "olefactory seizures and psychiatric disorders with olefactory hallucinations." In other words, if he finds a case where the sense of smell is involved in any fashion, then he chops out the amygdala on the grounds that it is involved in smell perception and elaboration. This is the same amygdala that Balasubramaniam mutilates on the grounds that it is involved in aggression. Again and again we will find this phenomenon—that the psychosurgeon picks out the symptom that he wants to focus upon, then destroys the brain's overall capacity to respond emotionally, in order to "cure" the symptom which he focused upon, completely neglecting that he has simply subdued the entire human being.

One of Chitanondh's patients is a nine-year-old boy whom he thinks has an olefactory hallucination but who is obviously involved in a behavioral struggle with his parents. This patient has a "habit" of running away from home, allegedly to smell engine oil in cars!

"Chief complaint of an obsessive smelling habit. For two years before admission he had a strong compulsion to smell engine oil. . . . He would not give any reason why he had to do this. The parents punished the patient but he would not give up the peculiar habit." P. 192.

Despite the boy's denial that he was hallucinating, the neurosurgeon performs this "sedative neurosurgery" and of course the boy no longer runs away to smell engine oil.

In a rare show of public disagreement, the discussants quoted after this report seem piqued at their colleague's assault upon this child. One, a neurosurgeon, says: "If the neurosurgeons move psychosurgery from the frontal lobe to the temporal lobe (amygdala), we need to know some elementary psychiatry." P. 196.

Does this mean, as it seems, that it is not necessary to know elementary psychiatry if the neurosurgeon sticks to the frontal lobes — literally the heartland of man's highest and most subtle functions?

Another discussant of Chitanondh's work, a Japanese, warns that he, unlike the Thal, only operates on the mentally retarded! In a sentence he thus condemns his own methods as too gross or too inhumane for children of normal intelligence, while at the same time condemning the mentally retarded to sub-human status.

The Japanese have been doing both frontal lobotomies and the newer amygdalotomies (temporal lobotomies) steadily without going underground during the late 1950's and the 1960's. They publish their work in English language journals and influence the International and American movement.

Narabayashi and Uno of Tokyo report in 1966 on a follow-up of 27 children ages *five to thirteen* who have had amygdalotomies. They operate on: ". . . children characterized by unsteadiness, hyperactive behavior disorders and poor concentration, rather than violent behavior; it was difficult to keep them interested in one object or a certain situation." P. 168.

Here is a description of the *best* results as achieved in five of their many cases: "(They) have reached the degree of satisfactory obedience and of constant, steady mood, which enabled the children to stay in their social environment, such as kindergarten or school for the feebleminded." P. 167.

Sano, also in Tokyo, reports on 22 cases beginning with the youngest *age four*. His *best* results? "Emotional and personality changes: the patient became markedly calm, passive and tractable, showing decreased spontaneity." P. 167.

Remember these descriptions when we examine related surgery being performed on depressed people, obsessive neurotics and a raft of others in the United States. Again and again we will find a kind of "tunnel vision" that allows a psychosurgeon to obliterate the liveliness and spontaneity of the individual while acting as if he is merely attacking a symptom or specific "illness" such as depression or obsessive neurosis.

Professor Sano is not an incompetent whose hypothalotomy operations cannot be trusted for technical expertise. He is an Honorary President of the International Association for Psychosurgery. Sano will be joining several American psychosurgeons (W. H. Sweet, Frank Ervin, Vernon Mark and others) at a large upcoming conference on violence and its treatment at the Texas University Medical School on March 9–11 in Houston (98).

The Japanese have not given up the more traditional frontal lobotomy. From the recent Second International Conference, Kalinowsky comments

"An impressive clinical report of 519 patients was given by the Japanese neuropsychiatrist S. Hirose, who prefers the orbitoventromedial undercutting procedure." This is a more limited, modified frontal lobotomy, involving cuts where they will do the most, in the brain pathways which lie toward the midline underside of the frontal lobes.

I have a summary of Hirose's talk given at the Second International in the summer of 1970 in which he describes 119 cases that he has done since 1957. He says that he operates on neurotics and psychotics, individuals with "protracted emotional tension states, over-sensitivity, excessive self-consciousness, and obsessive states."

Much as he did in his 1965 *American Journal of Psychiatry* report, he continues to recommend mutilating the brains of people who are: "delicate, warm-hearted, conscientious, enthusiastic, perfectionistic . . ."

This is important — that even the old-fashioned lobotomists are now advocating their gross forms of intervention for more normally functioning human beings. "A kind of plastic surgery of mental states," Hirose calls it in 1965.

Moving away from the Far East, we find that the West Germans are very active.

Hassler and Dieckmann have been operating on the thalamus of children — 13 cases reported in this article — in order to reduce "aggressiveness, destructiveness and agitation."

They also believe they can "treat" specific psychiatric illnesses when they attack and destroy sections of the brain. Their psychiatric rationalizations are extremely crude; "Obsessive-compulsive neuroses are comprised as well of the perpetual repetition of non-sensical ideas as also of the psychomotor phenomenon of compulsion . . . (*sic*) Thus the irrational activation of thought may result from functional disturbance of the intralaminar nuclei."

The notion that specific neurotic disorders might be traceable to a disturbance in a nucleus within the brain is so crude that even the Russian, Khachasturian, with his own lack of sophistication, was able to dismiss it two decades ago.

The gross destructiveness of this kind of surgery, despite all apologies to the contrary in the literature, is again indicated by Hassler and Dieckmann's report that it can produce severe amnesia which lasts up to six weeks after surgery. In their minds, this is not an untoward side-effect, but an important aspect of the treatment which *helps* the therapeutic result.

This is in fact a common theme — increased damage leads to increased result — in the early lobotomy literature of Freeman and Watts (1950). Freeman (1959) suggests that it is good to damage the intellectual capacity of the neurotic because the neurotic thinks too much (p. 1526); and similarly the West Germans boast of: "alleviation of impulsion and over-subtle reasoning in all cases."

One of their patients became dangerous and attacked two nurses after surgery.

Still in West Germany, F. D. Roeder experimented with lesions in the hypothalamic region in an effort to cure "sexual deviation." The written report is only 25 lines long but the pathology slide takes up half a page, in typical psychosurgical reverence for technology. This is what he accomplished: "Potency was weakened, but preserved. . . . The aberrant sexuality of this patient was considerably suppressed, without serious side-effects. One important feature was the patient's incapacity of indulging in erotic fancies and stimulating visions . . ."

He boasts in addition that there was a disappearance of homosexual impulses and that psychiatric commitment could therefore be avoided. Psychiatric commitment avoided by obliterating a man's fantasy life.

Now for the English-speaking world.

In Sidney, Australia, a group including Harry Bailey and John Dowling has published a report of 50 cases of cingulotomy with mention of 50 more on the way. The patients include a wide variety of people with depressions, including psychotics and obsessive-compulsive neurotics, and the cases were purposely selected to limit them to individuals with "basically sound personality structure" rather than to hopelessly deteriorated individuals.

The Australians report "excellent" results in the form of a statistical outline of psychological test results and impressions of post-surgical adjustment, including comments on the return of professional people to a successful professional life. But there is only one very short clinical description, and we must take their statistics on faith.

Nor can we trust their assertion that many return to professional work, since Freeman (1959) and Sargant and Slater (1964) have already disclosed that modified lobotomies return individuals to professional work but that they function with less sensitivity toward others and even with ruthlessness.

This Austrian study also displays the typical lobotomist preference for women: 64% according to a small print footnote to a chart. These psychosurgeons lament public resistance to their work which apparently limits their access to patients. For some unexplained reason, they label this public resistance "the Ben Casey effect."

Nearer to home in the English speaking world, the Canadians are becoming active again. In recent years the old-fashioned modified prefrontal lobotomy has been used on a variety of non-schizophrenic patients by R. F. Hetherington, P. Haden and W. Craig, Departments of Surgery, Psychiatry and Psychology, Kingston Psychiatric Hospital and Queens University, Kingston, Ontario. Their report to the Second International Conference in 1970 admits that the hospital refused to allow them to operate on males because of the unfavorable publicity given to lobotomies in Canada after the negative follow-up studies of McKenzie and Kaczanowski. But they were allowed to operate on women, 17 in number.

Still in Canada, we find Earle Baker, Assistant Professor of Psychiatry, University of Toronto, reporting in 1970 on "A New Look at the Bimedial Prefrontal Leucotomy." (Leucotomy, or "cutting of the white matter," is used as a synonym for lobotomy.) He describes 44 cases with "hard core functional psychiatric illness," including *six with personality disorders* and *twenty-five with neuroses,* who have been lobotomized between 1958 and 1968!

The article is fairly typical of the older literature with the exception of its more modern claim that lobotomy offers something for everyone: ". . . Safe and effective method of reducing the symptoms of excessive tension, anxiety, fear, or depression in patients with a wide variety of illnesses, including anxiety neurosis, phobic psychoneurosis, obsessional neurosis, neurotic or psychotic depressive reactions and schizophrenia. This operation should be considered in such neurotic, personality and psychotic illnesses when medical treatment has failed." P. 37.

Baker openly acknowledges that the operation produces an organic brain syndrome—a sign of generalized damage to the entire brain. In this instance, it is characterized by "some disorientation, apathy, silliness and denial," lasting up to two or three weeks and sometimes longer. In addition, as in the old days, there are "occasional changes in moral code, anger, sexuality, or interpersonal relations," which the authors admit are permanent.

Women are their main targets, too, 27 females and 17 males, age 20–58, and as we continually see, the women "do better," 12 of 25 women accounted for declared to have an "excellent" result, while *only* 4 of the 17 men accounted for have an "excellent" result. That's 48% against 23%, but the investigators involved do not even mention this enormous discrepancy. It must be taken out of a chart!

Baker and his associates give us some fascinating vignettes to support their contemporary use of the frontal lobotomy. Case #1 is a suburban housewife who is promiscuous, runs away from home and becomes suicidal on occasion. After her lobotomy she is no longer promiscuous and becomes a faithful partner in her marriage.

These modern lobotomists describe considerable changes in the lives of their patients and make facile moral judgments about these changes. One man sold the family business that he never wanted; one middle aged man went out dating for the first time in his life; two couples came to blows for the first time; and three marriages broke up—all of which the authors put their approval upon as signs that the operations made the patients "more open" and "less dependent."

One of their patients became so liberated that he went on to rob a bank. The judge gave him an extra heavy sentence, presumably to compensate for the moral obtuseness produced by the surgery.

Moore wrote a response to the *Canadian Medical Association Journal* stating that the judge was wrong in giving the longer sentence because the patient's moral code would be unaltered by an "indefinite jail sentence," as a result of his surgery.

Unlike the Far Eastern and some European psychosurgeons, the English by-and-large have retained an *unabated* preference for mutilating the frontal lobes.

The English total is now reaching or surpassing the 20,000 mark. Tooth and Newton took a national census of England and Wales and came up with an official count of 10,827 as of 1954—but even this figure excluded the several hundred done in general hospitals, as well as the unknown hundreds done before 1942.

Extrapolating from Pippard's official count of 400 plus in the year 1961, Sargant and Slater estimate a total of 15,000 by 1962. If that rate remained constant, we would now be reaching a grand total of 18–19,000 in 1972. But the rate seems to be accelerating! The British surgeon, Geoffrey Knight, for example, presented statistics on 1,050 cases of his own at the 1970 Second International, and much of his work originates after 1960.

I can only give a small sampling of the English literature, for England appears to have led the world since the relative decline of the lobotomy in America.

Knight and his associates seem to be the most busy, at least in the published literature. I add this qualification because Walter Freeman told me of one British surgeon who had done 4,000 without any follow-up studies, published or unpublished! But to return to Knight, his original method is described as a bimedial lobotomy with orbital area undercutting of the frontal lobes, really the old-fashioned modified frontal lobotomy which so many psychiatrists think has been long dead. It is an extensive mutilation of the brain, involving a narrow longitudinal 2 cm. wide by 6 cm. deep cut at the midline of the frontal lobes at about the level of the eyes, or orbits. His first series included 550 patients, many of them with depressions.

It is impossible to judge the effects of his surgery, since he is a statistical lobotomist who offers practically no data about the people involved. Even a surgeon reporting on a new technique for removing an appendix is likely to tell us something about the general condition of his patients as well as the exact kind of appendix he is talking about, purulent, ruptured or whatever. But in taking out pieces of the brain, Knight tells us nothing or next to nothing about the nature of the individuals involved either before or after surgery. It is no surprise then that Kalinowsky, in a phone conversation with me, said that some psychosurgeons read Knight's own data completely differently than he does, in this instance favoring the results of his older methods to his new radiation implants.

Knight's new radioactive technique, again applied to hundreds of patients, is simply a more sophisticated method for destroying frontal lobe tissue. He plants radioactive seeds in the areas he might otherwise attack surgically (57, 58, 83). But the actual effects upon the personalities of his patients cannot even be guessed at—except on the basis of our general knowledge about the effects of lobotomy. All we can find in Knight's many journal articles are meaningless lists of one or two word diagnoses paired statistically with equally meaningless categories of improvement.

Knight tells us in a 1966 report that he was inspired to action after reading about the increased admission rate of old people to the state hospitals. What is his solution? Rehabilitation centers? Better housing and more social opportunities for the old? No. His answer is increased lobotomizing of older people, and he has done exactly that.

An article by Sykes and Tredgold follows up another series of 350 patients, some of them apparently done by Knight. Again we have empty statistics, and the general impression that the lobotomy never had a bad side-effect on anyone, or hardly anyone. But one statistic tells us a great deal about the mentality of the lobotomist—only 59 of these 350 patients had a serious trial of psychotherapy before being subjected to surgery.

What is Knight's theoretical justification? It is the same old "reduction of intensity of emotional reaction," Knight tells us in 1969. His elaboration of the theory behind this is crude and simplistic beyond belief: "Since primitive emotions are damaging emotions, it might be deduced empirically that the interruption of connections from primitive cortical areas would contribute to the results obtained." P. 257.

This theory amounts to nothing more than a *bias*—that strong emotions are bad. He calls these emotions "primitive," when in fact they may be the highest expression of our human development. Indeed, the frontal lobes are integral to all of man's most sensitive, subtle and human qualities—love, empathy, creativity, abstract thinking and such (25, 26, 34, 92). Severing the connections between these lobes and the lower brain does not bleach the lobes of their primitive influences, but in fact ruins the function of these lobes. The lower portions of the brain are no more "primitive" in function than the heart and lungs which phylogenetically pre-date much of the brain's development.

Knight supports the theoretical basis for his operation, entirely from animal experiments—as if the whole body of lobotomy literature did not exist. But what he says is what the lobotomists have been saying all along anyway. Animal psychosurgery succeeds in producing "quiescence and tameness."

Post and his colleagues are again representative of the statistical lobotomist, reporting on 52 patients in middle and later life who are allegedly helped (40% of them) by the old-fashioned bimedial frontal lobotomy.

Marks and his colleagues somehow came up with twenty-two cases of "agoraphobia"—fear of open spaces—and lobotomized them, again with the bimedial frontal lobotomy. They present no case material, so we can't judge what they mean by "agoraphobia" or why they would destroy a person's brain to cure such a symptom. In fact, agoraphobia as an isolated symptom is so rare that one must distrust their clinical judgment in its entirety. People crippled by such a symptom almost invariably demonstrate a complex of psychiatric symptoms, as do almost all individuals who are psychologically crippled.

The absurd becomes obscene in an unsigned editorial comment in 1969 in the *British Medical Journal* calling for brain surgery for sexual disorders (5). The editorial comment praises German investigators for destroying a portion of the brain (hypothalamus) of three male homosexuals, resulting in "a distinct and sustained reduction in the level of sexual drive," and all other drives of course, though they are unmentioned.

This editorial considers the "need to protect the public," but also suggests that voluntary consent should be obtained. But voluntary consent is a myth when the individual involved is a social deviant subject to the alternative of prison or involuntary mental hospitalization (13).

But why call this editorial obscene? Because the writer brings up the alternative of castration for homosexuals and argues that castration is "open to question on ethical grounds," while lobotomy is not. This Englishman would rather lose his brains than his testicles.

The *Manchester Guardian,* April 2, 1968, reports that a gambler who has stolen money has been sent from court into psychiatric custody for "voluntary" brain surgery to cure his gambling. The psychiatrist involved was Harry Fleming, senior consulting psychiatrist, Winwick Hospital.

Dr. Fleming did not go uncontested. Another psychiatrist, F. R. C. Casson wrote into the medical journal, *Lancet,* to complain: "I have not previously heard of leucotomy being suggested as a remedy for compulsive gambling. By its reduction of moral inhibitory factors, one would imagine that it might facilitate irresponsible gambling behavior." P. 815.

II. Current Psychosurgery in the United States

Petter Lindstrom, who has many hospital appointments around the country, including the Children's Hospital and Adult Medical Center in San Francisco, estimates that 400–600 psychosurgical operations are performed each year in the United States, and he personally accounts for 250 in the past five years in a recent letter to me. H. T. Ballantine, a psychosurgeon at the esteemed Massachusetts General Hospital, writes to me that he agrees with this estimate and that he has done 160 since 1965. Both Jack Lighthill and M. Hunter Brown in Santa Monica, California, also agree with the estimate and personally account for 110 cases in the past five years.

All the psychosurgeons who have written to me agree that the current rate is going up rapidly and that we are, in the words of one of them, approaching a "second wave" of psychosurgery.

No one knows for sure how many persons were mutilated in the "first wave". Walter Freeman, America's dean of lobotomy, has given me a personal and probably reliable estimate of 50,000. Most chronic mental hospitals — and there are hundreds in the country — have a caseload of old lobotomy patients. The past literature contains hundreds of articles, and many lobotomists and hospitals accounted for several thousand at a time. Freeman, for example, says that he did about 4,000.

Freeman, formerly Professor of Neurology, the George Washington University School of Medicine in Washington, D.C., has come out of retirement with invitations to speak at national and international conferences, including his appointment as an Honorary President of the new International Association for Psychosurgery. In a very recent (late 1971) article in the *British Journal of Psychiatry* he advocates operating upon schizophrenic patients early in their illness rather than as a last resort. This will open the way for another phase of massive institutional lobotomization of young people.

Speaking at the Washington, D.C. academy of Neurosurgery in 1965, Freeman accurately describes the effects of his surgery when he points out that lobotomy leads to some of the same results as the last stages of deteriorating schizophrenia. When such a patient is so demoralized and deteriorated by institutional life that he no longer gives the ward any trouble, then there's no purpose to giving him surgery. Says Freeman: ". . . a deteriorated schizphrenic looks and acts the same with or without his frontal lobes. When the progress notes of such a patient read, "Gives no trouble on the ward," it is generally too late to expect any substantial result from operation." P. 157.

Lothar Kalinowsky, Professor of Psychiatry, New York Medical College in New York City, has written numerous books on somatic therapy, and more recently has spent considerable time on promotional for psychosurgery, including the *Psychiatrist News* article, plus a published panel, and at least one unpublished panel on the West Coast.

In the published panel discussion Chairman Kalinowsky is again touting lobotomies for "intractable and disabling neuroses, chronic depression unresponsive to other treatments." Panel member Henry Brill, a very well known state hospital psychiatrist from Pilgrim State, Long Island, where several thousand lobotomies were once done, spoke with indignation when he defended this treatment as prematurely discarded and "cast aside too cavalierly." Brill also let on that "informal communications with American psychiatrists indicate that the operation has not been abandoned as completely as one might imagine from a casual reading of the literature."

Fritz Freyhand of St. Vincent's Hospital, James Cattell of the department of psychiatry at Columbia P and S, and Joseph Ransohoff, from Bellevue, in New York City, participated in the panel. Dr. Ransohoff mentioned that he'd done 35 lobotomies in the past five years.

Kalinowsky himself refused to give me an estimate on the phone or by mail concerning the number of lobotomy referrals he had done in the past few years. Only a few, he kept protesting, but with further questioning he admitted to having seen three patients in the last week (May 3, 1971) as possible candidates for lobotomy, one or two of whom he said would probably end up under the surgeon's knife.

E. A. Spiegel, Professor Emeritus at Philadelphia's Temple University, has been active as President of the International Society for Research in Stereoencephalotomy and as editor for the annual review called *Progress in Neurology and Psychiatry*. For the first time in many years, in 1970 he allowed psychosurgery to appear in his review book in the form of a three page survey.

Spiegel and his Philadelphia colleague, Henry T. Wyeis, are pioneers in stereotaxic brain surgery, but they have done only a few psychosurgery or psychiatric cases in recent years. Wyeis reporting at the Second International on four "compulsive neuroses" operated on during the previous four years (79).

Spiegel's *Progress in Neurology and Psychiatry* is not the only annual review to resurrect psychosurgery in America. *The Yearbook of Psychiatry and Applied Mental Health,* edited by Wortis, abstracts an article I will review in this section. The American psychiatrist, Francis J. Braceland adds an editorial comment: "It is interesting that psychosurgery is once more being considered. . . . The followup study is encouraging. . . . Nevertheless, these procedures should be used only as a last resort, and after all other methods have failed."

Another major promotional figure in American psychosurgery, William B. Scoville of Hartford Hospital and Yale University, is President of the new International Society for Psychosurgery. In *Medical World News* he reports doing about two a month, (57) and in a letter to me he notes the demand is going up now. This Associate Clinical Professor of Neurology at Yale uses orbital undercutting, a frontal lobotomy not unlike that used by the dean himself, Walter Freeman, so many years ago.

Writing in 1969, Scoville recommends lobotomy for depressions and for anxiety states, especially in the aged, much as Knight recommends. He also lists some cases of conversion neurosis, severe obsessive-compulsive neurosis, and certain forms of schizophrenia, even though he says the delusions may get worse. And going contrary to many other lobotomists, he suggests it for some drug addicts.

Most important is his recommendation for depression, since depression is one of the most common problems in any psychiatric practice, especially in the elderly for whom he strongly favors lobotomy. His comments are particularly dangerous because he favors lobotomy over repeated courses of electroshock, stating: "More than one or two courses of shock treatment probably causes more diffuse brain damage than the newer fractional lobotomies." P. 153.

He repeats this allegation about electroshock in his promotion of lobotomy in *Medical World News* in January 1971. It is important because electroshock is used so very widely, tens of thousands of patients every year, so that any trend to replace it with surgery would vastly increase the lobotomy population, a trend already apparent in England.

Still in his 1969 article, Scoville argues that all forms of psychosurgery accomplish the same basic mutilation, partial destruction of the "limbic system" or emotional regulating connections between the midbrain and frontal lobes, with a resultant disruption of the emotional component of the mind.

As he succinctly puts it: "All prefrontal surgery probably benefits by a blunting function." P. 456.

Consistent with this, he says: "It is apparent to this writer that different types of mental disease do not require different areas of ablation or tract interruptions. There appears no need to vary location of operation in the neuroses, cyclical depressions and schizophrenia." P. 456.

He adds that the lower down the cut, the more specific the suppression of emotion, while the higher the cut, the more intellectual impairment.

I agree with Scoville that the mind functions as a whole and is disrupted as a whole, and that the basic goal and the basic consequence of psychosurgery are always one in the same—to blunt, tame, quiet, sedate, or otherwise submerge or partially destroy the individual's unique emotional responsiveness.

In *Medical World News,* Scoville is said to have performed over a thousand lobotomies.

J. M. C. Holden, Associate Professor of Psychiatry and Physician Superintendent of the St. Louis State Hospital Complex, offers one of the most extensive and candid reviews of frontal lobotomy in late 1970 in *The American Journal of Psychiatry,* reporting on over 400 cases done some time ago in the St. Louis area. I wrote and asked about the numbers currently being done, and his colleague, L. Hofstatter, replied that the state hospitals no longer do them and that those being done are carried out in private practice.

Holden is very candid about the kind of damage done by the original lobotomy operations. "The frequent effect of such overoperation was irreversible change in mood, emotion, temperament, and all higher mental functions. The more extensive the section, the greater likelihood that such symptoms would develop. Postoperative mortality and morbidity, incidence and duration of confusion, urinary incontinence, unequal pupils, facial assymetry, convulsions, and other neurological sequelae were greater when the section had been more extensive. Excessive weight gain and temporary or permanent changes in performance on the rational learning test and conventional intelligence and personality tests after operation were also reported. . . . Some patients showed frank clinical deterioration that persisted after operation." P. 595.

He adds that not only did this prefrontal lobotomy destroy areas of the frontal lobe, but that the degeneration reached down into the thalamus.

Holden candidly describes the operation that mutilated tens of thousands in the English-speaking world alone, and then goes on to *praise it* as a necessary phase, a stepping stone, toward the newer, better surgery, and toward a better scientific understanding of the brain.

He recommends experimenting with more limited and localized surgery, but he himself admits that the areas attacked and destroyed — the hypothalamus, the nuclei of the thalamus, the amygdala — are all functionally *inter-related* "to mobilize the total body resources in stressful situations." "Interference with *any part* [my italic] of these circuits is reflected in changes in the homeostasis in others, but the nature of this interdependence and its precise relationship to behavior remains speculative." P. 593.

He acknowledges that some people have raised ethical objections, but he doesn't discuss these objections, and instead concludes that the modified *frontal lobotomy* should be continued in the United States as a "treatment" in neurotic and psychotic states characterized by a high degree of emotionality or tension.

Arthur Winter of East Orange, New Jersey, will soon be coming out with a book on lobotomies in collaboration with Scoville and Heath. Winter writes to me that he is doing "stereotaxic prefrontal lobotomies," limited to one side of the frontal lobes, in some instances at least. He would not tell me how many cases he had done, but sent me a detailed report on one 33-year-old man with a diagnosis of schizophrenia on whom he had operated in 1969. A photograph provided by him in *Medical World News* shows a good size "1 cm." obliteration looking as large as a walnut squarely in the middle of one frontal lobe.

Winter bases his work in large part on the Shobe and Gildeas article in the *Journal of the American Medical Association,* October 7, 1968, a report which describes "excellent" follow up results with a group of largely older private patients with agitated depressions. There are no control groups and insufficient clinical data.

The use of prefrontal lobotomy on individuals with agitated depressions opens the way to massive lobotomization of large segments of the population. The individual with an agitated depression is typically an older woman (18 females to 9 males in Shobe's study) who becomes depressed, hypochondriacal, obsessive and generally tense during her midlife and menopause. This person has always been a target for whatever current "therapy" someone wishes to push—insulin shock, electroshock, anti-depressants, tranquillizers, and now, lobotomy.

Petter Lindstrom of San Francisco has been reporting for many years on the use of destructive ultrasonic energy as a substitute for the surgeon's knife in frontal lobotomy. He calls it PST for Prefrontal Sonic Treatment. In *Medical World News* he is reported to have done 475 patients over the past twelve years, from children age eleven to elderly people age eighty, suffering from just about everything—anxiety, depression, obsessive neuroses, phobias, hypochondriasis, addictions and pain.

In a recent, as yet unpublished paper, presented at the Second International Conference on Psychosurgery (1970), Lindstrom presents this case: "A 13-year-old schizophrenic girl became disabled by progressive anxiety and psychosomatic symptoms in spite of drugs and psychotherapy, and was unable to go to school. Following the PST she was able to return to school and now has attended school regularly for four years, achieving passing grades. She has been helping with the work at home. Both the patient and the parents are pleased with the progress."

Writing in 1964 and talking about a series of 60 psychotics and 154 neurotics, he drops that typical statistic without remarking upon it—72% females among the psychotics, and 80% females among the neurotics.

Lindstrom apparently balks at being called a lobotomist. He says that he has been able to titrate his doses of energy so that he can reach a point where the damage is not grossly perceptible and hence does not constitute a lobotomy. But if he's getting a behavioral effect, he's done a lobotomy, even if it's merely a lobotomy by disruption of the brain chemistry. Otherwise it's a placebo.

Lindstrom, Winter, Scoville, and other lobotomists are making direct attacks on the frontal lobes. This is still among the most popular approaches to the psychosurgery of American patients.

H. T. Ballantine, Jr., is performing cingulotomies at perhaps the most prestigious general hospital in the world, The Massachusetts General of Boston. Scoville says that this type of surgery represents a "fractional lobotomy (77, 78). Ballantine also notes that the operation, when done on monkeys, produces "tameness and placidity," which certainly puts it in the class of the lobotomy in this regard.

Scoville, in his introduction to the unpublished Transactions of the Second International, believes that cingulotomy surgery is only successful because it is inaccurate and inadvertently cuts directly into some of the fiber tracts of the frontal lobes.

Ballantine makes references to other surgeons with series of 52 and 16 patients, and briefly describes his own series, mostly psychotics, ages fifteen to eighty-three with that typical distribution, 20 females, 14 males. He tells us virtually without explanation, that 22 were usefully improved, 10 were failures and 8 became *symptom free.*

Only dead people are symptom free.

Ballantine writes me that he is still active and has operated on 160 patients since 1965.

M. H. Brown and Jack Lighthill of Santa Monica, California, report in 1968 on another group of patients who have had their cingula obliterated. They have done 110 cases, 71% women. Two thirds of them had intractable neuroses, and 91.9% are considered good results, with little explanation of how this evaluation was arrived at. "Destructive emotional forces were removed," they tell us, including a reduction in anxiety, phobias, depression, hostility and obsessive thinking.

In recent personal correspondence with me, Dr. Lighthill sent copies of letters from other psychosurgeons applauding a "second wave" of psychosurgery around the world. He agreed with Lindstrom, as I mentioned, that 400–600 operations are being done a year in the United States, and said that his own group had operated on 110 patients before 1966, and an equal number, 110 *since* 1966.

Lighthill writes to me and Brown mentions at the Second International that they see a bright future for operating on criminals, especially those who are *young* and *intelligent,* a promise you will see being fulfilled in Mississippi.

Neurosurgeon Glenn Meyer and psychiatrists at the University of Texas Medical Branch in Galveston have also been experimenting with cingulotomies for the past several years, with a total of 27 performed on "alcoholics" and "drug addicts," as reported in an unsigned front page article in *Psychiatric News,* the official newspaper of the American Psychiatric Association, December 16th, 1970 (71). A psychiatrist, Winston Martin, reports on the data in this article entitled "Psychosurgery Hailed in Experimental Texas Study." The report speaks of results that are "nothing short of spectacular." "The procedure either helps or completely rids the patient of his emotional illness." No side-effects are found whatsoever, but it is noted that 15% of the patients have seizures post-operatively. Their press release announces that a "cure" has been found (71).

Vernon Mark, Frank Ervin and his associates from Boston City Hospital report in 1970 the details of one case of depression in which the psychosurgical operation was a great success but the patient killed herself.

Briefly here is the story. A woman with a long and difficult psychiatric history is brought in for psychosurgery, specifically a thalamotomy, mutilation of an emotion regulating portion of the brain. Her mother is heavily involved with her and with the psychiatrist and surgeon, and is probably a significant force in getting her to submit to surgery. The patient gets obviously worse after the first mutilation is performed, so she is done again with the convenience of her implanted electrode. After the second mutilation she becomes enraged at her psychiatrist and her neurosurgeon, and refuses to talk with or deal with her neurosurgeon any more. Nor will she ever submit to a suggested *third* operation. Her electrodes are therefore removed, but her rage is dismissed as "paranoid" by V. H. Mark and his associates.

Her mood then improves, as we are told, until she reaches a state of "high spirits." She is allowed out of the hospital to shop whereupon she goes directly to a phone booth, calls her mother to say "goodbye," takes poison and kills herself.

Her suicide is not seen as the vengeful act of a mutilated soul against her mother and her physicians. Instead, her suicide is interpreted as a sign that she was getting over her depression, a "gratifying" result of the operation—the word gratifying cropping up several times. All this is based upon the simplistic notion, sometimes taught to beginning psychiatric residents, that the occasionally observed phenomenon of suicide in the midst of an apparent recovery can be explained by a hydraulic conceptualization of increased energy permitting the patient to suicide before the depression is fully over. This explanation overlooks the individual dynamics, which cry out in this case.

This is the *only* detailed case report I have found in the entire current lobotomy literature, and I am grateful for this one instance in which enough material is provided for an independent judgment of the "gratifying" effects of psychosurgery.

But I have left something considerably more disturbing for my last detailed report—the mutilation of very young children for the admitted purpose of making them more manageable at home, at school or in the hospital.

Led by Congressman Gallagher's committee hearings, there has been a public outcry against the *drugging* of hyperactive children. Now we have physicians performing mutilating *surgery* upon hyperactive children, sometimes with multiple operations that can lead to gross intellectual deterioration. Surgery, unlike medication, is always permanent! And while only one center in the United States is known to be pursuing this work at the present time, there is the *current* precedent of psychosurgery on hyperactive children around the world (8, 9, 19, 62, 64, 75) as well as a past precedent for multiple severely mutilating lobotomies on children in the United States by Freeman, Watts and Williams (25, 94). In addition, Ballantine has operated on children as young as fifteen and Lindstrom on children as young as eleven. I also have had personal communications with one well-known American professor of psychiatry who advocates lobotomy on children but feels that "irrational" public resistance would prevent it at the present time, and Brown and Lighthill want to operate on young psychopaths.

O. J. Andy, Professor and Department Director of Neurosurgery at the University of Mississippi School of Medicine in Jackson is currently active in operating on hyperactive children. He is assisted by a psychologist, Marion Jurko, but lists no psychiatrists on his team. In 1966, he describes his surgery as "under the charge of I. S. Ravdin, Professor Emeritus of Surgery at the University of Pennsylvania and James D. Hardy, Professor and Chairman, Department of Surgery at the University of Mississippi in Jackson.

In a personal letter to me dated May 28, 1971, Andy writes that he has operated on 30–40 patients ages seven through fifty, the *majority* children. In another personal letter to me, his colleague, Jurko, writes that the age range begins at *five*. The goal is frankly stated by Jurko—to "reduce the hyperactivity to levels manageable by parents"!

Andy and his colleague, Jurko, reported their work at the Second International Conference on Psychosurgery, as well as in American and international journals, but nonetheless Andy appears wary of the accusation that these children have "psychiatric problems." These are not psychiatric cases but "behavioral problems," presumably with neurological causes, he writes to me. But he admits that he can find nothing neurologically wrong in many of these children, except something as meaningless as difficulty in a specific form of wrist coordination (alternating pronation and supination) which any anxious child might fumble with.

Despite his protests about the non-psychiatric nature of these childrens' problems, he goes on to describe them as suffering from "some form of hyperactivity, aggression and emotional instability." He makes this quite specific: the triology of symptoms is hyperactivity, aggression and emotional instability. As we'll see, *all* of his patients suffer from very well-defined psychiatric problems, and his surgery, thalamotomies and a few cingulotomies, is aimed at nothing more nor less than controlling aggression in difficult children. Andy writes to me: "In relation to the operative results, the category under aggression appears to be alleviated to a much greater extent than the other two categories [hyperactivity and instability]."

As Freeman and Watts discovered years earlier in *Psychosurgery* and as Williams and Freeman report in their study of lobotomized children, it can be very difficult to control a child surgically. But you can usually mutilate him repeatedly until he stops bothering anyone. Quoting Andy's letter: "On the other hand, although a child who is somewhat retarded and nonproductive can also undergo a very dramatic change from an extremely aggressive and hyperactive individual to one who is cooperative and easily managed, although still not productive." (sic)

Just how hard it is to control a child is illustrated in a case which he reports on two occasions. In 1966 he describes J. M. as follows: "A boy of 9, had seizures and behavioral disorder (hyperactive, combative, explosive, destructive, sadistic)." [His parentheses.]

In the tradition of Freeman's mutilation of children and aggressive adults, he simply operates and operates and operates until the child causes no more trouble. He begins with a bilateral mutilation of the thalamus, and repeats it on one side nine months later. The patient's behavior then "improves" and he can return to special education. After a year, though, "symptoms of hyperirritability, aggressiveness, negativism, and combativeness slowly reappeared," so he was brought back and operated on more extensively, this time mutilating the fornix. Now the patient gets worse and shows signs of brain damage from the surgery in the form of the loss of recent memory. So the child's brain is mutilated a fourth time. Now, Andy tells us, "the patient has again become adjusted to his environment and has displayed a marked improvement in behavior and memory."

Because Andy repeats the same four cases in a 1970 report, we find out that J. M., this little boy of 9, had about as bad an outcome as we might have imagined. He is of course still easy to manage. "Intellectually, however, the patient is deteriorating."

Andy operates in Jackson, Mississippi, but does not tell us the race of the children he has operated on. [Subsequently, we located three children, who were black.]

Andy does not limit his brain surgery to children. The adolescents upon whom he operates, according to Jurko's letter, often have criminal records, with "explosive, impulsive and unpredictable behavior." Thus they are fulfilling Brown and Lighthill's hope for a great future for psychosurgery operating on people with criminal behavior. Jurko does not say, however, whether these adolescents are young and intelligent, as Brown and Lighthill would hope for their surgery candidates.

In the absence of an outraged response from the medical and lay public, we will probably be in for a tide of psychosurgical mutilations of children, much as we already have in India, Thailand and Japan!

Andy also operates on adults. Here is how his colleague, Jurko, pictures these adults in a letter to me: "The adults are average to above average in intelligence. Many have held jobs of responsibility prior to and even during their years of increasing discomfort (2–10 years). Most of them have a constant pain syndrome, face, chest quadrant, etc. . . . Most of them will tell you that they are tense, nervous, anxious, depressed, and have strong suicidal thoughts. Many show high specific anxiety and some have evidence of "free-floating" anxiety.

These people sound remarkably like very many psychotherapy patients prior to successful therapy.

Andy's case reports in the literature, so limited in number and simplistic in presentation, yield similar thumbnail sketches: in one case, "alcoholism, drug addiction, attempted suicide, aggressive and destructive outbursts, nervousness, and emotional instability," or in another case, "nervousness, spells of shaking all over, explosive anger, attempted suicide."

Earlier we found Brown and Lighthill advocating the use of psychosurgery for young criminals, and now we find Andy and Jurko are operating upon young individuals with criminal records. And at the time that I am making this report, a project has been uncovered in the California prison system aiming at one use of psychosurgery for the control of prison inmates (66)! A sharp condemnatory response from the press, congressional interest, and the work of the Berkeley Medical Committee for Human Rights (Edward Opton, Jr.) has caused the project to be temporarily tabled.

III. Newest Advances in Mind Control

The psychosurgical techniques in Part III seem especially suited to totalitarian application on a large scale for a wide variety of citizens, and so I have separated them out for special attention. Each of them has been developed for the specific purpose of controlling the individual without requiring prolonged hospitalization and without preventing him from returning to his family and his work.

The first study involves the direct use of "psychotherapy" by psychiatrists to monitor the gradual, progressive lobotomization of the individual. It first appeared in 1963 in *Current Psychiatric Therapy,* a widely read American yearbook, and it is still continuing. The work, described as "progressive leucotomy," is reported by three Britishers, H. J. Crow, R. Cooper and D. G. Phillips, Burden Neurological Institute and Frenchay Hospital, Bristol, England. The technique involves a carefully organized management of the individual patient as he undergoes progressive electrical frontal lobotomy over a period of half a year or more under the direct supervision of a "psychotherapist."

The targets of the new technique are people with "anxiety-tension states" and "obsession syndromes," particularly individuals "of good intelligence and personality," who "sometimes have heavy responsibilities." The goal is a carefully titrated lobotomy which blunts the individual's emotional responsiveness without incapacitating him in the performance of these responsibilities.

The technology utilizes 24–36 tiny electrodes which produce small coagulations of tissue when the current is turned on. After they are implanted within the frontal lobes through two holes in the skull, they can then be left in place within the brain for up to seven months, taped to the scalp in a hidden fashion which permits the patient to walk around and even to leave the hospital between his treatments. His physicians can then talk with his family and with the ward staff to evaluate how "good" his behavior has become, before subjecting him to further partial lobotomies.

That these physicians are not talking about minor damage to the brain is indicated by the admission that they "overdid it" in one of their fourteen cases, though they do not tell us what happened to the victim.

As a psychiatrist, I am haunted by one aspect of this technique, the participation of the "psychotherapist," who literally sits beside his patient conducting an interview with him while the neurosurgeons gradually turn up the electrical current. In this manner the "therapist" monitors and titrates the amount of tissue destruction required to change the patient's ongoing emotional reactions. The patient cannot tell when his brain is being coagulated, but the therapist can tell immediately, since destruction of frontal lobe tissue is immediately reflected in a progressive loss of all those human functions related to the frontal lobes—insight, empathy, sensitivity, self-awareness, judgment, emotional responsiveness, and so on.

When Freeman and Watts (1950) operated on their patients without general anesthesia, the patients sometimes cried out that they were dying from the surgery as they felt their vital mental functions being cut away. The surgeons would then tell them to pray or to sing patriotic songs or simply ignore them while going on with the cutting.

The newer methods of these Britishers are much more subtle, but basically the same. The patient is fussed over and given reassurance. The process is so gradual and remote—controlled electrically with no obvious intervention taking place—that the patient never realizes what is happening to him. In fact, the patient gets so much attention from the ward team that other patients on the ward, who cannot discern the gradual extinction of his human qualities, ask if they can have the treatments, too.

H. J. Crow reports again on his work in 1965, and his report is noteworthy as a typical lobotomist article, all technology, a few sparse statistics about his successes, many diagrams, and *not one sentence* that could be called a clinical or human description of a patient. He continues to use "up to 34 separate small electrodes widely spread like a net across each frontal lobe," and has added electrodes in the anterior portion of the cingulum for patients with "obsessional" symptoms, thus performing both lobotomies and cingulotomies on some of his patients.

This article not only leaves out any descriptions of the patients beyond these one and two word diagnoses ("all anxiety syndromes, some having obsessional features"). It also seems to leave out that one disastrous case which they admit they "overdid" in the first article. Thus Crow says, "Of the first 25 cases . . . all have returned to a social life which is more or less normal."

We are told that individual and group psychotherapy goes on during the progressive lobotomization and then that intensive forms of therapy continue afterward for years. What we see described is a very directive influence, the sort we might expect would work with someone who had been brain damaged:

"From my experience, patients at this stage are amenable to, and eagerly seek advice about their future. Common-sense planning of their work and leisure, and advice about more ordinary attitudes in personal relationships, allows them to get started in a workable pattern of new life which they soon stamp with their own new and individual characteristics. They often need reassurance that an appropriate anxiety about, say, health or money is not a sign of returning illness. After an intensive course of advisory therapy an interview, often short, every month or two for half a year with lengthening intervals thereafter, is usually sufficient to help the patient to make and keep his readjustments."

He then says that some of these patients "require support for a long time," and goes on to describe social work, welfare, rehabilitation and psychological services, all of which may be brought to bear upon the patient.

Their lobotomized patients are thus given extensive often long-term services probably made available to very few if any other patients in Great Britain, certainly not to patients suffering from "anxiety syndromes," and yet they never once mention the possibility that whatever useful effects they achieve may be due entirely to these massive efforts mobilizing psychiatry, social work, welfare, rehabilitation and psychological services. Typically, they have no control groups with patients who are given these services without lobotomies!

If the patients are not brain damaged, why do they need such intense supportive help in the management of the details of their everyday life? Why would regular psychotherapy be contra-indicated as "unnecessary and unprofitable at this stage, and will at best delay intrapsychic and social adjustments"? Freeman and Watts also found that lobotomy patients needed daily guidance and were poor candidates for psychotherapy, but the reason was obvious in their case — the surgically damaged patients had lost the capacity for insight and judgment.

Crow reassures us that there are no bad side-effects, specifically no "insensitivity in social relationships." But a few pages after this reassurance, he tells us that the surgery sometimes produces "an over-optimistic attitude to his own capacities and to others' good will."

He also seems to imply that this may often be a "permanent euphoria" typical of brain damaged patients: "This can, of course, be a permanent euphoria, but I have seen cases where it has been a transient phenomenon and seemed to be a true joyfulness of release."

This kind of euphoria from brain damage is apparent in the two largest American studies from the 1950's: Greenblatt, Arnot and Solomon, and Freeman and Watts. Freeman and Watts' book is filled with case histories that read like classic studies of brain damaged individuals. In the other study, Harry Solomon in the introduction speaks of a "joyfulness" much as Crow does, but in a remote portion of the book the psychologist says the clinicians are too biased to be trusted and that the patients are actually brain damaged and "slap-happy." Many followup studies have found severe brain damage and deteriorating states years after lobotomy (23, 59, 61, 93).

Crow has sent me a page summary of his report at the Second International Conference on Psychosurgery, August 1970, in which he reports that he has done 103 patients since 1958. He summarizes a very naive and crude psychophysiological theory to justify his surgery, in which a specific region, "the anterior para-cingulate," is "involved in retaining mental items in consciousness, and thus to obsessionalism." Unlike some other lobotomists, he is unwilling to admit the inter-relatedness of human brain and mind functions, and the general blunting function of all psychosurgical interventions.

Implanting electrodes into the brain is at the heart of all of what is called ESB, or Electrical Stimulation of the Brain. The "stimulation" can be mild and probably reversible, or permanently destructive, depending upon the strength of the electrical current.

One of the most active ESB psychosurgeons is Robert G. Heath, Chairman and Professor of the Department of Psychiatry and Neurology at Tulane in New Orleans. He will soon be publishing a new book as part of the revival of psychosurgery.

According to *Medical World News,* which provides a disturbing photograph of one of his patients "wired up," Heath holds this record of 125 electrode implantations at one time, a brain turned into a human pincushion. These tiny electrodes are attached to wires or injection catheters which must also pass through the brain tissue.

Heath claims that these implantations are "harmless," but in an aside he lets on that they are in fact so traumatic that "studies were not initiated until a minimal period of six months following operation, assuring elimination of any variation introduced by operative traumas, e.g., edema, anesthetic effects." 1963, p. 572. Six months is a very long recovery time for a non-traumatic procedure. But since Heath will let a patient remain wired up for years, six months may not seem a long duration to him.

The justification for this trauma to the brain is "therapy," and Heath claims that it is never done for any reason except "therapeutic." But if you read his articles, you will find *almost nothing* about therapy in them. Sometimes he doesn't even mention what disease the patient is supposed to have! And many of his "results" offer nothing more than a sentence or two about a curious response of some scientific interest elicited by an obviously non-therapeutic stimulation exercise. And in keeping with this, and typical of most modern psychosurgical literature, his emphasis is almost entirely on developing a new technology. There are pages and pages about technique for every few lines about its effects upon the patient.

In "Electrical Self-stimulation of the Brain," Heath describes individuals who wear their own self-stimulation units on their belts, transisterized packets, which they can take with them as they walk around, even as they go to work outside the hospital. These experiments often involve research into "pleasure centers" within the brain, and sometimes patients will indulge themselves at the rate of more than one thousand stimulations an hour.

In one case a man pressed one of his several buttons in a "frantic" fashion because it built him up toward a feeling of orgasm that he was never quite able to consummate. This particular man's problem was "narcolepsy," a tendency to fall asleep unexpectedly in inappropriate situations, and since he wore his pack on his belt, his friends or other patients could simply press his "wake up" button for him when he began to doze off.

Electrodes can be implanted in pain centers as well as pleasure centers. The totalitarian potential is beyond belief—a permanent set of buttons for pain and pleasure which *other people* can control. And as we'll see when we get to Delgado, these portable stimulators can be manipulated by *remote control,* even by computers at a distance!

As we will also see in Delgado's work, sexual responses seem particularly easy to elicit by ESB. Another of Heath's patients was so subject to this kind of control that he would make a sexual reference whenever one particular electrode was activated. And though Heath gives us no clinical details about this or any other of his patients' experiences, *Medical World* reports that Heath has used these techniques to treat homosexuals and frigid women.

On rare occasions Heath elaborates a philosophical basis for his work. Writing in *The Journal of Neuropsychiatry,* for example, he takes a strong moral stand that Einstein's level of thought was better than Christine Keller's, the woman who created a scandal around her sexual activities with British politicians in 1963. Heath explains that Einstein's thought was of a higher level because Einstein's thought was less pervaded with "emotion and wishes." It is an exact equivalent of Knight's statement that "primitive emotions" are bad emotions. Not much justification for coagulating, radiating, slicing up or stimulating the brains of their patients.

Heath's concerns go far beyond the laboratory. He was elected President of the Society for Biological Psychiatry in May, 1969, at their Miami Beach annual meeting. In his presidential address, published as "Perspectives in Biological Psychiatry," he takes the stand that *all* the significant advances in psychiatry have been biological, and he postulates that so-called mental patients suffer from "inappropriate anxiety." Therefore the cure—"instantaneous replacement of irrelevant anxiety with positive pleasure feelings" by psychosurgical techniques.

He becomes quite specific in his presidential address when he talks about drug addiction. Is the root of the problem poverty and racism, since drug addiction around the world and in America is overwhelmingly a problem of the poor! No, it's not that. Is the new phenomenon of drug addiction among middle class youth related to the disaffection of youth from the society? No. Does it relate to the tremendous profits made by criminal groups from promoting drugs among the poor? No. What then is the problem of drug addiction according to Dr. Heath? Drug addiction, he says, is an attempt at self-medication for pleasure in people who have a *neurological defect in their pleasure centers!* His cure then is corrective surgery or a better, more efficient pleasure producing compound.

Three or four years ago (1968B), Heath had already reported psychosurgical operations on 58 patients, at least 44 with psychiatric illnesses. By now he has most likely done many more. But the influence of his work goes far beyond the clinical through his positions of leadership within the psychiatric world, including his directorship of the Department of Psychiatry and Neurology at Tulane.

Perhaps the first of the new batch of books on electrical psychosurgery is *Depth-Electrical Stimulation of the Human Brain* by Mayo Clinic trained C. W. Sem-Jacobsen, who has returned to Norway, where he is Medical Director, Gaustad Sykehus, Oslo. Sem-Jacobsen's book is a classic of technology devoid of human considerations. The book can be read from cover to cover without ever gaining a clear idea what purpose all this psychosurgical gadgetry will serve. His discussion of ethics is limited entirely to *medical* considerations, such as not causing undue pain, avoiding unnecessary surgery, showing concern for the patient, and the like, all admirable, but hardly inclusive when dealing with physical control of the human mind.

We learn more about Sem-Jacobsen's work from his unpublished report to the Second International Conference on Psychosurgery, and from a description of it in *Medical World News*. He has operated on at least 132 patients for various psychiatric problems. Feeding half a dozen or more electrodes through a single hole in the skull, he can elicit, he says, almost every mood and emotion — depression, wild euphoria, grave fright, irrational confusion. His methods for treating people involve stimulating the brain electrically until the unwanted behavior is located, and then coagulating the area with electricity.

Though technologically exacting, this method must rank as one of the most anachronistic, considering the outmoded theory behind it — that so-called mental illness can be reduced to foci of disordered brain tissue. That theory was outmoded and even an embarrassment to lobotomist Freeman (1950) when Moniz first proposed it in 1935 to justify the very first mutilations on a large scale. But since Sem-Jacobsen doesn't report anything about his patients' lives — not even the usual thumbnail sketches — in his book or in any sources available to me in the literature, we have no idea what his psychosurgery is actually doing to his clients.

The political potential of lobotomy and electrical stimulation of the brain is promoted outright by Jose M. R. Delgado, Professor of Physiology at Yale University and author of the recent book *Physical Control of the Mind,* "Toward a Psychocivilized Society," published in 1969 and available in paperback. Delgado was brought to America from Spain by John Fulton, an American physiologist whose animal lobotomy experiments and whose enthusiasm for experimenting on the human brain inspired Moniz and Freeman and whose book, *Frontal Lobotomy and Affective Behavior,* praises Moniz for his courage in defying the outrage of the medical community against his brain mutilations.

Delgado's goal is nothing less than physical exploration and physical control of the mind for the advancement of civilization: "The thesis of this book is that we now possess the necessary technology for the experimental investigation of mental activities, and that we have reached a critical turning point in the evolution of man at which the mind can be used to influence its own structure, functions and purpose, thereby ensuring both the preservation and advance of civilization. The following pages contain a discussion of what the mind is, the technical problems involved in its possible control by physical means, and the outlook for development of a future psychocivilized society." P. 19–20.

Note that he is specifically talking about tampering with the "structure, functions, and purpose" of the mind and "its possible control by physical means."

After pages of documentation about what has already been done by a few investigators working with very little funds, he then proposes a giant billion dollar government investment in mind control: "National agencies should be created in order to coordinate plans, budgets, and actions just as NASA in the United States has directed public interest and technology, launching the country into the adventures and accomplishments of outer space." P. 259.

He advocates a complete educational program, from infancy and nursery through adulthood and mass education for the indoctrination of the people into a respect for physical control of the mind: "The mass media must be mobilized for this purpose, and preparation of entertaining and informative programs should be encouraged and promoted by the neurobehavioral institutes." P. 262.

In his introductory remarks to the section on controlling "behaving subjects" he promotes the ideal of *remote control* of human beings by other human beings. He points out that we can open garage doors from a distance, adjust a television set without leaving our seat, and direct orbiting space craft from earth. Then he makes his point: "These accomplishments should familiarize us with the idea that we may also control the biological functions of living organisms from a distance. Cats, monkeys, or *human beings* can be induced to flex a limb, to reject food, or to feel emotional excitement under the influence of electrical impulses reaching the depths of their brains through radio waves purposefully sent by an investigator." P. 75. (My italic.)

But he is aware that this may disturb some of his readers, and so he denies time and again that human beings can be controlled in any "bad" ways, turning them into robots, or the like. But he says outright that the problem fascinates him and preoccupies him: ". . . we have the possibility of investigating experimentally some of the classic problems of mind-brain correlations. In addition to new answers, implanting of electrodes has introduced new problems: Is it feasible to induce a robotlike performance in animals and men by pushing buttons of a cerebral radio stimulator? Could drives, desires and thoughts be placed under the artificial command of electronics? Can personality be influenced by ESB? Can the mind be physically controlled?" P. 97.

Delgado is working on the ultimate lobotomy—direct long term physical control of human beings. He has even gone so far as to work it out cosmetically: "Some women have shown their feminine adaptability to circumstances by wearing attractive hats or wigs to conceal their electrical headgear, and many people have been able to enjoy a normal life as outpatients." P. 88.

Again, despite his denials that there is anything reminiscent of 1984 about all this, he has been working on remote control of humans by *computers* which can selectively inhibit various emotions as they are detected and recorded from brain waves: "A two-way radio communication system could be established between the brain of a subject and a computer . . . anxiety, depression, or rage could be recognized in order to trigger stimulation of specific inhibitory structures." P. 201.

While this is "speculative," it is by no means a remote possibility. Using the computerized remote control technique, they have been able to suppress the activity of a monkey's amygdala simply by putting an inhibitory or negative and painful stimulus into the brain every time the amygdala sent out any signs of activity (p. 92). The amygdala is that portion of the brain which the psychosurgeons cut out in order to tame human beings. There is no doubt that they will soon be able to do this to humans with computers and electrodes by remote control!

The experiments Delgado describes with monkeys have gone further than any he tells about with human beings, but the model can be easily transferred to human behavior. In groups of monkeys he has been able to activate the followers to depose the leaders, and to activate the leaders in more aggressive activities against the followers.

But he and his colleagues have already done enough to show us what is in store for mankind in the "psychocivilized" society. Not only do we have the work of Heath and Sem-Jacobsen with chronically implanted electrodes and human beings working and living with self-stimulator packs on their belts, but we have the reports of Delgado himself.

In one case, a 36-year-old woman was stimulated electrically: ". . . the patient reported a pleasant tingling sensation in the left side of her body 'from my face down to the bottom of my legs.' She started giggling and making funny comments, stating that she enjoyed the sensation 'very much.' Repetition of these stimulations made the patient more communicative and flirtatious, and she ended by openly expressing her desire to marry the therapist." P. 145.

This was a woman who had no interest in her therapist and who showed no unusual behavior when not under ESB. Another woman who was "rather reserved and poised" became "more intimate" with the therapist when under ESB: "This patient openly expressed her fondness for the therapist (who was new to her), kissed his hands, and talked about her immense gratitude for what was being done for her." P. 145.

In a third case, an 11-year-old boy who was otherwise normal in his behavior became so sexually excited about his male therapist while being stimulated electronically that he denied his identity and decided that he would rather be a girl: "Following another excitation he remarked with evident pleasure: 'You're doin' it now,' and then he said, 'I'd like to be a girl.'" P. 147.

Delgado is also able to control physical activity. In one case a patient is being stimulated and doesn't realize it, so that when the stimulation makes him turn and look around in robot-like searching behavior, he makes up explanations to justify what he is doing, such as "I heard a noise," or "I was looking under the bed" (p. 116). In another case where the client is being made to flex his hand, he is told to fight the impulse, but he cannot. He admits, "I guess, Doctor, that your electricity is stronger than my will."

In another example, Delgado shows that the subject's state of *anxiety* can sometimes be brought under the direct control of the psychosurgeon: "One could sit with one's hand on the knob and control the level of her anxiety." P. 135.

The degree of overall brain control is then alluded to in experiments which we can only imagine: "Often the patients performed automatisms such as undressing or fumbling, without remembering the incidents afterward. Some of our patients said they felt as if their minds were blank or as if they had been drinking a lot of beer." P. 174–175.

Delgado concludes his section on "Electrical Activation of the 'Will,'" with this portentious pronouncement: "We may conclude that ESB can activate and influence some of the cerebral mechanisms involved in willful behavior. In this way we are able to investigate the neuronal functions related to the so-called will, and in the near future this experimental approach should permit clarification of such highly controversial subjects as "freedom," "individuality," and "spontaneity" in factual terms rather than in elusive semantic discussions. The possibility of influencing willful activities by electrical means has obvious ethical implications, which will be discussed later." P. 189.

Delgado does discuss these ethical implications and invokes the model of involuntary psychiatric treatment and electroshock therapy (p. 216) as justifications for going ahead with ESB control.

The degree to which Delgado wants to control people comes out most clearly as he summarizes what's wrong with current therapy and how much more effective ESB can be. "Psychoanalysis requires a long time, and a person can easily withdraw his cooperation and refuse to express intimate thoughts." P. 216.

Even electroshock is no good in part *because he can't use it on normal people*: "Electroshock is a crude method of doubtful efficacy in normal people." P. 216.

Listen to what his methods have to offer compared to analysis or shock: "Although electrical stimulation of the brain is still in the initial stage of its development, it is in contrast far more selective and powerful; it may delay a heart beat, move a finger, bring a word to memory, or set a determined behavioral tone." P. 216.

He offers us a vision of generals and armies controlled by Electrical Stimulation of the Brain — in the interest of "preventing violence" of course (p. 176). And finally leads himself into sophistries about freedom and individually which undermine the basic tenets of western political freedom: "The individual may think that the most important fact of reality is his own existence, but this is only his personal point of view, a relative frame of reference which is not shared by the rest of the living world. This self-importance also lacks historical perspective, for the brief existence of one person should be considered in the terms of the world population, mankind, and the whole universe." P. 236.

He then goes on to *attack* the notion that man has "the *right* to develop his own mind," to develop his own unique potential "while remaining independent and self sufficient." As he concludes: "This kind of liberal orientation has great appeal, but unfortunately its assumptions are not supported by neurophysiological and psychological studies of intra-cerebral mechanisms." P. 239.

Delgado is the theoretician of the lobotomists, the great apologist for Technologic Totalitarianism (17), complete with an outright attack on "liberal" politics, meaning not the liberalism of the left, but principles of personal autonomy, independence and freedom, man's "inalienable rights" as annunciated in the Declaration of Independence.

IV. Conclusions and Recommendations

All forms of psychosurgery blunt the individual's emotions and make him more docile. Each technique attacks and mutilates brain tissue that has nothing demonstrably wrong with it, and each does this within the delicately balanced "limbic system" of the brain which harmonizes the most highly developed human capacities, including emotional responsiveness.

While the more advanced methods of brain stimulation have a greater variety of effects, to the extent that they destroy tissue within the brain, they will tend to reduce emotional responsiveness as "partial lobotomies." And of course they subject the individual to the control of others.

Scientifically, lobotomy and psychosurgery have no rational or empirical basis. Empirically, no study has ever been done involving matched control groups. That is, no one has ever taken two similar groups and subjected one to surgery and left one alone for comparison. This is the scientific method at its best and it is totally absent from the hundreds of pro-lobotomy articles in both the first and second waves of psychosurgery.

Three controlled studies have been done retrospectively matching as nearly as possible the surgical groups and the regular hospital populations upon which no surgery was done (Robin, Vosburg and McKenzie). In all three studies lobotomy was found to have no beneficial effect whatsoever. Vosburg, Moser and even pro-lobotomy followups such as Dynes and Miller found that the lobotomy surgery had left the patients with crippling brain damage. Vosburg found that the patients had surgically-produced brain damage as well as their initial psychiatric difficulties and that "In sum, they act as if they have been hurt."

The current literature is as woefully inadequate scientifically as the earlier literature, and in fact bases itself on studies by Shobe, Tooth and Newton and others which fall by every standard of scientific research.

The scientific *rationale* is no more solid than the empirical evidence. As we have seen, psychosurgery is a uniformly damaging operation—exactly what one would expect from mutilating normal brain tissue. There can be no rationale for "helping" an individual by blunting his highest adaptive mechanisms. This method simply hides the individual's failure to adapt by partially doing away with the individual's responsiveness. In every case we are dealing with the eradication of symptoms by partially eradicating the individual. To repeat the obvious, improvement in function cannot allow mutilation of the functioning brain.

In defense of psychosurgery, the alleged biological origin of "mental illness" is often raised. Elsewhere Thomas Szasz and I (14, 15, 17) have raised serious questions about the medical model for human problems. But this distinction is not even relevant here. If we grant that some problems may be biological, it makes even less sense to mutilate the biologic process. Since the brain is such a delicately balanced instrument with unimaginable interrelations, senseless mutilations of one part or another can only disrupt the harmony still further, resulting in a general subduing of the organism and a general malfunction of his adaptational processes.

Vidor describes how an artist can no longer create after the lobotomy, and the dean of lobotomists, Walter Freeman (1959), tells us how in the newer modified lobotomies creativity is still reduced to zero: "What the investigator misses the most in the more highly intelligent individuals is the ability to introspect, to speculate, to philosophize, especially in regard to the self." P. 1526. "Creativeness seems to be the highest form of human endeavor. It requires imagination, concentration, visualization, self-criticism, and persistence in the face of frustration, as well as trained manual dexterity. . . . Theoretically, on the basis of psychologic and personality studies, creativeness should be abolished by lobotomy. . . . On the whole, psychosurgery reduces creativity, sometimes to the vanishing point." P. 1534–5.

He then says that some businessmen can return to work, but that they too are impaired: "Although they may not become leaders in their professions, they serve adequately and comfortably." P. 1535.

This is not the writing of an anti-lobotomist, but the statements of the world's most experienced psychosurgeon, an Honorary President of the new International Association for Psychosurgery. The words are written as the definitive statement on psychosurgery in the prestigious source book, *The American Handbook of Psychiatry* (1959).

Ethically, psychosurgery is equally unsound. At best it blunts the individual, and at worst, it destroys all his highest capacities. As Freeman has said on many occasions, this amounts to destroying the "self" of the individual (1950, 1959). The "self" is the ethical foundation of many modern psychological theories, where it often appears in terms of "identity" or "self-insight," and other related concepts. Similarly, psychosurgery blunts or destroys the individual's capacity for autonomy and independence (14). Crow, a very modern British psychosurgeon, describes how his clients need careful guidance and support for years after their surgery in the most simple life problems. Psychosurgery offends the whole western ethical tradition of respect for the individual.

Politically, the dangers from psychosurgery are so vast as to defy summary. In his definitive text in 1950 we can see the political function of psychosurgery in the state hospital system in terms of Freeman's first four categories of success over a fifteen year period (p. 515):

First, "older patients."

Second, women more than men.

Third, Negroes especially, particularly Negro females, his most successful group.

Fourth, "simpler" occupations.

Thus he used the surgery to blunt those people whom the society found most vulnerable and most easily returnable to relatively non-functional or low level tasks within the society.

Greenblatt, Arnot and Solomon blithely sum up that "Freeman and Watts offer the opinion that results of prefrontal lobotomy are slightly better with females, Jews and Negroes." p. 21. Freeman and Watts did not say *slightly*.

Both Freeman and Watts and Greenblatt, Arnot and Solomon in their classic studies say that a major function of state hospital lobotomy is to make it easier and economically cheaper to keep the patients institutionalized! No wonder, as Greenblatt, Arnot and Solomon again quote their colleagues, "Freeman and Watts reported that patients showing the best post operative results were those who were confused, dull, and retarded for several days after operation," p. 23.

We are again seeing an attempt to revive the use of psychosurgery to blunt and control inmates — Andy with institutionalized children and the California prison system with difficult prisoners (66).

But the total political threat of psychosurgery is considerably larger than the institutional threat. In my newest novel, *After the War* (15), I describe a futurist use of psychosurgery for political control within the society. But while I was writing this novel, I had no idea that Delgado had already formulated a political program for the control of the society under an enormous NASA-like project for physical control of the mind. Nor did I know that he and others like Heath were already far along in experimenting with implanted electrodes for the longterm (years!) control of individuals — even by remote control! Nor did I know that a number of social, economic and political problems — drug addiction, alcoholism, homosexuality, depressions of old age — were being dealt with psychosurgically. The increasing application of these methods to "neurotics" and to people who are already well enough to work and to live with their families raises the specter of wide applications, particularly of women, who continue to be the majority of victims.

On a tape recording made for the archives of the American Psychiatric Association Museum and Library, Walter Freeman discusses the original outcry against lobotomy when it first began in Portugal (29). Dismissing this outcry, Freeman laughs and quips "Oh, there's plenty of Portuguese." This is an attitude which cannot be permitted to thrive again in America as it did in the 1940's and 1950's when 50,000 victims fell to psychosurgery. Russia outlawed lobotomy in 1950 (45). We are too far behind them in this regard.

While accepting these scientific, ethical and political objections to psychosurgery in general, some well-meaning physicians and laymen still see a use for psychosurgery in the relief of intractable pain and anxiety in terminal illness (96). But the use of psychosurgery for this purpose borders on euthanasia — a partial destruction of the responsive "self" or "identity" of the living human being — and therefore suffers from all the dangers inherent in euthanasia. But still more important, to allow its use for this one purpose opens up experimentation on thousands of dying patients and further promotes its future use for other more dangerous purposes.

Some individuals with a civil libertarian orientation also believe that, while psychosurgery is personally repugnant to them, it should nonetheless be left up to individual choice. According to this principle, involuntary psychosurgery would be abolished, but not voluntary psychosurgery. But the distinction between voluntary and involuntary becomes very blurred within psychiatry. We have already found examples of "voluntary" psychosurgery performed on a chronic gambler and upon sexual deviants who were under threat of criminal prosecution. The psychosurgery to be performed upon the prisoners in California was also suppose to be "voluntary." And as I have analyzed in some detail (13) and described at great length in my first novel (15), so-called voluntary treatment is often forced upon the psychiatric patient by threats and outright coercion even in the best of voluntary hospitals.

There is still another reason to prohibit voluntary psychosurgery, and that has to do with its mutilating effect upon the individual's mind. To the extent that psychosurgery "blunts" the individual, I personally feel that it partially kills the individual. If we accept this concept, then we can allow the person the right to suicide or partial suicide but we cannot allow a second party to aid him in the suicide. Just as it is against the law to take a person's life even with his consent, so it should be against the law to take *part* of a person's life, even with his consent.

For these reasons, I believe that all forms of psychosurgery should be outlawed in America as they were in Russia (45). [My views have changed concerning the outlawing of psychosurgery. See my introduction.]

The outlawing of psychosurgery can be accomplished directly by federal and state legislation. It can also be accomplished indirectly by taking psychosurgeons to court when this seems warranted. Suits might be based upon any tendency to make exaggerated claims, thus leading to "uninformed consent" on the patient's part. Other suits might be brought upon the grounds that the patient has been robbed of his civil rights by being deprived of his mental capacity to exercise them.

In the meanwhile, the public must apply the sort of pressure that has brought a temporary stop to psychosurgery in the California prisons. Psychiatric hospitals, institutions for the mentally retarded and general hospitals (where most are now being performed) must prohibit psychosurgery within their walls. Hospital review committees must set up where necessary to determine if questionable cases fall into the category of psychosurgery — brain surgery which mutilates healthy tissue for the purpose of blunting emotions and controlling personal conduct.

Well over 100,000 persons have already been subjected to psychosurgery around the world, including 20,000 in England, perhaps 50,000 in America, and many more thousands in Canada. We are now in the midst of a resurgence, including psychosurgery upon hyperactive children. It is time to take action before this revival takes on the proportions of the first wave that peaked in the 1950's.

BIBLIOGRAPHY FOR AUTHOR'S NOTE

1. Breggin, Peter R. "Psychosurgery for the Control of Violence," in *Neural Bases of Violence and Aggression,* edited by W. Fields and W. Sweet, Warren H. Green Publisher, St. Louis, Mo., 1975.

2. Breggin, Peter R. "Psychosurgery for Political Purposes," *Duquesne Law Review* 13:841–862, 1975.

3. Breggin, Peter R. *Electroshock: Its Brain-Disabling Effects,* New York: Springer Publishing Company, 1979.

4. Breggin, Peter R. "Brain-Disabling Therapies," in *The Psychosurgery Debate,* edited by E. Valenstein, San Francisco: W. H. Freeman, Publisher, 1980.

5. Breggin, Peter R. "Disabling the Brain with Electroshock," in *Divergent Views in Psychiatry,* edited by M. Dongier and E. Wittkower, Hagerstown, Maryland: Harper and Row, 1981.

6. Breggin, Peter R. "Psychosurgery as Brain-Disabling Therapy," in *Divergent Views in Psychiatry,* edited by M. Dongier and E. Wittkower, Hagerstown, Maryland: Harper and Row, 1981.

7. Breggin, Peter R. *Chemical Lobotomy: The Brain-Disabling Effects of Psychiatric Drugs* (tentative title), New York: Springer Publishing Company, 1982 (in press).

BIBLIOGRAPHY

1. Andy, O. J., "Neurosurgical Treatment of Abnormal Behavior," *Amer. J. Med. Sci.* (1966) 252:232–238. See reference 99.

2. Andy, O. J., "Thalamotomy in Hyperactive and Aggressive Behavior," *Confin. Neurol.* (1970) 32:322–325.

3. Anonymous, "Leucotomy Today," *Lancet* (1962) 2:1037–8.

4. Anonymous, "Standard Lobotomy. The End of an Era," *Canadian Med. Assoc. J.* (1964) 91:1228–1229.

5. Anonymous, "Brain Surgery for Sexual Disorders," *Lancet* (1969) 4:250–251.

6. Bailey, Harry; Dowling, John; Swanton, Cedric; Davies, Evan, "Studies in Depression: Cingulo-tractotomy in the Treatment of Severe Affective Illness," *Med. J. of Australia* (1971) 1:8–12.

7. Baker, Earle; Young, M. D.; Gauld, D. M.; Fleming, J. F. R., "A New Look at Bimedical Prefrontal Leucotomy," *Canadian Med. Assoc. J.* (1970) 102:37–41.

8. Balasubramaniam, V.; Kanaka, T. S.; Ramanugam, P. V.; Ramanurthi, B. "Sedative Neurosurgery," *J. Indian. Med. Assoc.* (1969) 53:377–381.

9. Balasubramaniam, V.; Kanaka, T. S.; Ramanugan, P. V.; Ramanurthi, B. "Surgical Treatment of Hyperkinetic and Behavior Disorders," *Int. Surg.* (1970) 54:18–23.

10. Ballantine, Jr., H. T.; Cassidy, Walter; Flanagan, Norris; Morino, Raul, Stereotaxic Anterior Cingulotomy for Neuropsychiatric Illness and Intractable Pain," *J. Neurosurg.* (1967) 26: 488–495.

11. Barhol, H. S., "1,000 Prefrontal Lobotomies—A Five-to-ten-year Follow-up Study." *Psychiat. Quart.* (1958) 32:653–678.

12. Batchela, Ivor, *Henderson and Gillespics Textbook of Psychiatry;* Oxford Medical Publishers, 1969.

13. Breggin, Peter Roger, "Coercion of Voluntary Patients in an Open Mental Hospital," *Arch. Gen. Psychiat.* (1964) 10:173–181.

14. Breggin, Peter Roger, "Psychotherapy as Applied Ethics," *Psychiatry* (1971) 34:59–74.

15. Breggin, Peter Roger, *The Crazy from the Sane* (a novel about hospital psychiatry); Lyle Stuart, Pub., 1971. A second novel, *After the Good War* (Stein and Day, 1973) deals in part with the politics of psychiatric technology including psychosurgery (paperback edition, Popular Library, 1974).

16. Breggin, Peter Roger, "Psychosurgery," *Medical Opinion and Review,* March, 1972; also, Breggin, Peter Roger, "Second Wave," in *M/H,* March, 1973.

17. Breggin, Peter Roger, "Psychiatry as Applied Utopian Ethics," for presentation and inclusion in the *Proceedings, 4th International Congress on Social Psychiatry,* May, 1972 (in press, *Mental Health and Society*).

18. Brown, M. Hunter and Lighthill, Jack, "Selective Anterior Cingulotomy: A Psychosurgical Evaluation," *J. Neurosurg.* (1968) 29:513–519.

19. Chitanondh, H., "Stereotaxic Amygdalotomy in Treatment of Olefactory Seizures and Psychiatric Disorders with Olefactory Hallucinations," *Confin. Neurol.* (1969) 27:181-1960.

20. Crow, H. J.; Cooper, R.; Phillips, D. G., "Progressive Leucotomy," in Masserman, Jules, *Current Psychiatric Therapies,* III, Grune and Stratton, 1963.

21. Crow, H. J., "Brain Surgery in the Treatment of Some Chronic Illnesses," a paper given at the British Council for Rehabilitation of the Disabled, Tavistock House (South), Tavistock Square, London, 1965. Published separately.

22. Delgado, Jose M. R., *Physical Control of the Mind — Toward a Psychocivilized Society;* Harper Colophon, 1969.

23. Dynes, John B., "Lobotomy — Twenty Years After," *Virginia Med. Quart.* (1968) 95:306-308.

24. Evans, Philip, "Failed Leucotomy with Misplaced Cuts: a clinico-anatomical study of two cases," *Brit. J. Psychiat.* (1970) 118:165-170.

25. Freeman, Walter and Watts, James, *Psychosurgery;* Charles C. Thomas, 1950.

26. Freeman, Walter, "Psychosurgery," in Arieti, S., *American Handbook of Psychiatry,* II; Basic Books, 1959.

27. Freeman, Walter, "Psychosurgery," *Am. J. Psychiat.* (1954) 121:653-655.

28. Freeman, Walter, "Recent Advances in Psychosurgery," *Med. Ann, D.C.* (1965) 34:157-160.

29. Freeman, Walter, A Taped Interview for the American Psychiatric Association Museum Library, April 17, 1968.

30. Freeman, Walter, "Frontal Lobotomy in Early Schizophrenia: Long follow-up of 415 cases," *Brit. J. Psychiat.* (1971) 119:621-4.

31. Gallagher, Cornelius, E., "Federal Funds of 283,000 to Harvard Psychologist B. F. Skinner," *Congressional Record,* H12623-12633, Dec. 15, 1971. A summary of investigations into "mind control."

32. Greenblatt, Milton; Arnot, R.; Solomon, H., *Studies in Lobotomy,* Grune and Stratton, 1950.

33. Greenblatt, Milton and Solomon H., eds., *Frontal Lobes and Schizophrenia,* Springer Publishing Co., 1953.

34. Group for the Advancement of Psychiatry, Lobotomy," in *Report #6,* 1948.

35. Hassler, R. and Dieckmann, G., "Stereotaxic Treatment of Compulsive and Obsessive Syndromes," *Confin. Neurol.* (1967) 29:153-158.

36. Heath, Robert G., "Development Toward New Physiologic Treatments in Psychiatry," *J. Neuropsychiat.* (1964) 5:318-331.

37. Heath, Robert G., "Development Toward New Physiologic Treatments in Psychiatry," *J. Neuropsychiat.* (1964) 5:318-331.

38. Heath, Robert G.; Stanley, John B.; Fontana, Charles J., "The Pleasure Response: Studies in Stereotaxic Technics in Patients," Kline and Laska, ed., *Computers and Electronic Devices in Psychiatry;* Grune and Stratton, 1968.

39. Heath, Robert G., and Guerrero-Figuroa, R., "Stimulation of the Human Brain," *Acta Neurol. Latinoamer,* (1968) 14:116-124.

40. Heath, Robert G., "Perspectives for Biological Psychiatry," Bio. Psychiat. (1970) 2:81-87.

41. Hirose, S., "Orbito-ventromedial Undercutting, 1957-1963," *Amer. J. Psychiat.* (1964) 121:1194-1202.

42. Holden, J. M. C.; Itil, T. M.; Hofstatter, L., "Prefrontal Lobotomy: Stepping-Stone or Pitfall?" *Amer. J. Psychiat.* (1970) 127:591-598.

43. Kalinowsky, Lothar, "Psychosurgery Panel," *Dis. Nerv. Sys.* (Feb. 1969) 30 suppl.:54-55.

44. Kalinowsky, Lothar, "Psychosurgery Said to Help in Certain Neuroses," *Psychiatric News* (1971) Vol. VI, No. 7, p. 7 (April 7).

45. Khachaturian, A. A., "A Criticism of the Theory of Leukotomy," *Nevro-patol. I. Psikhiatriya* (1951) 20:#1. Microfilmed English translation, Library of Congress, TT 60-13724.

46. Knight, Geoffrey C., "Stereotaxic Tractotomy in the Surgical Treatment of Mental Illness," *J. Neurosurg. and Psychiat.* (1965) 28:304.

47. Knight, Geoffrey C., "Intractable Psychoneuroses in Elderly and Infirm — Treatment in Stereotactic Tractotomy," *Brit. J. Geriatric Preceice* (1966) 3:7–15, 1966.

48. Knight, Geoffrey C., "Bi-frontal Stereotactive Tractotomy: An Atraumatic Operation of Value in the Treatment of Intractable Neuroses," *Brit. J. Psychiat.* (1969) 115:257–266.

49. Lewin, W., "Observations on Selective Leukotomy," *J. Neurol. Neurosurg.* (1961) 24:37–44.

50. Lindstrom, Petter A., "Profrontal Ultrasonic Irradiation — A Substitute for Lobotomy," *A.M.A. Arch. Neurol. and Psychiat.* (1954) 72:399–425.

51. Lindstrom, Petter A.; Moench, L. G.; Roynanek, Agnes, "Prefrontal Sonic Treatment," in Masserman, J., ed., *Current Psychiatric Therapies, IV,* Grune and Stratton, 1964.

52. Livingston, Kenneth, "The Frontal Lobes Revisited. The Case for a Second Look," *Arch. Neurol.* (1969) 20:90–95.

53. Manchester *Guardian,* April 2, 1968, p. 18.

54. Mark, Vernon H.; Barry, Harbert; McLardy, Turner and Ervin, Frank, "The Destruction of Both Anterior Thalamic Nuclei in a Patient with Intractable Depression," *J. Nerv. Ment. Dis.* (1970) 150:266–272.

55. Marks, I. M.; Birley, J.; Gleden, M. G., "Modified Leucotomy in Severe Agoraphobia," *Brit. J. Psychiat.* (1965) 112:757–769.

56. McKenzie, K. G., and Kaczanowski, G., "Prefrontal Leukotomy: A Five-Year Controlled Study," *Canad. Med. Assoc. J.* (1964) 91:1193–1196.

57. *Medical World News,* "Neurosurgeons Take Route V-90 to Lobotomy," January 24, 1968, pp. H3–H4.

58. *Medical World News,* "The Lobotomists Are Coming Again," January 15, 1971, pp. 34ff.

59. Miller, A., "The Lobotomy Patients — A Decade Later," *Canad. Med. Assoc. J.* (1967) 96: 1095–1103.

60. Moore, D., "Prefrontal Leukotomy," *Canad. Med. Assoc. J.* (1970) 102:876.

61. Moser, H. M., "A Ten-Year Followup of Lobotomy Patients," *Hosp. Community Psychiat.* (1969) 20:381.

62. Narabayashi, H.; Nagao, T.; Saito, Y.; Yoshido, M.; and Nagahata, M., "Stereotaxic Amygdalotomy for Behavior Disorders," *Arch. Neurol.* (1963) 9:1–17.

63. Narabayashi, H. and Uno, M., "Long Range Results of Stereotaxic Amygdalotomy for Behavior Disorders," *Confin. Neurol.* (1966) 27:168–171.

64. Narabayashi, H., "Functional Differentiation in and around the Vertical Nucleus of the Thalamus based on Experiences in Human Stereoencephalotomy," *Johns Hopkins Med. J.* (1968) 122:205–300.

65. *Newsweek,* "Probing the Brain," (Cover Story), April 21, 1971, pp. 60–77.

66. Opton, Jr., Edward, mimeographed communications on behalf of the Medical Committee for Human Rights, Berkeley, California, December 30, 1971. See also, "Doctor's Warning on Vacaville's 'Torture' Cures." The Berkeley *Barb* Dec. 2, 1971, and "Prison Reform, California Style," *d.c. gazette,* Feb. 9, 1972.

67. Personal Communication by letter.

68. Personal Communication by telephone.

69. Pippard, John, "Leucotomy in Britain Today," *J. Ment. Sci.* (1962) 108:249–255.

70. Post, F., "An Evaluation of Bimedical Leucotomy," *Brit. J. Psychiat.* (1968) 114:1223–1224.

71. *Psychiatric News,* "Psychosurgery Hailed in Experimental Texas Study," Dec. 16, 1970, p. 1. See also, *News Release,* U. Texas Medical Branch at Galveston, Sept. 9, 1970, 7 pages.

72. Rinkel, Max, *Biological Treatment of Mental Illness;* Farrar, Straus and Giroux, 1966. See p. 66 and p. 146.

73. Robin, A. A., "A Controlled Study of the Effects of Leucotomy," *J. Neurol. Neurosurg. Psychiat.* (1958) 21:262–269.

74. Roeder, F. D., "Stereotaxic Lesion of the Tuber Cinerium in Sexual Deviation," *Confin. Neurol.* (1966) 27:162–3.

75. Sano, K.; Yoshioka, M.; Ogashiwa, M.; Ishijma, B.; Ohye, C., "Postero-medical Hypothalamotomy in Treatment of Aggressive Behavior," *Confin. Neurol.* (1969) 27:164–167.

76. Sargant, W. and Slater, E., *Physical Methods of Treatment in Psychiatry;* Williams and Wilkins, 1964.

77. Scoville, William B., "Recent Thoughts on Psychosurgery," *Connect. Med.* (1969) 33:453–456.

78. Scoville, William B., ed., *Transactions of the Second International Conference on Psychosurgery;* Charles C. Thomas, in press. See reference 99.

79. Second International Conference on Psychosurgery, August 1970, Copenhagen, Denmark. Summaries furnished by participants provide the material cited. See Scoville above for in press source and *see* Kalinowsky (1971) for summary in print. Psychosurgeons from more than a dozen countries contributed. Now published as reference 99.

80. Sem-Jacobsen, Carl W., *Depth-Electrographic Stimulation of the Human Brain and Behavior;* Charles C. Thomas, 1968.

81. Shobe, Frank and Gildea, Margaret, "Long-Term Followup of Selected Lobotomized Patients," *JAMA* (1968) 206:327–332.

82. Slater, E., and Roth, M., *Clinical Psychiatry.* 3rd ed. Williams and Wilkins, 1969.

83. Smith, Aaron, "Selective Prefrontal Leucotomy," a letter, *Lancet* (1965) 1:765.

84. Solomon, P., and Patch, K., *Handbook of Psychiatry,* 2nd Ed., Lange, 1971.

85. Spiegel, E. A. and Wycis, H. T., *Stereoencephalotomy, I,* "Thalamotomy and Related Procedures," Grune and Stratton, 1962.

86. Spiegel, E. A., Presidential Address, list Meeting Amer. Br. Int. Soc. Res. Stereoencephalotomy, Atlantic City, 1968, *Confin. Neurol.* (1969) 31:5–10.

87. Spiegel, E. A., *Progress in Neurology and Psychiatry,* Grune and Stratton, 1970, see pp. 67–69.

88. Strom-Olson, R., and Carlisle, "Bifrontal Stereotactic Trackotomy: A Followup Study of Its Effects on 210 Patients," *Brit. J. Psychiat.* (1971) 118:141–154.

89. Sykes, H. K. and Tredgold, R. F., "Restricted Orbital Undercutting: A Study of Its Effects on 350 Patients Over the Years 1951–1960," *Brit. J. Psychiat.* (1964) 110:609–640.

90. Tan, E.; Marks, I. M.; Marset, P., "Bimedial Leucotomy in Obsessive-Compulsive Neuroses," *Brit. J. Psychiat.* (1971) 118:155–164.

91. Tooth, G. C., and Newton, M. P., *Leucotomy in England and Wales;* H. M. Stationery Office, London, 1961.

92. Vidor, R., "The Situation of the Lobotomized Patient," *Psychiat. Quart.* (1963) 37:97, 104.

93. Vosburg, R., "Lobotomy in Western Pennsylvania: Looking Backward Over Ten Years," *Amer. J. Psychiat.* (1962).

94. Williams, J. M. and Freeman, W., "Evaluation of Lobotomy with Special Attention to Children." *A. Res. Nerv. Ment. Dis. Proc.* (1963) 31:311.

95. Wortis, Ed., *The Yearbook of Psychiatry and Applied Mental Health:* Yearbook Medical Publishers, 1970. Review of Brown and Lighthill Article.

96. Fedio, Paul and Ommaya, Ayoub. "Bilateral Cingulum Lesions and Stimulation in Man with Lateralized Impairment in Short Term Verbal Memory." *Experimental Neurology* (1970) 29: 84–91. This psychosurgery is being carried on at the National Institute of Neurological Disease and Stroke in Bethesda, Maryland, apparently for the relief of terminal cancer patients, and represents a more conservative approach to psychosurgery according to my initial inquiries.

97. Vaernet, K. and Madison, Anna, "Stereotactic Amygdalotomy and baso-frontal tractotomy in psychotics with Aggressive Behavior," *J. Neurol. Neurosurg. Psychiat.* (1970).

98. Breggin, Peter R., "Psychosurgery for the Control of Violence: A Critical Review." Chapter XVI in *Neural Bases of Violence and Aggression,* edited by W. Fields and W. Sweet. St. Louis, Mo., Warren H. Green, Publisher, 1975.

99. Hitchcock, et al., *Psychosurgery,* 1972, published by Charles C. Thomas, is the latest most complete pro-psychosurgery compendium with articles by Andy, Mark, Ervin and Sweet and others. An article by Ruth Anderson describes the destructive effects of the latest operations. The papers are from the Second International Congress on Psychosurgery in 1970.

Vernon H. Mark

A Psychosurgeon's Case
for Psychosurgery

There is a compelling case to be made for psychosurgery. It is not so well known as the case *against* psychosurgery, which is part of a widespread movement against psychiatry in general. But psychosurgery is more rational, factual, and ultimately more humanitarian.

Psychosurgery may be broadly defined as brain surgery to correct mental and behavioral disorders. In my opinion, it should be used only if some recognized disease is the primary cause of a patient's unwanted and abnormal behavior, and if all other treatments have failed. Abnormal behavior that is not associated with disease should be dealt with by other means, such as politics, law, or education, and not by medicine.

The legitimate domain of psychosurgery, in other words, is narrow. Psychosurgery should not be used to improve any behavior whatsoever, nor is psychosurgery a proper treatment for every abnormality. The proposition that electrical brain stimulation and brain surgery should be used to improve every aspect of human life is wrong for at least two reasons. It assumes that we know much more than we actually do about the brain; and more important, it assumes that medical men are the best authorities on how to improve humanity "beyond the normal." The position that psychiatric neurosurgery should be used to correct any abnormal or undesirable behavior is also unacceptable, because current definitions of "abnormal behavior" may be purely social or political, and have little or nothing to do with disease states.

From *Psychology Today* 8 (July 1974):28, 30, 33, 84, 86. Copyright © 1974 by Ziff-Davis Publishing Company. Reprinted by permission.

An Absurd Split

The campaign against *all* kinds of psychosurgery appears irrational. Moreover, its loud public clamor has raised the gravest ethical and social issues. Before considering some of those issues, I must single out a prejudice endemic to the sciences of human behavior. It is the historical dichotomy between "purely organic" and "purely social" abnormalities. Specifically, physicians tend to categorize a few abnormal behaviors, such as paralysis, blindness and dementia, as neurological problems. At the same time, certain other abnormalities, such as depression and aggression, have found a hard niche within the domain of psychiatrists, sociologists and criminologists. Many of them view these behaviors as nothing but the reflections of particular environments. They tend to believe that brain function or dysfunction is not an important determinant of abnormal behavior. Even those few social scientists who admit that brain function might be important often believe that so little is really known about the brain that it is useless to spend time and money investigating it.

This division of labor has had absurd consequences, for *no* human behavior, normal or abnormal, comes from the brain alone without the environment. Nor can any behavior, whatever its environmental determinants, take place without the brain's function.

Perhaps the split between organic and environmental theories of behavior is a result of overspecialization within medicine. The neurologists are in one place while the psychiatrists and social workers are in another. Despite such difficulties, physicians must try to embed neurological diagnoses into a larger, more integrated view of human behavior. The present controversy over psychosurgery, however, indicates that the greatest threat to a more holistic view of behavior lies not in the possibility that social considerations will be slighted by neurologists, but rather that neurological considerations will be left out entirely.

Origins of Psychosurgery

In its classical sense, psychosurgery involves operations on the frontal lobes or their connections in the brain. The object is to relieve symptoms of intractable depression, agitation, compulsion, delusion, hallucination and paranoia in psychiatrically diseased patients with no known structural brain alterations. This kind of surgery is used only when treatments such as psychotherapy and drugs have failed.

Frontal-lobe surgery, initiated by the Nobel Prize winner António Egas Moniz in 1935, appeared effective in treating agitation and depression. Such operations became widely used in the United States in cases of agitated schizophrenia. Several studies have shown that radical frontal lobotomy and frontal lobectomy made it possible for patients to leave mental institutions and carry on better integrated lives.

But some of these patients paid too high a price for treatment. Emotions became blunted, and intellectual powers deteriorated. The subsequent development of drugs like Thorazine and Stelazine—which could accomplish many of the same therapeutic goals without surgery—brought an end to radical frontal-lobe surgery in the U.S.

In Great Britain, psychosurgery never achieved the popularity that it did in this country; but its more restricted use also made it less susceptible to replacement by drugs. Hugh Cairns and his associates at Oxford modified the original frontal-lobe operations. They initiated the operation of cingulotomy, in which the destructive lesion was restricted to a small bundle of fibers called the cingulum. Psychiatrists evaluated these patients before their operations and for years afterward. The evidence seems to indicate that carefully selected groups of patients can derive important benefits from restricted forms of frontal-lobe surgery.

Since the 1950s, psychosurgery has expanded beyond its classical meaning. Today the term includes any neurosurgical operation that affects human behavior, even if the patient has obvious brain disease. The most controversial patients in this expanded definition are those who have both intractable epilepsy and psychiatric symptoms, which may include abnormal aggression. These patients' symptoms have often been relieved by neurosurgery. They are the same patients who have been characterized as victims by irresponsible critics of psychosurgery.

In a sense, the brain responds as a whole to a given environmental stimulus. And yet we can localize portions of the brain that govern particular behaviors. It is this partial specialization of function according to structure that makes neurosurgery possible at all, for we can influence the function in a part of the brain without interfering with the entire organ.

One specialized portion of the brain, the limbic system, or limbic brain, tends to govern "fight or flight" behavior, as well as sexuality, appetite, and emotional tone. The limbic brain may be damaged by various abnormalities, including tumors, strokes, infection, head injury, and poison. One of the commonest diseases afflicting the limbic brain is focal epilepsy, which may be accompanied by a number of behavioral abnormalities. Occasionally, abnormal aggression is one of these—although episodes of catastrophic rage occur more frequently *between* than during epileptic seizures.

Drugs and psychiatric treatment sometimes relieve epileptic symptoms. In other cases the drugs fail, and when they do, surgical removal of the anterior portion of the temporal lobe (lobectomy) may be necessary. The operation involves the removal of several parts of the limbic brain.

X-Rays and Electrodes

Within the past few years, more precise techniques have been developed for selected patients. Less brain tissue needs to be destroyed. Surgeons implant small electrodes into the afflicted portion of the brain. These electrodes record or stimulate the brain's electrical activity; they can also destroy small amounts of tissue, thus relieving some epileptics of their disabling symptoms.

Critics of psychosurgery have argued that temporal-lobe epilepsy is extremely difficult to diagnose and that neurosurgeons, in effect, may be operating on patients with mild neurotic symptoms. Recent studies, though, indicate that most patients with this disease have definite and serious structural abnormalities in the temporal lobes of their brains that can be seen on special x-ray films known as pneumoencephalograms or in specimens of tissue removed during temporal lobectomy. One fifth of surgical patients with temporal-lobe epilepsy are reported to have brain tumors. Surgery, in short, may relieve up to 70 percent of otherwise untreatable epileptics of their seizures, abnormal aggressiveness, and other psychiatric symptoms.

Other brain abnormalities besides epilepsy may be related to violent behavior. Patients suffering from large tumors, excess spinal fluid accumulations, internal bleeding and various other diseases and injuries have in some cases become abnormally aggressive. Neurosurgery has relieved such patients of their emotional disturbance by treating the tissue abnormality.

This brief review illustrates the promise of neurosurgery for certain psychiatric disorders. It is our observation that a person whose brain is damaged (especially if the injury is in the limbic system) cannot respond as appropriately to environmental stress as a person whose brain is normal. The relative importance of environmental and organic factors must be evaluated in each case.

Spurious Charges

The opponents of psychosurgery have used my colleagues and myself as targets. The book I wrote with Frank R. Ervin, *Violence and the Brain,* has become notorious in some circles. Our discussion of violent epilepsy has been characterized, among other things, as a racist argument, since we suggested (in a 1967 letter to the *Journal of the American Medical Association,* and in our book) that some of the personal violence of urban riots may have been related to individual brain dysfunction. What is often overlooked is that we ascribed some of the violence during riots to the police and National Guard, and we pointed out that a diagnostic review should include them as well as the violent rioters.

Let me comment further on the charge of racism. First, the theory that *some* violence is related to brain disease would not cause us to look for such disease more searchingly in black ghettos than anywhere else. By contrast, the theory that personal violence is exclusively social in origin might very well direct our attention to black ghettos because that is where we see some of the worst social conditions in America. This second theory is of limited applicability, whereas the theory that violence is a sociobiological phenomenon causes us to look for brain disorders in every segment of the population. Moreover, empirical evidence suggests that the occurrence of individual violence is more common among whites in this country than is generally conceded. Consider the many thousands of people injured or killed in domestic quarrels or by automobiles; many of them are not only white but from the middle and upper socioeconomic classes. Often these tragedies are related to severe brain poisoning with alcohol. Our social and legal apparatus consider such violence, if at all, in a different category from that of the ghetto. Yet, in reality, the fruits of violence are the same in the ghetto as in the suburbs; only the style is different.

I do not wish to minimize the potential dangers in a theory of violence that looks for causes, among other places, in the individual organism. There is the real danger that state institutions where blacks are disproportionately represented may offer up their inmates as candidates for psychosurgery in order to keep them quiet or even to punish them. If this were to happen, then the charge of de facto racism would be justified.

A Place for Psychosurgery

We have to guard against such dangers in several ways. We should limit neurosurgery, in patients with abnormal aggression, to cases where pathological disorders of the brain are well defined. We must also observe strict rules as to informed consent. Finally, we should clarify the political and legal rights of prisoners. Under the present constraints of informed consent that exist in prisons, I think no one should perform psychosurgery on convicted felons.

Despite these restrictions, I still believe that psychosurgery (outside of prisons) can be an appropriate form of treatment. Critics have suggested that other, less radical, treatments are good enough. Yet the two main alternatives to psychiatric surgery—psychotherapy and drug therapy—may be ineffective or have serious side effects.

Environmental manipulation, psychoanalysis, behavioral conditioning, and other forms of psychotherapy may all be successful in relieving the symptoms of some patients. Psychotherapists, however, have pointed out serious methodological flaws in attempts to evaluate the results of psychotherapy. In cases of serious mental illness, there is no convincing statistical evidence that psychotherapy is better than any other mode of therapy, or even chance alone. Moreover, a recent report indicates a 10 percent complication rate (including death) in relatively normal students undergoing encounter group therapy.

Drug therapy raises other problems. Agents such as Thorazine, Stelazine and Haldol, which replaced frontal lobotomies, are certainly more effective in relieving symptoms than inert substances or conventional sedatives. But administration of such agents over a period of weeks or months may incur complications. A syndrome resembling Parkinson's disease is common, and some of these drugs may occasionally produce a fatal decrease in white blood cells. A more serious complication is the syndrome called tardive dyskinesia.

It consists of slow, rhythmical movements around the mouth, smacking of the lips, blowing of the cheeks, and side-to-side movements of the chin, plus other bizarre muscular activities. The condition becomes dangerous when it impairs breathing or motor coordination. There is no known treatment, and post-mortem pathological studies have indicated that it is accompanied by structural changes in the brain.

The dilemma of drug therapy for seriously ill patients received attention recently in a revealing editorial in the *Archives of General Psychiatry*:

"*Because of the lack of adequate substitutes* for the neuroleptic drugs in the treatment of psychosis, tardive dyskinesia has been accepted as an undesirable but occasionally unavoidable price to be paid for the benefits of prolonged neuroleptic therapy." (Italics added.)

An estimated 250-million people have taken neuroleptic drugs since their introduction in the 1950s. Tens of thousands of patients in the U.S. take them regularly. Only a few hundred patients a year undergo psychosurgery.

The Attack Upon Psychiatry

Implicit in everything I have said is the belief that psychosurgery is part of medicine, part of psychiatry, and, as such, one of many efforts to relieve human suffering. It strikes me as particularly unfortunate, then, that the main theme among critics of psychosurgery is not simply the belief that this limited tool is improper, but that *psychiatry itself*—including the techniques of drug treatment, electroconvulsive shock, and behavioral conditioning—is a threat to human dignity.

"Antipsychiatry" originated, I believe, when a vocal segment of psychiatrists abandoned the medical model of psychiatric disease in favor of a social or political model. The result of this abandonment has been a growing inability to decide who is mentally ill and who is not. Typically, it seems, antipsychiatrists waver between the idea that nobody is mentally ill, and the equally arbitrary notion that everybody is. The medical model of psychiatric disease, upon which psychosurgery rests, is more scientific, more cautious, and ultimately more humane than this sociopolitical alternative. It conforms to other kinds of medical practice in terms of theory and treatment. More important, it demands an accurate and thorough diagnosis for each patient before treatment.

The fundamental question raised by recent attacks on psychiatry concerns the accuracy of psychiatric diagnosis. Who is diseased and who is just a victim of circumstance? Questions of illness are difficult to decide in any field of medicine. But I contend that physicians, including medically oriented psychiatrists, are in a stronger position to answer this question accurately than are socially and politically oriented psychiatrists. In any case, a high incidence of faulty and arbitrary diagnoses is inevitable whenever medical criteria and thorough evaluations are ignored.

A recent experiment has demonstrated what happens when psychiatrists and psychologists fail to be diagnostically rigorous before applying psychiatric labels. David Rosenhan, a psychologist at Stanford, and seven other normal subjects presented themselves to psychiatric hospitals in various parts of the country with a single complaint that did not correspond to any known psychiatric disease. These pseudopatients were admitted without question and diagnosed as psychotic. The only people in these hospitals who recognized them as phonies were the other patients.

Hagop Akiskal and William T. McKinney, Jr. have described a "pseudoepidemic" of psychiatric disease in the U.S. and have suggested that some psychotherapists are treating many patients who are not really sick. These two writers call for a more honest assessment of potential psychiatric patients, with more frequent application of the diagnosis "no mental disorder."

"Sick Society"

Abandonment of the medical model and the resultant overdiagnosis of mental illness have allowed antipsychiatrists to thrive. Some members of this faction claim that there is no such thing as mental disease—that there is only a "sick society." One influential spokesman, Thomas Szasz, looks at the medically oriented, institutional psychiatrists as agents of an oppressive state. Another spokesman, Seymour Halleck, claims that all psychiatry must be political since it deals with the distribution of power and the maintenance of the status quo.

There are other dangers in the current antimedical philosophy. One of them is psychiatric misdiagnosis that fails to take note of brain abnormalities, such as tumors and other structural disease. Several years ago, a study of 18 patients who died in a mental hospital revealed that they had had tumors of the limbic system of the brain. Some of them died before the true nature of their illness was appreciated.

Another danger arises from the way certain antipsychiatrists face the possibility that some patients will attempt suicide. Thomas Szasz, for example, states that therapists should not interfere with a patient's "free will," if he wants to kill himself. The medical model is far more humane, for it views self-destructive tendencies, especially in drug-intoxicated or temporarily disturbed patients, as symptoms of disease that require some form of intervention.

Still another danger raised by the antipsychiatrists is that their theories could lead to the complete legal prohibition of all neurological surgery, neuropharmacological therapy, behavior-conditioning therapy, and neuroelectric therapy for psychiatric patients. Withdrawal of antipsychotic drugs would unmask symptoms of severe agitation in large numbers of mental patients. Many of them, currently treated as outpatients, would require hospitalization, but there are not enough hospitals to hold them all. A likely consequence would be chaos within many families and communities.

The suicide rate might rise dramatically if it were illegal to treat suicidal patients. Many suicide attempts are unsuccessful at first because of prompt medical treatment. Should these pathetic individuals be allowed to suffer and slowly die because of legal sanctions that prevent their receiving medical attention?

Unsound Theories

The sociopolitical doctrines of the antipsychiatrists lack empirical foundation. Whereas biological abnormalities that relate to mental disorders are often very clear, the theory that mental illness is purely sociopolitical in origin remains unsubstantiated. Robert N. Wilson, a social scientist at the University of North Carolina who has worked in the field of mental health, recently stated: "Our faith in an essentially social etiology of psychological disorder has been shaken by the paucity of clearly demonstrable causal patterns."

There has never been a society or culture without mental illness. From the right-wing government of Nazi Germany where mental patients were often killed, to communist countries where political psychiatry is a fine art, mental disease has remained a persistent phenomenon. And yet it is the avowed intention of some antipsychiatrists to work for the overthrow of the establishment in favor of a new political system that they presume would abolish mental illness.

After a thorough study of antipsychiatry, Sir Martin Roth, former president of the Royal College of Psychiatrists, concluded that this movement could not help mentally ill patients. An even more devastating criticism has been advanced by the psychologist and political scientist Peter Sedgwick. He suggests that the antipsychiatrists are attempting to block all forms of effective treatment for mentally ill patients in order to highlight the failure of our present forms of government to meet their social obligations. According to this analysis, untreated mental patients are hostages to the political aims of the antipsychiatry movement. If Sedgwick is right, the situation reveals a political cynicism and disregard for patients' rights that should propel the antipsychiatrists onto the center stage of public scrutiny. Up to this point, the antipsychiatric arguments have consisted only of criticisms. It is time for them to disclose a positive program, if they have one.

The antipsychiatrists and other critics of the medical model of psychiatry often construe human violence as the expression of free will. Accordingly, they think the medical correction of brain disease, which would stop violent episodes, has an unnatural and degrading effect on human dignity. This view is particularly inappropriate, not because free will is to be denied but because the quality of human life is to be prized. Many patients with focal brain disease associated with violent behavior are so offended by their own actions that they attempt suicide. They feel that their human dignity has been lost precisely because of uncontrollable behavior patterns which they find unnatural and repugnant. Because of the relationship in some patients between limbic brain disease and aggressive behavior, the correction of that organic condition gives the patient *more* rather than less control over his own behavior.

There is already enough knowledge of both environmental controls and psychoactive drugs to influence a vast segment of our population, without invoking brain surgery or electrical brain stimulation. The great hope of brain research is that it will free seriously ill, but presently untreatable, patients from their disabilities.

Stephan L. Chorover

Psychosurgery: A Neuropsychological Perspective

Introduction

We are still far from understanding how our brains give rise to the varied phenomena of our subjective experience. But despite our relative ignorance, we biologists and behavioral scientists stand today in a position comparable to that occupied by our colleagues in nuclear physics almost 30 years ago. In 1945, developments in that field led to the atomic bomb and ushered in a new world of ethical and social problems. During the past few decades, developments in the biobehavioral sciences have spawned a wide-ranging psychotechnology, a varied arsenal of tools and techniques for predicting and modifying human social behavior. The continued development and deployment of this psychotechnology has also engendered serious ethical and social problems that can no longer be ignored.

Psychosurgery is among the more controversial forms of psychotechnology. Also known as "psychiatric neurosurgery," "mental surgery," "functional neurosurgery" and "sedative neurosurgery," psychosurgery may be defined as brain surgery that has as its primary purpose the alteration of thoughts, social behavior patterns, personality characteristics, emotional reactions, or some similar aspects of subjective experience in human beings.[1] . . .

Psychosurgery for Violence

It has long been popularly believed that there is a close association between

From *Boston University Law Review* 54 (March 1974):231, 239–248. Reprinted by permission of the publisher and the author.

epilepsy and violence. The phrase "a fit of anger" nicely epitomizes this view. Over the years, a large number of clinical studies have dealt with this question. After reviewing the available literature and assessing the clinical experience of neurologists who have cared for many patients with seizure disorders, a recent study sponsored by the National Institute of Neurological Diseases and Stroke concluded that "violence and aggressive acts do occur in patients with temporal lobe epilepsy but such are rare, perhaps no more frequent than in the general population."[2]

Two of the best known cases of this kind are "Thomas R." and "Julia S." Their pseudonyms have entered the vocabulary of psychosurgery, their cases have been fictionalized in a best-selling novel,[3] and they continue to arouse public interest as purported successes of Drs. Vernon H. Mark and Frank R. Ervin, the authors of the controversial *Violence and the Brain*. Bearing in mind that the existence of a causal connection between epilepsy and violence remains an open question in the view of most neurologists, let us consider each of these cases in turn.

The Case of Thomas R.

The Presentation by Mark and Ervin. Thomas is introduced to Mark and Ervin's readers in the following passages:[4]

> He was a brilliant [*sic*] 34-year-old engineer with several important patients to his credit. Despite his muscular physique it was difficult to believe he was capable of an act of violence when he was not enraged, for his manner was quiet and reserved, and he was both courteous and sympathetic.

Despite a history of physical illness, Thomas managed to educate himself as an engineer.

> He was an extremely talented man, but his behavior at times was unpredictable and even frankly psychotic. He was seen and treated by psychiatrists over a period of 7 years with no effect on his destructive outbursts of violence.
>
> Thomas's chief problem was his violent rage; this was sometimes directed at his co-workers and friends, but it was mostly expressed toward his wife and children. He was very paranoid, and harbored grudges which eventually produced an explosion of anger. He often felt that people were gratuitously insulting to him. . . .

For example, during a conversation with his wife,

> he would seize upon some innocuous remark and interpret it as an insult. At first, he would try to ignore what she had said, but could not help brooding; and the more he thought about it, the surer he felt that his wife no longer loved him and was "carrying on with a neighbor." Eventually he would reproach his wife for these faults, and she would hotly deny them. Her denials were enough to set him off into a frenzy of violence.

Thomas was referred to Mark and Ervin by a psychiatrist who they say had concluded that "prolonged psychiatric treatment did not improve his behavior and . . . that his spells of staring, automatisms and rage represented an unusual form of temporal lobe seizure."[5] An electroencephalographic examination revealed electrical brain activity considered by them to be indicative of epilepsy, and additional tests suggested the presence of other brain abnormalities. After experimenting with a wide range of pharmacological agents, none of which proved therapeutic, they decided to proceed with stereotaxic surgery. Arrays of electrodes were implanted in both temporal lobes with their ends reaching the nucleus amygdala. The "optimal site for destructive lesions"[6] was sought through repeated stimulation and recording. Stimulation in one portion of the amygdala "produced a complaint of pain, and a feeling of 'I am losing control,'" two reactions that marked the onset of Thomas' periods of violence. However, stimulation of a portion of the amygdala just four millimeters to the side produced the opposite reactions of detachment, "hyperrelaxation" and a "feeling like Demerol."[7]

Mark and Ervin's account of how they obtained Thomas' consent to their proposed surgery is revealing both in terms of what is said and what is left unsaid. They viewed Thomas as keenly aware of personal insults and highly sensitive to threats, and found that "the suggestion that the medial portion of his temporal lobe was to be destroyed . . . would provoke wild, disordered thinking."[8] At this point in their discussion, they acknowledge in a footnote the physician's "extraordinary responsibility" of safeguarding the rights of the patient and of securing his free and informed consent.[9] But, they continue, "[u]nder the effects of lateral amygdala stimulation, [Thomas] showed bland acquiescence to the suggestion" that psychosurgery be performed.[10]

> However, 12 hours later, when this effect had worn off, Thomas turned wild and unmanageable. The idea of anyone's making a destructive lesion in his brain enraged him. He absolutely refused any further therapy, and it took many weeks of patient explanation before he accepted the idea of bilateral lesions [*sic*] being made in his medial amygdala.[11]

Since Mark and Ervin considered Thomas' rage inappropriate and were, by their own account, able to blunt it by lateral amygdala stimulation, it is perhaps not surprising to learn that Thomas finally "accepted the idea." Directly following this quoted passage, we are informed of the success of the procedure in these brief sentences: "Four years have passed since the operation, during which time Thomas has not had a single episode of rage. He continues, however, to have an occasional epileptic seizure with periods of confusion and disordered thinking."[12]

The reader, recalling Mark and Ervin's original assertion that Thomas' "chief problem was his violent rage"[13] and that he exhibited some preoperative seizures and confused or disordered thinking, may reasonably conclude from this account that bilateral amygdalectomy has not only improved Thomas' condition, but has also effected a specific and total cure of his chief complaint. The rage is allegedly gone, the other preoperative symptoms remain essentially unchanged, and no postoperative side effects are mentioned. In light of the devastating effects of bilateral amygdalectomy on the social behavior of nonhuman primates, the apparently successful outcome of Thomas' case seems remarkable indeed. The implied absence of any adverse social reactions appears especially unexpected. Is it sufficient, however, to rely on mere implications? Highly relevant information is not provided by the published case histories. Prior to his operation, Thomas was married and supported his family through his work as an engineer. It would seem that a full account of the effects of his psychosurgery should include, for example, information concerning his marriage and his employment.

Contradictory Reports. At the request of Thomas' family an independent follow-up of Thomas' case has been performed by Dr. Peter R. Breggin, a psychiatrist and well-known critic of psychosurgery.[14] Dr. Breggin interviewed the patient and his family, reviewed the hospital charts made before and after surgery and discussed the case with several well-informed individuals.

According to Dr. Breggin, Thomas was continuously employed through December 1965. During that year he began to have serious marital problems which prompted visits to his wife's psychiatrist. Breggin conducted a telephone interview with this psychiatrist during which he was told that Thomas' wife was indeed afraid of him, but that no actual harm was done to her.[15] Moreover, writes Breggin:

> [the] psychiatrist remembers that Thomas was depressed, but not sufficiently depressed to warrant electroshock or drugs. His memory is entirely consistent with the hospital records which report no hallucinations, delusions, paranoid ideas or signs of difficulty with thinking. In the charts, his most serious psychiatric diagnosis is "personality pattern disturbance," [a classification] reserved for mild problems with no psychotic symptomatology.[16]

Finally, certain hospital charts state that "[h]e has never been in any trouble at work or otherwise for aggressive behavior."[17] In short, Dr. Breggin's account stands in sharp contrast to the published assertions of Drs. Mark and Ervin. Indeed, Breggin claims that the only incidence of violence mentioned in Thomas' hospital files were those provoked by Mark and Ervin themselves.

Thomas was treated by Mark and Ervin from October 1966 until his release from Massachusetts General Hospital on August 27, 1967. He subsequently returned with his mother to the west coast, unable to rejoin his wife and children because his wife had, during his treatment, filed for divorce. Eventually, she married the man about whom Thomas had allegedly been paranoid.[18] Shortly after the operation, it became apparent that Thomas was socially confused and unable to cope with the complexities of normal life. He was soon admitted to a west coast Veterans Administration hospital where he was placed on a locked ward and given heavy doses of medication. Breggin's account suggests that Thomas' new physicians did not have access to his medical records from Massachusetts General Hospital. Indeed, they regarded his comments concerning Mark and Ervin's procedures as evidence of his delusional state of mind.[19] After six months of confinement, he was discharged with a diagnosis of "schizophrenic reaction, paranoid type."[20] At present, Breggin claims, Thomas is totally unable to work, is incapable of caring for himself and must periodically be rehospitalized as assaultive and psychotic.

Dr. Breggin is not the only available source of information about Thomas' postoperative history. His follow-up study has recently been supplemented by a complaint filed in behalf of the patient[21] and is generally consistent with information the author has obtained from other sources.[22] In August 1972, Dr. Ernst Rodin, a Detroit neurosurgeon, visited Dr. Mark's project in Boston. Rodin, at that time a coauthor of a proposal to perform psychosurgery on involuntarily incarcerated individuals,[23] made the visit "to obtain the most up-to-date information on the results of surgery for aggressive behavior in human beings. . . ."[24] Hoping that this inquiry would strengthen his proposal, Rodin was all the more disturbed by the disparities he discovered between the published accounts and the information available at first hand. Specifically, Dr. Ira Sherwin, a neurologist involved with the project, told Rodin that "he was not aware of any genuinely successful cases"[25] and that Thomas R. "will never be able to function in Society."[26]

The Case of Julia S.

The Presentation by Mark and Ervin. Julia S., another one of Mark and Ervin's celebrated patients, is the daughter of a well-to-do physician. She is described as being "an attractive, pleasant, cherubic blonde who looked much younger than her age of 21."[27] Starting with an attack of encephalitis before the age of two, she had a long history of brain disease. Her epileptic seizures began at about the age of 10, some being grand-mal convulsions, but most appearing to be petit-mal, or psycho-motor, seizures characterized by "brief lapses of consciousness, staring, lip smacking, and chewing."[28] Between seizures, Julia's behavior was marked by "severe temper tantrums followed by extreme remorse."[29] She also experienced "racing spells," which began with terrifying feelings of panic and ended in her rapidly running aimlessly about the streets. At least 12 people are said to have been assaulted by her, and when she was 18, she seriously injured other women in two separate stabbing incidents.[30]

Because Julia failed to respond to extensive psychotherapy, drugs and electroshock, Mark and Ervin concluded that her case "clearly illustrates the point that violent behavior caused by brain dysfunction cannot be modified except by treating the dysfunction itself."[31] Accordingly, they explored Julia's brain, producing rage reactions with the aid of amygdala electrodes and a telemetry device called a "stimoceiver." Finally, lesions were made in the "appropriate

areas." *Violence and the Brain,* which was published two years after Julia's operation, contains the following evaluation by Mark and Ervin:

> It is still too early to assess the results of the procedure, but she had only two mild
> rage episodes in the first postoperative year and none in the second. Since she had
> generalized brain disease and multiple areas of epileptic activity, it is not surpris-
> ing that epileptic seizures have not been eliminated, or that her psychotic episodes
> have continued at the post-operative level.[32]

Contradictory Reports. The author is aware of no independent and detailed
follow-up studies that may have been made of Julia's case. However, a former
member of the project staff, a professional person who was particularly concerned about Julia and in a position permitting almost constant observation of
her, recalls that Mark and Ervin's treatments made Julia more despondent
and brought an end to her guitar playing and to her desire to engage in
intellectual discussion.[33]

Psychosurgery and Deviance Control

Results obtained in both animals and human beings raise serious doubts
about the purported merits of psychosurgery. The continued performance of
the procedure when its scientific foundations remain dubious and its therapeutic value has yet to be established may justifiably be considered questionable or even irresponsible. What is more ominous, however, is the increasing
promotion and practice of psychosurgery as a technique of deviance control.
The development of psychosurgery is another example of the time-honored
practice of reducing complex social problems to the status of personal infirmities.[34] The authors of *Violence and the Brain* are among those who have advanced the view that social deviance and interpersonal violence in our society
may be attributable to some kind of "brain dysfunction." It follows from this
view that amygdalectomy may be an appropriate treatment for individuals
whose brain dysfunction results in "a low threshold for impulsive violence."[35]

Other psychosurgeons have also advocated their medical procedures as an
approach to social policy planning in the area of deviance control. At the Second
International Conference of Psychosurgery in 1970, for example, Dr. M. Hunter
Brown, a California psychosurgeon, urged his colleagues "to initiate pilot programs for precise rehabilitation of the prisoner-patient who is often young and
intelligent, yet incapable of controlling various forms of violence."[36] Jessica
Mitford has recently noted, however, that the increasing popularity of
behavior alteration programs among penologists is in part due to their interest
in suppressing those prisoners who interpret prison life in socioeconomic or
racial terms.[37] These suggested uses for psychosurgery clearly involve more
than medical considerations.

Foreign psychosurgeons, it would seem, have been at least as devoted to
deviance control as their American counterparts. During 1972, a group of

German neurosurgeons performed stereotaxic psychosurgery involving the destruction of a portion of the hypothalamus upon "22 male patients, 20 of them being sexual deviants, one suffering from neurotic 'pseudo homosexuality' and one from intractable addiction to alcohol and drugs."[38] According to their report, "15 of the sexual deviants obtained a good result which was in most cases excellent with complete harmonization of sexual and social behavior."[39] In only one case were poor results acknowledged, and no cases of serious side effects were reported. In an earlier report, however, these same researchers found that their first three patients suffered a postoperative "incapacity to indulge in erotic fantasies and stimulating visions."[40] This obliteration of the patients' fantasy lives inexplicably failed to qualify as an untoward side effect in the more recent description of the same operations.

Psychosurgery explicitly aimed at taming hyperactive children has been performed in India, Thailand, Japan and the United States. In a summary of 115 patients,[41] including 39 children under the age of 11, one team recently claimed that the destruction of the cingulate gyrus, amygdala and regions of the hypothalamus "proved to be useful in the management of patients who previously could not be managed by other means."[42] An American psychosurgeon who favors the selective destruction of the thalamus in such cases has claimed to have obtained "good" or "fair" results in a majority of operations.[43] It is impossible to assess his findings in an objective fashion because of his characteristically unilluminating case reports, of which the following is typical:

> A seven-year-old mentally retarded child had sudden attacks of screaming, yelling, running and beating his head against the wall. The walls were actually indented by the blows.
>
> Following thalamotomy three years ago, the patient did not display the wild, aggressive and screaming behavior. The improved behavior was an enjoyment for both the child and the parents.[44]

Conclusion

Because the weight of the available evidence indicates that limbic system psychosurgery produces a marked deterioration in behavior, serious impairments of judgment and other disastrous social adjustment effects, and because psychosurgeons have failed to provide balanced accounts of their cases, it would appear prudent for the medical profession and the relevant regulatory agencies of state and federal government to act promptly along the following lines. First, there should be an explicit recognition that psychosurgery is a highly experimental procedure and not a proven therapeutic one as is so often alleged by its contemporary proponents. Second, psychosurgery should not be performed upon children, prisoners, involuntarily held or committed mental patients, or those deemed to be mentally retarded. Third, a registry and assessment mechanism should be established to collect and disseminate information on present and past practices in psychosurgery. One function of such an agency might be the systematic psychological assessment of surviving psychosurgery patients and post-mortem examinations of their brain tissue when they die. Fourth, there should be a temporary moratorium on all further psychosurgical operations until the risks can be weighed against the benefits discovered by a systematic and impartial review of the field.[45] Finally, basic research on brain mechanisms and behavior should be supported and extended. Carefully pursued and properly interpreted, such research offers the only reliable course of action for increasing our understanding of human brain function and its relation to behavior. A better understanding of this kind, coupled with broader public education in the brain sciences, should ultimately provide the best possible defense against the simplistic theories upon which much of contemporary psychosurgery has been built.

It would be a mistake, however, to view psychosurgery in a social vacuum. Although it has unique characteristics, psychosurgery is, in terms of social policy, merely one of a large number of psychotechnological means that are continually being advanced to deal with troublesome individuals or groups. The relevant "target populations" are vaguely defined as "aggressive," "assaultive," "volatile," "acting-out," "disruptive," "incorrigible," "uncooperative," or "dangerous." The possibility that such behavior may be justifiable is generally ignored as are the social consequences of discouraging diversity. Indeed, the physical and chemical control of disruptive behavior has been suggested in every futuristic model of technological fascism. Insofar as the causes of social conflict actually lie in the domain of social affairs, psychotechnological treatment of deviants should be regarded as a perversion of medicine and a distinct threat to individual liberty. The time has come to examine the entire spectrum of psychotechnology and to question the prevalent ideologies of behavioral prediction, modification and control. We must try, most of all, to assess the impact and social consequences of psychotechnology in the broad contexts of politics and public policy. For to deny the power and political appeal of repressive psychotechnology is to expedite its encroachment, and to refrain from combatting it is to surrender not only our constitutional freedom, but also our human dignity.

NOTES

1. This is essentially the definition given by Dr. Bertram S. Brown, Director of the National Institute of Mental Health. *See Hearings on S. 974, S. 878 and S.J. Res. 71 Before the Subcomm. on Health of the Senate Comm. on Labor and Public Welfare,* 93d Cong., 1st Sess., pt. 2, at 339 (1973).

2. Goldstein, "Brain Research and Violent Behavior," 30 *Arch. Neurol.* 1, 28 (1974).

3. *See* M. Crichton, *The Terminal Man* (1972). Thomas appears to be the model for Harry Benson, the title character in Crichton's novel. Ellis, the fictional neurosurgeon in the book, expresses with some literary license Mark and Ervin's view that psychomotor epilepsy and other brain damage are major factors in contemporary social violence and that psychosurgery offers a rational approach to the prevention of such violence. In this connection, it is of interest to note

that Crichton has added a postscript to the paperback edition of the book which reveals: "In the face of considerable controversy among clinical neuroscientists, I am persuaded that the understanding of the relationship between organic brain damage and violent behavior is not so clear as I thought at the time I wrote the book." *Id.* at 282 (1973 ed.).

4. Mark & Ervin, *Violence and the Brain,* 93–94 (1970).

5. Mark & Ervin, "Is There a Need to Evaluate the Individuals Producing Human Violence?," *Psychiat. Opinion,* Aug. 1968, at 32, 33.

6. *Id.* at 33.

7. Mark & Ervin 96.

8. Mark & Ervin, *supra* note 5, at 34.

9. *Id.*

10. *Id.*

11. Mark & Ervin 96–97.

12. *Id.* at 97.

13. *Id.* at 93.

14. Breggin, "an Independent Followup of a Person Operated upon for Violence and Epilepsy" by Drs. Vernon Mark, Frank Ervin and William Sweet of the Neuro-Research Foundation of Boston, *Rough Times,* Nov.–Dec. 1973, at 8, col. 1.

15. *Id.* at 8, col. 3.

16. *Id.*

17. *Id.*

18. *Id.* at 9, col. 2. For a description of this aspect of his "paranoia" see Mark & Ervin 93–94.

19. Thomas' discharge summary from the Veterans Administration Hospital reads: "Patient stated that . . . Massachusetts General Hospital were [sic] controlling him by creating lesions in his brain tissue some time before. Stated that they can control him, control his moods and control his actions, they can turn him up or turn him down." Breggin, *supra* note 22, at 9, col. 2. *See also* Memorandum, note 14 *infra,* at 4.

20. Breggin, *supra* note 14, at 9, col. 3.

21. Kille v. Mark, Civil No. 681998 (Super. Ct., Suffolk County, Mass., filed Dec. 3, 1973).

22. Hunt, "The Politics of Psychosurgery," Part I, *Real Paper* (Boston), May 30, 1973, at 1, col. 1, *reprinted in Rough Times,* Sept.–Oct. 1973, at 2, col. 1; Hunt, "The Politics of Psychosurgery," Part II, *Real Paper* (Boston), June 13, 1973, at 8, col. 1, *reprinted in Rough Times,* Nov.–Dec. 1973, at 6, col. 1; Trotter, Violent Brains (unpublished manuscript written for Ralph Nader's Center for Responsive Law, Washington, D.C.); Memorandum from Dr. Ernst Rodin to Dr. J. S. Gottlieb, Aug. 9, 1972, submitted as Exhibit AC-4 in Kaimowitz v. Department of Mental Health, Civil No. 73-19434-AW (Cir. Ct., Wayne County, Mich., July 10, 1973).

23. This proposed research was ultimately blocked in Kaimowitz v. Department of Mental Health, Civil No. 73-19434-AW (Cir. Ct., Wayne County, Mich., July 10, 1973), discussed elsewhere in this symposium. *See* comment, "*Kaimowitz v. Department of Mental Health:* A Right to Be Free from Experimental Psychosurgery?", 54 B.U.L. Rev. 301 (1974).

24. Memorandum, *supra* note 22, at 1.

25. *Id.* at 4.

26. *Id.*

27. Mark & Ervin 97.

28. *Id.*

29. *Id.*

30. *Id.* at 97–98.

31. *Id.* at 98.

32. *Id.* at 107–08. As late as 1972, the authors were similarly uninformative: "It is still too early to assess the results of the procedure, but the frequency of both the rage attacks and epileptic seizures have been markedly decreased since operation." Mark, Ervin & Sweet, "Deep Temporal Lobe Stimulation in Man," in *The Neurobiology of the Amygdala, supra* note 23, [in the original text] at 485, 494. *See also* Trotter, *supra* note 22, at 12 [in original text].

33. The author is in possession of an extensive record of personal observations made by this member of the project staff, who wishes to remain anonymous.

34. *See* Chorover, "Big Brother and Psychotechnology," *Psychology Today,* Oct. 1973, at 43, 45.

35. Mark & Ervin 2.

36. E. Valenstein, *Brain Control: A Critical Examination of Brain Stimulation and Psychosurgery,* 255 (1973).

37. *See* Mitford, "The Torture Cure," *Harper's,* Aug. 1973, at 16. *See also* J. Mitford, *Kind and Usual Punishment* (1973).

38. Müller, Roeder & Orthner, "Further Results of Stereotaxis in the Human Hypothalamus in Sexual Deviations, First Use of This Operation in Addiction to Drugs," 16 *Neurochirurgia* 113 (1973).

39. *Id.*

40. Roeder & Miller, "Zur Stereotaktischen Heilung der Pädophilin Homosexualität," 94 *Deutsch. Med. Wochnschr.* 409 (1969).

41. Balasubramaniam, Kanaka, Ramanugam & Ramanurthi, "Surgical Treatment of Hyperkinetic and Behavior Disorder," 54 *Int'l. Surgery* 18 (1970).

42. *Id.* at 22.

43. *Hearings, supra* note 1, at 353 (testimony of Dr. Orlando J. Andy).

44. *Id.* at 348. *See also* Andy, "Neurosurgical Treatment of Abnormal Behavior," 252 *Am. J. Med. Sci.* 232, 236–37 (1966), *reprinted in Hearings, supra* note 1, at 417, 421–22.

45. *See* S.J. Res. 86, 93d Cong., 1st Sess. (1973). This resolution, introduced by Senator Beall, calls for a two-year moratorium during which the Secretary of Health, Education and Welfare would compile and analyze the available data.

David Avery

The Case for "Shock" Therapy

Jack Nicholson in the film *One Flew Over the Cuckoo's Nest* is punished with electroconvulsive therapy (ECT) for his high-spirited capers in a mental hospital. The scene demonstrates a popular misconception of ECT as a medieval torture inflicted on helpless or nonconforming mental patients. A group called the Network Against Psychiatric Assault has asked for a total ban on ECT, describing it as a "bogus, barbaric and destructive technological weapon." Some states have passed laws restricting ECT treatment in favor, as one California legislator said, of "more creative, positive treatments." Professionals who oppose it speak of its risks and dangers. Dr. John Friedberg argues (*Psychology Today*, August 1975) that it "obliterates memory," "damages the brain," and "has caused more suicides than it has prevented."

Yet, if we take a second look at "shock treatment," we find that the opponents such as Dr. Friedberg rely on opinion and anecdote and ignore the scores of controlled studies done in recent years to attest to its safety and effectiveness. Most importantly, the movement to abolish ECT disregards the thousands of patients for whom the treatments offer the only rescue from deep and often suicidal depression.

Four controlled studies involving over 1,000 depressed patients show a lower suicide rate with ECT compared with other treatments. ECT is particularly effective in the treatment of clinical depression, which, unlike situational sadness, is associated with a very high death rate from suicide, malnutrition, heart attack, and exhaustion. Data from 15 studies involving over 4,500 depressed

From *Psychology Today* 11 (August 1977):104. Copyright © 1977 by Ziff-Davis Publishing Company. Reprinted by permission of the publisher and the author.

persons indicate that the overall death rate is significantly lower with ECT than with psychotherapy. Although antidepressant medications are also effective in less severe cases, studies demonstrate that drugs take longer than ECT to act and may prolong the agony of depression.

Introjected Anger

We don't know why ECT works, but we do know that the punishment theory is mistaken. A popular opinion is that depression represents "introjected anger." According to this theory, the fright and pain from ECT satisfies the person's need for self-punishment, and recovery takes place. Yet, ECT is painless. The patient receives an anesthetic and is unconscious during the one or two minutes of treatment.

Controlled studies were devised to test the punishment theory. Some depressed people unknowingly received a sham treatment (a subconvulsive dose of electrical current) and did no better than the controls, while those who received a dose high enough to induce a seizure experienced marked improvement. These studies prove that a seizure is necessary for the treatment to be effective, not a painful experience that "shocks" a person back to health.

Why is seizure a *sine qua non?* Evidence suggests deficiencies of two neurotransmitters in the central nervous systems of depressed persons, norepinephrine and serotonin. Even though some animal studies show increased production of these substances during seizures, it is too early to formulate a mechanism to explain how ECT works. We don't know how aspirin works either, but that doesn't diminish the empirical evidence for its efficacy.

ECT has been proven an effective treatment for depression, but is it safe? Much is made of the risk of death during ECT use, but one survey done in Denmark reveals that only one person died out of a total of the 3,438 who were treated over a one-year period. Moreover, critics who emphasize the death risk do not mention that the risk of death within the year for a depressed person *not* receiving ECT is 300 times greater. The death and brain damage that *have* been attributed to ECT are nearly always complicated by significant life-threatening problems. In his *Psychology Today* article, for example, Dr. Friedberg cited the case, in 1942, of a 57-year-old man who died after ECT and attributed the brain damage found at the autopsy to the ECT. Dr. Friedberg neglected to mention that the man had a history of severe heart damage, and that neuropathologists found the cause of death to be a heart attack. Heart damage, not ECT, is a well-documented cause of brain cell death.

A recent review by neuropathologists concludes that neuronal damage due to ECT in a physically healthy person is unlikely. At least six studies show that animals given ECT have no destruction of neurons. In addition, since 1972, two animal studies using the most sensitive microscopic techniques revealed that seizure activity comparable to ECT caused no change in the ultrastructure of the brain.

Loss of Memory

The question of whether ECT causes significant loss of memory is complicated by the memory problems associated with depression itself. Half of the depressed patients who have not received ECT complain of memory problems and often have such difficulty concentrating that they do poorly on objective memory tests. ECT does cause a few minutes of confusion on awakening and a transient memory disturbance. People are occasionally unable the remember events that happened during the few weeks of treatment. However, they are able to recall as well as ever events from the more distant past and are able to learn and retain new information as well as, or better than, before. A recent study showed progressive *improvement* in short-term memory in depressed patients receiving ECT. In 1975, a study done six months after treatment showed that on six objective memory tests, ECT patients performed as well as recovered depressed people who did not receive ECT.

Sylvia Plath's *The Bell Jar,* Robert Pirsig's brilliantly reconstructed account of his past, *Zen and the Art of Motorcycle Maintenance,* and Mark Vonnegut's *The Eden Express* are hardly the products of damaged, enfeebled minds, even though the authors all received ECT *before* the books were written.

The ECT controversy reflects a tendency to see a natural antagonism between science and humanism. Many critics reject the treatment because they wish to see the mind as separate from the brain—free from the biological whims that affect every other organ of the body. Yet, much can be learned from both the recent biological data and the insights of humanism.

Elliot S. Valenstein

Science Fiction Fantasy and the Brain

Two criminologists recently proposed an unusual method for maintaining surveillance of paroled criminals and preventing them from repeating their
crimes. Barton Ingraham and Gerald Smith suggested that the authorities
could keep track of their locations and of their physiological states by monitoring signals transmitted from their bodies. Through a signal to electrodes in the
brain, bad behavior could be deterred by "adversive" effects and good behavior rewarded by pleasurable effects. Ingraham and Smith suggest the following
scenario: "A parolee with a past record of burglaries is tracked to a downtown
shopping district (in fact, is exactly placed in a store known to be locked up for
the night) and the physiological data reveal an increased respiration rate, a
tension in the musculature, and an increased flow of adrenaline. It would be a
safe guess, certainly, that he was up to no good. The computer in this case,
weighing the probabilities, would come to a decision and alert the police or
parole officer, so that they could hasten to the scene; or, if the subject were
equipped with an implanted radiotelemeter, it could transmit an electrical signal which could block further action by the subject by causing him to forget or
abandon his project."

This proposal is not written by two science-fiction writers. Smith and Ingra-
ham are evidently qualified professionals, and their article appeared in *Issues in
Criminology,* a journal published at the University of California, Berkeley.
There is little likelihood that anyone is going to permit them to try their scheme.
What deeply concerns me is that such exaggerated and distorted portrayals of

From *Psychology Today* 12 (July 1978):29–31, 37–39. Copyright © 1978 by Ziff-Davis Publishing
Company. Reprinted by permission of the publisher and the author.

the power of brain-stimulation techniques frighten the public and could lead to suppression of very valuable research that is beginning to yield new insights into the workings of the brain. Even more important, this type of thinking diverts energy away from finding more realistic solutions to such social problems as the ones posed by recidivist criminals.

The emergence of electrical and chemical techniques for modifying the human brain has clearly aroused mixed emotions. We are fascinated by these developments and what they might tell us about ourselves. But many of us are also anxious about their use in the future. The topic can hardly be avoided, as we are constantly exposed to popular accounts in newspapers, magazines, novels, TV shows, and movies — all depicting what is presumed to be the great power of brain stimulation to control behavior, emotions, and even thoughts.

Michael Crichton's *The Terminal Man* will probably have a greater impact than Mary Shelley's *Frankenstein* not because of its literary qualities but because it has convinced many people that computerized control of the human brain is possible now, or at least not very far off in the future. A story in *Esquire* described a government of the future, an "electroligarchy" in which class distinctions were based on the number of electrodes implanted in people's brains and the amount of free will thus remaining to them. According to the article, the lowest class, the "neutrons," would have 500 electrodes inserted in their heads and would be completely robotized. "They could dig ditches all day and love every minute of it," said the story (which, incidentally, was written by David Rorvik, whose recent book, *In His Image: The Cloning of a Man,* has created a stir).

Of course, some of these stories are meant only to amuse us, but that does not stop them from having an influence. Psychiatrists see patients these days who believe their thoughts and emotions are being controlled by devices implanted in their brains while they are asleep. Though such thoughts may be paranoid, they are not very far removed from what many normal people believe is possible.

Along with fears about the misuse of brain stimulation have come equally worrisome suggestions on how this power might be used to cure seemingly intractable psychiatric and even social problems. The potential for brain interventions to achieve desirable social goals was expressed, for example, by the social psychologist Kenneth Clark in his presidential address to the American Psychological Association convention a few years ago. Clark startled a number of people in the audience, myself included, with his suggestion that "we might be on the threshold of that type of scientific biochemical intervention which could stabilize and make dominant the moral and ethical propensities of man and subordinate, if not eliminate, his negative and primitive behavioral tendencies." Clark also suggested that all political leaders should be required to "accept and use the earliest perfected form of psychotechnological, biomedical intervention which would assure their positive use of power and reduce or block the possibility of using power destructively." The fact that this fantastic suggestion comes from a respected social scientist — a member of a minority group that is usually very reluctant to accept biological explanations and remedies for social behavior—indicates the widespread influence of the new developments in brain technology.

In order to discuss the problems raised by the new techniques realistically, it is essential to separate fact from fantasy. A closer examination of the results of some typical experiments may be the best antidote for the more common misconceptions. By now, José Delgado's demonstration in the bull-fight arena is well-known. An article in the *New York Times* was typical of the way the former Yale University researcher's experiment has been reported: "Dr. Delgado implanted a radio-controlled electrode deep within the brain of a *brave bull,* a variety bred to respond with a raging charge when it sees any human being. But when Delgado pressed a button on a transmitter, sending a signal to a battery-powered receiver attached to the bull's horns, an impulse went into the bull's brain and the animal would cease his charge. After several stimulations, the bull's naturally aggressive behavior disappeared. It was as placid as Ferdinand."

What really happened? After receiving the stimulus, the bull simply stopped charging and turned away from its target. The stimulation forced the bull to keep turning in the same direction. From popular accounts of this demonstration, it would be easy to conclude that we are close to being able to control aggression by modifying the activity of a specific brain area. In fact, there is no convincing evidence that the stimulation had a specific effect on the bull's aggressive tendencies. We can only conclude that the stimulus led to the stereotyped—repetitive—circling movement. (Patients who have had electrodes placed in this brain region—it is called the caudate nucleus—also respond to stimulation by exhibiting various types of motor responses, that is, movements.) In Delgado's demonstration, it would be closer to the truth to say the bull was *confused,* not pacified. But it is much more dramatic to talk about controlling aggression.

Aggression does not live in the caudate nucleus or in any other single brain area. When we speak of behavior as complex as aggression, it is clear that a large amount of the brain is involved. Moreover, any single area plays a role in many different kinds of behavior—some desirable, some undesirable, depending on circumstances and our own attitudes, at any given moment, about what is desirable. The belief that we can stimulate or destroy a given region of the brain and change one and only one type of behavior is sheer fantasy.

Let's look at another example. People often assume, even those who should know better, that it is possible to arouse distinct motivational states by electrical stimulation of specific areas of the brain. The experimental literature contains cases of animals that have supposedly been made hungry, thirsty, maternal, sexy, and so on, by brain stimulation. There is usually the implication that such natural motivational states can be turned on and off with a great amount of reliability and selectivity.

In my own laboratory, my collaborators and I have shown (in many different ways) that brain stimulation does not duplicate natural motivational states. Instead it evokes behavior that is *stereotyped and has a very compulsive quality*. For example, when an animal's brain is stimulated, it may start to eat food, but only one type of food and not another. A stimulated rat may not even eat the same food if the form of its meal is modified slightly, for example, if food pellets are served as a mash. More recently, Gary Berntson at Ohio State has demonstrated that hungry cats, when stimulated, may leave a dish of highly preferred liquid tuna fish and eat much less preferred dry cat chow. To put it simply, these stimulated animals do not behave as if they were hungry. Also, stimulation does not always produce the same behavior. A rat may eat only food when stimulated. Later, when stimulated again, it may start to drink, or show some other behavior, even though the intensity of the stimulation remains the same. This is quite different from the belief that stimulation at one brain site invariably makes the animal hungry, while at other sites it makes him thirsty, aggressive, maternal, sexy, and so forth.

If the response to brain stimulation is variable in inbred rats, it is certainly much more variable in monkeys, apes, and man. In monkeys, for example, brain stimulation may initiate drinking when the animal is confined to a restraining chair. But when the same stimulation is administered to monkeys who are in a cage and not restrained, they do not drink even though they may be sitting within inches of the water dispenser. Delgado recently described gibbons tested in his former laboratory at Yale that began to fight when stimulated in a particular area of their brain (central gray). However, when he moved the animals to an open field on Hall Island in Bermuda, the same gibbons would run into the bushes without expressing any hostility, even though the brain stimulation was identical in all respects. (Apparently, a Caribbean vacation can do much for the disposition of apes as well as man.) In both these examples, it is clear that environmental factors determined the results of stimulation.

In humans, brain stimulation may evoke general emotional states that are somewhat predictable, in that certain areas tend to produce unpleasant feelings and others more positive emotional states. Patients may report feeling "tension," "agitation," "anxiety," "fear," or "anger"; or they may describe their feelings as very "pleasant" or "relaxed." Different patients report different feelings from stimulation of what is presumed to be the same brain area, and the same person may have very different experiences from identical stimulation administered at different times. The impression that brain stimulation in humans can repeatedly evoke the same emotional state, the same memory, or the same behavior is simply a myth.

The brain is not organized into neat compartments that correspond to the value-laden labels we assign to behavior. A concept such as aggression is a man-made abstraction that does not exist as a separate entity in the nervous system. Aggression is clearly a heterogeneous concept, and many parts of the brain play a role in different aspects of its expression. And each of these parts also plays a role in other traits as well, including some we think of as having positive aspects, such as self-assertiveness and ambition.

The earliest information on the effects of brain stimulation on humans was obtained by neurosurgeons. They stimulated the brains of awake patients before surgery as a means of reducing the chance of damaging some area essential to speech or other important functions. More recently, doctors have implanted electrodes in the brains of patients—and left them there for months, in some cases—for both diagnostic and therapeutic purposes. Diagnostically, the electrodes are used primarily to find an abnormal brain locus that may be responsible for triggering epileptic seizures and to decide if it can be excised surgically. In therapeutic uses, doctors stimulate the brain in attempts to inhibit areas responsible for intractable pain, epileptic seizures, and certain severe spastic muscle conditions.

These treatments are new and controversial, but some success has been reported. Most controversial is the therapeutic use of brain stimulation on psychiatric patients. At Tulane University, Robert Heath claims that the procedure has significantly improved very severely disturbed schizophrenic patients. Reaction to Heath's work ranges from interest to disbelief and outrage; opinions vary, both among professionals and laymen, on how much of this work is justifiable and acceptable. But there is no reason to believe that brain stimulation will have wide application in the treatment of psychiatric disorders.

Explanatory models for psychiatric disorders vary greatly, and anyone who is smart will not choose sides. At one extreme is Thomas Szasz's position that mental illness is a myth, reflecting society's arbitrary labels for behavior it considers deviant. Others argue that at least some psychiatric illness—for example, schizophrenia—can be attributed to inherited enzyme deficiencies that result in abnormal brain chemistry. Somewhere in between are most of the behavior therapists, who argue that psychiatric disorders are not diseases but learned, maladaptive response patterns.

There is some validity to each of these positions, depending upon which psychiatric problem you are talking about. Nevertheless, there are certain people who feel there is something inherently evil in searching for biological causes.

It is well to recall that not so very long ago, our lunatic asylums, as they were called, were filled with people who were suffering from an unrecognized vitamin-deficiency disease, pellagra, but their symptoms—depression, dementia, and even hallucinations—were attributed to mental problems. One of the most common diagnostic labels in asylums around the turn of the century was GPI—general paralysis of the insane, or general paresis—a type of neurosyphilis. The maniacal outbursts, depression, or memory loss in such patients were considered mental problems; there were no other obvious symptoms of their infection.

We don't even have to go back as far as the turn of the century. An article in a recent issue of the *American Journal of Psychiatry* describes a number of patients who suffered from a contortion of the limbs or torso that was diagnosed as a conversion hysteria. Many were given psychoanalytic treatment for periods of up to two years without any success. It was subsequently discovered that they were suffering from an inherited form of the disorder called dystonia.

Parkinson's disease was also considered a conversion hysteria by the French neurologist Charcot, who attempted to treat it with psychotherapy. Victims of this disease exhibited movement disorders, tremors, but particularly an inertia—a difficulty in initiating motion. Although several researchers had reported peculiarities in specific regions of the brains after autopsies on Parkinson patients, most of what we know about the disease was put together in the last 20 years. Through brain-staining techniques, we now know a great deal about the biochemistry of different brain circuits. Swedish investigators had described a circuit in the brain that uses the chemical substance called dopamine for transmitting impulses from one nerve to the next. Most of the brain's dopamine was found to be concentrated in a relatively limited area. Interestingly, the circuit originated in a region called the *substantia nigra,* an area early neuroanatomists had suspected was abnormal in patients with Parkinson's disease. Cells in the *substantia nigra* normally contain a black pigment (thus the name), but the number of these pigmented cells—which contain dopamine, as we now know—were significantly reduced in Parkinson patients.

This dopamine circuit that originates in the *substantia nigra* terminates in the caudate nucleus—the brain region where Delgado placed his electrodes in the bull experiment. During the last 20 years, it was discovered in quick succession that (1) animals whose dopamine levels were reduced by biochemical techniques developed Parkinson-like symptoms, and (2) Parkinson patients had significantly lower levels of dopamine metabolites in their urine. In autopsies on Parkinson victims, researchers also observed that the levels of dopamine in the caudate nucleus were abnormally low.

A great number of these unfortunate people received some relief from the discovery of L-dopa, a precursor, or building block, that the brain can use to produce dopamine. L-dopa therapy followed quite naturally from advances in our knowledge of brain chemistry. It does not provide relief for all patients, but it has certainly relieved many more than would have been helped by psychotherapy.

Parkinson's disease is not simply a movement disorder. It is really a disorder that interferes with the integration of sensory and motor events. There are also emotional complications as well. The patients exhibit reduced responsiveness to strong stimuli and are often depressed. With an extra challenge, however, some patients suddenly show a remarkable reduction in symptoms. For example, some severely debilitated Parkinson patients cannot walk without help. But if white lines are painted on the floor and patients are asked to step over them, they often can step out briskly. Some of the patients carry bits of paper in their pockets that they can scatter in front of them and step on or over them. Other patients who have great difficulty walking have much less of a problem when confronted with the special challenge of mounting steps, dancing, or even swimming. In emergencies such as a fire, Parkinson patients may run quite well. Apparently, potent stimuli can induce an emotional reaction that makes movement possible. The dopamine system seems to play a critical role in regulating emotional arousal and this is somehow involved in the process that translates sensory input into motor output. Because this system is very markedly dampened in Parkinson patients, stimuli that are stronger than usual are required to arouse them emotionally and to generate action.

Although it may not be immediately apparent, our knowledge of the function of the dopamine system is helping us understand why brain stimulation evokes certain behavior patterns. In brain-stimulation experiments on animals, the electrodes are located in brain areas where they can *excite* this same dopamine circuit. The results, therefore, are opposite to those seen in the Parkinson patients. The animals become hyperactive and very responsive to external stimuli. Because the electrical stimulation activates the dopamine circuit on only one side of the brain, the animals tend to eat, drink, or attack another animal only if the stimulus (food, water, or a suitable prey) is presented to one side of their field of vision and not the other. This has been demonstrated most convincingly by John Flynn at Yale, who has shown that normally peaceful cats can be transformed by brain stimulation into mouse killers, but will attack a mouse only when it is visible to one eye and not the other. Although there is no convincing evidence that direct activation of dopamine pathways underlies *all* of the behavior evoked by brain stimulation, researchers have consistently found enhanced responsiveness to stimulation on one side of the body.

It is also possible to destroy the dopamine system on only one side of the brain by using electrolytic current or injecting selective neurotoxins that destroy dopamine-secreting nerve cells. Two physiological psychologists, John Marshall and Philip Teitelbaum, have shown that when the system is thus destroyed in animals, they do not respond to touch or smells presented to one side of their body, even though they respond normally to the same stimuli presented to the other side. Animals showing this reaction—which is called sensory-neglect syndrome—are relatively unresponsive to many different stimuli. They are lethargic and emotionally unresponsive; they eat much less food and are less interested in a sexual partner.

If an area of the brain near the dopamine circuit (the ventromedial hypothalamic area) is destroyed, the opposite occurs. The animals overeat and overrespond to stimuli. They tend to be hyperkinetic, irritable, hyperemotional, and even overly sensitive to tastes—that is why they are said to be finicky eaters. There is some evidence that destruction of this more medial brain area activates the dopamine circuit by removing a normal inhibitory influence.

Of great theoretical and clinical relevance here are the observations that amphetamine—which activates dopamine pathways—produces stereotyped behavior in animals and a heightened responsiveness to at least some stimuli.

Thus, a rat given amphetamines will almost always display a stereotyped sniffing or gnawing restricted to some specific part of its environment. Different species display other behavior in response to amphetamine injections. Cats will move their heads back and forth repeatedly. The reactions of monkeys and man are not as predictable, but each individual tends to repeat some idiosyncratic behavior pattern and commonly has heightened and distorted perceptual experiences. People who take large doses of amphetamines may have visual hallucinations. Others may experience the sensation of parasites under the skin and engage in uncontrollable scratching. "Speed freaks" have become thoroughly trapped in the performance of some repetitive act — taking apart a clock or rearranging a pocketbook — during which time they are unresponsive to other stimuli. This abnormal focusing of behavior has been called "punding" in the drug culture in Sweden and "knick-knacking" in San Francisco's Haight-Ashbury.

The stereotyped behavior and hypersensitivity of animals and people given large doses of amphetamine are considered a useful model for the study of schizophrenia. In fact, the drugs that are most effective in blocking amphetamine-induced stereotyped behavior in animals are generally the drugs most effective in reducing schizophrenic symptoms.

It is recognized that perceptual distortions such as hallucinations and heightened sensitivity to stimuli, as well as stereotyped behavior, are common features of schizophrenia. Indeed, only a short time ago, most psychiatrists had little experience with speed freaks and commonly diagnosed them as paranoid schizophrenics. Of course, thought disorder is a very important part of schizophrenia, but some researchers now suggest that such symptoms develop as a reaction to what has been referred to as the "perceptual onslaught" from an overwhelming sensitivity to stimuli. Perceptual distortions may be the *cause* of thought disorder, rather than the other way around, as has been traditionally argued.

It appears that Parkinson's disease and schizophrenia seem to reflect abnormal hypo- or hyperexcitement of a dopamine circuit. Although this is clearly an oversimplification, Parkinson patients have a deficiency of dopamine, are unresponsive to stimuli, and have difficulty initiating movement. Schizophrenic patients are hyperresponsive to stimuli, often display spontaneous stereotyped motor acts, and, at least judging by the effectiveness of anti-dopamine drugs, may have overactive dopamine circuits. No evidence of excessive dopamine has been found, but several investigators have reported an abnormally high number of dopamine receptors in the brains of schizophrenic patients, including a few who have not had any medication.

Increasing dopamine levels in Parkinson patients by giving them L-dopa sometimes causes hallucinations and other psychiatric complications. Dopamine-blocking drugs given to schizophrenics in large doses over long periods cause motor disturbances referred to as tardive dyskinesia. It would be an oversimplification, however, to conclude that Parkinson's disease and schizophrenia represent opposite processes. Several cases of patients who have both these disorders have been reported. The fact that there are actually several partially overlapping dopamine circuits has raised the possibility that one pathway may be more critical for Parkinson symptoms while the other may be so for psychiatric disorders.

Several investigators have reported that the antipsychotic drugs that are most effective in reducing the symptoms of schizophrenics — the phenothiazines and butyrophenones — are most effective in preventing dopamine release or in occupying dopamine receptors in a way that prevents their activation. In contrast, drugs that activate the dopamine system, such as amphetamine, precipitate psychoses in patients diagnosed as premorbid schizophrenics.

Philip Seeman and Tyrone Lee of the University of Toronto have recently shown a strong relationship between the relative effectiveness of different drugs in reducing schizophrenic symptoms and the capacity of these drugs to inhibit the release of dopamine in brain tissue slices containing dopamine neurons and to block the dopamine receptors in brain-tissue homogenates. All of this evidence (and there is much more) suggests that there are dopamine circuits that play a crucial role in normal and abnormal behavior by adjusting the responsiveness of sensory-motor systems.

Ultimately, if we have sufficient understanding of the brain, we will be in a better position to help those who need help in ways that everyone agrees are desirable. But the preoccupation with control rather than understanding could set back such efforts considerably.

I, too, recognize that there are dangers. Patients clearly need protection from unjustifiable exposure to innovative therapies, but it could be equally dangerous, I believe, to unnecessarily restrict biologically oriented research through government intervention.

Many people fear that the techniques of brain stimulation could be used to control political dissenters or militant minority groups. Some claim, for example, that poor people, blacks, and women are the principal recipients not only of brain stimulation but also psychosurgery. Such was the view in an often-cited article several years ago in *Ebony* magazine entitled "Psychosurgery: A New Threat to Blacks."

The charges are not true. Although research on humans should be continually scrutinized for possible abuses, the best data have shown that the poor, blacks, and other minorities are significantly underrepresented in this patient population.

There is no doubt that our present understanding of how an intractable psychiatric disorder can be changed by any physical intervention into the brain is extremely crude. Nevertheless, these techniques should be evaluated primarily on the basis of the possibility of their improving a patient's life, the risks of physical, emotional, and intellectual impairment, the alternative effective therapies that are available, and the consequences of "doing nothing." In such controversies, the evidence will not be convincing, and even experts will differ in their conclusions.

There is a great danger, however, in deciding these questions in the political arena, with hastily written legislation. For example, a bill recently proposed by Rep. Louis Stokes of Ohio would prohibit psychosurgery in federally supported institutions for purposes other than treatment of a brain disease that has already been diagnosed. Such is the looseness of the wording that it is not even clear whether electrical stimulation of the brain is included in the definition of psychosurgery. The bill would ban the use of brain surgery for "modification or control of thoughts, feelings, actions, or behavior." It speaks of the "awesome potential" of psychosurgery as a weapon for repression of minority groups, political dissenters, and the poor.

Again, the language is pure fantasy that exaggerates the power of the techniques and is based on unfounded fears. If passed, such legislation would establish the risky precedent of giving Congress or state legislatures the power to decide on the legitimacy and efficacy of any number of medical procedures which may affect us all.

We are all aware of the increasing concern over the ethical and social implications of scientific research. This is a very healthy and much-needed development. It would, however, be naive to believe that all the good motives belong with those who espouse so-called ethical causes, while all the bad motives belong to those they criticize. From my perspective, it does not seem that the people who are raising ethical issues are more immune to the lure of prestige, power, and prosperity than those engaged in research. We need muckrakers and gadflies to get issues on the agenda, but solutions will not come from the moral crusaders who insist on distorting the evidence and reducing complex issues to the simplistic level of the "good guys versus the bad guys."

Legislation that is hastily written in response to demands and demagogy and based on distortions may do more harm than the problem it is attempting to remedy. If we attempt to legislate iron-clad protections against every possible perversion of scientific knowledge — no matter how remote the danger — we are going to create such cumbersome controls that the most creative people will be driven out of the field. We must, above all, distinguish carefully between real and imagined dangers.

Suggestions for Further Reading

Psychosurgery, Electroshock, and Electrostimulation

Annas, George J. "Psychosurgery: Procedural Safeguards." *Hastings Center Report* 7 (April 1977):230-233.

Avery, David. "The Case for 'Shock' Therapy." *Psychology Today* 11 (August 1977):104.

Beresford, H. Richard. "Legal Issues Relating to Electroconvulsive Therapy." *Archives of General Psychiatry* (August 1971):100-102.

Blachly, P. H. "Attitudes, Data and Technological Promise of ECT." *Psychiatric Opinion* 14 (1977):9-12.

———. "New Developments in Electroconvulsive Therapy." *Diseases of the Nervous System* 37 (June 1976):356-358.

Brady, John P., and Brodie, H. Keith, eds. *Controversy in Psychiatry*. Philadelphia: W. B. Saunders Co., 1978, Chs. 3 & 4.

Breggin, Peter R. *Electroshock: Its Brain-Disabling Effects*. New York: Springer, 1979.

———. "Psychosurgery for the Control of Violence — Including a Critical Examination of the Work of Vernon Mark and Frank Ervine." *Congressional Record* 118 (March 30, 1972):E3380-E3386.

———. "The Return of Lobotomy and Psychosurgery." *Congressional Record* 118 (February 24, 1972):E1602-E1612.

———. "The Second Wave." *Mental Hygiene* 57 (1973):10-13.

Bridges, P. K., and Bartless, J. R. "Psychosurgery: Yesterday and Today." *British Journal of Psychiatry* 131 (September 1977):249-260.

Burt, Robert A. "Why We Should Keep Prisoners From the Doctors: Reflections on the Detroit Psychosurgery Case." *Hastings Center Report* 5 (February 1975):25–34.

Coleman, Lee. "And Now, Medicare for Psychosurgery?" *Inquiry* (February 5, 1979):11–14.

Crichton, Michael. *The Terminal Man.* New York: Bantam Books, 1972.

"Debate Over Psychosurgery." *Journal of the American Medical Association* 225 (August 20, 1973):913–920.

Delgado, José M. R. *Physical Control of the Mind: Towards a Psychocivilized Society.* New York: Harper & Row, 1969.

———. "Psychocivilized Direction of Behavior." *Humanist* (March-April 1972):10–15.

"Electrical Stimulation of the Brain" and "Electroconvulsive Therapy." In Reich, Warren T., ed. *Encyclopedia of Bioethics* Vol. I. New York: The Free Press, 1978, pp. 356–361.

Fried, Samuel, ed. *Psychosurgery: A Multidisciplinary Symposium.* Lexington, Massachusetts: D. C. Health and Co., 1974.

Friedberg, John. "ECT as a Neurologic Injury." *Psychiatric Opinion* 14 (January-February 1977):16–19.

Gaylin, Willard M., Meister, Josel S., and Neville, Robert C. *Operating on the Mind. The Psychosurgery Conflict.* New York: Basic Books, 1975.

Hodson, John D. "Reflections Concerning Violence and the Brain." *Criminal Law Bulletin* 9 (October 1973):684–702.

Holden, Constance. "Psychosurgery: Legitimate Therapy or Laundered Lobotomy?" *Science* 179 (1973):1109–1112.

Kieffer, George H. *Bioethics: A Textbook of Issues.* Reading, Massachusetts: Addison-Wesley Publishing Co., 1979, pp. 262–283.

Laitinen, Lauri V., and Livingston, Kenneth E., eds. *Surgical Approaches in Psychiatry.* Baltimore: University Park Press, 1973.

London, Perry. *Behavior Control.* New York: New American Library, 1977.

———. "Legislating the Brain: The Citizen as Patient." *Columbia Forum* 1 (1972):2–7.

Mark, Vernon H. "Brain Surgery in Aggressive Epileptics." *Hastings Center Report* 3 (February 1973):1–5.

Mark, Vernon H., and Ervin, F. R. *Violence and the Brain.* New York: Harper and Row, 1970.

Mark, Vernon, and Neville, Robert. "Brain Surgery in Aggressive Epileptics." *Journal of the American Medical Association* 226 (November 12, 1973): 765–772.

Miller, Henry. "Psychosurgery and Dr. Breggin." *New Scientist* 27 (July 1972): 188–190.

Murphy, Jeffrie G. "Total Institutions and the Possibility of Consent to Organic Therapies." *Human Rights* (Fall 1975):25–45.

"Physical Manipulation of the Brain." *Hastings Center Report* (Special supplement, May 1973).

"Psychosurgery." In Reich, Warren T., ed. *Encyclopedia of Bioethics* Vol. III New York: The Free Press, 1978, pp. 1387–1392.

Restack, Richard M. *Premeditated Man: Bioethics and the Control of Future Human Life.* New York: Penguin Books, 1977, Ch. 1.

Robinson, Mary F., and Freeman, Walter. *Psychosurgery and the Self.* New York: Grune & Stratton, 1954.

Salzman, Carl. "ECT and Ethical Psychiatry." *American Journal of Psychiatry* 134 (September 1977):1006–1009.

Schwitzgebel, Robert L., and Schwitzgebel, Ralph K., eds. *Psychotechnology: Electronic Control of Mind and Behavior.* New York: Holt, Rinehart & Winston, Inc., 1973.

Scovern, Albert W., and Kilman, Peter R. "Status of Electroconvulsive Therapy: Review of the Outcome Literature." *Psychological Bulletin* 87 (March 1980):260–303.

Shapiro, Michael H., and Spece, Roy G., Jr. *Bioethics and Law.* St. Paul, Minnesota: West Publishing Co., 1981, Chs. 4, 6.

Shuman, Samuel I. "The Emotional, Medical and Legal Reasons for the Special Concern About Psychosurgery." In Frank J. Ayd, ed. *Medical, Moral and Legal Issues in Mental Health Care.* Baltimore: The Williams & Wilkins Co., 1974, pp. 48–80.

————. *Psychosurgery and the Medical Control of Violence.* Detroit: Wayne State University Press, 1977.

Smith, J. Sidney, and Kiloh, L. G., eds. *Psychosurgery and Society.* New York: Pergamon Press, 1977.

Smith, W. Lynn, and King, Arthur, eds. *Issues in Brain/Behavior Control.* New York: Spectrum Publications, 1976.

Synder, Solomon H. *Madness and the Brain.* New York: McGraw-Hill, 1973.

Spoonhour, J. M. "Psychosurgery and Informed Consent." *University of Florida Law Review* 26 (Spring 1974):432–452.

Valenstein, Elliot S. *Brain Control: A Critical Examination of Brain Stimulation and Psychosurgery.* New York: John Wiley & Sons, 1973.

————. "Science-Fiction Fantasy and the Brain." *Psychology Today* 12 (July 1978):38ff.

————, ed. *The Psychosurgery Debate: Scientific, Legal, and Ethical Perspectives.* San Francisco: W. H. Freeman, 1980.

Winter, A., ed. *The Surgical Control of Behavior.* Springfield, Illinois: Charles Thomas, Publisher, 1971.

8. Controversial Behavior Control Therapies
Drugs, Behavior Modification, and Sterilization

Introduction

There is little doubt that psychotropic drugs have helped to revolutionize the quality of care and the quality of life presently available to patients in mental hospitals, as Gerald L. Klerman points out in the opening essay of this section. Although other factors have been involved, such as economics and heightened sensitivity to human rights, little doubt exists that drugs play a major role in enabling hundreds of thousands of former mental patients to be released from, and to be maintained outside of, mental hospitals during the past 25 years. Klerman reviews the major types of psychotropic medication currently in use in mental hospitals and explores both their strengths and limitations. Among their limitations, we find that although most are not addictive, some are. They do not cure, but offer only chemical maintenance. However, without pejorative connotations, the same may be said for insulin shots administered to diabetics, kidney machines for renal failures, and pacemakers for those with coronary problems. There are some mental disabilities for which no effective chemotherapies have yet been developed. Drugs may be, and often have been, used improperly as "chemical strait jackets" rather than in their therapeutic capacity to restore high functioning and enhanced rational autonomy. Inadequate testing has left the safety and effectiveness of many psychotropics in doubt. The antipsychotics may have highly undesirable long-term side effects such as tardive dyskinesia. This is an iatrogenic disease, i.e. one caused by long-term medical treatment itself. When high doses of antipsychotic medication are administered for two years or more, especially in combination with anticholinergic agents, irreversible and incurable brain damage may occur which manifests itself in rhythmic involuntary movements and loss of muscular control. This usually begins with facial muscles and spreads to limbs, trunk, and occasionally to muscles which control breathing, swallowing, and speaking. It may affect up to forty percent of chronic institutionalized patients. However, medications often involve trade-offs, and, on reflection, many persons might be quite willing to accept some of this in exchange for many years of high functioning which would not be available otherwise. New preventive measures are also being developed for tardive dyskinesia. Over-medication has become a problem in recent years; but on the whole, if properly used, psychotropic drugs seem to measure up quite well by the criteria of acceptability given in the introduction to the preceding section.

Almost everything that happens to patients in mental hospitals is called "therapy," all of which is supposedly directed toward solving the patient's "problem." Different schools of psychology tend to have radically different conceptions of what a patient's problem really is. Some see the problem as a functional "mental illness" underlying strange behaviors and belonging to the realm of the "psychological." Some see strange behaviors as being caused by environmental stresses, particularly in the patient's family situation; and that is regarded as his problem. Others view the problem as organic and locate it in abnormal brain structure and chemistry. Still others insist that all of the above are irrelevant and that the aberrant behavior itself is the problem. The behavioristic school of psychology takes this view, and much of the behavior modification therapy developed in recent years has emerged from this theoretical perspective. Behavior modification attempts to get at the "real problem" in a direct, quick, and economical way, without appeal to mysterious mental causes or nonexistent organic abnormalities, and without objectionable bodily interventions or years of expensive and ineffective talk-therapy. Theodore Ayllon explores the therapeutic and ethical advantages and disadvantages of a number of behavior modification techniques widely used in institutions, such as desensitization, token economies, aversive conditioning, and others. He insists that behavior modification techniques ought never dehumanize the patient by violating basic legal and moral rights, though this has not always been observed. In guaranteeing a patient's right to the basic necessities of a dignified human existence, therapists are forbidden to employ some powerful human motivators: e.g., the deprivation of food, drink, shelter, safety, privacy, and the like. But the potential for patient abuse unless certain fundamentals are assured is so overwhelming that this price must be paid. Ingenious behavior modifiers still have enormous room for therapeutic maneuvering even after the essential patient rights have been assured.

Sterilization is one of the most controversial therapies used on the mentally ill and the retarded. Recent federal regulations have made the use of this procedure on low income persons almost impossible, as Rosalind Petchesky indicates. In the past, it has been widely used and is still available to higher income families who do not depend upon federal financing. Petchesky examines the many reasons for prohibiting it, such as its typical imposition without non-coerced informed consent, failure to provide or advise less restrictive alternatives, and the discriminatory manner in which it is applied. Most sterilized persons have been women. Even if it were true that mentally retarded persons make poor parents, we do not sterilize *all* poor parents. And even if there are genetic factors involved in mental illness and retardation, we do not sterilize *all* persons with physical and mental genetic diseases that are equally debilitating, costly to society, and have equal probabilities of genetic transmission to offspring. If population pressures some day force our society to adopt a program of involuntary eugenics, justice would still require that we afford persons with mental disabilities *equal* protection under the law, which we clearly have not been giving them in the past.

Gerald L. Klerman

Psychotropic Drugs as Therapeutic Agents

Concern over psychotropic drugs is among the oldest and newest of civilization's preoccupations. At the dawn of civilization, in the ancient Middle East, alcoholic ferments were widely utilized, having been developed at about the same time as the domestication of animals, the discovery of agriculture, and the creation of the first cities. Almost every society since has developed various potents, brews, and remedies aimed at changing mood and behavior, be it disturbed or normal. The ancient Greek Homeric legends contain discussions of various drugs which today we would consider psychotropic. In Western society, scientific interest in psychotropic drugs emerged in the middle of the nineteenth century when pharmacology and psychology developed as distinctive scientific disciplines. In France, Austria, England, and the U.S.A., interest grew in the opiates, in hashish, and in other derivatives of cannabis and in cocaine as Western European scientific and intellectual circles became increasingly aware of drugs used for psychotropic purposes in the cultures of South America, the Middle East, and the Orient.

Psychopharmacology did not emerge as a distinct science, however, until the decade after World War II. The term psychopharmacology had been used in the 1940s and 1950s in a few scientific articles, but it was not until the discovery of LSD by Hoffman in 1943 and the synthesis and clinical introduction of chlorpromazine by French pharmacologists that a systematic, scientific investigation of drugs which affect the mind reached self-conscious and organized proportions. The pace quickened rapidly after Laborit, Delay, and

From *Hastings Center Studies* 2 (1974):81–93. Copyright © 1974 by The Hastings Center. Reprinted by permission of the publisher and the author.

Deniker introduced chlorpromazine in 1952. In the next few years, the pace of development rapidly accelerated. Dozens of new compounds were developed for therapeutic investigational use, various national and international societies were formed, and federal and other support emerged.

In large part, the rapid growth and wide impact are consequences of the recent development of pharmacologic compounds which alter mental functioning and of the reevaluation of previously used substances such as alcohol and cannabis in the light of advanced psychopharmacologic techniques. The findings from neurobiology, neurochemistry, and neurophysiology have also made it increasingly possible to relate the psychological effects of psychotropic drugs with normal biological mechanisms of action upon the brain.

Now, in the early 1970s, in the public arena as well as in scientific circles, there is widespread interest in psychotropic drugs, those which influence the mind and alter behavior, mood, and mental functioning. The science of psychopharmacology is growing rapidly and serves often as the interface between psychiatry, psychology, pharmacology, and neurophysiology, and the field is coming to have implications for education, law, religion, and sociology.

Today, the science of psychopharmacology encompasses the study of a wide range of compounds, only some of which are being used for therapeutic purposes.[1] Reevaluating previously used compounds in light of new discoveries of the relationship between the brain and behavior, it is possible to regard psychotropic drugs as falling into three main groups depending on the purpose for which the drug is used. These groups are:

1. *Therapeutic agents.* Those psychotropic drugs such as antipsychotic, antidepressant, antianxiety agents used for treatment of psychiatric disorders. The success of these compounds has contributed greatly to the changes in the therapy of mental illness and to man's greater awareness of the potentialities of psychopharmacology.

2. *Drugs used for nontherapeutic purposes* — recreation or personal enjoyment. It is indicative of the ambivalence of our society towards these compounds that no generally agreed upon term exists for this use of psychotropic drugs. Included in this group are alcohol, hashish, marijuana, and other derivatives of cannabis, the various hallucinogens (also called psychomimetics) and psychedelics, including LSD, psilocybin, and mescaline, and the various opiates including morphine and heroin. These drugs have in common the capacity to alter the normal mood state in a way that subjects find pleasurable and seek repeated experience without being directly involved in treatment of defined mental illness of psychological disturbances.

3. *Drugs to enhance performance and capabilities.* Although, at the present time, there are relatively few drugs which have the demonstrated capacity to enhance performance, this area probably represents the future scope of psychotropic drugs. Currently, drugs such as caffeine, and at times amphetamines, are used to counter fatigue and to alter the decrement of performance associated with drowsiness. The hope for the future is to develop drugs which will

enhance normal performance by improving memory, learning, sexual ability, and intellectual functioning.

This paper will deal predominantly with the current therapeutic use of psychotropic drugs. Despite current criticism of the medical model both within and without psychiatry and the behavioral sciences, it is my conviction that the best way to initiate analysis of these problems is from the vantage point of medical practice and biomedical research. However, it soon becomes evident that one must go beyond the concerns of therapeutic practice. Use of these drugs generates controversy and conflict in society since we have not yet determined the modes by which individuals and groups should regulate and control consciousness, emotional states, or behavior by use of psychotropic drugs.

Classes of Psychotropic Drugs Used as Therapeutic Agents

The treatment of mental illness has been dramatically changed, if not revolutionized, since the mid–1950s when pharmacotherapeutic agents had their first impact. During a brief period, four new types of drugs were introduced into therapeutic practice: chlorpromazine, rauwolfia, meprobamate, and imipramine. The dramatic effects of these drugs on a wide variety of mental and other illnesses not only has influenced therapeutic practice but also has led to increasing sophistication in the evaluation of these compounds. Because of initial skepticism about their efficacy, considerable effort was expended to develop new research techniques, and new methods evolved such as the double-blind and placebo-controlled trials, advanced descriptive techniques, psychometric evaluation, and multivariate statistical techniques dependent upon computer technologies in the evaluations. As a further consequence, the demonstrations of the therapeutic efficacy of these compounds generated questions about their modes of action on the brain and precipitated a vigorous interchange between clinical investigators in neurochemistry and neurophysiology.

In this section of my paper, I will describe the main class of drugs used as therapeutic agents, their range of efficacy, and their place in modern psychiatry.

It is conventional to divide the main classes of drugs used as therapeutic agents into three groups: *antipsychotic drugs* (those used in the treatment of major mental illnesses, including schizophrenia and related syndromes such as paranoia and catatonia); *antidepressant drugs*; and *antianxiety drugs*.

Antipsychotic Drugs[2]

1. The *phenothiazines* are the largest group and the most widely used. Chlorpromazine, the prototypic drug, was the first compound established as efficacious for psychoses and remains the reference compound. There are at

least a dozen other phenothiazines available for use in the United States, but their similarities are so great that most generalizations can encompass the whole group. Existing differences are related mainly to dosage, side effects, and pharmacologic properties. Included in this group are chlorpromazine (Thorazine), promazine (Sparine), thioridazine (Mellaril), perphenazine (Trilifon), trifluroperazine (Stelazine), and fluphenazine (Prolixin).

2. The *thioxanthines* (Taractan and Narvene) are closely related to the phenothiazines in their chemical structure, pharmacologic actions, and range of clinical effects; but they have not yet achieved wide popularity, as indicated by the number of prescriptions written. Some clinicians report that the thioxanthines may have greater sedative-hypnotic and mood elevating effects than the phenothiazines, and thus advocate them for the treatment of agitated depression and mixed anxiety-depressive states. These claims, however, have not yet been fully substantiated.

3. The *rauwolfia derivatives* are of considerable historical and research interest. Their current use derives from the experience of Indian medicine and the subsequent isolation by Swiss pharmacologists of the active ingredients from the Indian snake roots plant. In current American psychiatric practice, they are not widely prescribed, but they are used extensively in the treatment of hypertension.[3]

4. The *benzoquinolines* are compounds included for their chemical and pharmacologic completeness. Although tetrabenazine, the prototypic compound of the series, had shown some clinical utility, it is not used in the United States. The benzoquinolines are of interest mainly to research psychopharmacologists because they share some of the properties of reserpine, including the capacity to deplete brain amines.

5. The newest group of antipsychotics are the *butyrophenones*. Only recently introduced into the United States, they were developed in 1959 by Janssen in Belgium, and since then a large number of derivatives have been synthesized and studied extensively in Europe and North America. They are highly potent compounds and share with the rauwolfia derivatives many clinical properties including the potential for inducing depression. They produce a high percentage of extra-pyramidal side effects; but in contrast with the phenothiazines, they produce autonomic side effects in only a small percentage of patients. While many Europeans feel they have greatest value in severely paranoid, withdrawn, or hallucinating patients, debate continues over whether they offer more than the phenothiazines for these patients. The butyrophenones seem specific and highly effective for patients with the rare and dramatic de Tourette's syndrome, a children's disorder marked by motor tics and outbursts of explicatives and cries.

Clinical experience indicates that similarities in effects among these five classes of antipsychotic compounds are far greater than their differences. These drugs do not cure schizophrenia, paranoia, mania, or hebephrenia in the same way that antibiotics cure central nervous system infectious disease; the antipsychotic drugs are more like agents used in general medicine since they suppress symptoms, reduce the period of hospitalization, and facilitate the patient's community adjustment. This form of their therapeutic action has necessitated maintenance therapy for prolonged periods of time, often at a reduced dose. Consequently, the prolonged maintenance approach generates considerable need for aftercare programs and for provision of social service and medical support for the large numbers of patients being discharged from mental hospitals into the community.

Antidepressant Drugs

While schizophrenia and other psychoses are the most severe and dramatic of the mental illnesses, the affective disorders, especially depression, are far more widespread. The advent of effective antidepressant drugs has reduced the need for hospitalization, and has allowed increasing numbers of patients to be treated in the community. Currently, depressed patients are increasingly diagnosed in the milder forms which allow treatment on an ambulatory basis. The use of convulsive therapy ("shock treatment") has decreased dramatically although it has not been completely eliminated.

There are three classes of compounds with what are generally regarded as specific antidepressant properties. These are: the psychomotor stimulants, the monoamine oxidase inhibitors, and the tricyclic derivatives of imipramine.

1. The *psychomotor stimulants,* of which amphetamines are the most widely known, have limited, if any, value in the clinical treatment of most depressions. While they do produce mood elevation in most normal and depressed persons, these changes are of short duration and of limited therapeutic value. In medical practice, the amphetamines are most widely prescribed for the treatment of obesity, but even here their value is in question. The most important questions facing the use of the amphetamines currently involve their potential for abuse and their tendency to produce psychic dependency and toxic states when used for prolonged periods.

In an attempt to find psychomotor stimulants without the adverse effects of amphetamines, a number of related compounds have been developed, the most significant of which are methylphenidate (Ritalin) and phenmetrazine (Preludin). Unfortunately, these new compounds have not been free of the dependence and abuse characteristic of the amphetamines.

Mention should be made of the demonstrated value of the psychomotor stimulants (including amphetamines and methylphenidate) in the treatment of children with hyperkinetic learning disorders. This use has caused widespread public controversy. While there are questions raised about the social consequences and possible misuse of these compounds in some school systems, their clinical efficacy does not seem to be in question for a real, but still not fully defined, group of children with the association of learning difficulties and motor overactivity.

2. The *monoamine oxidase (MAO) inhibitors* were introduced in 1957 with

much public interest and drama. Included in this group are Marsilid, Nardil, Niamid, and Parnate. Their value in clinical practice has decreased because of two factors: their relatively high toxicity, especially the liver damage, the hypertensive episodes associated with the ingestion of cheese, wine, and other food stuffs; and relatively less clinical efficacy compared to the tricyclic compounds. Nevertheless, they retain an important role in the treatment of depression, especially for those patients who do not respond to other drugs or those patients with recurrent depressions whose previous responses seem to be specifically related to this group of compounds. They also have considerable research interest since they provide an important investigational tool by which pharmacologists can influence levels of brain amines by inhibiting monoamine oxidase, a major enzyme for the metabolism of brain monoamines.

3. The most important specific antidepressant drugs are the *tricyclic derivatives derived from imipramine.* In the United States, a number of these compounds are marketed, including Tofranil, Elavil, Aventil, Pertefrane (also known as Norpramine), and Sinequan. These compounds have a wide range of uses, including efficacy in mixed anxiety-depressive states. They have a wide dose range and are relatively safe. Considerable disagreement exists in determining characteristics of patients who respond best to antidepressant drugs, but there seem to be good correlations of improvement with age, symptom pattern, absence of precipitating events, and other features described in the psychiatric literature as the "endogenous" form of depression.

It is important to acknowledge that while these classes of drugs are grouped as antidepressant, in clinical practice depressed patients are treated with a wide variety of drugs, including various phenothiazine derivatives, sedative hypnotics, and "minor tranquilizers." This practice is based on the fact that most depressive patients experience associated symptoms of anxiety, insomnia, and tension which are often helped by these other psychotropic compounds.

There seems widespread recognition of the extent to which depression exists in industrial society, and it may well be said that whereas the 1950s were seen as the age of anxiety, the 1970s will be known as the age of depression, or as a return of the age of melancholia. It is not clear whether this is due to a true increase in the incidence and prevalence of depression or to a greater recognition of the variety of clinical states associated with the disorder.

Antianxiety Drugs

In this group are included the barbiturates, the nonbarbiturate sedative-hypnotics, meprobamate, and its derivatives, and the diazepoxide series (Librium, Valium, and Serax). As mentioned previously, there are problems in the terminology of this group of compounds. They are often called "minor tranquilizers" to distinguish them from the phenothiazines and related compounds used in the treatment of psychoses. Originally, one motive for introducing the term tranquilizer was to distinguish meprobamate and the newer compounds from the older barbiturates, usually called sedative hypnotics; yet pharmacological and clinical experience now indicate that these distinctions were more useful for advertising claims than for investigation of their pharmacological and clinical properties. Considerable research has established that the new compounds, meprobamate, and its derivatives, and the diazepoxide derivatives (Librium and Valium and Serax), are closely similar pharmacologically to the oldest barbiturates and sedative hypnotics. Moreover, their common pharmacologic properties are qualitatively different from the antipsychotics. The antianxiety drugs are not effective in the treatment of psychoses. Antianxiety agents do not produce extra-pyramidal side effects, and they have little effect on autonomic nervous system functions. They raise the convulsive threshold while the antipsychotics lower it. They do produce psychic dependence and have a tendency to be abused, which is not true of the antipsychotics and antidepressants.

There seems to be a general agreement on the rank order of this group of compounds based on their clinical and pharmacological effects. This order is as follows: (1) barbiturates, (2) meprobamate and its derivatives, (3) diazepoxide derivatives. This rank order corresponds to relative efficacy: the barbiturates are a little more effective than placebo, with the meprobamate group next, and the diazepoxides best established in the treatment of anxiety, tension, and related states. This action must be seen against the background of the high spontaneous improvement rate and great degree of placebo response rate for most anxiety and neurotic symptoms, particularly for symptoms associated with situational stress.

This rank order also corresponds with their toxicity. The barbiturates have a low safety margin and are the most widely used instrument for suicide in the United States (probably second to the automobile). On the other hand, few or no deaths from overdose have been reported with diazepoxide series. The same rank order applies in the treatment of epilepsy, the barbiturates being the most effective. This rank order also corresponds to their tendency to produce dependence, habituation, and addiction. The barbiturates are the most addicting of the group, and the barbiturate withdrawal syndrome can be fatal. Dependence and addiction can occur with the meprobamate and diazepoxide series, but it tends to occur less frequently and to be much less dangerous than dependency upon the barbiturates.

There are significant groups of psychoneuroses for which these compounds are not effective. Obsessive-compulsive states, dissociative states, conversion hysteria, and phobias are not influenced by antianxiety drugs. There are no drugs effective for forms of these psychoneurotic conditions.

Antianxiety drugs are of value in the treatment of anxiety and tension associated with situational states and stress. They seem to be of most value for short-lived episodes of neurotic symptoms, and experienced clinicians discourage their use beyond a number of weeks. They are widely prescribed and their high rate of prescription generates important questions about the boundaries between psychopathological forms of anxiety and tension and the emotional changes associated with the stresses of everyday life. Lively controversy exists about the moral implications of the use of these compounds in American society, and the concerns about whether or not we are becoming "a medicated society" with an excessive tendency to rely upon drugs as modes of coping. I will return to this issue later.[4]

Social and Moral Consequences

As in the case of most technological advances, the advent of new drugs produces an impact upon our institutions' cultural orientation and values. The introduction of effective psychotropic drugs for clinical treatment of mental illness has had immediate and direct, important consequences for mental health care. There has been a shift from hospital to community-based programs. The deleterious effects of hospitalization has been minimized and, in some instances, eliminated by the use of open door techniques and restriction of adverse practices such as seclusion and restraint, by the shortened period of hospitalization, by the decreased stigma attached to mental illness, and by the broadened definition of mental illness. Moreover, large segments of the population are seeking help from mental health professionals. Much social deviance, previously regarded as legal, is being redefined as mental health; and it is hoped that psychopharmacologic agents will prove useful in altering behavior deviance such as alcoholism, drug addiction, and perhaps even crime and delinquency.

These changes have had consequences not only for the health care system but for the legal system—especially for the definition of deviance itself and the type of stigma to be attached to various forms of deviant behavior. I have identified a number of moral and social issues which I believe we must face, in particular four issues: (1) the "right" to treatment, (2) the dilemmas of involuntary treatment of mental disorders by drugs and other techniques, (3) the emergence of new forms of social disability and chronicity for mental patients in the community, and (4) the controversy over whether or not we are becoming an overly medicated society.

The Right to Treatment

A number of court rulings are establishing the right to treatment for patients hospitalized in public mental institutions. The availability of effective therapeutic techniques has accelerated a dramatic shift in orientation of mental institutions from purely custodial care to active treatment and the question is being raised whether any patients should be admitted to these hospitals without demonstration that active treatment will be provided. These court cases have highlighted a long-term conflict in the relationship of mental hospitals to the larger society, the conflict between their custodial and therapeutic functions. Too often, psychiatric institutions have been used as disguised or even overt forms of social control. In the late eighteenth and nineteenth centuries, the emergence of mental hospitals for this purpose represented a major humanitarian advance and so long as there were not active effective treatments, the distinction between these two functions was not as clear as it has now emerged. Psychotropic drugs have contributed greatly to the reduction of custodialism and to the liberalization of institutional practices. There has been a rise in therapeutic optimism among professions, and a rise of expectations among patients, their families, and most significantly, the legal system that treatment will be provided. If the right to treatment is established and incorporated in law, then the number of questions will rise about the adequacy of resources made available for treatment programs and about alternative procedures that will need to be established for handling socially deviant and illegal behavior by persons with mental illness.

The Dilemmas of Involuntary Treatment

Closely related to the issue of the patient's "right" to treatment are the dilemmas associated with involuntary treatment in psychiatry. Unlike other medical specialties under certain conditions, psychiatry has the legal power and social sanction to coerce patients to accept treatment. This is not an absolute power since it has been controlled by the process of legal commitment. In recent decades, the commitment power and the attendant ability to coerce treatment have been under attack. Currently, the leading spokesman for critics of involuntary treatment is Thomas Szasz, who has both challenged the procedures of involuntary treatment on intrinsic moral grounds and pointed out various abuses.

It is valuable to separate the issue of occurrence and extent of abuse from the intrinsic moral issue. It must be acknowledged that abuses of these powers have and do occur, particularly in the procedures for involuntary hospitalization and in the use of some biological treatments, particularly the convulsive treatment (shock) and the psychosurgery techniques, including lobotomy. Currently, it is likely that there are abuses in the use of psychotropic drugs.

The intrinsic moral issue arises from the fact that certain forms of antisocial and deviant behavior are the direct consequences of mental illness, whether these illnesses are the manifestation of established brain disease, personal development, or unknown etiology. Such behaviors, to cite two difficult cases, are found in the deluded and paranoid patient who is hostile, angry, destructive, or threatening, for which psychotropic medication will provide calming and normalizing effect; and in the intensely depressed and suicidal patients where treatment with drugs or convulsive therapy reduces the suicidal drive and ameliorates the severity of depression. In these two situations, the moral dilemma arises when the psychiatrist and other staff assume responsibility for decision making and treat the patient even though the patient may expressly deny wanting treatment or may attempt to avoid it. Underlying society's delegation of this authority to psychiatry is a view of human nature held by society at large and embodied in our legal code, and specifically a belief that there are exemptions to the general principle that adults have individual free will and the right of self-determination for their actions. Where antisocial and disturbed behaviors are regarded as the manifestation of mental illness, however defined, our society exempts the person from certain sanctions and responsibilities when treatment is provided. The other restriction on self-determination occurs with suicidal behavior, particularly when associated with mental illness such as depression.

The advent of psychotropic drugs as effective treatments has intensified these dilemmas. It is noteworthy that the debates over these issues arise at a time when commitment and involuntary hospitalization is decreasing and when increasing proportions of patients are being treated voluntarily, especially in psychiatric units in general hospitals and in community mental health centers. The relative importance of the large public mental institution in the mental health system is declining and its restrictive practices and custodial atmosphere are rapidly being eliminated and there are indications that the transformation of these institutions is in prospect. With more effective treatments as may be expected in the future, the moral issue may become more intensified as the occurrence of abuses decreases.

A problem related to involuntary treatment arises when "informed consent" is advocated. Under what circumstances can psychiatric patients be considered to have "rational" knowledge, understanding, and free will to give truly informed consent in regard to accepting or refusing treatment? These issues will become more intensified as new drugs become available with a wider range of indications, particularly those which may reduce aggressive behavior or modify sexual activity or procreation. As psychiatric treatments have become more effective, the tendency has grown to widen the definition of mental illness, particularly in the nonpsychotic conditions whose only manifestations may be changes in emotional states such as increased anger, or depressive mood, anxiety states, or behavior which deviates from social norms. There is likely to be a further blurring of boundaries between conventional definitions of social deviance and mental illness. We have already seen this process occur in alcoholism, in drug abuse, and increasingly in juvenile delinquency and criminal behavior, as predicted by Samuel Butler in his utopian novel *Erewhon*. Many fear that the power of involuntary treatment will be granted to custodial families in the name of "mental health" and that psychotropic drug treatment will be used as a form of social control. Since abuse of these powers has previously occurred in the United States and probably is occurring in other nations such as the U.S.S.R., political dissent and social nonconformity, it is feared, will be defined as mental illness and treated coercively with medication.

There are genuine dilemmas in these issues. In clinical experience, there are circumstances where the patients' refusal of treatment, especially by paranoid and suicidal patients, need to be countervened. We must acknowledge the moral conflict when the psychiatrist has the power to coerce his patients into treatment for any such power affords opportunities for abuse.

New Forms of Chronicity

Another set of consequences arising from the therapeutic success of psychotropic agents is the emergence of new forms of chronicity in the lives of patients formerly hospitalized but now discharged and residing in the community. The issue is to ensure the quality of life being lived by these patients. The fear has been expressed that the decline in the numbers of patients in public mental hospitals is only a statistical artifact, not a true gain. Whereas these patients were formerly living lives of quiet desperation as chronic patients in mental institutions, similar patterns of chronic illness and social impairment are being lived by these patients in nursing homes in the case of the aged, or in rooming houses and other marginal residential facilities in the case of chronic psychiatric patients. The effectiveness of the psychotropic drugs has contributed to these trends since the available agents, particularly the antipsychotic drugs, ameliorate the patients' severe disturbances, particularly their psychotic thinking, sufficiently so as to allow discharge into the community but the patients are left emotionally blunted, occupationally impaired, and socially isolated.[5]

An Overmedicated Society?

Whereas most of the issues described above apply to the use of psychotropic drugs for psychotic or depressed patients, the most publicized recent discussions have concerned the use of psychotropic agents by relatively normal or mildly neurotic persons with anxiety, tension, depression, insomnia, and related symptoms often associated with the stresses of everyday life in modern industrial society.

This issue has gained prominence, in part, because of the growth in rates of prescription and utilization of psychotropic drugs, particularly the anti-anxiety agents ("minor tranquilizers"). For example, recently available statistics indicate that the production and distribution of psychotropic drugs have become a major component of the pharmaceutical industry. It is estimated that in 1967 almost 180 million prescriptions for psychotropic drugs were written at a cost of almost $700 million. Interestingly, the single most prescribed compound in the United States is chlordiazepoxide (Librium) with gross sales of $150 million. Prescriptions of this compound represent about seventeen percent of all prescriptions written. When prescriptions of all psychotropic drugs are tallied, they account for twenty-five percent of all prescriptions.

Other data reveal that seventy percent of all psychotropic drug prescriptions are written by general practitioners, internists, and surgeons, not by psychiatrists or neurologists. Nevertheless, psychiatrists and neurologists have higher rates of prescription of these drugs than other medical specialties. Since they represent a minority of medical practitioners, they do not produce the majority of prescriptions. Further data from a California study indicates that about seventeen percent of adults report frequent use of psychotropic drugs, the figure being twice as high in women as in men. The heaviest drug use occurs in the age group 40–59. Interestingly enough, men are more likely to use stimulants in the 30's age group, tranquilizers in the 40's and 50's, and sedatives in the 60's and older. About thirty percent of the sample reported use of some psychotropic drug within the past twelve months. Related to the use of drugs by prescription are the wide number of nonprescription agents (OTC: Over the Counter) which are advertised for relief of headache, tension of everyday life, insomnia.

Figures such as these are impressive because they indicate a wide use of drugs to relieve emotional distress within the population at large. Whether or not this practice constitutes a moral crisis in our society is under debate since many individuals feel that the use of medication for such purposes is misuse. This debate has uncovered a conflict which I have identified between two extreme value orientations: pharmacological calvinism and psychotropic hedonism. The pharmacological calvinist view involves a general distrust of drugs used for nontherapeutic purposes and a conviction that if a drug "makes you feel good, it must be morally bad." The dominant American value system condones and sanctions drug use only for the therapeutic purposes and then only under professional supervision by physicians and pharmacists. In this view, abstinence is the highest ideal, the purest route to pharmacological salvation. The history of Western society reveals resistance to each compound introduced for such usage. For example, when tea and coffee and tobacco were introduced in Western Europe, their use was accepted only after considerable debate and resistance. Attempts at prohibition of alcohol failed, as is likely to be the outcome of the current attempt at prohibition of marijuana.

Pharmacological Calvinism

It is of note that mental health professionals, especially in the field of psychotherapy, have their own variant of these calvinist views. Especially among psychoanalysts and other psychotherapists there is the view that any drug use is a "crutch" and that the best way to cure schizophrenia, neurosis, depression is through psychotherapeutic means using verbal insight. The conviction is often held that the use of psychotropic drugs in psychiatric treatment is morally wrong, independent of its efficacy, because it promotes gradual dependency. Drug therapy is thus a secondary road to salvation, the highest road to salvation is through insight and self-determination. This view, although held only by a minority of psychiatrists, is also embodied in the popular media's current attempts at drug-abuse education. Thus, if a drug makes you feel good, it not only represents a secondary form of salvation but somehow it is morally wrong and the user is likely to suffer retribution from either dependence, liver damage, or chromosomal change, or some other form of medical-theological damnation. Implicit in this theory of therapeutic change is the philosophy of personal growth, basically a secure variant of the theological view of salvation through good works.

While this view may still represent the dominant theme, it has undergone considerable weakening and erosion of support. One source of erosion is the strain resultant from the exemption of alcohol, caffeine, and tobacco from these prohibitions. There is conflict between our espoused values on abstinence and actual behavior. American society's stance on tobacco and alcohol contrasts sharply with its attitudes on marijuana and this inconsistency contributes to the current generation gap and distrust among young people when adults discuss drugs. A related source of strain derives from advertising, where there has been commercialization of drug terminology, especially from the psychedelic culture. By using the drug trappings, the media glamorize the drug culture and contribute to the view of drug-taking as attractive, desirable, and efficacious. In large part, the motivations of the pharmaceutical and advertising industries are economical, their intent is to widen the size of the drug-user market by extending the rationale of drug use to include relief of minor symptoms related to emotional stresses. They recently have attempted to reduce the stigma attached to the use of psychotropic drugs by identifying the viewer with drug-taking, by depicting use in the ad, and by making the drug user seem as attractive and "normal" as the viewer himself, rather than deranged and abnormal.

The most serious challenges to pharmacological calvinism, however, have come from the youth culture. The current youth culture distrusts adults' authority in the drug area and regards drug-taking as part of its general hedonistic view. Achievement is valued less than the immediacy of personal relations and the use of drugs which enhance such relations, as may be the case with marijuana or minor tranquilizers, is not regarded as wrong in any moral or value basis.

Given the likelihood that further advances in pharmacology will increase the effectiveness of drugs in this realm, the value conflict of society is likely to become more intensified.

Implications for the Future

Looking to the future, the easiest predictions to make are those which foresee the development of more efficacious therapeutic agents for the already defined forms of mental illness. New agents will be developed for the treatment of schizophrenia, paranoia, mania, depression, obsessions, and other mental illnesses whether psychotic or neurotic in degree. There will be relatively little moral dilemma in these instances since the use of drugs for these conditions represents an extension of conventional medical treatment.

The more significant future issues are likely to be consequent to the development of drugs for improvement of human capabilities and for the enhancement of personal pleasure and enjoyment. As knowledge of the relationship of brain and behavior increases, it is likely that we will develop knowledge of the neurochemical and neuropharmacological bases of memory, learning, mood, aggression, appetite, and sexual lust. For example, there will be chemical agents developed which will enhance memory which may in fact reduce or eliminate the development of senile dementia in the aged. With greater knowledge of the chemistry of learning, it may be possible to develop drugs which will accelerate the learning of children and allow a different timetable of learning than the current one. Clearly this development would have implications for education and child development.

Suppose pharmacologists do in fact derive drugs which promote memory and learning. The possibility arises that the beneficial effects of these drugs are only operative while drug ingestion continues and in order to maintain memory improvement and accelerated learning continued drug treatment is required. If such be the case, what would be the social and moral dilemmas in the field of education and in the care of the aged?

Mention has already been made of the widespread use of existing drugs to reduce anxiety and tension and to avoid insomnia. As more effective drugs become available, it may well be that American and other industrial societies will redefine the "right to life, liberty, and the pursuit of happiness" to guarantee the right of absence of guilt, anxiety, tension, depression, and insomnia. If this is the case, dilemmas described above will intensify. Most of the drugs currently available for the relief of anxiety and tension carry some danger of dependence, habituation, and addiction. What if the drugs to be available had even lower potential for these complications than currently the case with diazepoxide derivatives?

The controversy following the recent presidential address by Kenneth Clark before the American Psychological Association highlighted the moral dilemmas associated with the possible development of drugs to reduce hostility and aggression. In part, this controversy rests on a purely empirical question. What would be the consequences of such drugs on levels of drive, assertiveness, aggression, and achievement? It may be that the neurophysiological substrata of hostility and destructive behavior is inexorably linked with the sources of initiative and assertiveness. If this proves to be the case, the availability of pharmacologic agents which influence these drives would pose immense moral dilemmas, particularly given the widespread concern over increased crimes and acts of violence and long-standing debate over the sources of man's aggression, whether manifested by individuals or in social groups.

Difficult as these moral dilemmas will be when drugs are available to enhance performance, even greater difficulties will arise with the development of drugs which promote personal enjoyment. We have seen a forerunner of such difficulties in the controversy over LSD and the emergent psychedelic movement in the 1960s. The toxicity associated with LSD and other psychedelic drugs obscured the moral issue raised by the ideology espoused by Leary and Alpert and their followers. Let us assume that drugs become available which could induce euphoria, pleasantness, expanded states of awareness, and feelings of well-being without producing the toxic reaction associated with LSD or the dependence and addiction associated with opiate derivatives. Would our society be willing to accept use of such drugs for purely hedonistic purposes akin to the way in which tobacco and alcohol have now been accommodated?

This is a period of rapid change in the drug field, not only technologically but also in social attitudes. The ability of the pharmaceutical industry to synthesize new compounds will produce substances with a wide range of therapeutic activity and more likely with the capacity to enhance performance and improve personal enjoyment. These technological advances are likely to have profound consequences on values, particularly beliefs around the relationship between future achievement, immediate enjoyment, and the nature of the good life.

NOTES

1. Psychopharmacology refers to the scientific field which studies drugs that affect the mind, behavior, intellectual functions, and mood. Psychotropic drugs are those compounds which influence the psychic functions and behavior. Not all psychotropic drugs are therapeutic. For example, heroin, alcohol, LSD are psychotropic drugs with considerable social and research interest, but currently they have no demonstrated therapeutic value in the treatment of established mental illness.

2. There are some semantic problems to be identified. Although there is imprecision about the use of the term antipsychotic for this category of drugs, it has a considerable advantage over the initially advocated term, "tranquilizer," which unfortunately, since 1950, the professional press has tended to emphasize. The word tranquilizer is now seen as a misnomer since it implies a clinical utility only in patients who are excited and require calming. Experience has shown that these drugs have significant effects upon disturbed thinking as occurs in schizophrenia psychoses, but that they are unlikely to influence significantly any excitation and overactivity without the presence of disturbed thinking.

Widespread usage distinguishes major tranquilizers, such as the phenothiazines, from the minor tranquilizers, such as the meprobamate series and the diazopoxide derivatives. In my opinion, this latter group is related more closely to the sedative-hypnotics than to antipsychotics such as the barbiturates. The major tranquilizer–minor tranquilizer distinction is inadequate and inaccurate. It implies that the meprobamate-barbiturate group is basically similar to the phenothiazine group, but contains weaker pharmacologic compounds. This is not accurate and it is far better to see these two classes of compounds as qualitatively different.

A different set of semantic problems arises in communication between the Anglo-U.S. approach and the French school of psychopharmacology. The French school, whose views are most influential in Western European and South American psychiatry, reserves the term "tranquilizer" for sedative hypnotic drugs of the meprobamate diazopoxide series. The French school uses the term "neuroleptic" for the group of drugs which are called antipsychotic or major tranquilizers in the United States. The French employ this term because they feel that the effectiveness of these drugs in treating psychoses is related to their capacity to influence the extra-pyramidal nervous system. They postulate the theoretical view that the *sine qua non* of these drugs' effectiveness against psychoses derives from their actions upon the basal ganglia and subcortical centers which regulate the extra-pyramidal system. Without elaborating upon the technicalities of this debate, I should acknowledge that the situation is complex. All classes of antipsychotic drugs produce varying degrees of extra-pyramidal side effects, and moreover, recent biochemical findings do suggest common actions of these drugs upon dopamine metabolism. These are promising clues for further investigations on the mode of actions of these drugs, and they also suggest possible biochemical links to the causation of schizophrenia.

3. If the rauwolfias were the only antipsychotic drug available, however, most clinicians would conclude that they constituted a major therapeutic advance since they are superior to placebo or other control groups. They have demonstrated effectiveness in approximately the same range of patients as do the phenothiazines, but they seem to lack the phenothiazines' "clinical punch." A significant side effect of the rauwolfias is their tendency to produce depression in upwards of ten to fifteen percent of patients. This effect is best documented with the treatment of hypertension. The rauwolfias have had important research impact because of their tendency to influence brain levels of amines, and research with the rauwolfias has contributed greatly to our knowledge of neuropharmacology and has stimulated hypotheses about the relationships of neurochemistry to mental disorders.

4. While the three classes of drugs described above represent the main classes used as the therapeutic agents in mental illness, mention should be made of two other clinical states in which drug therapy has produced highly valuable results. Lithium has been successful in the treatment of mania and recurrent affective disorders, and psychomotor stimulants have had good results for hyperkinetic children. See the paper by Paul Wender in *Hastings Center Studies* 2 (1974).

5. A related consequence is the concern over the possible impact upon families and local communities of the presence of these discharged patients who are improved but not well. This concern is especially true for the impact of discharged, psychotic mothers and fathers upon family-life and children. Whether one believes in a genetic transmission of severe mental illness, especially schizophrenia, or in the role of social-cultural factors, the presence in the home of intermittently psychotic or borderline patients constitutes a potential danger to children and increases the likelihood of transmission of mental illness across generations.

In large part, these issues are largely empirical since insufficient data are available as to the extent to which the trends described above do occur. Here further research should clarify many of the issues. Were it in fact true that these consequences do occur, the moral issue would be as to which life style is desired, and what resources our society is prepared to allocate to improve the quality of life for patients discharged into the community but not capable of complete self-sufficiency. A more difficult moral dilemma arises in the issue of attempting to interrupt, by family planning and birth control, the transmission of mental illness across generations and the possible desirability of advocating conception along with maintenance antipsychotic, psychotropic drug treatment.

Teodoro Ayllon

Behavior Modification
in Institutional Settings

The major premise underlying behavior modification techniques is that behavior is governed largely by environmental events.[1] A major avenue, therefore, for acquiring new behavior patterns is through either structured or unstructured learning in response to such events. Using established procedures in the area of social learning to set the conditions under which this new learning, and hence new behavior, will be acquired, the behavior therapist can attempt to structure behavior.

This approach has three distinguishing characteristics. First, instead of attempting to explain a psychological problem or emotional conflict in abstract terms, the behavioral therapist examines the individual's unique behavior in relation to his immediate social environment. Second, treatment is then tailored to the individual, and evaluation of treatment effectiveness is accomplished using predetermined criteria based on the individual's unique characteristics. Finally, if evaluation shows that the procedures are ineffective, the treatment is restructured. Thus, the procedures are self-correcting. The approach of behavior modification is, therefore, more pragmatic and empirical than other, largely theoretical, psychological approaches.

Treatment of a child who does not want to go to school may serve to exemplify the behavioralist's approach. Instead of defining the child's psychic conflict as "school phobia," the problem would be behaviorally defined as low or zero school attendance.[2] The advantage of such a tactic is real; it is not a mere exercise in semantics. Evaluation of treatment effectiveness is well advanced

From *Arizona Law Review* 17 (1975):3–19. Copyright © 1975 by the Arizona Board of Regents. Reprinted by permission of the publisher and the author.

when the problem can be set in a readily observable and quantifiable domain, as opposed to a reified, mentally-based domain. Thus, 90 or 100 percent school attendance becomes the performance criterion of treatment effectiveness against which the child's progress is measured. Opening the problem and evaluation criteria to quantification and direct observation allows the behavioral therapist to determine whether or not particular techniques change the behavior problem.

Major Techniques of Behavior Modification

Systematic Desensitization

Among the most often used techniques in behavior modification are token economies, aversive conditioning, and systematic desensitization. The last technique is particularly useful in inducing behavioral change in an individual whose unadaptive or neurotic behavior was acquired in an anxiety generating situation.[3] Systematic desensitization therapy amounts to systematic elimination of the anxiety response associated with a given stimulus.[4] For example, phobias in general, such as acrophobia, the fear of crowds, and other psychological problems associated with emotional inhibition,[5] have been treated through systematic desensitization.[6]

The therapy has several distinguishing characteristics. The patient is first put into a state of deep relaxation. While in this state he identifies the different situations that might give rise to his neurotic reaction, and then, if there are more than one, he ranks them in order of the probability that they might trigger the neurotic reaction.[7] The result is a graduated hierarchy of situations that produce anxiety in the patient. By exposing the patient to the least offensive situation and then gradually working up the hierarchy, the therapist can desensitize the subject.[8]

The Token Economy

Another major technique in behavior modification therapy is the token economy.[9] A quasi-economic system is established within the institution, and desired behavior is rewarded with tokens. Specifically, this set of complementary procedures is characterized by three features. First, as in other behavior modification techniques, the behavior that is the major focus of the treatment is defined in performance rather than psychic terms.[10] Second, a contractual arrangement is established between the patient and the hospital administration setting forth the rewards and penalties associated with certain conduct. For ease of operation, a currency system using tokens is instituted.[11] Third, as motivation to induce the target behaviors, a wide range of backup rewards, privileges, and items are made available to the patient in exchange for tokens.

By reducing the time lag between payments of tokens and the purchase of rewards, the currency system can maintain an optimal level of motivation.

The token economy technique has been used in a variety of situations. In mental hospitals the technique has had a series of successful applications. This in large measure due to the fact that the token economy has been used to eliminate symptoms. For example, auditory hallucinations, hypochondriasis, and chronic refusal to eat have been eliminated using token economies.[12]

The token economy system has been used in schools for both retarded and normal children. In the case of retarded children, treatment objectives have included teaching academic skills such as reading, writing, and arithmetic, as well as social skills such as speech fluency and good eating habits.[13] Schools for normal children have used the system for eliminating discipline problems, raising attention and concentration levels,[14] and enhancing academic performance.[15]

The token economy system has recently been applied to the field of criminal corrections. These efforts have involved institutionalized delinquents,[16] youthful offenders,[17] and adult offenders.[18] Treatment objectives have included improving educational and vocational performance, controlling discipline problems, and the rationalized management of detained delinquents.[19] In addition, the token economy has been used to prevent delinquent behavior through placement of predelinquent boys in residential, home-style living arrangements.[20] Treatment objectives in this residential placement program have included modification of undesirable social behavior, development of new behavior in the community, development of self-control, and instillment of responsibility for one's behavior.

Aversive Conditioning

Another method of behavior modification is aversive conditioning.[21] It has been defined as "an attempt to associate an undesirable behaviour pattern with unpleasant stimulation or to make the unpleasant stimulation a consequence of the undesirable behaviour."[22] Aversive conditioning decreases inappropriate or maladaptive behavior by using negative stimuli. For inappropriate behavior, such as when an autistic[23] child bangs his head, a negative stimulus, such as electric shock to the thigh, would be the consequence. For maladaptive behavior, such as homosexuality, the negative stimulus is paired to a stimulus that produces the maladaptive response. For example, the homosexual would be shocked whenever he is sexually aroused by a photo of a nude male. These negative stimuli should decrease head-banging by the autistic child and sexual arousal by the homosexual. The problem, however, is that while these behaviors have been broken, no new adaptive behaviors have been established in their place.[24] Thus, in order to be used effectively, aversive conditioning should be used in conjunction with therapy that will provide positive reinforcement and thereby build appropriate and functional behavior.

Aversive conditioning is typically reserved for behavior problems which will not decrease through any positive conditioning or where the client involved has agreed to this method of treatment. For the most part, aversive conditioning has been used with the most difficult of populations to work with, autistic children. Here, aversive stimuli, such as shock, have been used to save a child's life.[25] This method also has been used with homosexuals, transvestites, and people with fetishes who have agreed to undergo such therapy in a laboratory or a clinic.[26] Aversive conditioning, in the form of shock or chemicals which produce a bad taste, has also been used with alcoholics, drug addicts, and excessive smokers.[27] In general, these techniques are used only with behaviors which are highly resistant to change by any other type of procedure.

One of the major criticisms of aversive conditioning is that it produces bad side effects such as avoidance, escape, fear, and various other emotional responses. In treatments performed by very competent therapists, however, these negative side effects were not produced in autistic children.[28] Parents, teachers, and some professionals who do not have such competency have clearly produced inappropriate behavior, including anxiety, truancy, stealing, lying, and various nervous habits. Aversive conditioning, therefore, should be used only as a last resort, after all positive programs to change behavior have failed. Even then, it should be carried out only with the greatest of care and only if the persons administering the treatment are accountable for their actions.

Further, the use of aversive conditioning should always be well monitored.[29] The technique of defining behavior in measurable terms, as previously mentioned, is helpful once again, for the degree of success of the aversive therapy can be carefully observed. In this manner, the therapy can be precisely administered, avoiding application of aversive stimuli in unnecessary amounts, and thereby minimizing the collateral production of inappropriate behavior.

Alternatives to Aversive Conditioning

Because of the problems[30] associated with the use of aversive stimuli, other less objectionable techniques have been developed. Some procedures try to minimize reinforcement of inappropriate behavior. Total withholding of reinforcement is termed extinction.[31] For example, when the class clown starts to disrupt his classroom to get attention, the teacher and other students, using extinction therapy, would totally ignore his antics, thereby refusing the reinforcement he seeks. Withholding reinforcement for brief periods is termed time-out therapy.[32] For example, in one study an autistic child seeking social reinforcement of his tantrums and self-destructive behavior was placed alone in his room for 10 minutes whenever he exhibited such behavior.[33] Similarly, to the prison inmate who views group association as rewarding, placement in solitary confinement also may be considered a form of time-out therapy.[34]

Another alternative to aversion therapy is the response-cost technique. Certain bad behavior will entail a "cost" to the patient; something of value to him is removed from his environment in response to inappropriate behavior.[35] Thus, a cartoon show is turned off when a child sucks his thumb,[36] or a patient in a token economy must return tokens if he engages in inappropriate behavior. In most large settings, such as mental institutions or schools, response-cost and time-out have been used. Response-cost is a particularly useful procedure in settings with a large number of individuals since it can be carried out within the framework of a token economy system.

Although response-cost, time-out, and extinction therapies usually produce less severe side effects than standard aversive therapy, these procedures have certain limitations. They are usually slow in decreasing the target behavior, and, as with aversive conditioning, some undesirable emotional responses may be produced. Therefore, as with other aversion therapy, these techniques should be used in conjunction with a program which builds positive behavior through the use of rewards.

Suggested Guidelines for the Practice of Behavior Modification in Institutions

To ensure a proper respect for the ethical problems inherent in behavior modification[37] and to ensure that the inmate receives those legal rights to which he is entitled,[38] it is imperative that rehabilitation therapy be done with the patient's informed consent and be subject to scrutiny throughout the treatment.[39] In this way the patient participates in and is responsible for his own retraining; he is doing, not being done to. The patient, the therapist, and society gain when the manner of rehabilitation is agreeable, satisfying, and growth producing. Consistent with this view, this article recommends eight guidelines for the behavior therapist in administering treatment.

1. The patient should be informed of the possible outcome of the treatment.[40] The therapist should try to impart as clear an understanding of the anticipated behavior changes as is possible under the circumstances. One method for accomplishing this objective would be through the use of some form of written agreement.[41] If the skills that are expected to be acquired are spelled out in an agreement, there would be evidence of compliance with the goal of full disclosure. By using these "contracts," the mutual expectations on the part of both the subject and the therapist would be greatly clarified. A comprehensive therapy contract is now in use[42] which sets forth the expected behavior objectives of the treatment, the nature, methods, and duration of the treatment, and the specific criteria and social values that will be used to evaluate and measure the success of the treatment.[43]

2. The patient should be informed of the procedures that will be used in the treatment.[44] While the outcome may be desirable, the means used to achieve this result may be so personally distasteful as to make the individual's voluntary participation unlikely. For example, given the choice between a treatment using a reward system or one using drug-induced vomiting,[45] it is unlikely that a patient would choose the latter method.

3. The patient should be made to feel that he is free to choose whether or not to participate in a program.[46] This issue is of special concern with prison inmates or with involuntarily-committed mental patients who may feel that participation is necessary to achieve parole or release. Every effort should be made by the therapist to remove such implicitly coercive influences and to dispel any individual fear of retribution. Indeed, coercion could have adverse long range consequences since coercion may lead to extreme resentment on the part of the unwilling participant and intensify a desire for vindication against society upon his release.[47]

Freedom of choice does require that the patient be mature enough to make the choice and cognizant of what he is doing. The latter qualification, however, must not be extended too far. The patient should not be so protected by the requirement of informed consent that even when he knows what procedures will be used and accepts them, he is not allowed to participate in a rehabilitative program. The case of *Kaimowitz v. Michigan Department of Mental Health*[48] is an example of such overprotection. Because of the experimental nature of the treatment, the court refused to allow involuntarily-detained mental patients to consent to certain neurosurgical procedures. This is carrying the doctrine of parens patriae to a ridiculous extreme. Essentially, *Kaimowitz* assumed that the patient was not sufficiently mature or aware to know what he wanted for himself. In particular, the criminal patient, such as in *Kaimowitz*, may wish to jeopardize his health in the interest of science, perhaps as a way of repaying a debt to society, as Leopold did with malaria research.[49] The decision should be his.

4. The patient should be able at any time to discontinue his participation in a program without incurring prejudice or penalty. What was acceptable to the patient on paper may in fact turn out to be quite unacceptable in practice. Here again, the therapist must safeguard this right. Neither the therapist's rigor nor administrative convenience should be allowed to contravene the individual's wishes.

5. As an adjunct to the right to discontinue treatment, information necessary to make such a decision should be given the patient. He should be informed of his individual progress as often as he desires and in terms that he can readily understand.[50] False hopes of progress may induce continued participation in a program beyond the point at which the patient might otherwise wish to withdraw. Merely evaluating progress before and after treatment is insufficient, and withholding information for the sake of experimental rigor is unacceptable.

6. The patient is entitled to the treatment, rehabilitation, or education which is suited to his individual needs.[51] Requiring conformity to a single type of treatment or the intentional withholding of treatment through placement in an experimental control group is unacceptable. The need to foster individuality and to facilitate growth toward wholeness and self-actualization must be emphasized. The goal of a penal system, for example, if it is to be truly rehabilitative, should be to assist the development of self-esteem through the

active encouragement of unique talents. Decisions should not be made for the patient regarding what he will learn while in the institution.

7. The patient should be given the opportunity to express his feelings, views, and attitudes toward a program. While formal assessment before and after the program is acceptable here, the individual must be given the opportunity to express his opinions at any time during his participation. Often, the counseling group is ostensibly used for this purpose, but it is more honored in breach than in practice.[52] For example, there is often great reluctance on the part of prison inmates to go beyond a superficial level of discussion because of the fear that expression of negative feelings might compromise "good behavior."[53] This is unfortunate since group catharsis may serve a valuable function as a tension releasing mechanism, thereby keeping resentment at a minimum and avoiding future Atticas. Thus, if the inmate is to verbalize openly the feelings he is having in a given program, there must be an acceptance of these views by the staff and an absence of fear of retaliation in the inmate. In short, the patient's full participation in a program should be encouraged. His "good boy" docility should not be the primary concern.

8. Only behavioral techniques that enrich the patient's environment beyond a base guarantee of certain social and personal rights should be employed. An individual choosing not to engage in the rewarded activity should simply experience the absence of reward as opposed to coercion to conform to a given behavior. In general, neither sensory nor social deprivation should be considered as standard procedures to influence the individual's conduct. For example, in the START program[54] which took place in Springfield, Missouri, involuntary prison participants were prohibited from possessing reading material or otherwise using any educational, religious, or political material. They were denied the opportunity to view television or listen to a radio, and their actions were under continual surveillance.[55] In other words, the START program totally altered the confinement conditions of the prisoners and forced them to earn back what had rightfully been theirs upon admission into the institution. These kinds of sensory and social deprivations are not standard practices in behavior modification.[56] Further, such heroic means for changing behavior have typically failed to show that alternative techniques were inadequate.

Recommendations for the Use of Behavior Modification in Institutions

Compliance with the guidelines outlined above should provide assurance of effective treatment and awareness of situations of grave ethical concern. In addition to the guidelines, however, certain recommendations regarding methodology in general and the application of specific techniques can be made.

On the Token Economy and Community Mental Health

The most promising avenue for assuring full protection of the patient's rights may be found in the method of community mental health, which strives to maintain, as extensively as possible, the patient's exposure to his natural environment to ensure that the individual's expectations of himself and society are continued. The token economy system is just such a method since it attempts to maintain the continuity of social expectations and responsibilities that characterize the "natural" contingencies of the outside world.

Nothing will maintain the patient's freedom and responsibility for his own behavior as much as a system that functions as does a token economy — as an extension of the society from which the patient comes. Such an extension guarantees the patient's learning to cope with the demands and responsibilities expected of individuals outside the institution, thereby preventing disculturation. Further, normalization of social interaction is greatly dependent upon a system that enables individuals to exchange goods for services, favors, and other goods. An exchange system[57] helps the parties involved to assess precisely each other's expectations and the rewards or consequences for meeting or failing to meet these expectations.

Careful attention must be given the method and operation of a token economy. A token economy program is characterized by its empirical definition of target behaviors and the results associated with their achievement. Typically, the "rules" of behavior are explicitly and publicly stated, as are the rewards for observing those rules and the benefits which may be obtained in exchange for tokens. This procedure ensures that all individuals have the basis for exercising an informed choice.[58]

The aspect of choice in the token economy is of crucial importance. Choice, to be meaningful, must allow the person to achieve the consequences attendant upon choosing one thing over another. Once the individual discovers that, irrespective of his desires, he will be made to conform to institutional routine, his responsibility for his own actions is terminated. On the other hand, when the individual discovers that his desires will be respected, he will learn that he must bear the consequences of his own choice, and he will, in turn, learn responsibility for his own actions.

Thus, after the consequences of alternative choices have been outlined to the individual it is crucial that his choice be respected, since only in this manner can demeaning and eroding the individual's self-respect and dignity be avoided and responsibility for his own actions assumed. Acceptance of the consequences of one's own choices, however, will require at least a minimum of exposure to the consequences of other choices. Otherwise, the individual will not have an informed basis for choice.

A corollary of the need for individuals to exercise the free choice that is normally associated with community practices such as a token economy is the necessity for patients to have the right to voluntarily assume their own management. This action might include the patient seeking supervised work opportunities in positions which are both useful to the institution and therapeutic to the patient in terms of increased self-confidence and individual responsibility. It must be borne in mind that when patients are treated in mental institutions as if they were in medical hospitals, the objectives of social reeducation often are confused with those of physical restoration. Behavioral reeducation requires that the social environment in which the patient is living resemble closely that of the environment to which he will return. Therefore, if no expectations or demands are made of the patient in the institution, his reentry to a normal environment will only eventuate in failure because of his unpreparedness for such an experience.

To be sure, behavioral techniques enable the patient, upon commitment, to be shielded from all the demands and social pressures that led to his hospitalization. But gradually and systematically, as the patient improves, he is exposed to greater demands so that he learns to cope with most of the situations that he will encounter in the community. While it is appropriate to protect the patient from labor exploitation,[59] it also must be remembered that such protection must be balanced with efforts to keep the patient optimally motivated so as to improve his condition, to allow him to assume responsibility for his own actions, and eventually to permit his return to society.

On Rewards and Incentives

The major aspect of behavior modification is incentives and their use. While the notion of incentives dates from time immemorial, the sophisticated technology associated with their use is recent. Essentially, it is now known that incentives work under certain, and now well-researched, conditions and fail to work when these conditions have not been met. Current technology eliminates the uncertainty in the use of incentives. The naive notion that incentives ought to work has been rejected through research indicating that under certain conditions incentives may have the opposite effect from that expected.

Incentives intended to encourage certain behavior should only be employed after the display of that behavior. For example, if it is desired to encourage participation in a rehabilitative program, incentives should be used only when the individual has demonstrated some participation. Further, incentives must be meaningful to each individual. Since "one man's meat is another man's poison," it is basic to a behavioral approach to discover and develop meaningful incentives. Refusal to do so indicates failure.

What needs to be emphasized is that there are endless permutations and combinations of ways in which the patient may enjoy the rights given to him. For example, one patient may never make a phone call, even if he has the right to make one weekly, but another patient may wish to make a call daily. It is far too easy to standardize the rights of the individual in the institution. What is more difficult is to minimize regimentation, dependence, and eventually apathy. In an effort to enhance individual choice, variability, and differences, in contrast to conformity and regimentation, highly varied opportunities for self-motivation should be used as incentives to help the patients in their own rehabilitation and to reinforce their right to be different.[60]

While standardization of the rights and privileges used as incentives should be avoided, providing certain basic rights and privileges for all patients, such as food, lodging, ground privileges, and privacy, is legally required.[61] These rights and privileges constitute a floor below which guarantees may not drop.[62] Thus, contingent rewards should be made available in addition to those comforts and pleasures already guaranteed to the individual.[63] For example, if all individuals have been assigned a given room and bed, the reward could be the freedom to select the type of room or bed from among a wide range of choices. This effort would be consistent with developing responsibility for making choices. Additionally, withdrawal and return of personal property and privileges already permitted, though not required as basic, should not be the source of rewards. Regaining the possession of one's personal articles or privileges does not meet the contingent-rewards guideline since it is not an additional incentive. By insisting that rewards be additional to those rights and privileges already guaranteed or granted in an institution, deprivation of rewards will be avoided and enrichment of incentives ensured. As a general rule, it would be both effective and legally defensible to use rewards on a contingent basis so long as these rewards go beyond the minimum rights and privileges enjoyed by the patient. In so doing, the result will be an enriched environment that is not limited to the rights and privileges granted the patients.

On Seclusion

The solitary confinement of a patient in an empty room is still a treatment commonly used in institutions.[64] To justify the use of this procedure it is necessary that such use be constantly evaluated in terms of its effectiveness and that an additional program based on positive rewards be used concurrently with seclusion. By so doing, the cooling off or confinement period will result in a reduction of disturbed or aggressive behavior as the patient experiences the gross difference between seclusion and his interaction with the rewarding environment.

On Use of Aversive or Noxious Stimuli

Only when the patient's actions present a clear and imminent danger to his own or other's physical integrity may aversive or noxious stimuli be justified.[65] As was the case with seclusion, the patient must be concurrently exposed to a treatment based primarily on positive rewards. In addition, continuous checks must be made on the effectiveness of aversive procedures. Perhaps the best model for such procedures was pioneered in the use of aversive techniques to develop language and social skills in speech-free and self-abusive autistic children.[66] Unquestionably, the objective was desirable. In addition, the relative effects of a mild electric shock delivered to the child upon his displaying self-mutilation were evaluated. When the child ran to the arms of the investigator, the shock was terminated. The fact that this procedure generated an interest in people was considered a notable achievement since autistic children are characterized by their total social detachment. Finally, a socioeducational program based on positive rewards to ensure that the social gains would in time be self-sustaining was administered.

This work demonstrates the proper technical rationale for the use of aversive procedures. Whenever a shock was delivered to the child, care was taken to provide the child with an opportunity to extricate himself from the situation or to terminate the shock by engaging in a learned behavior. This procedure differs from the use of punishment in that the period of punishment is predetermined; it cannot be terminated by the subject. In using aversive stimuli, the individual subjected to it learns how to terminate it and how to avoid it in the future. This gives the subject control over both the onset and the termination of the stimuli. From a therapeutic viewpoint, generating interest in self-protection may well be the lowest level of motivation upon which the therapist can build complex adaptive behavior.

Conclusion

A new technology of behavior modification is rapidly emerging in the areas of therapy and prison rehabilitation. Conclusions may now be drawn as to the effectiveness of specific procedures. Rewards are most effective when they enrich rather than reduce the individual's range of incentives in an institution. Further, aversive procedures are most effective when they are used concurrently with a system of rewards. Because of ethical problems and limited effectiveness, however, aversive procedures, such as electric shock, should be used only in those cases where the individual is physically endangering himself or others. Indeed, heroic procedures such as electric shock are not standard and are of limited value since they teach an individual only what not to do, rather than what to do.

Research shows that it is possible to foster in patients and inmates new behaviors and to develop self-control and responsibility through a motivational system known as the token economy. This system restores to the individual the rights and social obligations found outside the institution. In so doing, the token economy preserves a modicum of social contact between the individual and society at large. Thus, behavior modification, by systematically exposing the individual to rewarding experiences, attempts to teach new and effective ways of meeting the demands of a socially complex world.

NOTES

1. Indeed, environmental events shape our character throughout life. The only difference

between behavior modification and other approaches to changing behavior is one of degree. Aversive conditioning is common in experience; for example, the child who learns to fear fire after being burned. By systematic application, however, behavior modification succeeds where other approaches fail. *See* Roos, *Human Rights and Behavior Modification*, 12 MENTAL RETARDATION, June 1974, at 4.

2. Ayllon, Smith & Rogers, *Behavioral Management of School Phobia*, 1 J. BEHAVIOR THERAPY & EXPERIMENTAL PSYCHIATRY 125, 126 (1970).

3. *See generally* Paul, *Outcome of Systematic Desensitization*, in BEHAVIOR THERAPY: APPRAISAL AND STATUS 63 (C. Franks ed. 1969); Russell, *The Power of Behavior Control: A Critique of Behavior Modification Methods*, 30 J. CLINICAL PSYCHOLOGY 111, 117-18 (1974).

4. *See generally,* J. WOLPE, PSYCHOTHERAPY BY RECIPROCAL INHIBITION (1958). Joseph Wolpe pioneered the technique. The historical origin and development is traced in Paul, *supra* note 3, at 64-66.

5. Some examples would be insomnia, shyness, homosexuality, and frigidity.

6. Systematic desensitization has been applied in mental health settings such as clinics and hospitals and in general practice.

7. The procedure is described in detail in Paul, *supra* note 3, at 68-70. The necessity for relaxation is in dispute.

8. For an exhaustive listing of medical articles on systematic desensitization, see W. MORROW, BEHAVIOR THERAPY BIBLIOGRAPHY 1950-1969, 156-57 (1971).

9. The token economy was developed in a ward of chronically psychotic female patients at the Anna State Hospital in Illinois. T. AYLLON & N. AZRIN, THE TOKEN ECONOMY: A MOTIVATIONAL SYSTEM FOR THERAPY AND REHABILITATION at v, 16 (1968) [hereinafter cited as THE TOKEN ECONOMY]. The literature on token economies is now extensive. *See* Davidson, *Appraisal of Behavior Modification Techniques with Adults in Institutional Settings*, in BEHAVIOR THERAPY: APPRAISAL AND STATUS 220, 229-35 (C. Franks ed. 1969); Kazdin & Bootzin, *The Token Economy: An Evaluation Review*, 5 J. APPLIED BEHAVIOR ANALYSIS 343 (1972). The legal problems have been exposed in Wexler, *Of Rights and Reinforcers*, 11 SAN DIEGO L. REV. 957 (1974) [hereinafter cited as Wexler, *Of Rights and Reinforcers*]; Wexler, *Token and Taboo: Behavior Modification, Token Economies, and the Law*, 61 CALIF. L. REV. 81 (1973).

10. While the performance objectives are often assumed to be clear-cut, the fact is that they are typically couched in terms that are abstract, mental, or largely unobservable. Therefore, for such objectives to be amenable to evaluation, further refinement towards objective definition is necessary.

11. Specially designed tangible items such as points, green stamps, credit cards, and similar symbols have been used as tokens.

12. Ayllon & Azrin, *The Measurement and Reinforcement of Behavior of Psychotics*, 8 J. EXPERIMENTAL ANALYSIS OF BEHAVIOR 357 (1968); Ayllon & Haughton, *Control of the Behavior of Schizophrenic Patients by Food*, 5 J. EXPERIMENTAL ANALYSIS OF BEHAVIOR 343 (1962); *see* Atthowe & Krasner, *Preliminary Report on the Application of Contingent Reinforcement Procedures (Token Economy) on a "Chronic" Psychiatric Ward*, 73 J. ABNORMAL PSYCHOLOGY 37 (1968); Lloyd & Abel, *Performance on a Token Economy Psychiatric Ward: A Two-Year Summary*, 8 BEHAVIOR RESEARCH & THERAPY 1 (1970). *See generally* THE TOKEN ECONOMY, *supra* note 9; Kazdin & Bootzin, *supra* note 9.

13. *Cf.* Birnbrauer, Wolf, Kidder & Tague, *Classroom Behavior of Retarded Pupils with Token Reinforcement*, 2 J. EXPERIMENTAL CHILD PSYCHOLOGY 219 (1965).

14. O'Leary, Becker, Evans & Saudargas, *A Token Reinforcement Program in a Public School: A Replication and Systematic Analysis*, 2 J. APPLIED BEHAVIOR ANALYSIS 3, 8-11 (1969).

15. Ayllon & Roberts, *Eliminating Discipline Problems by Strengthening Academic Performance*, 7 J. APPLIED BEHAVIOR ANALYSIS 71, 74-75 (1974); Lovitt & Curtiss, *Academic Response Rate as a Function of Teacher—And Self-Imposed Contingencies*, 2 J. APPLIED BEHAVIOR ANALYSIS 49, 52 (1969). In one study with disturbed adolescents, however, a token economy designed to increase productivity in classwork resulted in an increase in quantity but a decrease in quality. Cotler, Applegate, King & Kristal, *Establishing a Token Economy Program in a State Hospital Classroom: A Lesson in Training Student and Teacher*, 3 BEHAVIOR THERAPY, 209, 214-17 (1972).

16. Burchard & Tyler, *The Modification of Delinquent Behaviour Through Operant Conditioning*, 2 BEHAVIOUR RESEARCH & THERAPY 245 (1965).

17. H. COHEN, J. FILIPCZAK & J. BIS, AN INITIAL STUDY OF CONTINGENCIES APPLICABLE TO SPECIAL EDUCATION (1967).

18. Milan & McKee, *Behavior Modification: Principles and Applications in Corrections*, in HANDBOOK OF CRIMINOLOGY (D. Glaser ed. 1974); Boren & Colman, *Some Experiments on Reinforcement Principles Within Psychiatric Ward for Delinquent Soldiers*, 3 J. APPLIED BEHAVIOR ANALYSIS 29 (1970).

19. Again, one of the major problems in the application of behavioral technology to prisons is definition of the inmates' problems and the objectives of the prison. While the inmates' problems have often been conceptualized in a psychological manner involving pathological aggression toward society, this approach limits evaluation of a treatment's effectiveness. A behavioral redefinition of the inmates' problems involves pinpointing the areas of social interaction that require specific skills. A step in that direction is reflected in the selection of behaviors to be taught to the inmates while in prison. In selecting vocational, educational, and social objectives for therapy or treatment, the prison becomes associated with rehabilitative and educational efforts rather than with custodial goals.

20. This program included boys who were in trouble with their school or community or who were largely uncontrollable. Phillips, *Achievement Place: Token Reinforcement Procedures in a Home-Style Rehabilitation Setting for "Pre-Delinquent" Boys*, 1 J. APPLIED BEHAVIOR ANALYSIS 213, 213–14 (1968). Phillips, Phillips, Fixsen & Wolf, *Achievement Place: Modification of the Behaviors of Pre-Delinquent Boys Within a Token Economy*, 4 J. APPLIED BEHAVIOR ANALYSIS 45, 45–46 (1971).

21. *See generally* S. RACHEMAN & J. TEASDALE, AVERSION THERAPY AND BEHAVIOR DISORDERS: AN ANALYSIS (1969); Rachman & Teasdale, *Aversion Therapy: An Appraisal*, in BEHAVIOR THERAPY: APPRAISAL AND STATUS 279–320 (C. Franks ed. 1969). *See also* W. MORROW, *supra* note 8, at 154–55 (collecting sources).

22. S. RACHMAN & J. TEASDALE, *supra* note 21, at xii.

23. Autism is a form of childhood schizophrenia characterized by acting out and withdrawal. The autistic child is apt to perform acts of self-mutilation and head banging. Developmental language disorders and a marked inability to adjust socially are also characteristic. DORLAND'S ILLUSTRATED MEDICAL DICTIONARY 168 (25th ed. 1974).

24. Neither homosexuality nor heterosexuality fills the vacuum created when the other is extinguished. *Money, Strategy, Ethics, Behavior Modification, and Homosexuality*, 2 ARCHIVES OF SEXUAL BEHAVIOR 79 (1972) (editorial). It has been suggested that the proper way to extinguish homosexuality is to reward the subject with a homosexual experience after he achieves a heterosexual experience. Gradually, the number of heterosexual experiences needed to achieve a homosexual experience is increased until the frequency of homosexual activity is minimized or extinguished. *Id.* at 79–80.

The necessity of shock therapy to reduce homosexuality has been questioned. It has been observed that a male homosexual must be "strongly motivated toward change . . . to subject himself to a series of such shocks after visit. . . . [I]f other forms of psychotherapy were limited only to such a select group of exceptionally motivated homosexuals the results also would be better than average." Marmor, *Dynamic Psychotherapy and Behavior Therapy*, 24 ARCHIVES OF GENERAL PSYCHIATRY 22, 25 (1971).

25. In a laboratory setting, elecric shock has been delivered to children who climb to dangerous heights. Risley, *The Effects and Side Effects of Punishing the Autistic Behavior of a Deviant Child*, 1 J. APPLIED BEHAVIOR ANALYSIS 25–30 (1968). Shock also has been delivered to autistic children who engage in severe head banging and self-mutilation. Lovaas & Simmons, *Manipulation of Self-Destruction in Three Retarded Children*, 2 J. APPLIED BEHAVIOR ANALYSIS 143 (1969).

26. *See* Marks & Gelder, *Transvestism and Fetishism: Clinical and Psychological Changes During Faradic Aversion*, 113 BRITISH J. PSYCHIATRY 711 (1967).

27. *See generally*, A. BANDURA, PRINCIPLES OF BEHAVIOR MODIFICATION 501–54 (1969).

28. *See* Lovaas, Schaeffer & Simmons, *Building Social Behavior in Autistic Children by Use of Electric Shock*, 1 J. EXPERIMENTAL RESEARCH IN PERSONALITY 99, 106–08 (1965); Risley, *supra* note 25, at 21, 32–34.

29. *Accord,* Roos, *supra* note 1, at 5.

30. *See* text & note 37, *infra.*

31. Ayllon & Michael, *The Psychiatric Nurse as a Behavioral Engineer,* 2 J. EXPERIMENTAL ANALYSIS OF BEHAVIOR 323 (1959). *See generally* Sherman & Baer, *Appraisal of Operant Therapy Techniques with Children and Adults,* in BEHAVIOR THERAPY: APPRAISAL AND STATUS 192, 215-16 (C. Franks ed. 1969).

32. *See generally* Sherman & Baer, *supra* note 31, at 212-13.

33. Wolf, Risley & Mees, *Application of Operant Conditioning Procedures to the Behavior Problems of an Autistic Child,* 1 BEHAVIOUR RESEARCH & THERAPY 305, 311 (1964). In another study, children who broke rules applicable to playing pool with other children were isolated for brief periods. Tyler & Brown, *The Use of Swift, Brief Isolation as a Group Control Device for Institutionalized Delinquents,* 5 BEHAVIOR RESEARCH & THERAPY 1, 2 (1967).

34. A recent United States Supreme Court case has held, however, that prisoners may not be placed in solitary confinement without procedural due process guarantees. Wolff v. McDonnell, 418 U.S. 539, 563-67 (1974).

35. Legal strictures require, however, that certain basic rights, food, and privacy not be removed. Wyatt v. Stickney, 344 F. Supp. 373 (D. Ala. 1972), *aff'd sub nom.,* Wyatt v. Aderholt, 503 F.2d 1305 (#th Cir. 1974), *noted in* 51 B.U.L. REV. 530 (1971), 86 HARV. L. REV. 1282 (1973), *and* 25 U. FLA. L. REV. 614 (1973).

36. Baer, *Laboratory Control of Thumbsucking by Withdrawal and Representation of Reinforcement,* 5 J. EXPERIMENTAL ANALYSIS OF BEHAVIOR 525 (1962). *See* Sherman & Baer, *supra* note 31, at 212.

37. The ethical issues involved in behavior modification have been widely discussed. *See, e.g.,* B. SKINNER, BEYOND FREEDOM AND DIGNITY (1972); Bengelman, *Ethical Issues in Behavioral Control,* 156 J. NERVOUS & MENTAL DISEASE 412 (1973); Cooke & Cooke, *Behavioral Modification: Answers to Some Ethical Issues,* 11 PSYCHOLOGY IN THE SCHOOLS 5 (1974); Halleck, *Legal and Ethical Aspects of Behavior Control,* 131 AM. J. PSYCHIATRY 381 (1974); Roos, *supra* note 1. Behavior modification has been attacked as repressive, dehumanizing, and perhaps even part of a conspiracy to control those citizens who deviate from social norms. Halleck, *supra* at 381. Not all practitioners agree. One psychiatrist remarked that "[o]nly in rare and extreme situations are many people excessively concerned about the minutiae of patients' rights . . . ." Cole, 131 AM. J. PSYCHIATRY 927 (1974) (letter to the editor). In response, it has been charged that such statements are "dangerously naive." Halleck, 131 AM. J. PSYCHIATRY 928 (1974) (letter to the editor).

After arguing that behavior modification techniques contain no new power over mankind, one practitioner interestingly concludes that since there can be no meaningful debate about the ethics of methods that do not work, a discussion of the ethics involved in psychological control is now rather academic. Russell, *supra* note 3, at 132. Even so, this argument is premised upon a misconception—that behavioral techniques are due to a Hawthorne or placebo effect. In other words, whatever behavioral change might follow therapy is not due to the therapy, but to pre-existing forces. Those who would advance this point argue that behavioral experiments use no controls and that it is therefore a logical fallacy to assume that the cause of the modified behavior was necessarily the therapy. *See* Opton, *Institutional Behavior Modification as a Fraud and Sham,* 17 ARIZ. L. REV. 20, 22 (1975). In behavioral experiments, however, each person is his own control. The effects of behavior modification can be evaluated by terminating the behavioral procedure and observing whether there is reversion to the sort of behavior that the procedures had attempted to change. This on-off experimental design, called ABA design, is used in all behavioral experiments. *See, e.g.,* Tyler & Brown, *supra* note 33. Indeed, from an ethical standpoint, it is far better to use an ABA design for control than to let a group of patients sit idle, without treatment, merely to constitute a scientifically pure control group.

One more point should be made about the efficacy of behavioral techniques. Opponents argue that it is widely recognized that patients in a token economy eventually will decline to do jobs that are not paid and will request assignment to jobs that do pay. "Crazy they may have been, but not that crazy." Opton, *supra* at 25 n.17. This both misses and makes the point. Indeed, such behavior is not crazy. The people involved in these programs, however, have never exhibited such behavior before. In the example given, the token economy has taught the principle of economic utility to persons who never before acted in such a manner. This normal behavior was learned.

Certain ethical problems may be irresolvable. For instance, it is difficult to say what one does with a claustrophobic patient who pleads to be released from confinement, assuming he has previously agreed to treatment precisely outlined. Begelman, *supra* at 417. Of course, the patient should be released. The therapy, however, never gets a chance to work. Perhaps the solution lies in more innovative techniques and more gradual treatment.

38. These include all constitutional rights in general and, in particular, the rights to a residence unit with a screen, a comfortable bed, a locker, a chair, a table, nutritional meals, and social interaction, and the rights to have visitors, attend religious services, wear one's own clothes, have clothes laundered, and exercise outdoors. In general, there is a right to the least restrictive conditions necessary to achieve the purposes of commitment. Wyatt v. Stickney, 344 F. Supp. 373, 379–86 (M.D. Ala. 1972), *aff'd sub nom.*, Wyatt v. Aderholt, 503 F.2d 1305 (5th Cir. 1974).

39. Legally, however, consent is not required in all circumstances. *See* Friedman, *Legal Regulation of Applied Behavior Analysis in Mental Institutions and Prisons,* 17 ARIZ. L. REV. 39, 68–69 (1975).

40. *See* Wyatt v. Stickney, 344 F. Supp. 373, 380 (M.D. Ala. 1972), *aff'd sub nom.*, Wyatt v. Aderholt, 503 F.2d 1305 (5th Cir. 1974); Halleck, *supra* note 37, at 384; Roos, *supra* note 1, at 5.

41. These agreements appear to be contracts in the legal sense. There is mutuality of consideration—the therapist develops a treatment plan and the patient agrees to a fee. Failure of performance by the therapist, that is, failure of treatment, results in a reduced fee. Legal problems, however, remain. Should the patient fail to use his best effort to comply or if he terminates the treatment, it is not clear whether the therapist has a claim for his full fee. Neither is it clear whether the therapist, by contracting, has guaranteed certain results.

42. An example of such a contract is reproduced in Ayllon & Skuban, *Accountability in Psychotherapy: A Test Case,* 4 J. BEHAVIOR THERAPY & EXPERIMENTAL PSYCHIATRY 19, 22–23 (1973).

43. While this contract is, of course, intended for therapy rather than penal rehabilitation, it also could be used in a prison, thus paving the way for accountability in our prisons.

44. Wyatt v. Stickney, 344 F. Supp. 373, 380 (M.D. Ala. 1972), *aff'd sub nom.*, Wyatt v. Aderholt, 503 F.2d 1305 (5th Cir. 1974); *cf.* Halleck, *supra* note 37, at 384.

45. In the case of Knecht v. Gillman, 488 F.2d 1136 (8th Cir. 1973), a vomiting inducing drug called apomorphine was injected whenever certain behavioral requirements were not met, such as getting up on time and working. Although the objectives may be desirable, the extremely negative method of achieving them cannot be justified behaviorally since such behaviors can more easily be developed through positive means such as rewards.

46. *See* Wyatt v. Stickney, 344 F. Supp. 373, 380 (M.D. Ala. 1972), *aff'd sub nom.*, Wyatt v. Aderholt, 503 F.2d 1305 (5th Cir. 1974).

47. For example, in Springfield, Missouri in October 1972, a rehabilitative program called START (Special Treatment and Rehabilitative Training) began. This program involved inmates who were arbitrarily denied regular prison conditions without a hearing. For discussions of START, see Friedman, *supra* note 39, at 92–94; Wexler, *Of Rights and Reinforcers, supra* note 9, at 963–64.

48. 42 U.S.L.W. 2063 (C.A. 73-19434-AW, Cir. Ct. Wayne County, Mich., July 10, 1973) (partial report).

49. N. LEOPOLD, LIFE PLUS 99 YEARS 305-38 (1958).

50. Any evaluation index, such as a grade or performance rating, must be made known to the patient or inmate so that he can take part in the decision-making body regarding his terminating or continuing a given program.

51. *See* Wyatt v. Stickney, 344 F. Supp. 373, 384–86 (M.D. Ala. 1972), *aff'd sub nom.*, Wyatt v. Aderholt, 503 F.2d 1305 (5th Cir. 1974).

52. E. WRIGHT, THE POLITICS OF PUNISHMENT: A CRITICAL ANALYSIS OF PRISONS IN AMERICA 61 (1973).

53. Indeed, there is little to indicate that group counseling has made any significant difference to most inmates. *Id.*

54. See discussion note 47 *supra*.

55. The right to be free from unreasonable search and seizure, the right to privacy, the right against cruel and unusual punishment, and the freedoms of religion, speech, and association were alleged to be abridged. *See* Clonce v. Richardson, 379 F. Supp. 338, 352 (W.D. Mo. 1974).

56. Halleck, *supra* note 37, at 384.

57. Any arbitrary unit of exchange, such as gold, silver, blankets, shells, or cigarettes, could be used.

58. Since an individual choosing not to engage in the rewarded activity would simply experience the absence of reward as opposed to coercion to conform to a given behavior, the requirements of the eighth guideline in the previous section are satisfied. *See* text accompanying notes 54–56 *supra*.

59. This could be accomplished with a job rotation rule requiring that a patient not be allowed to hold the same job without interruption for more than a week at a time. *See* THE TOKEN ECONOMY, *supra* note 9, at 200–03.

60. *Cf.* N. KITTRIE, THE RIGHT TO BE DIFFERENT (1971). The methodology to achieve such objectives is available in the token economy. See text & notes 9–20 *supra*.

61. *See* discussion note 38 *supra*. Since many chronically ill patients may forego such rights, there is need for procedures which ensure that patients enjoy them. In this way, the danger of being deprived of items that are self-reinforcing would be avoided. *See* THE TOKEN ECONOMY, *supra* note 9, at 88–103.

62. Such free access to privileges and incentives is consistent with the priming rule describe in THE TOKEN ECONOMY, *supra* 9, at 91–93.

63. Wexler, *Of Rights and Reinforcers, supra* note 9, at 968–69. Idiosyncratic pleasures, such as feeding kittens, are the most effective reinforcers. Atthowe & Krasner, *supra* note 12, at 38.

64. Roos, *supra* note 1, at 5 (suggesting that a distinction should be drawn between time-out, which is therapeutic, and seclusion, which is long term and merely for the convenience of the staff).

65. For example, head banging, self-mutilation, and violent assaults on others would justify such therapy. Further, punishment and the use of noxious stimuli require the technical supervision of a trained professional since these techniques are easily subject to misuse and abuse.

66. *See* Lovaas, Schaeffer & Simmons, *supra* note 28; Lovaas & Simmons, *supra* note 25.

Rosalind Pollack Petchesky

Reproduction, Ethics, and Public Policy: The Federal Sterilization Regulations

On March 8, 1979, the Department of Health, Education, and Welfare's rules governing federal financial participation in sterilization programs went into effect.[1] Issued after six months of public hearings and in a climate of heated controversy, the federal regulations were welcomed by community, health, and professional groups for whom involuntary sterilization has become a pressing social issue.[2] But they also have met resistance from those who strongly favor sterilization as a means of population control. The regulations attempt to formulate a government policy for some difficult ethical questions: the meaning of "voluntary consent," the boundary between justifiable protection from abuse and unjustifiable paternalism, and the rights of those judged "incompetent to decide." Before examining the regulations themselves, it is important to understand the issues that generated them.

I. Ethical and Social Issues

Surgical sterilization is a procedure that renders a person permanently unable to bear children. While the ethics of a biomedical procedure are never determined by technology alone, the virtually irreversible nature of surgical sterilization makes the choice a more drastic one than it might be otherwise.[3] The question of "voluntariness" becomes more problematic and the conditions under which the decision is made—including the social, economic, institutional, and sexual conditions—require critical scrutiny.

From *The Hastings Center Report*, 9 (October 1979):29–41. Copyright © 1979 by The Hastings Center. Reprinted by permission of the publisher and the author.

A. What Is Reproductive Freedom?

Whether sterilization is moral or immoral in itself may be debated among theologians and ethicists. For the purposes of public policy and of this article, however, it is the *social arrangements* in which the procedure is embedded — the degree to which those arrangements allow for full participation and consciousness of the person being sterilized, and respond to that person's concrete social and biological needs — that are critical. The value of any method of contraception must be determined not only with regard to effectiveness and safety for the user (risks),[4] but also with regard to *reproductive freedom* (autonomy). This means the degree to which the form and the social relations implied by a particular birth control method allow the user fully to understand its medical consequences, actively to control its use and nonuse, and consciously to integrate its use with thoughtful decisions about the meaning of sexuality and childbearing in her or his own life and in society. In this view, *sterilization abuse* (or any form of involuntary sterilization) is wrong because it subverts the need of a person to control her or his own body and to decide, in a fully informed and conscious way, what sort of interventions may be made into bodily processes, including the biological capacity to procreate.

Thus, the basic issue involved in reproductive freedom is a principle that has very old roots in the tradition of radical individualism,[5] but that has been particularly espoused by the contemporary women's liberation movement: the need to control one's own body, or "bodily self-determination." It is primarily this value, and not any "right to procreate" per se, that informs the aim of reproductive freedom — the freedom to determine when, whether, and under what conditions one will or will not bear children. Along with intellectual development, control over one's own body is an essential aspect of personality development and hence of the means by which individuals live out their connections to social groups and social purposes. The principle has had a particular meaning for women historically, since women's bodies have frequently been objectified for the sexual and reproductive ends of others — for example, through forced marriage, rape, and state-sponsored population control programs. In this regard, it is important to note that most documented instances of coerced sterilization in the United States involve women.

A second principle underlying the claim of women particularly to reproductive freedom refers to the culturally determined position of women with regard to children. Because it is predominantly women who must bear the social consequences of pregnancy — a historical condition that could change if men shared equally in childrearing — feminists assert women's need to control the technical and material conditions of contraception, pregnancy, and childbearing.

Involuntary sterilization is an invasion of a woman's bodily integrity and identity for ends that usually accommodate the needs of others in disregard of her own needs, and that pre-empt her bodily self-determination. This is not to say that the need for control over one's body and reproductive capacities is absolute or exists in isolation from one's connections to other people. Individuals exist as social beings whose needs are defined by family, class, and racial as well as gender identities. Individual women exercise, limit, or lose their capacity to bear children in relation to others to whom they are responsible and who are responsible for them—sexual partners, parents, children; and wider communities beyond the family. But in the last analysis these social connections and responsibilities do not abrogate the necessity, in any morally acceptable system of "fertility control," to maximize the consciousness and participation of the individuals whose fertility is directly involved.

"Maximize" is a key word here, since the very capacity to make "informed and conscious" decisions, and thus to exercise bodily self-determination, is in some circumstances at issue. In the case of persons for whom this capacity is very limited (for example, the severely retarded), the need for bodily self-determination does not cease to exist; its potential for satisfaction simply has very particular requirements and limits.

B. Voluntary and Involuntary Sterilization

A social view of reproductive freedom requires an analysis of the conditions that structure individual decisions about sterilization, contraception, and childbearing. Most people most of the time make choices "freely" as conscious moral agents, but within a social framework of conditions and constraints that is not of their own making and that they themselves, as mere individuals, are powerless to change. Seen from this perspective, the concept of "informed consent" cannot be seen merely as a formal procedural requirement, but must take into account and attempt to mitigate the institutional and social pressures that may undermine such consent in practice.

This socially oriented concept of "voluntary consent" is implicit in the new federal sterilization regulations. In particular, the regulations are concerned with cases of sterilization abuse arising out of the disparities in knowledge and power between clinicians and (particularly poor) patients. Many other conditions, however, structure the social context of sterilization as a birth control option for people. These include economic conditions, such as equal access, regardless of class, to all family planning and health services; or a level of income and job security that makes it possible to raise children decently. They also include cultural conditions, such as a socially developed morality that acknowledges the sexual needs of women as well as men and the contraceptive and childrearing capacities and responsibilities of men as well as women. Such conditions are related to the ethics of sterilization and birth control because their persistent absence defines the existing social limits on most people's reproductive freedom.

The push to regulate federally funded sterilization occurs within a larger demographic context: the sharp increase in the use of sterilization worldwide as a form of contraception. The trend toward "voluntary sterilization," or the now common, medically recommended use of sterilization as a method of birth control, is of very recent origin. Demographic analyses of the latest data on United States fertility and contraceptive use show that sterilization has become the most frequently used form of contraception in the world; and next to the pill, the second most frequently used among Americans.[6] This represents a threefold increase since 1970—the largest increase for any method of contraception—with the result that, by 1976, 30 percent of all widowed, divorced, and separated women and single mothers aged fifteen to forty-four in the United States had been surgically sterilized; and nearly that number among all currently married couples (wife aged fifteen to forty-four) had had at least one of the partners sterilized.[7] In total, nearly 10 million persons in the United States (excluding those who have had hysterectomies) had been sterilized by 1977, according to figures published by the Association for Voluntary Sterilization (AVS)—approximately one million each year since 1974.[8]

The overall increase in surgical sterilization has taken place differentially depending on sex, race, class, and age. For example:

While vasectomies are an important form of contraception among white middle-class and upper-middle-class men, sterilizations in the United States, especially among low-income and minority groups, are performed more frequently on women—especially if hysterectomies are counted. According to the AVS figures, tubal ligations have steadily increased in proportion to vasectomies. Whereas in 1971 they represented only 20 percent of sterilizations compared to 80 percent for males, the proportions in 1977 were 40 percent male and 60 percent female.

Among married couples, sterilizations are still more likely to occur among black, Hispanic, and Native American women than among white women, particularly in certain regions and cities.[9]

Among low-income couples of all races, sterilizations have increased the most among those aged twenty-five to thirty-four; whereas the increase in sterilization of higher-income couples occurs among those aged thirty-five and older. (One unexamined factor that needs further analysis is the tendency of low-income women to begin childbearing at an earlier age.) Thirty-seven percent of all low-income white married couples aged twenty-five to thirty-four have had one partner sterilized, and these are mostly women.[10]

Do these disparities reflect merely a variety of "personal tastes"? Or does the rise in sterilizations raise ethical and social questions about the conditions of "reproductive choice" and the line between "voluntary" and "involuntary"? Critics of these disparities argue that, because of the irreversible nature of surgical sterilization, the statistical evidence of its prevalence among more vulnerable groups in the population—low-income and minority women—in itself creates a suspicion of involuntariness. An analysis of the general social conditions confronting most women who become sterilized reinforces this presumption. Such an analysis would include:[11]

Economic shifts, such as the rise in the labor force participation of married women with children; the rise in female-headed families;[12] and further cuts in (already inadequate) social services (child care, health care, welfare benefits), which intensify women's need for absolutely reliable means of birth control.

The serious health hazards or other inadequacies of alternative methods of birth control, particularly the pill, resulting in a drop-off in their use among most groups of women.[13]

The all-out political and legal attack on abortions, resulting in the practical unavailability of abortion as an option for many women—particularly low-income women—in most states.[14]

The bias in both public and private health insurance coverage toward fully reimbursing sterilization while covering abortion and nonsurgical means of contraception either very restrictively or not at all.[15]

Since 1970, the conscious, publicly espoused policy of medical and family planning professionals favoring sterilization as the most "efficacious," technically reliable form of contraception for all women, regardless of age or number of children.[16] The liberalization and promotion of sterilization has been an outgrowth of population control (as distinct from individual birth control).[17] It seems clear that this policy has influenced people's contraceptive behavior on a broad scale (rather than merely reflecting a "response" to "consumer demand").

These social and economic conditions raise questions about the increase in sterilization as a "method of choice." Clearly, even when voluntary, sterilization is often chosen in a context of heavy structural constraints. Moreover, there are more elusive cultural and ideological influences that encourage the trend toward sterilization, such as changes in sexual ideology and the popular image of sterilization as an avenue toward "sexual freedom."[18] This is not to deny that sterilization may be a very real and important way, within existing economic constraints and sexual relations, for women to gain some control over their sexual and reproductive lives, particularly given the minimal responsibility most men assume for contraception and childbearing. Nevertheless, the argument here is that all of the forces described together create a social climate that is helping to legitimate a return to the eugenic sterilization laws of the 1920s and proposals for the *involuntary* sterilization of certain groups, particularly poor and retarded women. For, if "voluntary sterilization" is widely growing, and presented in the media as "liberating" in itself, then coerced sterilization may more easily appear as "benevolent."

A number of involuntary sterilization proposals and actual incidents of involuntary sterilization under both state and federal programs have been widely publicized.[19] These proposals have distinct historic roots. In the early decades of this century, American upper-class social reformers, politicians, and academics campaigned to subject hundreds of thousands of the nation's poor, immigrant, and institutionalized populations to forced sterilization on eugenic grounds, succeeding to a startling degree, particularly among the so-called "feeble-minded" in institutions.[20] Judicial authorization for state eugenic sterilization laws came in Oliver Wendell Holmes's famous 1927 decision in *Buck v. Bell,* which maintained a "compelling state interest in preventing the procreation of children who will become a burden on the state," and which is still controlling law today in similar cases.

Many such cases have come to light since the early 1970s. The most famous involved the Relf sisters and other poor, teenage black women in a federally funded clinic in Alabama. The federal district court in 1974 found that:

> Over the past few years, an estimated 100,000 to 150,000 low-income persons have been sterilized annually under federally funded programs. . . . There is uncontroverted evidence in the record that minors and other incompetents have been sterilized with federal funds and that an indefinite number of poor people have been improperly coerced into accepting a sterilization operation under the threat that various federally supported welfare benefits would be withdrawn unless they submitted to irreversible sterilization.[21]

Other cases have involved a young married woman who discovered that her parents, because of her sexual activity, had previously had her sterilized through a court order without her knowledge;[22] indiscriminate sterilizations of institutionalized women;[23] and the current attempt to use eugenic sterilization statutes to facilitate the deinstitutionalization of retarded persons,[24] or the involuntary sterilization of retarded persons who have not been institutionalized.[25] At present, legislation authorizing the involuntary sterilization of the mentally incompetent or other groups on so-called "eugenic" grounds exists in some twenty-five states. Attempts to apply such laws, and proposals for extending them, are indistinguishable from their historical predecessors — in the eugenicist ideology to which they subscribe, and in their racist and sexist undertones. Those at whom the proposals are aimed (the "beneficiaries") are still primarily low-income, black or other minorities, and female; and their alleged "unfitness" is associated with mental disability and/or poverty. Those enunciating the proposals are still primarily white and upper-middle-class and often wear the hats of helping professionals, moralists, or fiscal reformers. The exception to this pattern is the growing appeal by associations made up of parents of the retarded, many of whom have come to see sterilization as an answer to their personal caretaking problems.

C. Sterilization Abuse

In sum, those who look critically at the pervasive use of sterilization are concerned about the incidence of sterilization abuse. Sterilization abuse occurs whenever surgical sterilizations are performed under conditions that, *de facto* if not *de jure,* pressure an individual into agreeing to be sterilized, or obscure the risks, consequences, and alternatives associated with sterilization. The term "abuse" is meant to suggest forms of pressure short of blatant coercion, which nevertheless are unfair or arbitrary. Thus abuse would include, for example, not only failure on the part of physician or provider to acquire written or formal consent, but failure to explain clearly, in the patient's own language, the irreversibility of the procedure and the existing contraceptive alternatives; threatening or implying loss of welfare or medical benefits as a consequence of refusal to consent; or making sterilization the condition for performing an abortion.

The publicity given to the *Relf* case generated a chain of sterilization abuse exposés, most of them involving poor and minority women. In 1976, the General Accounting Office found "that 3,000 female sterilizations had been performed in a four year period in the federally funded facilities of the Indian Health Service," using consent forms which were "not in compliance with . . . regulations."[26] Physicians themselves acknowledged the common practice in teaching hospitals of performing elective hysterectomies on poor black and Hispanic women as part of standard training in obstetrics and gynecology. Court cases began to reveal instances of abuse—such as the South Carolina rural doctor who for years had refused medical treatment to his female, financially dependent patients when they declined sterilization after their third child.[27] Finally, a number of radical political organizations—such as the Committee to End Sterilization Abuse and the Committee for Abortion Rights and Against Sterilization Abuse—emerged, whose main purpose has been to publicize and organize against sterilization abuse in the legislatures, the courts, hospitals, and communities.[28]

This is the climate that first produced guidelines in New York City upon which the federal regulations are based. (The New York City rules are broader in scope than the federal rules, since they apply to private as well as public programs.) After months of required testimony in all of DHEW's ten regions, agency policymakers had to weigh the testimony of women's and community health groups on the one hand and family planning and medical professionals on the other. Their aim was to develop a set of rules that would both "encourage access to the use of (sterilization) services," and guarantee "that receipt of such services be voluntary, and that no one be sterilized in the absence of full knowledge or against one's will."[29]

II. Substance of the Regulations

More than anything else, the federal sterilization regulations are intended to prevent the involuntary or indiscriminate sterilization of groups who are especially vulnerable to abuse—the poor, minors, and the mentally disabled. This goal is to be balanced with the DHEW policy of maintaining and supporting "access to sterilization services," and is reflected in the regulations' detailed procedures for assuring voluntariness and noncoercion in the relations between providers and consumers.

The most important provisions include:

Requiring that voluntary informed consent be obtained, using a mandatory, standardized consent form provided in the patient's preferred language;

Prohibiting any overt or implicit threat of loss of welfare or Medicaid benefits as a consequence of nonconsent;

Prohibiting the obtaining of consent during labor, before or after an abortion, or while a person is under the influence of drugs or alcohol;

Abolishing the distinction between "contraceptive" and "noncontraceptive" (or "therapeutic") sterilizations for purposes of federal regulation;

Prohibiting hysterectomies for sterilization purposes in federally funded programs;

Requiring a thirty-day waiting period between consent and operation (with waivers for early delivery and emergency abdominal surgery);

Requiring that complete information be provided, also in the patient's language, orally as well as in writing, regarding the irreversibility of sterilization, all risks and side effects, and alternative methods of contraception;

Imposing a moratorium on all federally funded sterilizations of persons under twenty-one, involuntarily institutionalized, or declared legally incompetent; and

Providing for federal auditing of sterilization programs in the ten states where most federally funded sterilization procedures are performed.

The following comments group these provisions by the larger policy issues that they address: (a) the meaning of "sterilization," that is, what is to be regulated; (b) the meaning of "informed consent" to sterilization; and (c) cases in which informed consent is considered unobtainable under existing circumstances.

A. What Is Surgical Sterilization?

The regulations define "sterilization" in such a way that certain common abusive practices are now made more difficult or prohibited altogether. In particular, this applies to indiscriminate counseling of sterilization for "therapeutic reasons" and the common practice of performing hysterectomies for "contraceptive purposes."

First, the distinction between "therapeutic" and "nontherapeutic" sterilizations, that is, those that are "medically indicated" as opposed to those that are performed for "contraceptive purposes only," has been eliminated. The Department believes that classifying a procedure as "therapeutic" can become a way for physicians to "avoid the restrictions of the regulations." It emphasizes that, wherever sterilization is performed in a situation where "other medical options exist," sterilization represents an irreversible choice to terminate childbearing; and that choice must be made within the safeguards of the regulations.[30] In practice, it is hard to see how *any* tubal ligations could be exempt from the regulations, since the procedure has no therapeutic value in itself and would scarcely be the only option for avoiding medically contraindicated pregnancies. Moreover, family planning specialists often acknowledge that the distinction is very difficult to maintain in practice, since many sterilizations are done for a combination of contraceptive and medical reasons (for example, diabetes, hypertension, or heart condition). Thus, given the growing proportions of tubal ligations that are classified as "therapeutic" rather than "contraceptive," this provision may help to prevent unnecessary "medical" sterilizations that might be regretted later.

Second, the regulations prohibit federal funding for hysterectomies done for sterilization purposes. Technically, the regulations define "sterilization" as "any medical procedure, treatment, or operation for the purpose of rendering an individual permanently incapable of reproducing." But in a separate section they provide explicitly that the DHEW "does not consider hysterectomy an appropriate method of sterilization, since compared to other forms of sterilization, hysterectomy is a risky, painful, and expensive procedure."[31] This is significant, given evidence of a rise in hysterectomies for "contraceptive purposes" and their preponderance among black and Hispanic women.[32]

B. What Are the Conditions of Informed Consent?

Following the precedent set by federal guidelines regulating research on human subjects, the federal sterilization regulations set out to establish the necessary preconditions that will assure that consent to sterilization be given in a manner that is truly informed and voluntary. As those who have pressed for a larger public role in the definition of "informed consent" are aware, the reality of informed consent has a social basis; in other words, it arises out of the actual relations of communication, authority, and power that exist between providers and the people they are serving.

Among the most controversial provisions is a mandatory thirty-day waiting period between the date of informed consent and the date of sterilization. Two exceptions are allowed: in cases of early delivery or emergency abdominal surgery, the waiting period may be reduced to a minimum of seventy-two hours (between the time of consent and sterilization) in order to avoid additional hospitalization. Over two-thirds of the comments received on this issue in the hearing process were absolutely or conditionally opposed to the mandatory thirty days. Opponents voiced concern that such a requirement "would discriminate against the poor" (since people seeking sterilizations through privately funded sources do not have to wait); that it would create a "barrier to access" for rural residents, migratory workers, and others; and that it would "constitute excessive regulation of medical practice."[13] DHEW rejected these arguments, resisting pressure from the obstetricians, gynecologists and other groups, and argued that, since "there is no such thing as an 'emergency' sterilization," there is no reason to hurry the procedure. Rather, the purpose of the 30-day waiting period is not just to prevent coercion but to insure, insofar as possible, that the individual reflects carefully on the consequences of the proposed sterilization and makes a decision that he or she will not later regret, since the procedure must be considered to be irreversible.[34]

Moreover, the comments on the thirty-day provision suggests that "careful reflection" is a matter, not only of "sufficient time," but also of counteracting the pressures of "an intimidating environment or stressful situation (such as during hospitalization)."[35] The waiting period thus responds to institutional realities by preventing situations in which a hospital setting or medical authority may put pressure on people to agree to sterilization. The mandatory thirty days was thought sufficient to give patients a chance to consult relatives, friends, and others before making the decision to get sterilized. Rather than a bureaucratic barrier, the waiting period may be seen as a precondition of voluntary consent, since "abuse appears likely to occur when persons are pressured or rushed into a decision."[36]

Other informed consent provisions also attempt to increase the resources and knowledge of patients. For example, they place much of the responsibility for "informing" on the provider. Not only must the person be given information about "available alternative methods of family planning and birth control," a complete explanation of the procedure to be used and all of its known risks and benefits, and explicit notice of its irreversibility, but this information must be provided orally, in the person's preferred language, and in a mode accessible to blind, deaf, or otherwise handicapped individuals. It is hoped that this provision will remove the kinds of cultural, class, and other barriers that often impede the communication process.

Further, informed consent as defined by the regulations means that no element implicit in the authority or power of the provider, or in the social or medical situation of the client, should become a subtle or overt means of coercion. Implicitly, this is an acknowledgment of the vulnerability many women feel in their relations with obstetricians or social workers. Thus, the regulations provide that consent may not be obtained while a "person" is "in labor or childbirth" or "seeking to obtain or obtaining an abortion." This is particularly important, given the routine practice in the past of requiring sterilization as a condition for performing abortions on low-income women utilizing public or teaching hospital service. Similarly, the provision that prohibits sterilization providers from threatening denial of medical services or welfare payments if a person refuses sterilization is an effort to prevent one of the most blatant forms of past abuse.

Attached to the regulations is a consent form to be used by all federally-funded providers. Among other things, it states prominently:

YOUR DECISION AT ANY TIME NOT TO BE STERILIZED WILL NOT RESULT IN THE WITHDRAWAL OR WITHHOLDING OF ANY BENEFITS PROVIDED BY PROGRAMS OR PROJECTS

RECEIVING FEDERAL FUNDS. . . . I UNDERSTAND THAT THE STERILIZATION MUST BE
CONSIDERED PERMANENT AND NOT REVERSIBLE. I HAVE DECIDED THAT I DO NOT WANT
TO BECOME PREGNANT, BEAR CHILDREN OR FATHER CHILDREN.

C. Under What Conditions Is Voluntary Consent Unobtainable?

The DHEW has continued its moratorium on sterilizations of certain groups for whom voluntary consent may be problematic. These include minors (under age twenty-one), institutionalized persons, and persons declared mentally incompetent.

It is important to be clear about the reasons for the moratorium, since its application to mentally incompetent persons in particular has become a major target of opposition to the regulations. Traditional common law grounds for exempting certain categories of persons from contractual rights and obligations have been based on the assumption that such persons (the traditional "lunatics, imbeciles, and infants") were irrational and hence incapable of knowing their own minds. The thrust of the moratorium, however, is not a claim about the inherent capacity or incapacity to consent to any of the groups mentioned. Rather, it is a statement of policy concerning the existing social and institutional conditions in which those groups presently find themselves, and the constraints on voluntary consent created by those conditions. This can be seen most obviously with regard to the prohibition on sterilizations among institutionalized persons.[37] The moratorium acknowledges that total institutions are "inherently coercive" environments and by definition contain a "potential for abuse" if sterilization of inmates is allowed.

The moratorium on sterilization of minors is based on evidence indicating a "higher rate of regret at being sterilized among younger women than among those who were sterilized at a later age." This tendency is not necessarily a reflection of an incapacity by younger persons to "understand the ramifications of the decision to be sterilized"; but may reflect the socially determined lack of autonomy that most teenagers have over their lives. Clearly, the motivation here is "protective": to guard young persons from being pressured into an irrevocable decision that they may later regret. The underlying emphasis is not on any characteristics assumed to be inherent in the status or personality of adolescents, but rather on the specific consequences of sterilization, its permanence, and the assumption that it is a graver matter for younger persons than older ones.

Most comments contesting this provision favored lowering the age limit to eighteen. While the moratorium on sterilization of minors has not stirred the same degree of legal and political controversy as the "mentally incompetent" issue, it could prove a major bone of contention in the future, especially in the context of the current public stir over "teenage pregnancy" and the abortion funding restrictions.

Along with the thirty-day rule, the most controversial of all the provisions in the federal regulations is the moratorium on funding for sterilizations of the mentally incompetent. While the regulations prohibit any form of involuntary sterilization, including of the mentally incompetent, or sterilization of any involuntarily confined persons, the difficulty comes in the increasingly common legal distinction between *competence* and *capacity* to consent. Courts and spokespersons for the mentally retarded have held that such capacity may exist for specific purposes even though a person has been declared generally incompetent.[38] They argue that many noninstitutionalized, legally incompetent persons may nevertheless have the capacity to consent to sterilization, in the sense of an "ability to understand the procedure and its effects." The majority who, in the public testimony, opposed the moratorium for such persons, invoked the principle of "reproductive freedom," citing the "right (of mentally incompetent persons) not to have children" and their right "of access to sterilization." *Whose* rights exactly were being put forward here, however, is unclear since the most frequent objections seemed primarily concerned with the problems of caretakers and parents.

The moratorium on the mentally incompetent is based on two considerations. As with the moratorium on minors, the intention is to avoid *prima facie* judgments about the inherent capacities of mentally incompetent persons as a category and instead to assess the concrete conditions under which such persons live either in existing institutional or "deinstitutionalized" settings. First, the comments oppose sterilization of mentally incompetent persons on the ground that such persons may be "only temporarily incompetent," and that medical and legal judgments about the permanence of incompetence are susceptible to error and difficult to monitor. The "normalization," or "developmental," view of retardation as an often changeable, ameliorable, rather than a fixed, condition is implicit in this view. Second, and most important, the Department recognizes the danger that caretakers, including parents, may "be tempted to consent to sterilization" as a way of avoiding the more difficult responsibilities of sex education, training in other forms of birth control, or alternatives to sterilization, "irrespective of the 'best interests' of the individual," and that this "could lead to abuse."[39] While parents have tended to consider this conclusion a dismissal of their needs and concerns, it could be seen as an acknowledgment of existing social realities—for example, the lack of sufficient training and community support services for mentally incompetent individuals, which increases the burden on parents and pressures them to seek sterilization for their retarded child.

There is, however, a loophole in the prohibition on federally funded sterilizations of the mentally incompetent. According to the regulations, a mentally incompetent person could seek a court judgment and be separately "readjudicated" competent for the purposes which include the ability to consent to sterilization."[40] (This, of course, does not apply to institutionalized persons under any circumstances.) In addition, the informed consent provisions require that the person securing consent and the physician performing the sterilization certify that "the individual to be sterilized appear mentally competent." After such certification and with court approval, a mentally incompetent person could be sterilized under federally funded programs without violating the regulations, since the sterilization would be legally voluntary.

At a meeting with consumer and community group representatives in the fall of 1978, Dr. Irvin Cushner, Deputy Assistant Secretary for Population Affairs at DHEW, emphasized the commitment of then-Secretary Califano to effective enforcement of the federal regulations. This was clearly a response to complaints by such groups in the past regarding the inadequate enforcement of the earlier (1974) regulations. Establishment of rigorous monitoring and enforcement mechanisms will ultimately determine whether the protections provided in the regulations will have any practical impact. As they stand, the regulations contain no regular means of communication between potential victims of abuse and regulatory agencies, nor is there information provided in the consent form telling consumers where to go or what to do if an abuse occurs. Further, it is not clear from the regulations at what point a pattern of abuse will result in federal sanctions, such as the withdrawal of funds. Finally, it is unclear how or whether the regulations themselves will be publicized among the general public, so that people in the community, health care workers and professionals concerned to prevent sterilization abuse can participate actively in the enforcement process.

All these weaknesses point to the need for local public enforcement and monitoring boards that broadly represent public health workers, community groups, women's groups, and consumer organizations, particularly groups who have tended to be victims of sterilization abuse in the past or who have made reproductive freedom their special concern. Even if effectively monitored, however, the regulations cannot guarantee against the sorts of economic and social pressures that often lead women to sterilization, especially in the context of cutbacks in abortion funding.

III. The Ethics of Sterilization Regulation

When New York City passed its guidelines regulating sterilization in the city's hospitals in 1976, a group of obstetricians and gynecologists immediately filed suit, charging that the guidelines violated both the individual's "right to choose" sterilization *and* the doctor's First Amendment rights; and further that they "impeded access" to sterilization services.[41] That suit was later dropped, but opposition to sterilization regulations continues. At present, rather than challenging the regulations directly, opponents are seeking to sidestep them — for example, through actions in the state courts invoking state eugenic sterilization laws, particularly with regard to the mentally incompetent. Clearly, those for whom "access" to sterilization is being most energetically sought are not middle-class women but those who are or may become state dependents.

Who are the groups opposed to the new regulations and what values do they represent? Along with the American College of Obstetricians and Gynecologists and the American Medical Association, the opponents of regulation consist of groups whose major concern is population control, such as Planned Parenthood and the Association for Voluntary Sterilization. While the population-oriented groups invoke caveats against "paternalism" and "government interference in the right to choose," their money, resources, and literature have for many years been directed at "stabilizing world population," reducing the birth rate in the United States, and targeting particular populations—the rural and urban poor in the Third World and in the United States—for family planning programs that feature sterilization. Some members of such groups couch their support of both abortion rights and sterilization in terms of arguments for "cutting the welfare rolls," particularly appealing in this period of economic crisis and political conservatism.

Opponents of the sterilization regulations make two different kinds of cases. First, there is the argument that regulation creates obstacles to the exercise of "free choice" by consumers and patients. This echoes the current argument from conservatives in Congress and in business to "deregulate" many areas of federal protection affecting consumers, workers, women, and minorities (for example, affirmative action, environmental protection, broadcasting). Sometimes this argument comes from people concerned with expanding birth control options, but more often it is an undisguised claim for the immunity of the medical profession from publicly imposed standards. Second, there is the argument that the state (through the courts) ought to sanction the involuntary sterilization of certain groups, especially retarded persons, in the interests of caretakers, taxpayers, parents, future children, or the retarded themselves. This argument too supports a range of agendas: from sincere concern for the consequences of pregnancy among persons unable to raise children, to a neo-eugenicist impulse to minimize the number of state-dependent or "unfit" people.

The first argument sees any attempt to create procedural safeguards against abuse—such as the thirty-day waiting period or the moratorium—as infringing on individuals' rights to make family planning choices "without government interference"; "protection" is viewed as inherently "paternalistic," a usurpation of moral autonomy. On the other hand, the second argument does not question the legitimacy of government regulation per se, but rather seeks the extension of government authority to impose involuntary sterilization on certain categories of people. The claim behind it is that sterilization will be "rehabilitative," that is, it will make the individual more "fit" to function in society, and that this value should take precedence over individual choice. This view thus challenges not only the moratorium but also the underlying policy of the regulations that all federally sponsored sterilizations must be strictly voluntary.

In practice, both positions, while appearing philosophically at odds, reach the same end: widening the terrain in which sterilizations may be performed unrestricted. (As usual, supporters of deregulation make no objection to government *subsidies,* for example, to the private medical sector through Medicaid).

Nonetheless, the debate between supporters and opponents of the federal sterilization regulations does raise two important questions: (1) what are the limits of justifiable protection? and (2) what are the limits of voluntary consent?

A. "Paternalism" and the Limits of Protection

Laws intended to protect the "vulnerable" and the "weak" from harm have no doubt been used as a pretext to exclude certain persons from full membership in society; many instances of protective labor legislation for "women only" are a case in point. It would appear that the only way to distinguish justifiable from unjustifiable "protective" laws and rules — that is, those that provide the necessary preconditions for moral and social autonomy from those that paternalistically deny such autonomy — is to look concretely at who is being protected and from what. (Another clue is to ask who is demanding protection, and on whose behalf — a political question.) In the case of sterilization regulations, opponents argue that the thirty-day waiting period and other procedural requirements attached to informed consent provisions are "paternalistic" and "discriminatory" because they "deny poor people's right to decide for themselves" and they "limit access to services." Whether these charges are true can best be determined by looking at what happens when no such protections exist.

The critical thing about sterilization, as DHEW recognizes, is its irreversibility. While those seeking sterilization may be inconvenienced by having to wait thirty days or fill out a rather long consent form, such inconvenience is hardly of the same magnitude as the experience of Norma Jean Serrena, a Native American woman, or the ten Chicana woman who have sued the Los Angeles Medical Center, or the Relf sisters, or others who have been permanently sterilized without knowing or understanding and who regret it deeply. The bodies and reproductive capacities of these women have been invaded and irrevocably altered; whereas, given access to alternative forms of birth control, a delay in the sterilization process could hardly have resulted in comparable distress. In sum, the concrete evidence of abuse — particularly against low-income and minority women — seems far in excess of the evidence for "denial of services." In this context, appeals to the "rights of the poor and migratory workers to be sterilized" seem discordant.

Complaints that the federal (and New York City) regulations "overprotect" individuals and infringe upon their "right to choose" sterilization, are not borne out by the facts. For example, recent data released by the New York City Bureau of Maternity Services and Family Planning show that, since sterilization guidelines have been in effect in the city, the number of sterilizations has not declined over previous years.[42] On the contrary, whether or not fewer women choose sterilization as a result of the regulations, it is not *their* "right to access" that is really being defended, but rather the medical profession's privileged autonomy and the "right" of providers to process people through sterilization procedures as expediently as possible. Protection against sterilization abuse is justifiable protection, insofar as it provides a necessary condition for avoiding undue pressure and being able to deliberate carefully about an irreversible procedure. The thirty-day waiting period and the other requirements attached to informed consent do not prevent anyone who wishes to do so from undergoing a sterilization program.

In contrast, we might look at the reasoning of those who oppose the federal regulations on benevolent-protective grounds. Whose interests are they protecting, and from what sorts of harm? Recent statements in favor of loosening the moratorium on sterilization of the mentally incompetent argue that sterilization is necessary — is, in fact, the most efficient means to protect retarded persons from sexual exploitation and abuse.[43] Indeed, many parents of the retarded who are deeply concerned about their disabled children's well-being and ability to function outside of institutions look to sterilization as an answer. But the problem with this approach is that, while mentally retarded women are frequently the victims of rape and sexual abuse, sterilization is no remedy against it whatsoever; all that sterilization protects against is pregnancy, but a sterile woman can still be raped. Indeed, it could be argued that sterilization may make retarded women, particularly those in institutions or exposed to assault from male relatives, more vulnerable to sexual abuse, insofar as it eliminates the most visible evidence of such abuse, that which caretakers are most worried about, and provides an excuse for failure to offer real forms of protection (such as better counseling and management).

The same is true with regard to the concerns of parents of retarded young men, who are vulnerable to sexual stereotyping and suspicion. Sterilization will provide no guarantee against malicious accusations of sexual perversion or molestation, for the very simple reason that sexuality and fertility are not the same thing. But the fact that this obvious reality is ignored says something about the real fears of parents. Behind the argument about "protection from sexual abuse" is often the concern of caretakers — parents as well as institutions — to protect themselves from the burdens of a retarded woman's pregnancy or from being involved in a paternity suit. While such burdens are real, do they justify the severe "protective" measure involved in involuntary sterilization? If protection from sexual abuse is really an aim, would not more adequate staffing, training in self-defense measures, better supervision and safer transportation be more relevant? It would seem that "protection" here is a gloss for other concerns to which sterilization may be an efficient but inappropriate response.

Another "benevolent" pretext for sterilization of the retarded, with or without their consent (usually the unstated assumption of such proposals is that consent will be given by guardians or third parties), is that, "freed from pregnancy, childbearing, and childrearing," they may thereby enjoy "an active heterosexual life."[44] Again, however, this assumption rests on a deep-seated fallacy, one which equates sterility with sexual pleasure (not so different from the equation of sterility with sexual safety). There is no evidence to suggest that sterilization is a necessary or a sufficient condition for sexual enjoyment, for the retarded any more than for anyone else. The only sense in which this might be true is the extrinsic one imposed by the perceptions and requirements of caretakers (if you become sterilized, then you will be allowed sexual privileges). A genuine concern for the sexual expression of retarded persons ought to focus, not on sterilization, but on the institutional and social conditions that most retarded persons experience, except those lucky enough to be in the most privileged families or the most progressive, experimental programs. More pertinent to "an active heterosexual life" for such persons would be commitment to programs involving sex counseling, body awareness, sex-integrated activities, private bedrooms, and many other basic conditions that are presently inaccessible to many retarded people (and many teenagers as well).

It would seem that the sexuality of retarded persons becomes real for parents and guardians only when it becomes visible, that is, if pregnancy occurs; conversely, if pregnancy can be avoided, it also becomes possible to avoid the conflicts and issues involved in teenage sexuality, to pretend they do not exist.[45] The tendency to use sterilization to dispose of all the complex problems regarding sexuality, sex education, and birth control among the retarded would seem to be a form of denial. Its implications for the retarded themselves are potentially dangerous, not so much because it deprives them of their "childbearing rights," but insofar as it rationalizes the neglect of basic needs and services necessary for their full sexual expression. In this context, the federal moratorium offers a measure of protection that may open the way to more socially useful changes.

B. Capacities and the Limits of Voluntarism

Proposals for involuntary sterilization, particularly of the mentally incompetent, rest on the premise that such persons lack a capacity to exercise voluntary consent. For those who oppose the federal regulations, especially the moratorium, claims on behalf of the mentally incompetent have tended to dominate those on behalf of interested others, such as parents and potential children of the retarded. Clearly, the courts have been more favorably disposed to benevolent-protective arguments than to utilitarian ones where involuntary sterilization is concerned.[46] In both cases, however, the claims are supported by assumptions or assertions about the inherent characteristics of mentally incompetent persons as a group—their capacity to use alternative forms of birth control and to exercise consent, as well as their capacity to bear and raise children (these issues are often and unjustly conflated).

What are the real limits on the capacity of retarded persons to participate in their own reproductive and sexual decisions, and how should these limits be determined? A full discussion of this question lies outside the bounds of this article, but certain general issues may be considered without venturing into debates about the etiology of retardation. Two main points, widely accepted by specialists in developmental disabilities, need emphasis: first, the tremendous range in both functional and cognitive abilities represented by different degrees of retardation, and particularly within the largest classification, the "mildly retarded"; and, second, the necessity of taking "each case on its own merits rather than on generalized emotion or blanket legal solution."[47] While the American Association on Mental Deficiency's classifications of mental retardation into "mild," "moderate," "severe," and "profound" are based primarily on IQ levels, it is important to remember that IQ—for "retarded" as for "normal" persons—is only a crude measure at best; that the functional capacities of persons with similar IQ levels may differ greatly depending on the quality of training, services, and care to which they have had access; and that IQ levels themselves may be increased through environmental ameliorations. Indeed, as one geneticist of retardation points out, the retarded are in fact "simply those individuals at the tail end of the normal distribution of intelligence and differ quantitatively rather than qualitatively from the remainder of the population."[48] Functional variation is particularly broad among those approximately 5.25 million persons classified as "mildly retarded" (indicating an IQ range of 68 to 52 on the Stanford-Binet Scale), who in fact represent well over three-fourths of all the retarded. But even among those whose disabilities place them in the "moderate" or "severe" category, counselors working in the field attest that there are some who develop an ability not only to function sexually and to use contraceptives but to understand what they are doing.[49]

In contrast, state involuntary sterilization laws and opponents of the moratorium rely on a set of assumptions about the origins of retardation and the inherent incapacities of retarded persons as an abstract category. These assumptions commonly include the following: (1) that retardation is in most cases genetically determined;[50] (2) that most *mildly* retarded persons are "incapable of managing temporary forms of birth control";[51] (3) that most mildly retarded persons are incapable of raising children, although they may be capable of marrying or otherwise engaging in sexual activity;[52] and (4) that the capacity of retarded persons to understand and consent freely to contraceptive planning, including sterilization, is negligible or nonexistent. The logical conclusion to such views was unceremoniously drawn in a recent newspaper column by George Will: "It is arguable that the right of the retarded to procreate . . . is problematic. And it is arguable that the state should—let us speak bluntly—license procreation."[53]

Leaving aside for a moment the issue of parenting capacity (and Will's "blunt" proposal), all of these assumptions are highly questionable, particularly when applied to the mildly retarded. First, there is little scientific basis for assuming a strict genetic determinism in most cases of mental disability, or that its incidence in the population could be "significantly" affected by preventing the retarded themselves from propagating. There are a few disorders that are known to be genetically transmitted, such as Down Syndrome and Tay-Sachs disease. In such cases, it is possible to use genetic counseling and diagnosis to prevent unwanted births. For the most part, however, it would seem truer to view mental disability as simply one tail of a bell-shaped curve. Like all variations in intelligence, its sources represent a complex set of interactions between genetic and environmental determinants; the genetic determinants of intellectual abilities cannot be isolated, since these are themselves affected by environmental conditions.[54] The evidence suggests, moreover, that a large proportion of mental deficiencies are associated with environmental conditions such as poverty, malnutrition, low birth weight, poor health care, or exposure to toxic substances such as lead or radiation, usually experienced prenatally and leading to permanent brain or central nervous system damage.[55] And these are the conditions, of course, that characterize the lives of lower-class and minority people, and many people working in hazardous occupations. Clearly it is cheaper and more politically expedient — particularly in a period of economic crisis and neoconservatism — to sterilize retarded persons rather than dealing with the economic, nutritional, medical, and environmental conditions that are known threats to healthy mental development. But such eugenics programs, based on totally faulty scientific premises, can never work even on their own terms; and their "blame-the-victim" connotations are morally obnoxious.

While little is known about the ability of mildly retarded persons to use alternative forms of birth control, much is taken for granted rather than empirically verified. As one rather cautious authority points out, in this as in any other area of functional behavior, the "capacity" of mildly retarded persons will vary greatly depending on the individual user's level of cognitive and functional ability; the presence of necessary counseling and education programs, including clinicians, parents, and personnel trained and sensitive in this particular area; and a cooperative state social service agency.[56] In the absence of such clinical and social conditions, we have little basis for assuming anything about the potential capacity of "many" or "most" retarded persons to adjust to temporary forms of birth control. On the other hand, there are reports of experimental programs that are attempting to provide retarded persons in group homes with sexual counseling services, birth control counseling and methods, and regular opportunities for a variety of sexual experiences (homosexual and auto-erotic as well as heterosexual). These pilot projects indicate that such programs, when offered seriously and with sensitivity and follow-up, may be quite successful (result in a high degree of self-regulation, low pregnancy rates, and satisfying social and sexual lives). Retarded persons involved in such programs, when given the necessary training and supervision, have been able to manage nonpermanent forms of birth control.[57] The point is not that other forms of birth control are always "better" for retarded persons than is sterilization (the pill, for example, has been associated with far more serious risks to health), or that they will always work. Rather, it is that access to a variety of options and services to enhance their reproductive and sexual experience is a necessary condition for retarded persons (or any persons) to develop the capacity to engage actively and voluntarily in such experience. Until programs of this kind are widely available and taken seriously, we will not really know much about the potential capacity of the mildly retarded either for sexuality or for self-administered birth control.

The assumption that many mildly retarded persons will be incapable of exercising sufficient foresight and responsibility to raise children independently may well be valid under existing social conditions. Yet even here it is important to point out the absence of empirical data. There are no studies reported that compare the behavior and effectiveness of retarded and nonretarded parents. Moreover, the argument voiced by advocates of the retarded is persuasive: that summary denial of the childbearing rights of retarded persons is discriminatory. What about other categories of "social deviants" whose behavior or condition may be detrimental to their children but whose legal right to raise their children is not challenged *a priori* (alcoholics, neurotics, emotionally disturbed persons)? Why are the issues any different in these cases?[58] Again, it would seem necessary to deal with the question of childbearing capacity in terms of an individual situation rather than on a wholesale basis through procedures that provide adequate guarantees of due process and effective advocacy.

This discussion might be clarified if we could separate the issue of child-rearing capacity from that of capacity to give informed consent. Social welfare workers and mentally disabled persons themselves have convincingly argued that many, perhaps most, persons classified as "mildly retarded" are capable of understanding the issues involved in decisions about sterilization and birth control, and at the same time may feel undesirous or incapable of raising a child.[59] In fact, the federal regulations do allow for such a possibility by leaving it open to the courts and clinicians to determine whether a particular mentally incompetent individual may be competent to exercise informed consent in reproductive matters and thus to become voluntarily sterilized under federally funded programs. How this will work out in practice, and whether the courts can be relied upon to assure that the "voluntary consent" of retarded persons is genuine and not manipulated, remains to be seen. Presumably, the "readjudication of capacity to consent" would *not* mean third-party consent, and would require that the retarded person herself or himself be adequately represented by an independent counsel or advocate.

The issue that remains, and to which the moratorium allows no exceptions, is that of profoundly or severely retarded persons who are not capable of voluntary consent, who may be unable to use temporary forms of birth control, who are at risk of pregnancy, and for whom such a pregnancy would be all objective standards present a real hardship. It seems altogether likely that, given both the sexual underdevelopment of such persons and their vulnerability, the vast majority of such pregnancies are the result of rape or incest.[60] This raises, once again, the point made earlier—the danger that introducing sterilization as a "solution" in such cases may encourage neglect of adequate staffing, services, and other protections to guard against incidents of sexual assault. I know of no study that systematically documents pregnancy rates among populations of retarded women, institutionalized as well as deinstitutionalized, much less the circumstances in which those pregnancies arise (which are often not known, since the victims usually do not know how to report). One might agree that, for certain severely retarded persons, sterilization would be a better alternative for the individual involved than anything else available, and therefore not be morally objectionable. However, under existing conditions the position of the federal regulations seems reasonable: that lifting the moratorium even in these cases would create a greater danger, since it would allow sterilization as an alternative to the development of decent care and social programs that maximize the potentialities of *all* persons, even the most disabled.

IV. Conclusion

The current debate about sterilization abuse and the federal sterilization regulations cannot be removed from the particular political and social context in which it is occurring — a context that includes fiscal crisis, anti-black and anti-feminist backlash, and the revival of biological determinism and eugenics. In this context, the likelihood that "modest" proposals for involuntary sterilization will be extended to large numbers of women, for purposes that have little to do with their own well-being and much to do with the concerns of racists, demographic and social planners, and fiscal managers, is a realistic concern. A political system for "licensing childbirth" in this society would reflect the dominant values of policy-makers, physicians, and judges about what sorts of people ought to be born. Predictably, it would give preferential treatment on the basis of class, race, sex, and a very class-biased view of "mental normality." It is interesting in this regard that the proposals already put forward in the *Hastings Center Report* and elsewhere apply not only to the severely retarded but to the mildly retarded, who number in the millions and include a high proportion of low-income and minority people.

Finally, it is no accident that proposals for the involuntary sterilization of the retarded have been raised, and linked to the more difficult question of capacity for childrearing, just at the time when abortion rights in the United States are undergoing political and legal erosion. For retarded women as for all Medicaid-dependent women, the restriction of abortion funds and the availability of sterilization funds makes sterilization a more compelling alternative. Indeed, many of the obstacles that mentally disabled women face to sexual and reproductive freedom are merely the extreme end of a continuum that affects many women in this society: the inadequacies of birth control methods, education, and reimbursement; the lack of adequate incomes and residential privacy; disproportionate burdens for the risks of pregnancy; and the persistent threat of sexual objectification and sexual assault. Involuntary sterilization is a diversion from these problems, not a solution to them. If effectively enforced, the federal sterilization regulations will help to dampen the enthusiasm for sterilization as a way to control populations rather than improving the quality of life.

REFERENCES

This paper owes a great deal to the research collaboration and ideas of Ann Teicher, and the collective support of the Committee for Abortion Rights and Against Sterilization Abuse. I would also like to thank Iris Lipner, Ruth Roemer, and Karen Stamm for their valuable insights and criticisms; and Irvin M. Cushner and Marilyn Martin, of the Office for Population Affairs, DHEW.

1. *Federal Register* 43:217 (Nov. 8, 1978), 52146-175. The applicability of the federal regulations is limited to programs or projects funded in whole or in part through federal grants (through the Title XX Social Services Program or the Public Health Service), or to individuals receiving Medicaid. Thus sterilization programs not funded through federal monies, including many done through private hospitals and clinics, are under no obligation to comply with the regulations, except with regard to their Medicaid patients.

2. Final publication of the regulations climaxed a series of earlier statutory and administrative rulings. The DHEW issued the rules that preceded the new regulations on April 18, 1974 (*Federal Register* 39:76, p. 4730). Title V of the Social Security Act, Title XIX (the "Medicaid" provisions), as well as Title X of the Public Health Service Act, authorizing federal planning family services, require that such services be "voluntary." See also the U.S. District Court's ruling in *Relf v. Weinberger,* C. A. No. 74-1797 (D.C. Cir. 1977).

3. Cf. Onora O'Neill, "Begetting, Bearing, and Rearing," in Onora O'Neill and William Ruddick, eds., *Having Children: Philosophical and Legal Reflections on Parenthood* (New York: Oxford University Press, 1979), p. 37.

4. Tubal ligation presents greater physical and psychological risks than its proponents sometimes admit. See Barbara Seaman and Gideon Seaman, *Women and the Crisis in Sex Hormones* (New York: Bantam Books, 1977), Ch. 17; and W. P. Black, "Sterilization by Laparoscopic Tubal Electrocoagulation: An Assessment," *American Journal of Obstetrics and Gynecology* 3:7 (Dec. 1, 1971), reporting a follow-up study done among 300 patients in Scotland during 1967-71 and warning against the serious respiratory and cardiac complications that may result if surgeons performing the procedure lack sufficient "experience and skill."

5. See, for example, the discussion of the Leveller concept of "property in one's person" as a notion integral to the seventeenth century radical idea of individual rights, in C. B. MacPherson, *The Political Theory of Possessive Individualism* (London: Oxford University Press, 1962), p. 140.

6. Kathleen Ford, "Contraceptive Use in the United States, 1973-1976," *Family Planning Perspectives* 10:5 (Sept./Oct. 1978), p. 268; Sidney H. Newman and Zanvel E. Klein, eds., *Behavioral-Social Aspects of Contraceptive Sterilization* (Lexington, Mass.: D. C. Heath, 1978), pp. 1-2; and Charles F. Westoff and Elise F. Jones, "Contraception and Sterilization in the United States, 1965-1975," *Family Planning Perspectives* 9:4 (July/Aug. 1977), p. 155. According to Ford's data, pill use has declined since 1973 among all groups in the population except white women aged twenty-five and under.

7. Kathleen Ford, "Contraceptive Utilization in the United States: 1973 and 1976," *Advancedata,* National Center for Health Statistics, DHEW, No. 36 (Aug. 18, 1978), Table 1; and "Contraceptive Utilization Among Widowed, Divorced, and Separated Women in the United States: 1973 and 1976," *Advancedata,* National Center for Health Statistics, DHEW, No. 40 (Sept. 22, 1978), Table 1.

8. The AVS figures are derived from an annual survey of private physicians and clinics (both public and private) conducted by AVS independently. Estimates cited here are those published in September 1978. It should be noted that these figures and percentages combine so-called "noncontraceptive" with "contraceptive" sterilizations, but this seems a more accurate representation of the sterilization picture than if "contraceptive" sterilizations alone are considered. While the ratio of "noncontraceptive" to "contraceptive" sterilizations is growing steadily, most family planning experts agree that the distinction is a very murky one in practice. Sterilizations reported as "noncontraceptive" in intent are often performed for a combination of reasons, including contraception. Moreover, it is extremely ambiguous what purely "medical indications" might exist for a tubal ligation.

9. Ford, *Advancedata,* No. 36, Table 1; Ad Hoc Women's Studies Committee Against Sterilization Abuse, *Workbook on Sterilization and Sterilization Abuse* (Bronxville, N.Y.: Sarah Lawrence College, 1978), pp. 12-14; and Paul J. Placek, "The Incidence of Sterilization Following Delivery of Legitimate Live Births in Hospitals: United States," *Monthly Vital Statistics Report,* National Center for Health Statistics, DHEW, June 17, 1977, p. 2.

10. Ford, *Family Planning Perspectives* 10:5, Tables 2 and 3 and p. 268.

11. For a much greater elaboration of this social analysis, see Rosalind P. Petchesky, "Sexual Freedom or Final Solution? — A Social Analysis of Female Sterilization in the Contemporary United States," forthcoming.

12. See U.S. Department of Labor, Women's Bureau, *1975 Handbook on Women Workers;* U.S. Department of Labor, Bureau of Labor Statistics, *U.S. Working Women: A Databook,* 1977; and Heather L. Ross and Isabel V. Sawhill, *Time of Transition: The Growth of Families Headed by Women* (Washington, D.C.: The Urban Institute, 1975).

13. Robert Hoover *et al.,* "Oral Contraceptive Use: Association with Frequency of Hospitalization and Chronic Disease Risk Indicators," *American Journal of Public Health* 68:4 (April 1978), 335–41; Judith Blake, "The Pill and the Rising Costs of Fertility Control," *Social Biology* 24:4 (Winter 1977), 269–80; and Charles F. Westoff and Norman B. Ryder, *The Contraceptive Revolution* (Princeton: Princeton University Press, 1977), pp. 46–49. By July 1977, "only 29% of men and 25% of women believed the pill to be safe" (Blake, pp. 271–72).

14. The implications of the bias in government policy are spelled out in Committee for Abortion Rights and Against Sterilization Abuse (CAR-ASA), *Women Under Attack: Abortion, Sterilization Abuse and Reproductive Freedom,* 1979 (pamphlet, available from CARASA, P.O. Box 124, Cathedral Station, New York, N.Y. 10025).

15. Charlotte F. Muller, "Insurance Coverage of Abortion, Contraception and Sterilization," *Family Planning Perspectives* 10:2 (March/April 1978), 71–77.

16. See Westoff and Ryder, *op. cit.;* Harriet B. Presser and Larry L. Bumpass, "Demographic and Social Aspects of Contraceptive Sterilization in the United States: 1965–1970," in Charles F. Westoff and Robert Parke, Jr., eds., *Demographic and Social Aspects of Population Growth* (Washington, D.C.: U.S. Commission on Population Growth and The American Future, 1972), p. 566; and Editorial, *Journal of the American Medical Association* 204:9 (May 27, 1968).

17. Helen Wolfers, "The Incidence of Psychological Complications After Contraceptive Sterilization," in Newman and Klein, *op. cit.,* pp. 137–138. See also Linda Gordon, *Woman's Body, Woman's Right: A Social History of Birth Control in America* (New York: Penguin Books, 1977), who develops the distinction between "birth control" and "population control" historically and theoretically.

18. A currently popular rock song from England celebrates "The Big V" — vasectomy — as the emblem of the cool, hip male. See also Samuel J. Barr, *A Woman's Choice* (New York: Rawson, 1977), pp. 128–29; and Evan McLeod Wylie, *All About Voluntary Sterilization: The Revolutionary New Birth-Control Method for Men and Women* (New York: Berkley, 1977), p. 74: "Take away tension. Take away conflict. Eliminate fear, resentment, frustration, worry and anger. Replace them with a sense of security and an ability to relax. The result is a new sexual freedom." In a similar vein, the *New York Times* story covering the opening of Planned Parenthood's new "minilap" out-patient sterilization clinic in New York City was featured on the "Style" page; Jane Geinesse, "Clinic to Provide Sterilization Using Simpler Technique," *New York Times,* March 20, 1979, p. C5.

19. See "Sterilization of the Retarded: In Whose Interest?" articles by Michael Bayles, Travis Thompson, and Robert Neville, *Hastings Center Report* 8:3 (June 1978); George F. Will, "Sterilization and the Retarded," *Washington Post,* Dec. 3, 1978, p. C7; Medora S. Bass, "Surgical Contraception: A Key to Normalization and Prevention," *Journal of Mental Retardation* (December 1978); and Gloria S. Neuwirth *et al.,* "Capacity, Competence, Consent: Voluntary Sterilization of the Mentally Retarded," *Columbia Human Rights Law Review* 6:2 (Fall-Winter, 1974–75), pp. 447–53.

20. The most complete critical histories of the early twentieth century eugenics movement are Allan Chase, *The Legacy of Malthus* (New York: Alfred A. Knopf, 1977); and Mark M. Haller, *Eugenics: Hereditarian Attitudes in American Thought* (New Brunswick, N.J.: Rutgers University Press, 1963).

21. *Relf* v. *Weinberger,* p. 1199; and *Workbook on Sterilization,* p. 18.

22. *Stump* v. *Sparkman,* 435 U.S. 349 (March 28, 1978).

23. *Wyatt* v. *Aderholt,* 368 F. Supp. 1383 (M.D. Ala., 1974); *In re Sterilization of Moore,* 289 N.C. 95 (Sup. Ct., N.C., 1976); *North Carolina Assoc. for Retarded Children v. State of N.C.,* 420 F. Supp. 451 (M.D.N.C., 1976).

24. See cases cited above, as well as *Cook v. State of Oregon,* 9 Ore. App. 1972.

25. *Ruby* v. *Massey* (D.C. Conn., 1978); and Michael Bayles, *op. cit.,* pp. 37–41.

26. *Workbook on Sterilization,* p. 20.

27. *Walker* v. *Pierce,* 560 F. 2d 609 (4th Cir. 1977).

28. The important role of feminists and health activists, both within the New York City Health and Hospitals Corporation, in health advocacy groups based in New York and Washington, and within DHEW, in initiating the city and federal guidelines cannot be overestimated.

29. *Federal Register* 43:217, p. 52147.

30. *Ibid.,* p. 52149.

31. *Ibid.,* p. 52163.

32. "Sterilization in the United States: Preliminary Findings from the National Survey of Family Growth: 1973," paper presented at the annual meeting of the Population Association of America, Seattle, Washington, April 1975, p. 5 (mimeo).

33. *Federal Register, op. cit.,* p. 52150.

34. *Ibid.,* p. 52151.

35. *Ibid.,* p. 52150.

36. *Ibid.,* p. 52151.

37. The definition of "institutionalized individual" in the regulations includes: "a person who is (1) involuntarily confined or detained under a civil or criminal statute, in a correctional or rehabilitative facility including a mental hospital or other facility for the care and treatment of mental illness, or (2) confined, under a voluntary commitment, in a mental hospital or other facility for the care and treatment of mental illness." This includes institutionalization in "halfway houses," reform schools, and other involuntary arrangements even where the restriction is not total. (*Ibid.,* p. 52156.)

38. See Bayles, *op. cit.;* Neuwirth et al., op. cit.; Paul R. Friedman, *The Rights of Mentally Retarded Persons* (New York: Avon, 1976); and President's Committee on Mental Retardation, *Mental Retardation: Century of Decision,* Report to the President (U.S. Government Printing Office, Washington, D.C., 1976), pp. 58–59.

39. *Federal Register* 43:217, p. 52154.

40. *Ibid.,* p. 52155.

41. Patricia Donovan, "Sterilizing the Poor and Incompetent," *Hastings Center Report* 6:5 (October 1976).

42. Karen Stamm, "City Releases Sterilization Data," *CARASA News* 2:11 (December 7, 1978), p. 11.

43. See Thompson, p. 30; *Cook* v. *Oregon* and *Ruby* v. *Massey.*

44. Neville, pp. 33–36.

45. Cf. Frank F. Furstenberg, Jr., "The Social Consequences of Teenage Parenthood," *Family Planning Perspectives* 8:4 (July/August 1976), p. 150.

46. See cases cited in notes 23–24.

47. On this point, see Isabel P. Robinault, *Sex, Society, and the Disabled* (Hagerstown, Md.: Harper & Row, 1978), p. 67; Friedman, *passim;* President's Committee on Mental Retardation, pp. 58–59; and Patricia M. Wald, "Basic Personal and Civil Rights," in Michael Kindred *et al., The Mentally Retarded Citizen and the Law* (New York: The Free Press, 1976), p. 5.

48. Irving I. Gottesman, "An Introduction to Behavioral Genetics of Mental Retardation," in Robert M. Allen *et al., The Role of Genetics in Mental Retardation* (Coral Gables, Fla.: University of Miami Press, 1971), pp. 50 and 62.

49. Oral interviews with I. Lipner, Developmental Center, Maimonides Hospital, and Karen Wolf, Garfield Manor Group Residence, Brooklyn, New York, January and February 1979. The views stated are based on the clinical experience of those interviewed and do not necessarily reflect agency or professional policy. See also, Winifred Kempton, "Sexual Rights and Responsibilities of the Retarded Person," *Social Welfare Forum, 1976* (New York: Columbia University Press, 1977).

50. Bass; Will; *Cook* v. *Oregon;* and *North Carolina Assc. for Retarded Children.*

51. Neville, p. 33; Bass, pp. 399–400; *Ruby* v. *Massey; North Carolina Assc. for Retarded Children.*

52. Neville, pp. 33 and 35; Bass, pp. 401–402; *Cook* v. *Oregon;* cf. President's Committee on Mental Retardation, p. 63.

53. Will, "Sterilization and the Retarded." I am grateful to Dr. Irvin Cushner for calling my attention to Will's article. Will approvingly summarizes the articles by Neville and Thompson in the June 1978 *Hastings Center Report,* using these as the basis of his argument.

54. See, for example, Gottesman, p. 50, who in the earlier part of his article presents this complex, multi-dimensional view of "causality" quite clearly, even though he later draws conclusions that are completely inconsonant with it (e.g., "that the voluntary restriction of fertility by retarded individuals would have a marked effect on reducing their own and society's burdens").

55. For a particularly thorough treatment of the existing empirical data in this area and its legal and social implications, see John R. Kramer, "The Right Not to Be Mentally Retarded," in Kindred *et al.,* pp. 31–59.

56. Robinault, pp. 63–64.

57. *Ibid.,* reporting on programs in Eastern Pennsylvania and Washington, D.C.; Kempton; "Sexuality and the Mentally Retarded," *Hospital Tribune,* February 1979, pp. 3–6; Winifred Kempton, Medora S. Bass, and Sol Gordon, *Love, Sex and Birth Control for the Mentally Retarded: A Guide for Parents* (Philadelphia: Planned Parenthood Association, 1971); and interviews cited in n. 49.

58. This argument is made strongly by S. John Vitello, "Involuntary Sterilization: Recent Developments," *Journal of Mental Retardation* (December 1978), p. 406; and Friedman, *op. cit.,* p. 122, who concludes: "Although we lack adequate predictive tools to distinguish beforehand between suitable and unsuitable parents, the absence of such refined techniques does not justify discriminating against mentally retarded parents in custody matters."

59. Opposition to involuntary sterilization of the mentally handicapped was expressed unanimously by a group of retarded persons attending a workshop on the "Childbearing Rights of the Mentally Handicapped" at a Conference on Childbearing Rights, sponsored by Low-Income Planning Aid, in Worcester, Mass., November 18–19, 1978, and attended by the author. Some among the group were parents, some had been voluntarily sterilized, and at least one woman reported having been molested by her father. Their strong consensus was that, while they themselves might individually prefer sterilization or decide that raising children would be too burdensome, they and most mildly retarded persons are competent to participate fully in making this decision.

60. *Ibid.* and sources cited in note 49; of necessity, the evidence here is anecdotal rather than documented.

Suggestions for Further Reading

Psychotropic Drugs and Drug Therapies

Advances in the Drug Therapy of Mental Illness. Albany, New York: World Health Organization, 1973.

Appleton, William S., and Davis, John M. *Practical Clinical Psychopharmacology.* Baltimore, Maryland: Williams and Wilkins, 1973.

Ayd, Frank J., Jr. *Rational Psychopharmacotherapy and the Right to Treatment.* Baltimore, Maryland: Ayd Medical Communications, 1975.

————. "Ethical and Legal Dilemmas Posed by Tardive Dyskinesia." *International Drug Therapy Newsletter* 12 (1977).

Bassuk, Ellen L. *The Practitioner's Guide to Psychoactive Drugs.* New York: Plenum Medical Books, 1977.

Berger, Philip A. "Medical Treatment of Mental Illness." *Science* 200 (May 26, 1978):974–981.

Brady, John P., and Brodie, H. Keith, eds. *Controversy in Psychiatry.* Philadelphia: W. B. Saunders, Co., 1978, Chs. 5, 6, 7.

Brecher, Edward, ed. *The Consumers Union Report: Licit and Illicit Drugs.* Boston: Little, Brown & Co., 1972.

Clark, Matt, et al. "Drugs and Psychiatry: A New Era." *Newsweek* (November 12, 1979):98–104.

"Controlling Behavior Through Drugs: Papers Prepared for the Institute Conference on Behavior Control Through Drugs, May 20–21, 1972. *Hastings Center Studies* 2 (January 1974):65–112.

Duster, Troy. *The Legislation of Morality: Law, Drugs and Moral Judgment.* New York: The Free Press, 1970.

Feldman, Harold S. "Psychopharmacology and the Law: A Forensic Psychiatrist's Viewpoint." *Journal of Clinical Pharmacology* 16 (October 1976): 577-580.

Goldsmith, William. *Psychiatric Drugs for the Non-Medical Mental Health Worker.* Springfield, Illinois: Charles C. Thomas, 1977.

Grinspoon, Lester, and Singer, Susan B. "Amphetamines in the Treatment of Hyperkinetic Children." *Harvard Educational Review* 43 (November 1973): 515-555.

Hollister, Leo E. *Clinical Uses of Psychotherapeutic Drugs.* Springfield, Illinois: Charles C. Thomas, 1977.

Iversen, Susan D., and Iversen, Leslie L. *Behavioral Pharmacology.* New York: Oxford University Press, 1975.

Jackson, Ian V., et al. "Treatment of Tardive Dyskinesia with Lecithin." *American Journal of Psychiatry* 136 (November 1979):1458-1460.

Kazamatsuri, H., et al. "Therapeutic Approaches to Tardive Dyskinesia: A Review of the Literature." *Archives of General Psychiatry* 27 (1972):491ff.

Kieffer, George H. *Bioethics: A Textbook of Issues.* Reading, Massachusetts: Addison-Wesley Publishing Co., 1979, pp. 283-306.

Klein, D. F., and Gittelman-Klein, R., eds. *Progress in Psychiatric Drug Treatment.* New York: Brunner/Mazel, 1975.

Klerman, Gerald L. "Psychotropic Drugs as Therapeutic Agents." *Hastings Center Studies* 2 (1974):81-93.

———. "Psychotropic Hedonism vs. Pharmacological Calvinism." *The Hastings Center Report* 2 (September 1972):1-3.

Lion, John R. *Art of Medicating Psychiatric Patients.* Baltimore, Maryland: Williams and Wilkins, 1978.

London, Perry. *Behavior Control.* New York: New American Library, 1977.

Opler, Lewis A., et al. "Tardive Dyskinesia and Institutional Practice: Current Issues and Institutional Guidelines. *Hospital and Community Psychiatry* 31 (April 1980):239-245.

Parry, Hugh J., et al. "National Patterns of Psychotherapeutic Drug Use." *Archives of General Psychiatry* 28 (June 1973):769-783.

Physicians' Desk Reference. Oradell, New Jersey: Medical Economics Company, reissued annually. See Drug Classification Index under: Antidepressants, Anti-Parkinsonism Drugs, Ataractics, Barbiturates.

Rust, Mildred D., and Hopper, Kim. "Issues in Behavior Control: An Exchange of Views." Man and Medicine 4 (1975):23-24 and 30-36.

Scull, Andrew. *Decarceration, Community Treatment and the Deviant: A Radical View.* Englewood Cliffs, New Jersey: Prentice-Hall, Inc., 1977, Ch. 5.

Silverstone, Trevor, and Turner, Paul. *Drug Treatment in Psychiatry.* Boston: Routledge & Kegan Paul, 1978.

Snyder, Solomon H. "Mending Shattered Minds." In *Science Year.* Chicago: World Books-Childcraft International, 1981, pp. 128-139.

Sterling, Peter. "Psychiatry's Drug Addiction." *The New Republic* (December 8, 1979):14-18.

Stimmel, Glen L. "Clinical Implications of Dopaminergic and Cholinergic Effects of Neuroleptic Drugs." *Hospital Pharmacy* 11 (1976):50–56.

Szasz, Thomas S. "The Ethics of Addiction." *American Journal of Psychiatry* 128 (November 1977):541–546.

"The Right to Refuse Psychoactive Drugs." *Hastings Center Report* 3 (June 1973): 8–11.

Valenstein, Elliot S. "Science Fiction Fantasy and the Brain." *Psychology Today* 12 (July 1978):28ff.

Veatch, Robert M. "Drugs and Competing Drug Ethics." *Hastings Center Studies* 2 (1974):68–80.

———. "Value Foundations for Drug Use." *Journal of Drug Issues* 7 (Summer 1977):253–276.

Wender, Paul H., and Klein, Donald F. "The Promise of Biological Psychiatry." *Psychology Today* 15 (February 1981):25–41.

Zander, Thomas K. "Medication and the Right to Refuse—Prolixin Decanoate: A Review of the Research." *Mental Disability Law* 2 (July–August 1977):37–42.

Behavior Modification Therapies

Arizona Law Review 17 (1975). Entire issue.

Ayllon, Teodoro, and Azrin, Nathan. *The Token Economy.* New York: Appleton-Century-Crofts, 1968.

Bandura, A. *Principles of Behavior Modification.* New York: Holt, Rinehart & Winston, 1969.

"Behavioral Therapies." In Reich, Warren T., ed. *Encyclopedia of Bioethics* Vol. I. New York: The Free Press, 1978, pp. 101–106.

Buckholdt, David R., et al. "The Underlife of Behavior Modification." *American Journal of Orthopsychiatry* 50 (April 1980):279–290.

Carrera, Frank, and Adams, P. L. "An Ethical Perspective on Operant Conditioning." *Journal of the American Academy of Child Psychiatry* 9 (1970):607–623.

Cotter, Lloyd H. "Operant Conditioning in a Vietnamese Mental Hospital." *American Journal of Psychiatry* 124 (July 1967):23–28.

Davidson, Park O., ed. *The Behavioral Management of Anxiety, Depression and Pain.* New York: Brunner/Mazel, 1976.

Erwin, Edward. *Behavior Therapy: Scientific, Philosophical, and Moral Foundations.* New York: Cambridge University Press, 1978.

Fordyce, Wilbert Evans. *Behavioral Methods for Chronic Pain and Illness.* St. Louis: Mosby, 1976.

Halleck, Seymour L. "Legal and Ethical Aspects of Behavioral Control." *American Journal of Psychiatry* 131 (April 1974):381–385.

Harris, S. L., et al. "Behavior Modification Therapy with Elderly Demented Patients: Implementation and Ethical Considerations." *Journal of Chronic Diseases* 30 (March 1977):129–134.

Hayer, Steven C., and Maley, Roger F. "Coercion: Legal and Behavioral Issues." *Behaviorism* 5 (1977):87–95.

Hersen, Michel, et al. "A Token Reinforcement Ward for Young Psychiatric Patients." *American Journal of Psychiatry* 129 (August 1972):228–233.

Holland, James. "Ethical Considerations in Behavior Modification." *Journal of Humanistic Psychology* 16 (Summer 1976):71–78.

Klerman, Gerald L. "Behavior Control and the Limits of Reform." *Hastings Center Report* 5 (August 1975):40–45.

London, Perry. *Behavior Control*. New York: The New American Library, 1977.

————. *The Modes and Morals of Psychotherapy*. New York: Holt, Rinehart, & Winston, 1964.

Martin, Reed. *Legal Challenges to Behavior Modification*. Champaigne, Illinois: Research Press, 1975.

McCarley, Tracey. "Issues of Autonomy and Dignity in Group Therapy." *Psychiatric Annals* (December 1975):35ff.

Roos, P. "Human Rights and Behavior Modification." *Mental Retardation* 12 (1974):3–6.

Rothman, David J. "Behavior Modification in Total Institutions." *Hastings Center Report* 5 (February 1975):17–24.

Schrag, Peter. *Mind Control*. New York: Pantheon Books, 1978.

Shapiro, D. "Legislating the Control of Behavior Control, Autonomy and the Use of Coercive Therapies." *Southern California Law Review* 47 (1974):237–356.

Stolz, Stephanie B., ed. *Ethical Issues in Behavior Modification*. San Francisco: Jossey-Bass, 1978.

Szasz, Thomas S. *The Theology of Medicine: The Political-Philosophical Foundations of Medical Ethics*. Baton Rouge: Louisiana State University Press, 1977, Ch. 5.

Ulmer, Raymond A. *On The Development of a Token Economy Hospital Treatment Program*. Washington, D.C.: Hemisphere Publishing Co., 1976.

Wexler, David B. "Token and Taboo: Behavior Modification, Token Economies and the Law." *California Law Review* 61 (January 1973):81–109.

Wheeler, Harvey, ed. *Beyond the Punitive Society—Operant Conditioning: Social and Political Aspects*. San Francisco: W. H. Freeman & Co., 1973.

Wilson, G. Terrence, and Davidson, Gerald C. "Behavior Therapy: A Road to Self-Control," *Psychology Today* 9 (October 1975):54ff.

Zeldow, Peter B. "Some Antitherapeutic Effects of the Token Economy." *Psychiatry* 39 (November 1976):318–324.

Sterilization

Burt, Robert A., and Price, Monroe E. "Sterilization, State Action and the Concept of Consent." *Law and Psychology Review* (Spring 1975):57–78.

Coburn, Judith. "Sterilization Regulations: Debate Not Quelled by HEW Document." *Science* 183 (1974):935–939.

Donovan, Patricia. "Sterilizing the Poor and Incompetent." *Hastings Center Report* 6 (1976):7–8.

Friedman, Paul R. *The Rights of Mentally Retarded Persons.* New York: Avon Books, 1976, pp. 115–121.

Gaylin, Willard, et al. "Sterilization of the Retarded: In Whose Interest?" *Hastings Center Report* 8 (1978):28–41.

Kieffer, George H. *Bioethics: A Textbook of Issues.* Reading, Massachusetts: Addison-Wesley Publishing Co., 1979, pp. 194–203.

Kittrie, Nicholas N. *The Right to Be Different.* Baltimore: The Johns Hopkins Press, 1971, Ch. 7.

Macklin, Ruth, and Gaylin, Willard, eds. *Mental Retardation and Sterilization: A Problem of Competency and Paternalism.* New York: Plenum Press, 1981.

McFadden, Charles. *Medical Ethics.* Philadelphia: F. A. Davis, 1967, Ch. 13.

McGarrah, Robert E., and Peck, Susan L. "Voluntary Female Sterilization: Abuses, Risks and Guidelines." *Hastings Center Report* 4 (1974):5–7.

Neuwirth, Gloria S., et al. "Capacity, Competence, Consent: Voluntary Sterilization of the Mentally Retarded." *Columbia Human Rights Law Review* 6 (Fall-Winter 1974–75):447–472.

Petchesky, Rosalind P. "Reproduction, Ethics, and Public Policy: The Federal Sterilization Regulations." *The Hastings Center Report* 9 (October 1979): 29–41. (See response in Vol. 10, No. 3, June 1980, pp. 4, 19.)

Robitscher, Jonas, ed. *Eugenic Sterilization.* Springfield, Illinois: Charles C. Thomas, Publisher, 1973.

Simonaitis, J. "The Right to Sterilization." *Journal of the American Medical Association* 226 (November 26, 1973):1151–1152.

Steinfels, Margaret O'Brien. "Involuntary Sterilization: The Latest Case." *Psychology Today* 11 (February 1978):124.

Sterilization: Implications for Mentally Retarded and Mentally Ill Persons. Ottawa: Law Reform Commission of Canada, 1979.

9. Responsibility, Criminal Competency and Commitment, and the Insanity Defense

Introduction

Several previous articles have touched upon the concept of responsibility and its relation to the concepts of blameworthiness and insanity. For instance, in section 2, Robert M. Veatch insisted that there could be no responsibility in a deterministic universe and that giving up this concept, along with all the other moral concepts and practices with which it has an essential logical connection, would be part of the price to be paid for adopting a deterministic metaphysic. The view that responsibility presupposes *free will* is widely held, but there is an alternative view that responsibility presupposes nothing more than a capacity for rationality. In section 2, Michael S. Moore denied that will power is relevant to responsibility and insisted on *rationality* alone, a position which determinists find extremely attractive. Taken as mutually exclusive, both views are probably correct in what they affirm and wrong in what they deny. If the debate over whether the mentally ill are responsible and blameworthy for their misdeeds is to make any progress, considerable conceptual clarification is required.

In the following selections, Herbert Fingarette develops the view that insanity involves irrationality and that we should not blame or punish the insane for their misdeeds, because they suffer from an inability to understand. His clear preference in the legal tradition is for the old M'Naghten test, which grants the insanity defense to those who suffer from "a defect of reason." He is much less sympathetic with subsequent legal tests that have recognized defects of self control as exculpatory conditions.

Fingarette rejects the often held position that responsibility involves that originative or creative causality which we call "free will." On this view, those who lack creative volitional autonomy cannot be considered blameworthy, precisely because they are not responsible for their immoral and illegal acts. Since we cannot freely choose an alternative unless we understand it, this position does not deny the importance of rationality. If mental health is rational autonomy, both rationality and autonomy are essential. There are ways of analyzing the concept of autonomy without introjecting free will, however. As Fingarette points out, we tend to excuse *psychotics* primarily because we believe them to be deficient in rationality; but it should be noted that we tend to excuse *neurotics* (who *know* what they are doing) mainly because they seem to be deficient in self-control or will power. They are compelled by powers in them which are not subject to conscious volition. Even when neurotics try to assume responsibility, they do so unrealistically and blame themselves for innumerable evil things far beyond their control. There is another meaning for "responsible" besides being subject to self-control, i.e., having and assuming duties or obligations. Neurotics may grossly exaggerate this sense of the term and assume obligations far beyond their powers, thus running the risk of excessive responsibility.

No astute determinist will concede that to adopt a deterministic metaphysic would require one to abandon the notion of responsibility as self-control, along with blameworthiness, the moral and legal practices of praising and rewarding, or blaming and punishing. Freedom of action (the ability to *do* what we want to do without external hindrance) still has an important place in a deterministic universe devoid of freedom of will (the ability to make originative choices).

The determinist typically holds (since the time of Jonathan Edwards) that a person is free and responsible for an act if:

(1) He knows what he is doing;
(2) He is adequately motivated to do it; and
(3) He chooses to do it in the absence of unusually powerful and imme-
    diate *external* constraints and restraints.

Fingarette emphasizes (1) but seems to presuppose (2) and (3). Though he may regard these conditions as necessary for responsible action, the indeterminist (the believer in free will) insists upon adding that:

(4) He makes an *internally uncaused* choice, at least in the sense that the
    causal conditions which make the choice possible are not sufficient for
    its occurrence, even if they are necessary.

On both views of responsibility, a person is a proper subject of blame or punishment if he or she is responsible for the act and the act is wrong. But if the agent is irresponsible, then a non-responsibility defense is warranted. The real question is, which concept of responsibility should we adopt, and why? Perhaps the free will issue is of little practical significance, since without it we could still adopt the deterministic concept of responsibility (1 through 3 above) and go right on about our business of dealing with moral and legal offenders.

Many persons who are charged with criminal offenses later find themselves hospitalized involuntarily in mental hospitals. Some are awaiting a determination of their competency to stand trial; others are being treated for restoration to such competency; and still others have been judged incompetent with little prospect of restoration to either competency or liberty. Some have actually been tried for their crimes, found "not guilty" because they were insane at the time of the crime, and yet they have been involuntarily institutionalized even though they are innocent. Although the two are easily and often confused, it must be clearly understood that the question of competency *to stand trial* is absolutely different from the question of sanity or competency *at the time of the crime.* Legally, the criteria for answering such questions are quite distinct. The former involves identifying abilities to understand the nature and circumstances of the offense and to cooperate with legal counsel in developing and presenting a defense, whereas the latter involves determining whether the offender knew and/or could control what he was doing at the time of the crime. Competency to stand trial is a very specific type of competency, quite distinct from one's competency to do such things as conduct business, make wills or contracts, marry, vote, or choose and refuse treatment. The courts consistently refuse to allow mental patients to be declared generally incompetent for everything. Indeed, theoretically, the presumption of competency in all respects remains fully intact for such persons until it is successfully challenged at formal competency hearings. Each competency hearing must be issue-specific, and the criteria used to determine competency to stand trial are explained in the selection entitled "The Nature of Competency to Stand Trial." In practice, it is occasionally difficult to distinguish between incompetency due to mental illness, and mere ignorance of the court system resulting from cultural deprivation.

Treatment designed to restore an individual's competence to stand trial frequently involves psychotropic drugs, and until quite recently most states had not recognized a person's right to refuse such medication. Even where such a right is recognized, the refusal may be questioned on the grounds that it is being used to evade the restoration of competency to stand trial which these drugs clearly facilitate. In the selection by Glenn C. Graber and Frank H. Marsh, it is contended that a defendant ought not to be drugged in order to stand trial. They object to "chemical competence" on many grounds. They seem to find the very idea abhorrent, perhaps ignoring the fact that ordinary competence depends upon normal brain chemistry, and that drug therapy can help restore normal brain chemistry. If properly used, drugs can also help restore memory, one's sense of personal identity, and normal rational functioning. This seems to have happened in the case the authors cite, despite their protests. If the defendant was extremely confused and out of control *before* the administration of drugs, competence either to consent to or to refuse therapy may be in doubt, and there certainly can be no unjustified infringements of autonomy where no autonomy exists. On the other hand, if the defendant refused further therapy *after* the drugs had restored his self-control and rational functioning, why is it less of a violation of "human dignity" to use drugs to restore rational autonomy than to use them to restore competency to stand trial? Furthermore, drug therapy, in conjunction with counseling, is definitely the method of choice for schizophrenia, instead of psychotherapy alone, which the authors advocate. No amount of talking will restore an imbalance in the dopamine circuit of the brain. The authors judge that it was in the patient's "best interest" not to stand trial; but it is not at all clear that it is better to be committed to indeterminate and often lifelong incarceration in a mental institution than to serve a fixed and frequently shorter sentence in a penal institution. Finally, the jury in this case apparently did fail to grasp the essential difference between competence at the time of the trial and sanity at the time of the crime; and it is doubtful that the ethics of this case would have attracted anyone's attention if that distinction had been properly appreciated.

In the final selection, June R. German and Anne C. Singer expose the incoherencies involved in punishing those who have been judged not guilty by reason of insanity. Theoretically, there are significant differences between *punishing* convicted criminals by putting them in penal institutions and *treating* in mental institutions those acquitted for crimes they may have committed under conditions of insanity. We punish convicted criminals for several reasons: to prevent and deter similar offenses, to rehabilitate, and to extract that sweet revenge which we dignify with the epithets of "justice" or "retribution." Though mental institutions aim at prevention, deterrence, and rehabilitation, they differ in theory from penal institutions in that it is improper to use them to extract societal revenge. In practice, however, there is often no difference between these two types of institutions in this crucial respect, as German and Singer explain. In their efforts to combine revenge with rehabilitation, even our penal institutions are dismal failures.

The case of John Hinckley is now forcing our society to rethink the logic of the insanity defense and the concept of non-responsibility.

Herbert Fingarette

Insanity and Responsibility

I

In the law we find a theme that is centuries old: Insanity is a condition precluding responsibility. The continuity through time, and the wide geographic
dispersion of this theme suggest that if we are to have an adequate critique of
the notion of mental illness, at least so far as this is a notion with the fundamental moral implication mentioned, that critique must be framed in a far
broader perspective than that of contemporary medical doctrine on mental
disorder. Medical doctrines about the nature and causes of mental disorder
have come and gone in the past several centuries; and at any one time there
has usually been a plurality of such doctrines, often incompatible with others.
Yet the theme of mental disorder as a condition precluding responsibility has
persisted nearly unchallenged. Therefore the task of the present study is to
identify and to state with a reasonable clarity a centuries-old and still current
notion of mental disorder as something that implies non-responsibility, a
notion which is *independent* of any of the different psychological or psychophysiological doctrines which have followed upon or co-existed with one
another during this long period.

I have already spoken of "insanity," "mental illness," and "mental disorder." I
could as well have used such terms as "mental disease," or "madness." The terminology varies, and the different terms have historically been used sometimes
interchangeably, sometimes with differing nuances. But somewhere within

From *Inquiry,* 15 (1972):6–29. Copyright © 1972 by Universitets Forlaget, Oslo, Norway.
Reprinted by permission of the publisher and the author.

the range of reference of these terms is a common core, a reference to an aberrant, unhealthy mental condition of a kind which precludes responsibility.

It is not in medicine but in law that we find the only sophisticated and reasonably continuous intellectual tradition in the matter. The thesis that there is such a thing as insanity, and that the insane person is, insofar as insane, not criminally responsible, has for long remained embedded in law. Yet even in the law, deeper questions about this thesis have remained troublesome. Debate and confusion have been persistent regarding the exact meaning of the key terms, the most appropriate form of insanity "test" to be used in criminal law, and — perhaps most obscure and least studied — the underlying legal and moral rationale for allowing insanity to preclude criminal guilt.

It thus becomes a matter of interest from a variety of perspectives to become clear about the meaning of insanity in the criminal law and the rationale for holding the insane non-responsible. One perspective from which such an inquiry is of interest is of course that of criminal law itself. In addition, a study of the law on criminal insanity can, I believe, illuminate the law generally as it is concerned in a variety of other criminal and civil contexts with mental incapacity and consequent impairment of responsibility. More broadly, and because the insanity plea in the criminal law has such a long and rich intellectual and practical tradition, a study of the concept of criminal insanity is also likely to throw light on the philosophical-moral concept of responsibility, and on the psychological-psychiatric concept of mental illness.

On the other hand, if we fail to study this long criminal law tradition about insanity, we probably fail to use the one central resource for any inquiry into the topic of mental illness and responsibility. And we are also likely to take quite the wrong road: The temptation has too often been to center the inquiry upon some contemporary empirical doctrine or theory in medical psychology. This is an understandable, common, but grievous error. Insanity, mental illness, mental disease — these are not medical concepts.[1]

II

In turning to the concept of insanity in the criminal law, we should note at once that we shift the focus of the inquiry as compared to many contemporary philosophical discussions of mental aberrance. The use of data illustrative of "neurosis" is typical of contemporary philosophical discussions of irrationality and illness. In the discussion which follows, however, the emphasis, at least initially, will be on data illustrative of "psychosis." The "psychosis" and "neurosis" labels derive from contemporary psychiatric doctrine, though they are not very precise or reliable in application. Consistently with my introductory remarks, however, I am not using these terms drawn from contemporary psychiatric terminology as the basis for the inquiry to follow. The context which actually guides the selection of illustrative case material will not be psychiatry but the criminal law on insanity. Nevertheless it is of practical use for the reader to be aware at once that the upshot of such selections will in fact be to focus inquiry on what is today called psychosis much more than on neurosis. Later on we will consider why this should be so, and some of the implications.

The kinds of persons who typically are defendants in the context of the insanity plea in criminal law are persons who commit a harm, forbidden by criminal law, where the harmful act seems to stem decisively from such conditions as: delusion (for example, of persecution); chronic, extreme, bizarre mood (for example, irrationally destructive depression); profound insensitivity, even in a rudimentary way, to moral injury, human suffering, and pain; failure to foresee the rudimentary practical (and in the relevant cases harmful) consequences of the act; chronic incapacity to act with reasonable foresight and responsiveness to the moral fabric of human relations. Such mental disorders fall roughly into the current psychiatric categories of paranoia, various schizophrenic and manic-depressive psychoses, and severe character disorders.

Let us begin by considering briefly the case of Daniel M'Naghten, out of which emerged the classic insanity test in Anglo-U.S. law. M'Naghten was under the delusion that there was a widespread Tory plot against him. He came to think that he could defend himself by assassinating the Tory Prime Minister. He therefore lay in wait, having ascertained which was the Prime Minister's carriage. When the carriage came by, he shot the occupant (not realizing that it was the Prime Minister's secretary, rather than the Prime Minister himself, who was in the carriage) and killed him.

Instead of being convicted of high treason, M'Naghten was held by the court to have been insane, and therefore not criminally responsible. The public outcry at this unpopular decision was such that the highest judges of England were formally requested by the Lords to present, as a collective body, an explicit statement and explanation of the legal grounds for acquittal by reason of insanity. This unusual though lawful request was acceded to, and the classic "*M'Naghten* test" for criminal insanity propounded by the judges was the result. They said that a person charged with a crime is properly held to have been criminally insane if at the time of the act he was

> laboring from such a defect of reason, from disease of the mind, as not to know the nature and quality of the act he was doing, or if he did know it, that he did not know he was doing what was wrong.

The *M'Naghten* test has dominated English and American law since then. In the course of time, the principal emendation of an obviously substantive nature in this test has been to add an alternative to the "lack of knowledge" clauses, a clause about lack of self-control. The "defect of reason" phrase has usually been dropped from later rewordings. The scope of "know" has in many versions of the test been made broader, and probably vaguer, by substituting words like "appreciate" or "understand." An element of degree has been introduced into what many considered to be the too inflexible, all-or-nothing wording of the original *M'Naghten* test. In recent times there has been a strong trend in the U.S. Federal Courts to adopt some variant of the insanity test formula proposed in the American Law Institute's *Model Penal Code*. The *Model Penal Code* in effect draws together a number of the refinements of *M'Naghten* just mentioned, and says that the defendant should be held to have been insane if, at the time of the conduct in question, "as a result of mental disease or defect he lacks substantial capacity either to appreciate the criminality of his act or to conform his conduct to the requirements of law." (Note that in this formulation the "defect of reason" phrase has been dropped.)

Perhaps the most controversial modern American ruling was in the 1954 *Durham* case, in which the court aimed to cut through the confusion and verbiage, and to treat the issue in what is supposed to be an "enlightened" and progressive way, that is, as an issue posing essentially a medical question. In *Durham,* the court required for a finding of insanity only that the unlawful act in question have been "a product of mental disease or defect." This apparently straightforward medical criterion had to be progressively revised and qualified with experience in using the *Durham* test, until *Durham,* as modified, had become within a decade or so surprisingly like the *M'Naghten* and the *Model Penal Code* formulations. This unexpected outcome is suggestive of the inherent force underlying the classic *M'Naghten* approach. The basic elements of the latter, though much maligned by medical men especially, have in substance and spirit shown remarkable durability — the principal substantive controversy remaining the question whether to include the lack of self-control clauses.[2]

Regardless of the doctrinal and practical difficulties which have been engendered, there has been a consistent consensus in the courts that it is essential to justice that we retain the principle that there are persons who are insane, who must be identified as such if charged with crime, and who must be exonerated of criminal guilt if the harmful deed was done by virtue of the insanity. What have the courts had in mind there? That is what we must seek to discover.

Who are the insane? Let us recall that we are not dealing with a notion rooted in some particular psychological or medical doctrine. Indeed the notion is often explicitly rejected as a non-medical one by psychiatrists. Insanity is, at bottom, a notion of everyday language, the language in which common men characterize individuals and pass moral judgments on them. It is this common notion which the law has embodied in substance though, as always, with refinements and specifications adopted to the distinctive purposes of the law.

Who are the insane? A few general, preliminary remarks may help to rough in an answer. The insane are madmen, crazy persons bereft of reason. They are persons whose conduct is irrational because they themselves are irrational persons.

To those who have ever observed an insane person, it is evident that such a person need not be mad in every respect — very few of the insane are. Nor need the person's loss of reason be continuous. Even in the respects in which a person is insane, the insanity may be manifest only intermittently.

But when the insane person's comportment manifests his insanity, we cannot in good conscience consider him responsible in comporting himself. Indeed it is more than a matter of conscience: it does not make sense to say that an insane person's comportment on a certain occasion was a distinctive manifestation of his insanity, and to assert that in so acting he was acting responsibly. Of course, even in insane comportment the person may manifest intelligence, skill, acuity of mind in one or another important respect; he need not act like a "wild beast" or "raving maniac," in a totally unintelligible or merely animal way. Such extremes of insanity are rare. Yet even though we see purpose, intelligence, skill, if we do nevertheless see the person as insane (as for example in M'Naghten's case), then we see him as not acting responsibly insofar as his conduct flows from his insanity.

III

Now I should like to take up these themes more systematically. There is a notion which lies at the heart of the idea of insanity — it is irrationality. I do not mean that insanity is simply irrationality. Insanity is more than that. But having seized upon the notion of irrationality, we have grasped what is the most distinctive element in insanity. The idea of irrationality is itself obscure in meaning, and that is part of the reason why the idea of insanity is obscure.

What basis is there for the thesis that the notion of irrationality is distinctive of (but not all there is to) insanity? I want to show that there is such a basis, at least enough to establish the plausibility of the thesis, and then to move to the next step in the inquiry. The next step will be to clarify the meaning of the obscure but key concept, "irrationality." Then I shall in turn move to consider what more there is in insanity besides irrationality. And having developed a reasonably full and clear analysis of the idea of insanity, it will then be possible to test and further confirm the whole analysis by applying the idea of insanity as so analyzed. We shall consider whether the analysis does set out what it is that leads men to see paradigm cases of insanity *as* paradigm, controversial cases *as* controversial, and insanity *per se* as inherently precluding responsibility.

The dictionaries tell us that the intimate linking of "insanity" and "irrationality" is indeed rooted in the language. Webster gives "irrational" as a synonym of "insane," and "rational" as a synonym of "sane." There are a number of other dictionary cross-references involving this entire family of terms, and they consistently confirm the close linkage. (The connection is more than English-linked. In French, we find that "fou" is defined as a matter of having "perdu la raison," or of being or acting "contraire à la raison." Similar close connections between sane and rational, and insane and irrational are found in other European languages.)

In law, from very early times on, it is common to use in this connection "loss of reason" or other idioms with the root-elements "reason" or "rational" coupled appropriately with qualifying terms or prefixes implying loss, breakdown, or absence. As has been noted, the classic *M'Naghten* test speaks of "defect of reason, from disease of the mind" as a necessary condition for criminal insanity.

It is only as we come toward the law in the twentieth century that we see the "defect of reason" element dropped as a component of the formal legal insanity tests, the notion of "mental disease" serving alone where *M'Naghten* had "defect of reason, from disease of the mind." Yet the history of the law, and the nature of the cases at issue, reveal that this omission has tended to coincide with an increase of confusion and controversy about criminal insanity, and reflects a partial loss of the original deep insight in the process of trying to square the legal language with contemporary psychological and psychiatric language.

The increased confusion comes about in this way. Terms like "reason" and "rational" have come to be used in a much more restricted way in contemporary psychology and psychiatry than in the long tradition of lay and legal usage. This narrower usage has to some extent infected contemporary lay and legal usage. Hence the original concept which was (and still is) central to insanity, i.e. irrationality, has become obscured for modern men. As a result, the concept of insanity itself has become more confused and controversial; and the task of displaying the meaning of that concept has become more difficult. What is the nature of this recent shift in meaning?

"Rational" and "irrational" have traditionally been terms which can apply to persons and to their acts, choices, demeanor, moods, emotions, beliefs, values, attitudes, desires—and indeed in connection with most of the basic categories in terms of which we characterize persons and their conduct. But in the narrower usage of contemporary psychology and psychiatry, the term "rational" and its cognates apply only to the intellectual operations, "cognitive functions" of the mind. Thus, for example, in this contemporary and narrow psychological usage, the logical manipulation of one's ideas about one's moods can be rational, but it makes no psychological sense to speak of the mood itself as being rational. Moods are phenomena connected with "drives," "tensions," "affect"— phenomena or processes supposedly external to those which constitute the activity of reason (intellect, cognition).

Thus although the psychiatric use is vague, it is still plainly much narrower than the (admittedly vague) traditional usage. This narrow use in turn leads to a strong tendency—even among those psychiatrists who insist that the mind is not (normally) "compartmentalized"—to insist, or at least to acknowledge, that a person's rational powers may be functioning at a rather high level of efficiency even when the person is gravely mentally ill. Perhaps certain types of paranoia—e.g. M'Naghten—are among the clearest examples of persons whose intellectual functioning can be in many important respects quite effective, whereas the person is plainly mentally ill. In contemporary psychological usage, M'Naghten's rational powers were quite good in most respects. In the traditional usage, M'Naghten was a paradigm of an irrational person.

Let us consider one further example. A woman is in a state of chronic and deep depression. She broods about the sin in the world and the sin in herself. She is so paralyzed by guilt that she remains helpless and motionless—until one day she rouses herself, goes to her children, kills them in order to save them from the awful destiny of all human beings, and then herself attempts suicide. Such a woman, at the time of the killings, could have a relatively intact reason in the narrow sense of that term as it is used by psychologists — since her purposeful and "rationalized" conduct at the end reveals that her capacity to make logical inferences was substantial. The psychologist would speak of a mood disorder, an affect psychosis, but not of a disorder of reason (intellect). However, in the traditional use, it is appropriate and natural to say that she was irrational, that her conduct was irrational, that her mood was irrational — that, in the language of the *M'Naghten* test, she suffered from a defect of reason.

In sum, then, it is my thesis that in order to understand the concept of insanity it is necessary to stay firmly with traditional usage of "rationality" and "irrationality," of "losing one's reason." It is this usage which I shall now try to make clearer by bringing out the considerations, in the context of insanity and responsibility, which guide us in using the language of "irrationality" as we traditionally have used it.

IV

What is irrationality — that is, in the sense requisite for insanity? It is intelligible to say in some types of cases — and so we must notice it in order to avoid later confusion — that a person's conduct was not rational but yet not irrational either. Typical instances would be chewing gum, whistling a song as one walks, moving one's foot in a quiet, rhythmic way as one sits cross-legged in a chair. It does seem forced to say that in doing these things one is being, or acting, or comporting oneself irrationally. We would not normally be inclined to call such conduct irrational. But in the context of a more theoretical discussion centering on the question of rationality, the fact that we are also inclined to resist classifying such conduct under the heading "rational conduct" leads us to raise the question of classifying, even to feel some slight inclination to classify, it as the contrary, i.e. irrational. And our resistance to classifying it as irrational elicits some inclination to classify it as rational. But our resistance to move unqualifiedly in either direction reflects our awareness that these two mutually exclusive categories are in some important way not exhaustive.

It is easy to see, as a result of recent studies which have appeared in the literature, that when we unqualifiedly call conduct rational, a necessary condition is that we see the conduct as somehow done for reasons. Just how this phrase "for reasons" is best further interpreted is a matter of some controversy which need not concern us here. It is enough for us here to see that failure to meet such a condition does not warrant calling the conduct "irrational." The gum-chewing and other examples mentioned can be *not* irrational and yet not call for *any* reason at all, even so empty a "reason" as "I wanted to" or "I felt like it." Then when is conduct definitely irrational?

Let us consider a number of different versions of the same basic illustration.

A (1) Jones has been walking in the woods, and has paused briefly. He idly picks up a stone, hefts it, eventually idly tosses it at a nearby bush.

A (2) Jones, having indulged idly once or twice more in the same activity as in A (1), is about to toss a stone again when Smith suddenly appears from out of the brush and directly in the line of fire. Jones does not throw.

A (3) Jones is idly tossing stones, and does not see Smith who is sitting, unaware of Jones, in the bushes directly in the line of fire. The stone hits Smith.

B. Jones has been walking in the woods and has paused briefly. He suddenly spies a rattlesnake nearby and moving toward him. Jones picks up a stone and throws it at the rattler to frighten it away.

C. Jones is strolling through the woods, enjoying the sun and air and the greenery around him. He casually stoops to pick up a rock which catches his eye, hefts it, and is about to toss it into the brush. Just then Smith comes into view in the line of fire. Jones recognizes Smith, a man he bitterly detests, and then, with hardly a break in his motion, but with the suspicion of a smile on his face, he completes the throw. Smith is hit by the rock. Jones rushes up to him and apologizes, assuring Smith that there had not been sufficient time to check the throw.

D. Jones is idly tossing rocks when Smith appears. Jones takes Smith to be slightly off to the side of the line of fire, and, without bothering to investigate more carefully, he throws. What Jones had not quickly enough grasped was that Smith did not see Jones and was moving toward the line of fire. Smith is hit.

E. Jones is stumbling through the woods drunk. He picks up a stone that catches his eye, stares at it glazedly, then sets himself to throw it. At that moment Smith appears out of the brush and directly in the line of fire. Jones sees Smith, hesitates in surprise, then throws the stone as previously aimed, i.e. directly at Smith. Smith is hit and falls to the ground. Jones stands, staring, perplexed, dazedly looks around, a bit startled by Smith's sudden disappearance. After a moment or two, Jones staggers off.

In case A (1), Jones just "feels like" tossing the stone as he rambles through the woods. Perhaps even "feels like" is too much of an accounting. As in the case of idly kicking one's foot when sitting cross-legged, Jones might deny that he "felt like" doing it and insist that he was just *doing* it. He might ask challengingly: "Why *not* do it?" "No reason," we respond, shrugging. Thus what is at issue here is a kind of conduct or comportment about which there was no good reason for him not to do it. Our reluctance to call his conduct irrational is strengthened and justified when, as we continue to observe him in A (2), we see that when Smith appears in the line of fire, Jones stops his throw in order not to hit Smith. In short, Jones is perfectly capable, as we normally presume, of grasping the relevance of aspects of his situation which are obviously relevant to what he is doing. When Smith appears in the line of fire, Jones instantly grasps the relevant spatial relationships, the human, moral, and even legal considerations relevant to his throwing the rock, and elects not to do so.

Nor do we consider Jones to be acting irrationally in A (3) just because, not realizing that Smith is seated, invisible behind the bush, he does throw the rock and hits Smith. Here it was not a case of failing to grasp the relevance of what was evidently relevant; it was a case of ignorance of fact. That is, what was relevant was not evident. So in A (3) we say Jones was ignorant, not irrational. Again, we feel confident about this because of A (2): when the relevant was evident, he grasped its relevance.

In case B, Jones's throwing the stone at the rattlesnake is not only not irrational, it is rational. He has good reason to throw the stone. But here, too, we see that another way one can characterize the situation is to say that he shows he can grasp the relevance of an evidently relevant feature of his situation. Here what is relevant is also his (good) reason for doing as he does.

In case C, Jones again grasps the evident relevance of Smith's appearance in the line of fire, and the relevance of certain moral (and legal) standards. In this case, however, the relevant standards are not (part of) his reason for throwing the rock; he acts as he does in spite of the wrongness and criminality of intentionally hitting Smith. But we can see that he grasps the relevance of these standards because we see how he attempts to conceal the criminal and immoral intent from Smith. Jones is rational but malicious. He could not be malicious — it would make no sense to call him malicious — if he had not grasped the relevance of the relevant moral standards.

In case D, Jones is not irrational; he is careless or reckless, throwing the stone without bothering to establish reliably whether Smith is moving toward the line of fire or not. He is mistaken about a matter of fact, it is true, but unlike Jones in A (3), who could not see Smith at all, this Jones sees Smith, grasps the relevance of the physical relations as he sees them, and he also grasps — we assume — the relevance of certain standards of caution when the physical relationships are as he sees them in relation to his conduct. Abiding by standards of caution would call for refraining from the throw because of the closeness of the calculation and the gravity of the possible harm. Since Jones elects not to abide by relevant standards of caution, we call him careless. (However if we assumed that he was incapable of grasping the relevance of elementary standards of caution to his situation, we would then be inclined to say it was not so much careless conduct as irrational conduct.)

In case E, a radically new element has been introduced. In this case, Jones is so drunk that although he is still capable of conduct — i.e. walking about, throwing stones — he fails to grasp (and indeed is incapable of grasping) the relevance of certain considerations which are evidently relevant to his conduct in this situation. Jones sees Smith. Jones neither intends to hit Smith nor is clear about what has happened after he does in fact hit Smith. He is too mentally confused to appreciate even the gross fact that if Smith is somewhere in the region of where the stone is going, Smith may be hurt. Jones is too befuddled to grasp the human, moral, legal implications of his conduct in this situation, even were he to have dimly appreciated that the stone would hit Smith, or even after the stone did hit Smith.

To *grasp the relevance* of evidently relevant aspects of one's situation — this notion requires emphasis and some brief elaboration.

Jones (in case E, intoxicated) might be able to answer questions as soon as he sobers up, or later in a trial:

Q: Where was Smith?
Jones: Right in front of me.

Q: Near enough to be hit by the rock?
Jones: Oh, yes, just a few feet away.

Q: You did see him there?
Jones: Oh, yes.

Q: Didn't you know you would almost surely hit him?
Jones: Well, of course, it's obvious that I would . . . but at the time, I just didn't really grasp it all. There he was . . . and I was throwing the rock there . . . but I was so befuddled it just didn't connect up. I was drunk. I think maybe I saw I would hit him, but . . . the significance of it just never came to me.

It is essential to note that at no time in the preceding discussion have we been concerned with relevance insofar as it has to do with subtleties, nuances, or details. We do not say Jones drunk is irrational because he did not appreciate nuances, subtleties, or details of the law or moral nuances. What is at issue is the kind of patent, rudimentary, fundamental relevance without which ordinary human intercourse breaks down. We do not say that Jones throwing a rock at the snake, or Jones throwing the rock maliciously at Smith, is rational because of the wisdom or moral depth of vision displayed. Both actions might in fact be rather foolish and perhaps both even morally wrong. No matter; these acts are not irrational acts. Jones is not irrational so long as Jones is capable of grasping what is patently, rudimentarily, and fundamentally relevant — that thrown rocks can hurt people, that hurting people and causing them to suffer are of themselves bad, that wilfully injuring people is generally a crime. . . . This kind of relevance I shall call, for the sake of brevity, essential relevance — i.e. the relevance which constitutes the essential warp and woof of the fabric of ordinary human intercourse.

It is this failure to grasp essential relevance that is what we see as irrationality in contexts related to insanity.

What is the difference between Jones's irrationality when he is drunk, and the irrationality of the insane? Jones is temporarily incapable of grasping the relevance of Smith's presence, and his temporary incapacity is caused by drink, that is, by an intoxicant whose effects are soon dissipated. (I shall here avoid discussion of the more complex case of the alcoholic whose capacities may in the long run be permanently or at least persistently affected.)

In the case of the insane person, we no longer see the irrationality as due to any such external causal agent with such plainly related direct and temporary effects. We see the person's mental makeup itself as being abnormal: By virtue of his mental makeup, the insane person has a propensity to act irrationally. That is, we see his mind as at least for a time such that he substantially lacks capacity to grasp the relevance of (at least some of) what is essentially relevant to his conduct in his situation. To the extent that we view the propensity to irrational comportment as due to factors other than his mind or personality, we do not call him insane. When there are fluctuations or limitations in the scope or duration of the disposition to irrational comportment (as there always are), we may take account of this in various ways, usage not being settled: We may say he is insane but does not show it always or in every aspect of his life; we may say he is insane only in certain ways, or only intermittently; we may speak of "remission" after a long period of recovered sanity; or we may say that the insanity was in fact never "cured." Choice of usage here depends upon many considerations including the psychological doctrines toward which one inclines. However for our present purposes such variants are of no fundamental significance. Our next task is to explore the bearing of the preceding account of insanity on typical types of mental disorder and the actual criminal law attitudes toward them.

V

In the classic case of Daniel M'Naghten we see that M'Naghten did suffer from "defect of reason" — he was under the delusion that the Tories were conspiring against him. To say it was a delusion is to say (a) he could grasp the relevance of any consideration that would show something to be compatible or incompatible with his delusion, but (b) anything relevant to an assessment of the force or weight of that consideration *independently* of whether it was compatible with his delusion was beyond his ken.

The merely stubborn but not delusory person does see the relevance of standards of assessment independent of conformity to his beliefs and he tries to use these standards for independently assessing the force of some consideration; but he tends to distort them, bend them to his purpose, apply them in biased ways, so that in the end it is conformity to his already established belief which is decisive. The insanely deluded person, however, has a radical blindness — what is relevant to independently assessing the force of considerations *pro* and *con* simply passes him by; he is unburdened by any concern except the test of consistency with his delusion. He recognizes inconsistencies, but freely introduces further assumptions which dissolve the inconsistencies, and his prime test of the truth of his new assumptions is that, if assumed, they do dissolve the inconsistency.

In the borderline cases, of course, we may be in doubt whether, for example, the "religious fanatic," is an exceptionally stubborn and biased person (one who has a sense of relevance but who perverts his standards in order to support his belief), or is a person subject to insane delusion (having no grasp of relevance beyond consistency with his delusion), or is a person whose vision differs so from ours, and whose sense of relevance is therefore so different from ours, that we wonder if he may be a true prophet.

Using the paranoid delusion as an example to work with can be misleading, for the person suffering from paranoid delusions can be an easy case to identify, especially when he commits bizarre crimes. The situation is more complicated when we turn to psychotic depressions.

The concept of the psychotic depression is the concept of a mood which, like the paranoiac's delusion, serves to preclude responsiveness to anything relevant to comportment which could give weight to any consideration independently of the dominance of the mood. The smile and helping hand of a neighbor have no independent probative force, even prima facie, as grounds for hope; they are perceived as guile, or as confirmation of the depressive's worthlessness.

A paralyzing lethargy of mind and body must be the end of an irrational depression gone to its logical end, since any policy or conduct, even purposeful tranquility, is inherently evil and doomed to failure. Only when the depression does not go to the most severe extent, or only in the periods before or after the depth of a psychotic depression does the depressed person have the motivation to engage in any enterprise of substance. The practical result, so far as criminal law is concerned, is that cases of harmful acts ascribed to psychotic depression tend to be somewhat more controversial, more difficult to identify as due to psychotic depression, than some paranoiac delusions. In such a case as M'Naghten's assassination attempt, however, the act is precisely the manifestation of the delusion in acute form.

As one might expect, there is in fact a certain unpredictability in jury findings, and a manifest uncertainty of legal doctrine in connection with psychotic depression as the basis for a plea of insanity. The situation is not helped by the tendency to put the issue on occasion in terms of "irresistible impulse," "compulsion," "loss of will," or "incapacity to conform." Putting the issue in these ways leads to pious philosophical affirmations about free-will, and suspect psychological debate over whether the defendant "knew" he was murdering someone but had "lost the power of will" to refrain.

The decision in such cases is made in practice, I suggest, by the trier of fact's making an estimate of the degree to which the defendant had capacity to grasp the relevance of moral, legal and practical considerations essentially relevant to what he was doing and even though these were incompatible with his mood. If the triers of fact in effect conclude that the defendant was blind to the relevance of such considerations, the finding will be that he was irrational, i.e. insane. If they find significant signs that the person grasped the relevance of such considerations, saw their force even when incompatible with his mood, but nevertheless acted consistently with his depressed mood and committed the unlawful act, then they will not find him insane. There is no simple way to decide such a question, of course. One must develop as full a portrait and history of the person as possible with an eye to discerning patterns of conduct and demeanor which reflect the capacity to apprehend what is essentially relevant. The triers of fact will not look for "will-power" but for signs that the person did really take some account of what was relevant. For the reason mentioned earlier, this decision is typically difficult to make in the case of depressives, the intermediate stages of depression presenting, in the nature of the case, conflicting signs with respect to the judgment to be made.

There has been great resistance in the U.S. courts to accepting the withdrawn, humanly estranged character evidenced by many schizophrenics as constituting insanity for purposes of the criminal law. The courts have usually held guilty the schizophrenic person who calmly plots and kills — in many cases in bizarre and horrible ways — and who makes attempts to hide his crime, and subsequently acknowledges that he knew it was a crime.

The debate has usually revolved around two main sorts of considerations. The theses in favor of the insanity finding are: (1) The defendant's grotesque act, bizarre motivation and estranged manner were so plain and extreme as to call forth intuitively the judgment that he was insane; (2) the defendant was diagnosed as schizophrenic, and this is a major "mental disease." The legal response has been, in effect, that "mental disease" does not of itself establish criminal insanity; the disease must have certain legally relevant consequences, for example, that the defendant didn't know he was acting criminally, or (in some jurisdictions) he could not control himself. And with respect to these legally relevant consequences, the facts often are that the schizophrenic killer acts and speaks in a way which shows he knew he was committing a crime (he says he knew it was a crime, and he tries to hide his tracks); and the planning and preparation which went into the complex course of conduct leading to the killing are inconsistent with the supposition that he could not control himself, that it was "an irresistible impulse" or an impulse of any kind at all.

In some jurisdictions, for example in California, there has been some tendency to reduce the seriousness of the charge in such cases, but to reject the plea of insanity. But the legal response has more typically been to reject the psychiatric position.[3]

I think we can see the meaning of this conflict more clearly by thinking of insanity, as I have proposed herein, as inherent mental irrationality, i.e. inherent mental incapacity to respond to what is essentially relevant. We then discover an ambiguity, an ambivalence, in the criminal law itself.

The kind of schizophrenic killer who has been sketched above is a person who does respond to the relevance of overt social prohibition — statutes, regulations, policemen as enforcers, etc. He grasps the relevance of the essentials of criminal law in its status as an expression of the will and power of the State and the emotional attitudes of the community. He can and often does take pragmatic self-protective action accordingly. Hence in these respects he looks like a "knowing" criminal.

But he does not respond to the relevance of those moral and humanitarian concerns which lie behind the law and which some would see as expressed *in* the law. Questions of moral evil or good, of human sympathy or antagonism, of human dignity, do not enter his ken. He is not morally evil or cruel—he is blind to this dimension of experience; there is nothing relevant here that he responds to as relevant. Unlike the malicious person, he does not grasp the moral relevance of what he is doing and act in spite of it, or out of a perverse delight in evil; he does not at all grasp the relevance of the morally relevant aspects of what he is doing.

The ambiguity in the criminal law is this: Is the fundamental responsibility of the citizen, so far as the criminal law goes, to this law in its status merely as an expression of State policy, or is it to the criminal law as a community expression of certain fundamental moral and humanitarian values? Those who deny or discount the latter are inclined to find such an estranged, schizophrenic defendant to be legally sane—i.e. responsible under criminal law (because capable of responding to the relevant statutes, sanctions, etc.). However, those who think of the moral dimension as inherent in the criminal law are inclined to hold that the person is criminally insane, or at least responsible in lesser degree (since, after all, he clearly is not responsive to the relevance of the moral dimension which is here held to be essential to the meaning of law).

Much the same sorts of considerations would apply in the case of the so-called "psychopathic personality" (or "sociopath") as apply in the case of the schizophrenic discussed above. I will not belabor the issue here, nor take time to introduce minor refinements of the discussion specifically required for application to the psychopathic personality.

Finally, we come to the general distinction between the neuroses and the psychoses. Why have the courts very generally refused to accept neuroses as insanity, and usually been willing to find insanity only in cases (but not in all cases) which in fact are diagnosed as psychosis?

VI

It is more the rule than the exception for psychiatrists who are speaking within the context of criminal law to state that only psychoses are "mental diseases" within the meaning of the legal insanity test formulae, all of which in U.S. law require "mental disease" as a necessary condition for a finding of insanity. Neurosis and character disorders are typically (but not uniformly) excluded from the category "mental disease," and hence they are in practice precluded as candidates for a finding of insanity. Yet this tendency among psychiatrists and courts to allow only psychoses as mental disease is strangely noteworthy. For (1) there is no authoritative medical definition or use of the phrase "mental disease"; (2) there is nothing in the official medical diagnostic manuals which says, or even says in effect, that only psychoses are mental diseases; and (3) there are no U.S. legal definitions of "mental disease" which specify that only psychoses can qualify. Thus there is no authoritative medical or legal basis for the limitation of mental disease to psychosis. Yet many a forensic psychiatrist confidently announces the proposition (or affirms plainly derivative propositions), both in sworn testimony and in less formal settings. And the courts typically accept it. Why should this be?

A review of the remarks often made in the context of such affirmations about psychosis and "mental disease" reveals that the reasons for this strange state of affairs are not simple. On the one hand, judges and lawmen generally tend to assume that the phrase "mental disease," which always occurs in the legal formulae, has a definite and acknowledged medical sense, or that at least ideally it should have one. Hence they have not explored the concept carefully, and have assumed that the burden for correct application of the concept is upon the medical expert once the phrase is invoked. On the other hand, the psychiatric medical experts seem to have been influenced by two sorts of consideration. First, in trying to make sense of the phrase "mental disease" (which, as has been noted, does not have a systematic or official role in medical doctrine) they have tried, for lack of adequate guidance from the courts, to interpret on their own initiative the intent of the law; or at least they have tried to estimate the practical limits of what courts would in fact be willing to accept as appropriate to justify absolving the defendant of criminal guilt. The psychiatrists have generally assumed (by and large correctly) that the mental aberration would have to be quite severe, and preferably bizarre, before the judges or juries would even consider lifting the burden of criminal responsibility. In casting about among authentic medical categories for something which might serve the purpose, they have seized upon the category "psychosis." The pragmatic estimate of the psychiatrists has usually been that to widen the range of "mental disease" beyond the psychoses to include neuroses would have no effect except to reduce the credibility of the expert in the eyes of the court. Since the psychiatrists have for such reasons offered "psychosis" as the meaning of "mental disease," the courts have tended to feel confirmed in the view that "mental disease" is a medically defined concept, and have tended in practice to accept what the psychiatrists affirm, assuming it to be based on medical grounds. Since the courts have tended to accept the thesis that only psychoses are mental diseases, psychiatrists have in turn tended to find this as confirmation that the doctrine is indeed the governing *legal* doctrine.

The upshot has been a rather wide consensus, arrived at through a variety of unwitting cross-purposes, among psychiatrists and lawmen. This consensus has persisted in the face of a number of more sophisticated and authoritative legal opinions insisting that "mental disease" in the insanity test formulae is a *legal* concept, and that *no* medical category, whether psychosis or any other, should be held to be decisive with respect to it.

It may seem odd that such a compounding of confusion, mutual misunderstanding, and usurpation of roles should have developed, persisted, and become in effect institutionalized without a legitimate basis ever being laid, and indeed in spite of significant and emphatic court decisions to the contrary. It is so, however.

I think this consensus is in fact a sound one, though arrived at in a thoroughly unorthodox way. It is its essential soundness which gives it its persistence in the absence of proper formal authority. I think its soundness can only be shown in a systematic way if we invoke the concept of criminal insanity as I have been developing it in the present discussion. Let us examine briefly, in the light of that concept, the differences between neurosis and psychosis. (I shall again omit discussion of character disorders, since the problems raised are not fundamentally different for our present purposes from those we will consider in the following discussion of psychosis and neurosis.)

Neurosis is a condition which, by definition, consists in some defect in capacity for rational conduct. The definition of neurosis in dynamic psychiatry always centers on the defensive process, i.e. a disavowal by the person (to self and others) of some impulse which the individual in fact has, and of any comportment motivated by that impulse. In psychiatry generally, the more eclectic definitions of the various neuroses in the official (U.S.) Diagnostic Manual of the American Psychiatric Association all include some form of irrationality as a central element. The defect in rationality may be relatively minor. It may be more severe and yet be socially adaptive, as in the case of a highly compulsive bookkeeper. It may be near-crippling in its gravity and social maladaptiveness, as in acute anxiety-neurosis, or in severe obsessional neuroses. Here the panic or phobia may be so intense and so easily triggered that the person in many situations cannot even appear to act rationally with respect to important social demands or norms. Nevertheless, it is in the nature of neurosis, as a matter of explicit definition for some schools of psychiatry, that although the condition involves irrational wishes and fantasies, often perceived in distorted fashion by the individual, the individual will not allow himself to indulge them overtly and explicitly. They are repressed; the person will not even admit them to himself. The reason, in technical terms, is that they arouse too much superego anxiety.

In paraphrase into ordinary English, the technical formulation amounts to saying: the neurotic does not indulge or even admit to himself his anti-social impulses because they arouse unbearable guilt in him; and they arouse this guilt by virtue of fundamental moral-criminal prohibitions whose relevance he grasps and whose governance he accepts. He adapts to his problem by means of a "split" in the psyche. There is a part of him which goes its way, irrational and covert. And there is a part of him (the more "reality-oriented" part) which retains responsiveness to the relevance of certain norms defining outer limits of social acceptability, for example, the limits embodied in the laws against murder, rape, incest.[4] It is a part of the concept of neurosis that this latter, reality-oriented part of him never loses its substantial and usually predominant influence over comportment with respect to such outer limits. Even in the case of severe neurosis, where violations of criminal law norms could on occasion occur, the neurotic difficulty does not stem from simple unresponsiveness to the relevance of those norms. On the contrary, the neurotic's *conflicts* arise just by virtue of his grasp of the relevance of moral norms and his intense concern and feeling of guilt at the prospect of violating them. The wrongful act of the neurotic is not the outcome of blindness to moral or legal norms, but to his undue concern for these norms; it is the result of the tangled web he weaves in attempting to reconcile his covert impulses with his sense of guilt for having them. Sometimes he gets tangled in his own web and is led to commit overt crimes. But insofar as he does incline to actual violations of criminal law as the outcome of his neurotic conflict, it is his keen sensitivity to the relevance of moral standards which makes the prospect of punishment, and of being held responsible, powerful sources of strength in his attempts to curb his lawless impulses.

Thus, using the definition of criminal insanity which I have been developing here, we find a psychiatric-legal rationale for the common, intuitively accepted practice in the courts according to which neurosis is rarely allowed as a basis for a finding of criminal insanity. And the neurotic and the public are generally likely to be safer the more keenly the neurotic feels he will be held responsible.

Psychosis, on the other hand, is often defined as essentially a break with "external reality," a "loss of contact with reality." The psychotic, unlike the neurotic, tends to indulge overtly the original forbidden impulse, and he may then "rationalize" this conduct by gross distortion of even the most patent of facts and norms in the "real world." He distorts so grossly because he is blind to certain kinds of essential relevance (whereas the neurotic's problem is to be unduly responsive).

The conduct flowing from the psychosis may happen to impinge on areas within the scope of criminal law. If it does, then the psychotic stands in direct contrast to the neurotic: the psychotic, because he flagrantly distorts facts and norms, and cannot correct these distortions, will be unable to take the law rationally into account.

Of particular importance in connection with assessing the psychotic's criminal responsibility is the fact that this diagnosis contains — unlike other generic psychiatric diagnoses — a built-in judgment of the gravity of the defect. Neurotic conditions can exist in a wide range of degrees of severity, from so mild and adaptive as hardly to be noticeable to cripplingly irrational and maladaptive. (The character disorders can also exist in a relatively mild degree or in extreme degree.) But psychosis is a concept which perhaps more than any other general diagnostic concept implies severity of mental disturbance. In the language I have been using, the psychotic defect in capacity for rational conduct is generally, therefore, a *substantial* defect.

VII

The preceding analysis of the distinction between neurosis and psychosis provides the basis for a more general characterization of mental disorder, which I would like to suggest freely in these last few paragraphs.

It is in connection with responsibility-impairment that I think such notions as "mental disorder," "mental disease," "mental illness," "insanity," "neurosis" *et al.* have their root significance. What is central to all these is the idea of irrationality, ascribed to the person rather than being viewed as due to an "external" influence; this irrationality is in effect understood as substantial impairment of capacity to respond to some kind of relevance which is distinctive in the basic ordering of human intercourse. (I use the phrase "distinctive in the basic ordering of human intercourse" as a way of capturing the vague but important distinction between what I have in mind here and the insensitivity to relevant matters which are, however, only subtly relevant, or which are relevant in relation to specialized or technical activities, or which are relevant in a way that can be grasped only by those with more than average sophistication or skill. The sort of relevance that is at issue here is that which is distinctive in such everyday and universal human kinds of human order as family, friendship, conformity to elementary date- and place-ordering practices, use of language and numbers in simple ways conforming to relevant usage, etc. Clearly the scope of the phrase will be not only indeterminate as we approach its plain limits, but also relative to the community in which we locate the person.)

If the terms have broad penumbras of vagueness, so does the concept of mental illness itself. Yet the concept is useful and important. It is useful and important just because it is critical in assessing a person's responsibility-status. If he is responsive to what is essentially relevant (has not "lost contact with reality"), then it makes sense to hold him responsible—we expect of him that he will on his own initiative abide by these norms, or if he does not, that he will have violated them in an understanding way and is properly subject to whatever policies we have with regard to those who knowingly violate the norms. On the other hand, if we see the person as not responsive to what is essentially relevant, then we recognize the pointlessness of the expectation that we can rely on the norms to be regulative with respect to his conduct generally. We realize that we must guide him rather than expect him to guide himself. He has not a minimal facility in the minimal ranges of activities which are generic to being human. We establish other basic relationships with him, for example, parent-child, guardian-ward.

In the case of neurosis, the lack of responsiveness is to relevance which, while not absolutely essential to the basic order of human intercourse, is still important and, as I say, distinctive of it. We do not establish a guardian-ward relation with respect to the neurotic person, but we do make pragmatic adjustments in appropriate areas of life where the neurotic is in fact unresponsive to relevance. In those areas we characterize him as "not in control," "compulsive," "obsessive," "suffering from other symptoms." Either we simply excuse him, hold him less responsible or non-responsible in specific contexts where we see he is irrational, or we take *ad hoc* steps to control and avert harmful conduct ("Don't let him get his hands on our best equipment; he is compulsively careless").

Individuals may and do vary greatly in temperaments and tastes, in personalities and abilities; they choose to act in different ways, for better or worse. But this is not the basis for classifying them as mentally healthy or not. The issue in this matter is whether in any or all of these respects they manifest irrationality, an incapacity to respond to what is essentially relevant, no matter how they ultimately elect to comport themselves in the light of what is relevant. It is not what they do, or whether we would do the same; it is whether they do it in the light of what is plainly relevant.

To speak in the broadest terms: Responsiveness to relevance is the condition of personal agency; it is the rationality of man as the rational animal. Comportment in the light of what is relevant is the root of responsibility, the essential condition of the agent's freedom, and is compatible with violation of the norm, foolishness, evil, irresponsibility (but not *non*-responsibility). In contrast, unresponsiveness to relevance constricts the scope of personal agency; it is the diminishing of rationality. Comportment which reflects unresponsiveness to relevance manifests fundamental limits of the agent's responsibility and hence of his freedom, too, and precludes the ascription of foolishness, evil, irresponsibility or their contraries. Mental health and mental illness are thus categories rooted in the spiritual: both the mentally healthy and the mentally ill suffer; but the suffering of the mentally ill is rooted in irrationality and hence impairment of responsibility. In more traditional language, a mind that is ill is a mind whose reason is defective. Rationality is mental health.

NOTES

1. For systematic discussions of this thesis, see the author's, 'The Concept of Mental Disease in Criminal Insanity tests', *University of Chicago Law Review*, Vol. 33 (1966), p. 239; and also *The Meaning of Criminal Insanity*, University of California Press, Berkeley & London, Spring, 1972.

2. The preceding account of the criminal law tests is highly condensed and simplified. It is intended merely as a general orientation for the reader not versed in the relevant law. For a full and systematic discussion of the legal and psychiatric background, with relevant citations, see the author's *The Meaning of Criminal Insanity*, op. cit. A comprehensive, lucid, and authoritative review of the field from a legal standpoint can be found in *The Insanity Defense*, by Abraham S. Goldstein, Dean of the Yale Law School (Yale University Press, New Haven, Conn. 1967).

3. A classic case bringing out all these features is *People vs. Wolff* (Supreme Court of California, 1964), in *Pacific Reporter*, 2d Series, Vol. 394, at p. 959.

4. A more precise, full, and systematic account of the defensive process—formulated both in non-technical and in psychoanalytic terms—is presented in the author's *Self-Deception*, Routledge & Kegan Paul, London 1969.

A. Louis McGarry

The Nature of Competency to Stand Trial

To be fit for trial, it is assumed that person must have minimal effective and cognitive resources available to him to assume the role of a defendant in court. Lacking these resources, the individual would be deprived of his due process right to testify in his own defense, to confront witnesses against him, and to maintain an effective *psychological presence* in court beyond his mere physical presence there. The issue of competency is thus an essentially legal issue, not a psychiatric issue. The criteria for competency to stand trial are concerned with the protection of the individual in the criminal system in order that he may be assured of a fair trial. No other area of the person's physical or emotional health is an issue. Whether or not the person has physical or psychological defects is irrelevant except to the extent that they substantially interfere with fitness for trial.

The common law criteria for competency are defined as (1) an ability to cooperate with one's attorney in one's own defense, (2) an awareness and understanding of the nature and object of the proceedings, (3) an understanding of the consequences of the proceedings. Within the framework of these criteria, a judgment must be made as to whether an accused person should stand trial without undue delay or whether the trial should be deferred until such time as the accused shall meet a minimal standard based on these criteria.

The determination of competency in the broadest sense must be based on some evaluation of these criteria. It must be a prediction because the judgment

From *Competency to Stand Trial and Mental Illness* Department of Health, Education, and Welfare publication no. (HSM) 73-9105, 1973. Copyright © 1973 by A. Louis McGarry. Reprinted by permission of the author.

of the actual performance of the defendant in the role of defendant has not occurred. An assessment of the defendant's ability to perform adequately at his trial must be made by individuals considered most expert to evaluate fitness for trial.

It is important that the assessment or evaluation of the defendant be made with a clear understanding of the requirements of the legal system. Psychological evaluation must be directed toward determining how well the individual will be able to meet the minimum requirements of the three common law criteria for competency. Issues such as legal responsibility for the offense or possibility of rehabilitation are not relevant considerations. Also, mental illness or pathology *per se* are not equivalent to capacity to stand trial, although such matters may be involved in a determination of competency.

The test which follows has been developed for the purpose of quickly screening defendants in order to make recommendations regarding their competency to stand trial.

*   *   *

COMPETENCY TO STAND TRIAL ASSESSMENT INSTRUMENT

		Degree of Incapacity				
	Total	Severe	Moderate	Mild	None	Unratable
1. Appraisal of available legal defenses	1	2	3	4	5	6
2. Unmanageable behavior	1	2	3	4	5	6
3. Quality of relating to attorney	1	2	3	4	5	6
4. Planning of legal strategy, including guilty plea to lesser charges where pertinent	1	2	3	4	5	6
5 Appraisal of role of:						
a. Defense counsel	1	2	3	4	5	6
b. Prosecuting attorney	1	2	3	4	5	6
c. Judge	1	2	3	4	5	6
d. Jury	1	2	3	4	5	6
e. Defendant	1	2	3	4	5	6
f. Witnesses	1	2	3	4	5	6
6. Understanding of court procedure	1	2	3	4	5	6

COMPETENCY TO STAND TRIAL ASSESSMENT INSTRUMENT
(continued)

7. Appreciation of charges	1	2	3	4	5	6
8. Appreciation of range and nature of possible penalties	1	2	3	4	5	6
9. Appraisal of likely outcome	1	2	3	4	5	6
10. Capacity to disclose to attorney available pertinent facts surrounding the offense including the defendant's movements, timing, mental state, actions at the time of the offense	1	2	3	4	5	6
11. Capacity to realistically challenge prosecution witness	1	2	3	4	5	6
12. Capacity to testify relevantly	1	2	3	4	5	6
13. Self-defeating v. self-serving motivation (legal sense)	1	2	3	4	5	6

Examinee _____ Examiner _____

Date _____

COMPETENCY TO STAND TRIAL: ASSESSMENT INSTRUMENT

Introduction

The instrument which this code book describes was designed to improve communication between the behavioral science disciplines (particularly psychiatry) and the law in an area of mutual responsibility — the determination of competency to stand trial. Prior attempts at such communication have suffered from the understandable tendency of each of these disciplines to adhere to the language and concepts of their own discipline. Thus the findings of the clinician have not been delivered in a form and language which are appropriate to the needs of the court. Insofar as clinical opinion has been delivered to the courts in this area, it has tended to be global, conclusional, and not substantiated by relevant clinical data.

We sought, therefore, to develop an instrument which delivered clinical opinion to the court in language, form, and substance sufficiently common to the disciplines involved to provide a basis for adequate and relevant communication. The purpose of the instrument is to standardize, objectify, and quantify the relevant criteria for competency to stand trial.

The Instrument

The instrument may be described as a series of thirteen functions related to an accused's ability to cope with the trial process in an adequately self-protective fashion. These functions or items were culled from appellate cases, the legal literature, and our clinical and courtroom experience. The total series is intended to cover all possible grounds for a finding of incompetency. The weight which the court may be expected to assign to one or another of the items will not be equal, nor is it intended to be. Neither will the weight assigned to a given item by the court in reaching a finding on competency for a particular defendant necessarily apply to the next defendant. For example, in the court's view, it may be far more critical to the defense of a particular defendant that he be able to "testify relevantly" than for another defendant whose attorney does not intend to put him on the stand. Considerations of the weight to be assigned a given item in the case of the particular defendant goes beyond the scope of what should be expected of the examining clinician. The task for the clinician is the providing of objective data, the import of which is the responsibility of the court.

This instrument is designed to reflect the competency status of a defendant at the time of examination. It is not a predictive instrument. Our experience indicates that with the passage of time and variations in clinical status, even from day to day, a given defendant will vary in the scores attained. This is particularly true of patient-defendants recovering from an acute psychosis.

It is important to note at the onset that the inability to function indicated by low scores on this instrument must arise from mental illness and/or mental retardation and not, for example, from ideological motivation. When there is doubt as to its connection with abnormal and mental processes, the item should not be scored and it should be indicated that the opinion does not reach reasonable clinical certainty on the particular item.

At the very least, individual items which are scored at one or two (out of a scale of five) should be substantiated by diagnostic and clinical data of adequate richness to establish a serious degree of mental illness or retardation and the manner in which such disability relates to the low degree of functioning in the particular item.

It should be noted that defendants with mental disability of a serious degree, including psychosis and moderate mental retardation, frequently are quite competent and may achieve high scores on any or all of the items. Mental disability is relevant to a competency determination only insofar as it is manifested by malfunctioning in one or more of the specific items of the instrument.

In the scoring of this instrument a basic assumption is that the accused will be adequately aided by counsel. A second basic assumption is that the professional who is using this instrument has at least a basic understanding of and experience in the realities of the criminal justice system.

Each item in the instrument is scaled from 1 to 5 ranging from "total incapacity" at one to "no incapacity" at five. If the instrument is used for outpatient or incourt screening purposes, a majority or a substantial accumulation of scores of three or lower in the thirteen items could be regarded as grounds for a period of inpatient observation and more intensive workup.

In our experience with patient-defendants who are in good contact, the examination and scoring, using this instrument, usually does not require more than one hour. Grossly psychotic or passive, concrete and under-responsive defendants obviously may require more extended examination. Care should be taken not to resort to leading questions. The device of offering two or three alternative choices to such defendants has been found to be useful.

In using this instrument interrater reliability can be significantly enhanced by frequent reference to the definitions of each item which follow and to the interview protocol and brief clinical examples of defendants functioning at different levels of each of the thirteen items.

A score of *one* on the instrument indicates that for the item scored a close to or total lack of capacity to function exists of the order of a mute or incoherent person or a severe retardate.

A score of *two* indicates that for the item scored there is severely impaired functioning and a substantial question of adequacy for the particular function.

A score of *three* indicates that there is moderately impaired functioning and a question of adequacy for the particular function.

A score of *four* indicates that for the item scored there is mildly impaired functioning and little question of adequacy for the particular function. An individual can be mildly impaired on the basis of lack of experience in the legal process or sociocultural deprivation with or without attendant psychic pathology.

A score of *five* indicates that for the item scored there is no impairment and no question that the defendant can function adequately for the particular function.

A score of *six* indicates that the available data do not permit a rating which is within reasonable clinical certainty.

*   *   *

Expanded Definitions with Sample Interview Questions
and Clinical Examples

1. *Appraisal of legal defenses:* This item calls for an assessment of the accused's awareness of his possible legal defenses, and how consistent these are with the reality of his particular circumstances.

Questions such as the following will yield data relevant to the scoring of this item:

How do you think you can be defended against these charges?

How can you explain your way out of these charges?

What do you think your lawyer should concentrate on in order to best defend you?

Clinical examples: An elderly paranoid man charged with assault and battery with a dangerous weapon (a golf club) on a neighbor, utterly denied that any attack had taken place and indicated that the "CIA had put him (i.e., the neighbor) up to it." He was unable to offer or agree to any alternative possibility of a defense. He received a score of 2, indicating severely impaired functioning and a substantial question of adequacy for this item.

A retired sailor living alone on inherited property is accused of murder. The victim was a young boy who was among a group of boys throwing stones at the defendant's house at the time of the alleged offense. The defendant reported that he had complained often to the local police about repeated harassments but that they ignored him. He further reported that he had written to the F.B.I., the U.S. Attorney General, and other authorities with no response. Although when he fired the shot he stated that he had shot over the heads of the boys, his theory of his proper defense was that a man in this country had the "inviolable constitutional right to protect his property with a gun," and he insisted that he would instruct his attorney to proceed with a defense only on this basis. Although insisting on his theory of defense, he did agree that his intent to fire over the heads of the boys should be put in evidence but that it was incidental to the main defense. He received a score of 3, indicating moderately impaired functioning and a question of his adequacy on this item.

A middle-aged man with a long history of criminal arrests, mostly for drunkenness, had been found guilty in lower court of four counts of larceny from his 83-year-old girl friend of a total sum exceeding $16,000. He received four sentences of two years each in the County House of Correction to be served "on and after," a total of eight years. His lawyer appealed and a new trial in the Superior Court had been scheduled. When interviewed, the defendant proved to be concrete, passive, and under-responsive. When asked the basis of his appeal he answered several times, "I don't know, my lawyer has all the facts." When offered the speculation that the lawyer may have appealed either on a legal technicality or because the sentence was too severe, the defendant answered, "He thinks it's too long. I hope to get two or three years." Later in the interview he stated that his girl friend was lying and that she had given him the money to "play the horses," and that she "was there," i.e., at the race track. However, he stated, "They wouldn't believe me because of my record." He received a score of 4, indicating mild incapacity and little question of adequacy on this item.

2. *Unmanageable behavior:* This item calls for an assessment of the appropriateness of the current motor and verbal behavior of the defendant, and the degree to which this behavior would disrupt the conduct of a trial. Inappropriate

or disruptive behavior must arise from a substantial degree of mental illness or mental retardation.

For this item, obviously observations as to the patient's manifest behavior are relevant and the content of the answers to questions less relevant. Questions we have used and found useful follow:

Do you realize that you would have to control yourself in the courtroom and not interrupt the proceedings?

When is the only time you can speak out in the courtroom?

What do you think would happen if you spoke out or moved around in the courtroom without permission?

Clinical examples: A young, male adult paranoid schizophrenic on two occasions (his arraignment and an earlier competency hearing) interrupts his attorney and addresses the court in loud tones, dismissing his attorney and insisting on voicing paranoid delusions to the effect that his attorney is part of a conspiracy by the F.B.I. to put him in prison because he is falsely believed to be a presidential assassin. On one occasion he struggled with court officers in an attempt to put "a petition to dismiss," which he had written, on the judge's desk. He was given a score of 2, indicating severely impaired functioning and a substantial question of adequacy on this item.

A manic defendant, although responsive to questions and in contact, is unable to remain seated during an examination for more than a few moments and moves distractedly about the room, lifting objects, pacing, rapping the walls. He received a score of 3, indicating that there is moderately impaired functioning and a question of adequacy for this item.

During the examination, a chronic schizophrenic, repeatedly grimaces, raises his right hand with three fingers extended, then places his index finger against his right temple. This recurs whether he is speaking or not. His hand is at rest only when he places it inside the belt of his pants. He was given a score of 4, indicating mildly impaired functioning and little question of adequacy on this item.

3. *Quality of relating to attorney:* This item calls for an assessment of the interpersonal capacity of the accused to relate to the average attorney. Involved are the ability to trust and to communicate relevantly.

The degree of trust and relevancy of communication which the defendant manifests with an examining psychiatrist is applicable here up to a point. Usually the defendant will have had at least one contact with his defense counsel and the questions we have found useful with this item are as follows:

Do you have confidence in your lawyer?

Do you think he's trying to do a good job for you?

Do you agree with the way he's handled or plans to handle your case?

Clinical examples: A middle-aged defendant with a diagnosis of involutional paranoid state is accused of killing a childhood acquaintance of his wife. He refused to see his court-appointed attorney and insists on handling his defense himself. His theory of defense consists of a claim of self-defense in that he and the victim struggled for possession of a gun and in the struggle the victim was shot accidentally four times. "I don't trust lawyers. They're all part of the criminal system. I'm going to tell my side of the story in my own way." He received a score of 2, indicating a severely impaired functioning and a substantial question of adequacy for this item.

A defendant is accused of the murder of his wife. He is cooperative with his attorney but insists, against the attorney's advice, that he will take the stand in order to tell "my side of the story." This consists of his continuing delusion that his wife had been poisoning his food and that this had resulted in his becoming impotent and "like a zombie." He received a score of 3, indicating moderately impaired functioning and a question of adequacy for this item.

A seventeen-year-old depressed black accused of assault and battery with a dangerous weapon is asked, "Do you have a lawyer?" and answers, "No, I have a public defender." When asked, "Do you have confidence in him?" he answered, "I don't know yet. I don't think he's very interested in my case." He received a score of 4, indicating mild incapacity and little question of adequacy on this item.

4. *Planning of legal strategy including guilty pleas to lesser charges where pertinent:* This item calls for an assessment of the degree to which the accused can understand, participate, and cooperate with his counsel in planning a strategy for the defense which is consistent with the reality of his circumstances.

Most frequently the issue here relates to plea-bargaining and agreement to settle for a guilty plea to a lesser offense. Less frequently strategic issues such as a change of venue, consideration of a plea of not guilty by reason of insanity, or the decision as to whether or not defendant should testify, arise and require some participation from the defendant. The essential question is whether or not the defendant can join with his attorney, even if passively, in planning (or accepting) appropriate legal strategy. Of concern here is the defendant who insists on irrational instructions to his attorney or insists on defending himself on the basis of an irrational theory of defense. Questions which have been useful on this issue are as follows:

> If your lawyer can get the District Attorney to accept a guilty plea to (manslaughter) instead of trying you for (murder—use examples relevant to the actual case, e.g., trespassing in place of breaking and entry, etc. would you agree to it?

> If your lawyer decides not to have you testify would you go along with him?

> Is there anything that you disagree with in the way your lawyer is going to handle your case, and if so, what do you plan to do about it?

Clinical examples: A grandiose, acute schizophrenic is accused of illegal possession of a fire arm. The defense attorney confers with the lower court judge who agrees to continue the case without a finding on the understanding that defendant would accept mental hospitalization. The defendant is willing to accept hospitalization but insists on a trial and "appeal all the way to the Supreme Court to expose the Fascist state we live in. I am L-4-C." He was given a score of 2, indicating severely impaired functioning and a substantial question of adequacy for this item.

An impotent man stabs his twelve-year-old daughter to death while she stands beside his bed because he "sensed evil in her that was rotting my life." He states that he would refuse to plead guilty to manslaughter if it could be arranged and insists on a trial for murder and "No lawyer would ever talk me out of it." He received a score of 3, indicating moderately impaired functioning and a question of his adequacy on this item.

A mental retardate with an I.Q. of 66 is accused of a homicide. He is highly suggestible and passive. His trust and dependency are easily obtained but he is capable of little or no independence of judgment and places himself uncritically and totally in the hands of his attorney. He received a score of 4, indicating mild incapacity and little question of adequacy on this item.

5. *Appraisal of role of:* a. Defense counsel
b. Prosecuting attorney
c. Judge
d. Jury
e. Defendant
f. Witnesses

This set of items calls for a minimal understanding of the adversary process by the accused. The accused should be able to identify prosecuting attorney and prosecution witnesses as foe, defense counsel as friend, the judge as neutral, and the jury as the determiners of guilt or innocence.

For this item a single question generally suffices and that is: *In the courtroom during a trial, what is the job of* . . . (here list the sub-items)? It is particularly relevant that the defendant be aware of the purposes of the prosecuting attorney.

Clinical examples: A young adult retardate (I.Q. 67) was asked "What is the job of the district attorney in court?" He answered, "He's a lawyer. Lawyers are supposed to help people." The defendant was then instructed about the actual role of the prosecutor, but on subsequent questioning it was clear that he was still unable to conceptualize the prosecutorial functions of the district attorney. He was given a score of 2, indicating that there was severely impaired functioning and a substantial question of adequacy for this sub-item.

When asked the job of defense counsel in court, a chronic paranoid schizophrenic with a fourth grade education, answered "My own lawyer is supposed to help the law." He was then asked, "And you too?" to which he answered, "Yes, a little." He was given a score of 3 on the "defense attorney" sub-item indicating moderately impaired functioning and a question of adequacy.

When asked about the job of the district attorney a poorly educated black who recently settled in Boston after an upbringing in the South, answered, "He's there to get out the truth." He was given a score of 4, indicating mildly impaired functioning, but with little question of adequacy on the "prosecuting attorney" sub-item.

6. *Understanding of court procedure:* This item calls for an assessment of the degree to which the defendant understands the basic sequence of events in a trial and their import for him, e.g., the different purposes of direct and cross examination.

An understanding of procedural niceties is not required here. Questions we have used to elicit relevant data here are as follows:

Who is the only one at your trial who can call on you to testify?

After your lawyer finished asking you questions on the stand, who then can ask you questions?

If the District Attorney (prosecutor) asks you questions, what is he trying to accomplish?

Clinical examples: A young adult, white, grandiose paranoid schizophrenic accused of indecent assault and battery on a minor refused counsel and insisted that he would conduct his own defense. He stated, "I will ask the questions. I will call the district attorney to the stand and expose their criminal black conspiracy against me." He received a score of 2, indicating severely impaired functioning and a substantial question of adequacy on the "defendant" sub-item.

A mildly retarded adult male (I.Q. 66) with a prior record of misdemeanors disposed of in lower court is charged with his first felony, breaking and entry in the nighttime. He states, "The judge will ask me questions to try to find out the truth. The lawyers are there to help me. They will ask questions, too." Attempts by the interviewer to explain the role of the district attorney in cross examination are met with partial success. The defendant subsequently states, "I understand that if the district attorney asks me questions he's trying to send me to jail." He received a score of 3, indicating moderately impaired functioning and a question of adequacy on this item.

A middle-aged man diagnosed as an inadequate personality is charged with incest. It is his first experience with criminal prosecution. He states, "I don't know anything about the law. I suppose my lawyer will take care of me. Yes, I used to watch Perry Mason." He was given a score of 4, indicating mildly impaired functioning and little question of adequacy on this item.

7. *Appreciation of charges:* This item calls for an assessment of the accused's concrete understanding of the charges against him, and to a lesser extent the seriousness of the charges.

What is required here should not be exaggerated. Basically a literal knowledge of the specific charge or charges is adequate. An understanding of the seriousness of the charges is of importance here only insofar as it might contribute to a perhaps cavalier or indifferent cooperation by the defendant in his defense. For example, if a manic defendant views an arson as a lark and is disposed to freely admit his action, there is question as to his self-protective capacity on this item. Questions useful in eliciting data here are:

What are you charged with?

Is that a major or a minor charge?

Do you think people in general would regard you with some fear on the basis of such a charge?

Clinical examples: A 19-year-old retardate (I.Q. 55) is accused of statutory rape of a 12-year-old girl. When asked why the police arrested him he smirks and waves his finger back and forth saying "No-no." When asked how old the girl was he says, "Not know, big girl." In an effort to establish the victim's age and sexual maturity in the defendant's eyes, pictures are drawn giving the defendant a choice between side views of women with very small, medium, and large breasts. With a mischievous and naughty facial expression he touches the picture with the very small breasts. He was given a score of 2, indicating severely impaired functioning and a substantial question of adequacy on this item.

A young adult catatonic schizophrenic is accused of arson of a church. When asked what he is accused of he states, "started a fire." When asked the seriousness of the charge, he answers, "No harm . . . (moan) stone won't burn." He was given a score of 3, indicating moderately impaired functioning and a question of adequacy on this item.

A manic defendant accused of successfully forging checks in the amount of $7,500 states, "They can't touch me. Any day now I'll be on the big board at the stock exchange. I'll cover the checks." He was given a score of 4, indicating mildly impaired functioning and little question of adequacy on this item.

8. *Appreciation of range and nature of possible penalties:* This item calls for an assessment of the accused's concrete understanding and appreciation of the conditions and restrictions which could be imposed on him and their possible duration.

Here, too, a concrete, simplistic understanding suffices. Generally, if the crime is a felony, the defendant should be aware that there is at least a potential state prison sentence even if such a sentence is unlikely in his circumstances. The potential sentence need not be known with precision. Of concern here is that the defendant have at least a gross understanding of what is at risk and a motivation to protect himself which is consistent with the risk. Relevant questions here are:

If you're found guilty as charged what are the possible sentences the judge could give you?

Where would you have to serve such a sentence?

If you're put on probation, what does that mean?

Clinical examples: A 19-year-old retardate (I.Q. 55) accused of statutory rape states, "No jail, me go home to mother." He was given a score of 2, indicating severely impaired functioning and a substantial question of adequacy on this item.

An elderly retired school teacher who had recently been widowed is accused of indecent assault and battery on the 7-year-old daughter of a neighbor. His diagnosis is senile dementia. He is irascible and insists that he simply "petted" the girl and that "no further prosecution is appropriate" and that there is no possibility of incarceration for such an "act" and "jail is for rapists and revolutionaries." He received a score of 3, indicating a moderately impaired functioning and a question of adequacy on this item.

A paranoid young woman who blames the mother of a former boyfriend for their breakup forces her way into the apartment of the mother. During an ensuing argument she picks up a poker and threatens the mother. The police are called and she is physically subdued. She is accused of attempted assault and battery with a dangerous weapon, breaking and entering in the nighttime, and resisting arrest. She states, "I suppose it's possible that they could send me to jail, but it's inconceivable. I've calmed down now. I will not further dignify that woman by responding to her trumped-up charges. The burden of these proceedings rests with her." She received a score of 4, indicating mild incapacity and little question of her adequacy on this item.

9. *Appraisal of likely outcome:* This item calls for an assessment of how realistically the accused perceives the likely outcome, and the degree to which impaired understanding contributes to a less adequate or inadequate participation in his defense. Without adequate information on the part of the examiner regarding the facts and circumstances of the alleged offense, this item would be unratable.

A police arrest report and/or communication from defense counsel or district attorney as to the real facts and circumstances surrounding the alleged offense are helpful here. If the patient irrationally perceives that there is little or no peril in his position and the case against him is strong, it might follow that he would have little or no motivation to adequately protect himself. Here, also, the psychotic person who, for irrational reasons, does not accept the criminal jurisdiction of the court might not adequately protect himself. Questions were used as follows:

What do you think your chances are to be found not guilty?

Does the court you're going to be tried in have authority over you?

How strong a case do they have against you?

Clinical examples: A middle-aged man diagnosed as involutional paranoid state is accused of the murder of his wife. He states, "This was an act of God. No temporal power has any authority over me. I will not participate in these proceedings." He was given a score of 2, indicating severely impaired functioning and a substantial question of adequacy on this item.

A paranoid young woman who blames the mother of a former boyfriend for their breakup forces her way into the apartment of his mother. During an ensuing argument she picks up a poker and threatens the mother. The police are called and she is physically subdued by them. She is accused of attempted assault and battery with a dangerous weapon, breaking and entering in the nighttime and resisting arrest. She states, "I suppose it's possible that they could send me to jail but it's inconceivable. I've calmed down now. I will not further dignify that woman by responding to her trumped-up charges. The burden of these proceedings rests with her." She received a score of 3, indicating moderately impaired functioning and a question of adequacy on this item.

A schizoid 20-year-old son of wealthy parents is accused of grand larceny from a mail order firm where he had worked as a shipping clerk. He states, "My father has hired the best lawyer in town for me. I don't have to lift a finger in there (i.e., the courtroom). The worst I could get is probation." He was given a score of 4, indicating mild incapacity and little question of adequacy on this item.

10. *Capacity to disclose to attorney available pertinent facts surrounding the offense including the defendant's movements, timing, mental state, and actions at the time of the*

offense: This item calls for an assessment of the accused's capacity to give a basically consistent, rational, and relevant account of the motivational and external facts. Complex factors can enter into this determination. These include intelligence, memory, and honesty. The difficult area of the validity of an amnesia may be involved and may prove unresolvable for the examiner. It is important to be aware that there may be a disparity between what an accused is willing to share with a clinician and what he will share with his attorney; the latter being the more important.

It is assumed that answers to questions on this item will not be available to the prosecution for purposes of incrimination and will be limited to the narrow question of the accused's competency. Here, too, the examiner should have adequate knowledge of the facts of the alleged offense from the police arrest report or counsel in order to record a valid score. Relevant questions are:

> Tell us what actually happened, what you saw and did and heard and thought before, during, and after you are supposed to have committed this offense.

> When and where did all this take place?

> What led the police to arrest you and what did you say to them?

Clinical examples: The alleged driver of a bank robbery getaway car is accused of armed robbery. In a high speed chase following the robbery an accident occurs and the defendant suffers a fractured skull and is unconscious for 12 hours. After emergency surgery for an epidural hematoma, the defendant complains of a retrograde amnesia from the time of the accident. He further asserts that he does not know his alleged confederate and states, "He must have made me drive at the point of a gun, but I don't remember." He was given a score of 2, indicating severely impaired functioning and a substantial question of adequacy on this item.

A State police sergeant 10 years from retirement is involved in a harrowing ghetto riot. His patrol car is surrounded by a mob which overturns the car while he is in it. He is subsequently rescued unhurt. Two weeks later, while driving home after a period of duty, he has an abrupt amnestic episode. Several hours later he is arrested by fellow police officers in a suburban home with a stolen car outside the home and two neighbors hand-cuffed to a pipe. He claims an amnesia except for isolated flashbacks. "I remember a scene with two people hand-cuffed to a pipe. I don't remember how I got there. The rest is blank. I last remember being on the freeway with my car." He was diagnosed hysterical neurosis, dissociative type and given a score of 3, indicating moderate incapacity and a question of adequacy on this item.

A 50-year-old catatonic schizophrenic is indicted for murder for the second time in his life. On the first occasion he was found not guilty by reason of insanity and subsequently released. He has been hospitalized for 10 years since the second alleged murder after having been found incompetent to stand trial. He is now in a stable remission from his illness on thorazine and wants to stand trial. On examination he states, "He (the victim) was a friend. We were in the kitchen. He leaned down to pick up something. I picked up the ax and hit him. I didn't plan it. It just happened. I didn't have any feelings." He was given a score of 4, indicating mild incapacity and little question of adequacy on this item.

11. *Capacity to realistically challenge prosecution witnesses:* This item calls for an assessment of the accused's capacity to recognize distortions in prosecution testimony. Relevant factors include attentiveness and memory. In addition there is an element of initiative. If false testimony is given the degree of activism with which the defendant will apprise his attorney of inaccuracies is important.

The relevant considerations turn primarily on the observations of the examiner regarding the perceptual abilities of the defendant during the clinical examination rather than on the content of answers to questions. Questions we have used are:

> Suppose a witness against you told a lie in the courtroom. What would you do?
>
> Is there anybody who is likely to tell lies about you in this case? Why?

Clinical examples: An elderly, paranoid man attacks his neighbor with a golf club. He is accused of assault and battery with a dangerous weapon. "The whole thing's a lie," he said. "If he (the neighbor) testifies I will stand up and tell the jury that he is a C.I.A. agent and that he is in a conspiracy against me. I will not allow him to testify." He received a score of 2, indicating severe incapacity and a substantial question of adequacy on this item.

A skid row alcoholic with organic deterioration is accused of breaking and entering and larceny. He states, "I don't remember things too good. Let them have it (i.e., the prosecution witnesses) their way. I was drunk. I don't remember taking anything." He was given a score of 3, indicating moderate incapacity and a question of adequacy on this item.

A mildly retarded (I.Q. 67) young, adult male who is passive and underresponsive, answers, "I don't know," to the question, "What would you do if a witness told a lie about you in the courtroom?" He is then advised that he should quietly get his lawyer's attention in such a situation and inform him of the lie. On subsequent questioning he shows that he has understood and that he would tell his lawyer. He received a score of 4, indicating mild incapacity and little question of adequacy on this item.

12. *Capacity to testify relevantly:* This item calls for an assessment of the accused's ability to testify with coherence, relevance, and independence of judgment.

Here again the relevant data arise primarily from the observations of the examiner regarding the defendant's ability to verbally communicate rather than specific content in the answers to specific questions. Affective as well as thought disorder considerations are of some relevance here, e.g., if the defendant is immobilized by anxiety or depression, or is manic, loose or regressed in his associations and responses. If questions, which might come up in direct and cross examination of the defendant, can be anticipated, given the facts and circumstances of the particular case, then this would of course be helpful but it is not essential for a valid rating on this item.

Clinical examples: A 40-year-old, homeless male diagnosed as a simple schizophrenic breaks into a rural food store. He eats some of the food in the store and then goes to sleep. In the morning the proprietor finds him. He is arrested and charged with breaking and entering and larceny. On being interviewed there are long pauses before he can answer questions and they must be repeated gently. "I had no money . . . I was hungry . . . I was cold . . . I went to sleep." He was given a score of 2, indicating severe incapacity and a substantial question of adequacy on this item.

A 30-year-old male schizophrenic (chronic undifferentiated type) is arrested after neighbors report that he has been shooting out of his window at dogs in his back yard. He is accused of illegal possession and unlawful discharge of a firearm. He insists on being tried to "clear the record" and refuses the alternative of mental hospitalization. He states that he was trying to "scare off" the dogs and had no intention of "hitting" them. However, he continues to talk after these objective answers to questions and rambles in a loosely associated, tangential, and circumstantial manner. He resists any interruptions in his discourses but can be stopped with some effort. He received a score of 3, indicating moderate incapacity and a question of adequacy on this item.

A mildly retarded young man (I.Q. 60) is accused, in his terms, of "first degree murder." He is concrete in his answers and has a very limited vocabulary. When pressed to elaborate on his answers or when vocabulary is used which he does not understand, he retreats to "I don't know." He can, given his limitations, nevertheless give an accurate and consistent, if simplistic, story of the events surrounding the alleged offense. He was given a score of 4, indicating mild incapacity and little question of adequacy on this item.

13. *Self-defeating v. self-serving motivation (legal sense):* This item calls for an assessment of the accused's motivation to adequately protect himself and appropriately utilize legal safeguards to this end. It is recognized that accused persons may appropriately be motivated to seek expiation and appropriate punishment in their trials. Of concern here is the pathological seeking of punishment and the deliberate failure by the accused to avail himself of appropriate legal protections. Passivity or indifference do not justify low scores on this item. Actively self-destructive manipulation of the legal process arising from mental pathology does justify low scores.

In this item the issue turns on the willingness of the accused to take advantage of appropriate *legal* protections even though he may feel that he should be punished. Will he, in other words, play the game; taking advantage of the rules built into the system for his protection. Relevant questions:

> We know how badly you feel about what happened—suppose your lawyer is successful in getting you off—would you accept that?
>
> Suppose the District Attorney made some legal errors and your lawyer wants to appeal a guilty finding in your case—would you accept that?
>
> We know that you want to plead guilty to your charge—but what if your lawyer could get the District Attorney to agree to a plea of guilty to a lesser charge—would you accept that?

Clinical examples: A 33-year-old paranoid schizophrenic is accused of murder. He is convinced that he will and should be executed since his is the "second messianic crucifixion." He declines a negotiated plea of manslaughter and attempts to instruct his attorney not to call any defense witnesses. He intends to address the court to request the death sentence since he "owes this to sinning mankind." He received a score of 2, indicating severely impaired functioning and a substantial question of adequacy for this item.

A middle-aged, unemployed house painter is accused of the murder of his eight-year-old daughter. At the time of the homicide, the defendant was convinced that the "end of the world" had come and that the "forces of the devil were at loose in the world," and that they were coming to "rape and murder my daughter." He was convinced he had to kill her to "be sure she would enter heaven without sin." After the homicide he is convinced that the devil had "taken over my body" but that he now "must make expiation." He insists on pleading guilty to first degree murder and he will be satisfied at nothing less than a "life sentence." He received a score of 3, indicating moderately impaired functioning and a question of adequacy on this item.

A chronic paranoid schizophrenic adult male with prior prison sentences sets a fire and turns himself into the police. He states, "I can't make it on the outside. They won't admit me at the State Hospital. I've got to get away for a while. I'd like to get 2 or 3 years." He received a score of 4, indicating mild incapacity and little question of adequacy on this item.

Glenn C. Graber and Frank H. Marsh

Ought a Defendant Be Drugged to Stand Trial?

A person who is charged with a crime cannot be compelled to plead to the indictment, be placed on trial, convicted, or sentenced while either insane or mentally incompetent. But how does this fundamental principle of American criminal jurisprudence apply to an individual who meets the standard of sanity or competence only when tranquilized with medication?

This question was recently at issue before the Tennessee Court of Criminal Appeals in the case of *State of Tennessee v. William Earl Stacy* [556 SW 2nd 552]. At the time of the appellate trial, several indictments were pending against the defendant Stacy in the lower criminal court, including a first-degree murder charge. Stacy was accused of fatally shooting a ticket agent at a bus station during what police theorized was an attempted robbery. In addition, Stacy was also accused of robbing a store shortly afterwards. Through his court-appointed counsel, the defendant filed a motion asking the court to find him mentally incompetent to stand trial.

At the preliminary hearing, the State's evidence indicated that Stacy behaved erratically at the scene of the crime. Witnesses testified that Stacy entered the bus station and approach the ticket agent in an unassuming manner, but suddenly became very belligerent and "wild acting," and killed the ticket agent. After his arrest later that same evening, he continued this "wild" behavior, and officials transferred him to a psychiatric hospital.

The attending psychiatrist there testified that Stacy was actively hallucinating when admitted: "He thought he saw ghosts, weird kinds of monsters—a

From *The Hastings Center Report,* 9 (February 1979):8–10. Copyright © 1979 by The Hastings Center. Reprinted by permission of the publisher and the co-authors.

black ghost appeared with two heads and a horn coming out of its nose. The ghost lit his cigarette from Mr. Stacy's and then extinguished the fire in his mouth." (*Tennessee v. Stacy,* at 555) The psychiatrist also reported that before Stacy's condition was stabilized with medication, he would "skip meals," experienced "difficulty in sleeping," and "voided on the floor for no apparent reason."

Stacy was diagnosed as a chronic, undifferentiated schizophrenic; but after he was given antipsychotic medication (Haldol in conjunction with Cogentin), he was able to function fairly well in the mental hospital. The hospital psychiatrist reported, for example, that Stacy "participated in many activities," "worked regularly and quite diligently," and that "his thinking was organized." Thus, in his opinion, the defendant would be able to understand the nature of the legal proceedings and to consult with counsel and participate in his own defense as long as he remained under medication. However, without the medication, the defendant would not meet the criteria for competence. The appellate court ruled that medication could be utilized and that the defendant could (and should) be tried in a state of synthetic competence. Nonetheless, Stacy's counsel entered an insanity plea.

On the specific point of law at issue in this case, the judges' conclusions are understandable. However, the case raises wider issues; and, from this viewpoint, we see significant dangers in the judicial findings.

Competence to Stand Trial

The question before the court was whether the defendant was competent to stand trial. For this, all that is required in Tennessee—as in most jurisdictions—is, first, that he be able to understand the nature of the charges against him and, second, that he be mentally capable of assisting his attorneys in preparing his defense against those charges.

These are modest requirements. The law does *not* require, for example, that the decisions made by the defendant be fully rationally defended, or even defensible. A given defendant can be allowed to stand trial even if he rejects particular advice of his counsel, advice that may be in his best interests. Further, the cause of his mental state at the time of the trial, the nature of his mental condition at the time of the crime, or even his guilt or innocence are not relevant to the question of competence to stand trial, as it is defined in law.

However, the precise nature of the defendant's mental state at the time of the trial is relevant. Was Stacy fully aware of the threat to his freedom that the charges against him represented? Was he capable of reacting to this threat with the same degree of emotion and interest as one whose mental state is not synthetically induced? To answer these questions, we need a good deal of information beyond the hospital psychiatrist's reports about his eating and work patterns. It is possible that, given the present state of knowledge, psychiatry cannot answer these questions; if this is so, then there are serious questions about the judicial findings on even this narrow point of law.

Concerns About Synthetic Competence

Uneasiness about the notion of "chemical sanity" or "synthetic competence" does not stem from the use of tranquilizing medications as such. Our society at present indulges in an almost endless consumption of prescribed and unprescribed medications. In the usual case, however, we judge ourselves to be within the limits of normality before taking the medication; thus we are not "chemically sane" or "synthetically competent" as a result of the medication. Concerns arise only when the medication is responsible for a transition from a state of insanity or incompetence to one of sanity or competence.

Beneath these concerns lies the general issue of personal identity. Can we say with assurance that the defendant was *the same person* at the trial (in his state of synthetic competence) as he was at the time of the alleged crime? If we take continuity of personality and memory to be the criterion of personal identity, serious questions may be raised on this point. Obviously, these questions have metaphysical aspects that would require extensive analysis that cannot be resolved here.*

Further, these questions may have practical aspects. An essential part of any criminal defense is the defendant's ability to remember and recall significant details and facts concerning the alleged crime, including events leading up to the incident and those occurring immediately thereafter. If the defendant was nowhere near the scene of the crime, for example, he will want to remember where he was. Even fairly minor details about the events might be important to the outcome of the case. A defendant who is in a state of synthetic competence may retain two or more distinct (although probably overlapping) sets of memories. It is possible that, in a drugged state of competence, a defendant would not fully identify with the persona who occupies the schizophrenic state and the memories associated with it. To satisfy the requirements of assisting with his defense, the defendant would have to maintain continuity of personal identity to enable him to connect his past with his present and both with his participation in the trial.

The fact that the defendant's mental state was synthetically induced is not relevant, in itself, to the legal point at issue. The question here is whether the source of his mental competence made a difference to the nature of his competence in a way that interfered with his functioning during the judicial process.

Although these matters may be irrelevant to the narrower point of law, they are surely relevant to the wider issue of justice. The rationale supporting the competence requirement embodies the important moral principle of respect for human dignity. Criminal punishment is to be adjudicated and dealt out only to persons who are aware of the process and can participate actively in it. Was the spirit of this principle of respect for the dignity of the defendant honored by bringing him to trial in a state of synthetic competence? The court pointed out the importance both of having the defendant's guilt or innocence established in a proper judicial procedure and of his right to a speedy trial. However, as important as these values are, they are fundamentally systemic values—that is, values created by the conceptual structure of the law. Was it just and humane to subject the defendant to the process of a trial in order to satisfy these procedural values? We think not.

Treatment Without Consent

Here lies the basic ethical problem: according to his lawyer's statements, the defendant was being treated without his consent, and one significant effect of this treatment was to subject him to a criminal trial that he would otherwise have escaped. Making him capable of standing trial appears to have been the sole motive of the State in forcing treatment upon him. If this is so, it was clearly an unjustified infringement upon his autonomy.

The role of the psychiatrist raises a related ethical problem. The issue of dual loyalties or the dual role of the psychiatrist has long been an acknowledged source of ethical dilemmas where an individual has been involuntarily committed to a mental institution. The role of the defendant's psychiatrist in this case raises an even more acute ethical problem. Not only was the State the psychiatrist's employer, it was also the prosecutor (as defender of the public good), and it had a strong interest in seeing the defendant brought to trial.

A psychiatrist in such a case might be forced to choose between two modes of therapy. One of them, psychotherapy, offers greater promise of long-term benefit to the patient, but would be less likely to make him competent to stand trial in the immediate future. The other would guarantee immediate competence to stand trial but would hold less promise of long-term benefit to the patient's mental condition. Caught in the grip of his dual loyalties, which therapy should the psychiatrist choose?

The issue of consent is complicated because making the defendant capable of standing trial was not the only effect of treatment. It cannot be denied that the treatment was partly therapeutic in its effects, at least in the short term. And the defendant's insistence that he wanted the treatment discontinued was no doubt influenced by his reluctance to stand trial. Surely if he had been offered the choice between treatment and nontreatment, both without liability to trial, he would have chosen treatment.

It is possible, of course, that he would have refused treatment even then, since the treatment carried significant risks and may have affected the quality of his consciousness in ways that he desired to avoid. In this case, then, it was certainly an injustice to force him to undergo the therapy.

Even if his refusal of treatment was motivated primarily by a desire to avoid prosecution, a further serious question is raised. Consider the following argument from the judicial opinion:

> The soundness of our ruling can best be illustrated by a reversal of the position of the parties. That is, if the State was alleging that Stacy was incompetent to stand trial, which it would have the right to do under existing law, but Stacy insisted

that he be tried on the merits and could show that he would be competent by taking tranquilizing medication, then unquestionably we would hold that he would have the right to be tried at his insistence, and it would be error not to proceed with his trial. Thus, we think the State has the same right to insist that Stacy be tried on the merits of the case so long as it can be shown that the medication administered will render him mentally competent, will not affect his health, and does not preclude him from receiving a fair trial (*Tennessee v. Stacy*, at 566).

The crucial difference between the hypothetical case raised by the court and the actual situation is that, in the hypothetical case, the defendant would be giving consent to the therapy.

The alternative to a criminal trial is civil commitment to a psychiatric hospital. In this case it is possible that the same therapy would be imposed without Stacy's consent after he had been civilly committed. However, one important difference between this alternative and his present situation is that the choices of therapy would be made on the basis of his best interest rather than on the needs of the judicial process. There might continue to be a question of the psychiatrist's dual loyalties; the pressures of economic efficiency and ease of management might incline him to make a decision not in Stacy's best interests. However, he would be freed from the pressure to bring his client into a mental state that would allow him to stand trial.

The Verdict

The defendant staked his defense on an insanity plea. The success or failure of this plea rested on the jury's ability to grasp the true picture of the defendant's mental state at the time the crime was committed. Thus, the manner and extent to which the jury came to know the defendant's condition was crucial to his acquittal on these grounds. Certainly if the jury had been allowed to see the defendant in his mental state when medication was withdrawn, they would have been likely to agree that his mental state at the time of the crime justified an insanity defense. When the defendant was in a synthetic state, the jury could only be informed about effects of the medication. Such information carried little if any evidential weight, and the defendant's insanity plea was much less likely to succeed.

There is, however, a distressing Catch-22 involved in the suggestion that the jury should have been allowed to view the defendant in his mental state when medication was withdrawn. Without this, the insanity defense was much less likely to succeed. However, if this had been permitted, the resulting mental state would have rendered him incompetent to stand trial; and thus the trial could not have proceeded until his synthetic competence had been restored. He was thus barred by the demands of the legal process from introducing a kind of evidence that was vital to his case.

The actual events of the trial prove the point. In his medicated state, Stacy sat quietly throughout the trial, demonstrating none of the disabling effects of his condition. Even though the jury was instructed at length about the defendant's medication, the synthetic stability that he manifested made it almost impossible for the jury to accept his insanity. No visual or mental connection could be made between the defendant's conduct at the trial and his conduct at the scene of the crime. The plea of insanity was disallowed and the defendant was found guilty.

NOTE

* Derek Parfit points out that one's view of the nature (as opposed to the logic) of personal identity may make a significant difference to his conclusions whether the same person is involved and, consequently, whether it is appropriate to punish him for the crime. See his essay, "Later Selves and Moral Principles," in Alan Montefiore, ed., *Philosophy and Personal Relations* (Montreal: McGill Queen's University Press, 1973), especially pp. 142–44.

June Resnick German and Anne C. Singer

Punishing the Not Guilty: Hospitalization of Persons Acquitted by Reason of Insanity

Introduction

In many states in this country, persons who are found not guilty of crimes by reason of insanity are in a worse position than if they had been convicted, sentenced, and imprisoned. One would reasonably expect a person not responsible for his criminal act to be removed from the criminal justice system and treated as dictated by his present mental condition. Instead, he is almost always hospitalized, either automatically or without the usual procedural safeguards afforded to civilly committed patients, locked behind barred doors of an institution looking more like a prison than a hospital, restrained beyond the time he would have been incarcerated if convicted of the offense charged, and released only through cumbersome judicial proceedings involving the prosecutor's office and other elements of the criminal justice system. Indeed, it is not unusual for an acquittal on insanity grounds to mire the "patient" in the criminal justice system for much of the rest of his life. Rather than being freed of the stigma of a criminal label, the acquitted patient finds himself doubly cursed as both "criminal" and "mental patient" and doubly neglected, for mental illness has been used to deny him the strict due process safeguards normally accorded prisoners, while his connection with the criminal justice system diminishes his chances for release when inpatient treatment is no longer medically indicated.

This paper concludes that commitment, treatment, and methods of release of persons found not guilty by reason of insanity ("NGIs") are unconstitutional,

From *Psychiatric Quarterly* 49 (1977):238–254. Reprinted by permission of the publisher.

violating the equal protection clause of the 14th amendment insofar as they differ from their counterparts in the civil commitment area. They also violate due process where they fail to provide adequate protection against deprivation of liberty, impose unfair burdens and standards of proof, and fail to provide meaningful treatment.

The terms "criminal commitment" and "civil commitment" are much misused and confused. Formerly, "criminal commitment" referred to any commitment originating out of an involvement with the criminal justice system, whether hospitalization was the result of an NGI acquittal, a finding of incompetency to stand trial, or a transfer of a convicted prisoner from a jail to a mental hospital. Many courts, however, have recently altered their terminology and now refer to the status of committed NGIs as "civil." Indeed, a "criminal" designation should be limited to those persons who are still involved in the criminal justice system at the time of their commitment. Thus, NGIs would not be considered to have been criminally committed. Nor would persons who have been committed at the end of a criminal sentence. On the other hand, a convicted prisoner transferred to a hospital from jail would fall into the "criminal" category of patient, as would a defendant found incompetent to stand trial. This article will not use the term "criminal commitment" in referring to NGIs.

Thus, commitment should follow an acquittal only if civil commitment would be appropriate after implementation of the procedures and applications of the standards established by state civil commitment legislation. Once committed, an NGI should be treated in a manner dictated by his mental condition, and should not automatically be sent to a maximum security hospital, currently a common practice in many states, solely on the basis of his status as an acquitted patient. Finally, time of release should be determined by improvement in mental condition rather than by the crime which initiated his involvement in the mental health system.

Commitment Procedures and Standards

With the exception of a few challenges, it was assumed until recently that one acquitted on insanity grounds would automatically be committed to a mental hospital. In fact, this seemed to be such a faultless procedure that some courts brushed off challenges to automatic commitment statutes with no more than a reference to NGIs as a "special class."[1]

Some jurists, however, spoke of a presumption of continuing insanity to justify automatic commitment.[2] Others dismissed challenges on policy grounds, stating that automatic commitment was a reasonable legislative means to discourage false pleas of insanity.[3] Some courts dismissed due process challenges on the grounds that once patients had been automatically committed, avenues were available to them to seek release.[4] Many seemed to find a kind of estoppel flowing from a defendant's insanity plea, preventing his later claim that he had since become well.[5] Still others assumed that because

NGIs had performed a criminal act they were more dangerous than other mental patients, and that this justified differences in treatment.[6] None of these grounds for denying NGIs the procedural and substantive safeguards afforded all other civilly committed patients, taken singly or together, can justify the discrimination sanctioned by these decisions.

Presumption of Continuing Insanity

Once a defendant has been found to have been insane at the time of the crime, this presumption serves to relieve the state of the burden of proving present insanity. This presumption has serious flaws, however. All that is determined by an insanity acquittal is that the patient either (1) was insane at the time of the crime, if the defendant must prove insanity as an affirmative defense, or (2) may have been insane, if the defendant need only establish a reasonable doubt as to his sanity.

These findings have no bearing on the defendant's mental capacity at the time of the trial. It is not unusual for many months to pass between the time of the act and the time of the trial. In most cases, if the defendant has been found to be incompetent to stand trial, this time is spent under treatment in a mental institution. Psychotropic medications, which have been available since the early 1950s, can effect dramatic relief of serious psychotic symptoms within a matter of weeks. In cases where the symptoms are less serious, the NGI may have been awarded bail while awaiting trial. He may have a job and be under outpatient therapy, visibly demonstrating his ability to function in the community. In either event, the defendant would have recovered enough to have sufficient mental competency to stand trial. Hence, the presumption is now more fiction than fact.

Moreover, the tests used for an acquittal by reason of insanity differ from the tests used for civil commitment. For example, in most jurisdictions an insanity acquittal is based on the M'Naghten test of whether the defendant knew right from wrong. Civil commitment, however, may be based on a test of danger to self or others as a result of mental illness. A person may not know right from wrong, but yet not require commitment, especially where the crime involved is not one of physical violence. The tests would similarly be different in other states where the criteria for civil hospitalization are whether the person's judgment is so impaired as to prevent his recognizing the need for care and treatment and whether hospitalization is essential for his welfare.

Legislative Policy to Discourage False Insanity Pleas

Automatic commitment, according to this rationale, is a legitimate legislative provision to discourage false pleas of insanity, because persons will not fabricate such a plea knowing freedom cannot be the outcome. However, this policy is just as likely to penalize those who are neither culpable for their past acts nor presently insane by confining persons who are not mentally ill and discouraging legitimate pleas of insanity by those who do not wish to trade a determinate jail sentence for the uncertainties of hospitalization. The policy also reflects a lack of faith in the jury's ability to separate past irresponsibility from present sanity. Furthermore, it fails to recognize that a court-ordered examination prior to trial is likely to flush out imposters.

Finally, automatic commitments may actually function more to encourage false insanity pleas than to discourage them. Frequently, the insanity defense is the result of a plea bargain. Where prosecutors and judges know that a defendant will be incarcerated even if not convicted, they are more likely to tolerate, or even encourage, an insanity acquittal, thereby saving themselves both the time involved in a full trial, and the risk of the defendant's release if he is not convicted.

Availability of Alternative Procedures for Release

Courts have dismissed the necessity for a hearing prior to commitment with the rationalization that paths were still open for the patient to obtain his release. This approach was approved even where statutes set a minimum length of hospitalization such as 6 months, 1 or even 2 years before the remedy could be invoked, and where the patient had to bear the burden of proof and meet a higher standard at the later juncture.

However, where the patient must shoulder obstacles such as the burden of proof, a higher standard of proof, or a lengthy minimum time to "serve" before release can be sought, neither habeas corpus nor a later release hearing is an adequate substitute for a full exploration of his mental condition prior to the initial hospitalization.

A Defendant is Estopped From Claiming Present Sanity
Once He Has Opted for a Insanity Defense

This rationale for automatic commitment presents the clearest example of a punitive orientation, for it justifies confinement solely on the fact that a criminal act was committed, ignoring whether there is any present need for treatment. It paints the insanity defense as a privilege, overlooking its historical rationale. By forcing a defendant to choose between incarceration in a mental hospital and a prison, it comes close to abolishing the insanity defense as a practical matter, and ignores the fact that by admitting commission of an act, a defendant has not admitted commission of a crime.

A Different Approach to NGIs Is Justified Because They
Are More Dangerous than Other Mental Patients

This belief is based upon the fact that NGIs have manifested antisocial conduct at the time of their crime, whereas dangerous conduct of others is often only anticipated. However, many persons obtain insanity acquittals for crimes which are not violent.

Discrimination based on past criminal conduct is particularly unwarranted when the NGI group includes those acquitted of nonviolent crimes and the civilly committed group consists of those found to be "imminently and substantially dangerous," the standard in some states. In fact, in these states, as in others, the civil patient may have actually engaged in criminal behavior but not have been charged with a crime because hospitalization was instituted instead.

The Supreme Court has held that the commission of criminal acts does not give rise to a presumption of dangerousness which can justify a difference in commitment procedures and confinement conditions for the mentally ill.[7] Rather, the act itself can only contribute to findings of dangerousness and mental illness. Furthermore, even if it were established that NGIs as a class were more dangerous, this fact alone would not justify confinement of any particular individual in the class without a specific finding of dangerousness.[8]

Not only is the presumption of dangerousness of NGIs no longer legally valid as a justification for denying them procedural and substantive rights; it is not medically supportable either. Studies indicate that mentally ill people who have committed criminal offenses do not as a group differ in treatment requirements or prognosis from those who have not been overtly antisocial. Both groups are afflicted with the same types of psychiatric disturbances and respond to the same therapeutic methods.[9] No empirical studies have been done that point the other way. It would seem that in light of the overwhelming hardships levied on NGIs in the name of dangerousness, the burden should be upon proponents of such discriminations to justify their position by hard data and not mere supposition.

In recent years, the United States Supreme Court has taken the first firm steps toward establishing that mentally ill persons involved in the criminal justice system are entitled to the same due process rights afforded others subject to involuntary hospitalization. In *Baxstrom v. Herold*,[7] a patient nearing the end of his prison term, was certified insane by a prison physician and transferred to Dannemora State Hospital, a maximum security mental hospital under the control of the New York Department of Correction. A hearing was held at which it was determined *ex parte* that Baxstrom would not be a suitable patient for a civil mental hospital, seemingly solely because of his prior criminal status. Thus, although his sentence would have expired on December 18, 1961, he was still being held in Dannemora when the Supreme Court decided his case on February 23, 1966.

The Supreme Court held that Baxstrom had been denied equal protection in that (1) the New York statutory procedure for committing persons at the expiration of a penal sentence denied jury review which is available to all other civilly committed persons in New York; and (2) he was retained in an institution maintained by the Department of Correction after his penal term expired although no judicial determination had found him "dangerously mentally ill," a necessary prerequisite to confining all other civil mental patients in such institutions. The Court rejected the state's argument that Dannemora was substantially like all other mental hospitals and, therefore, placement of a patient there was merely a matter of administrative discretion affecting no fundamental rights.

In a second case, *Humphrey v. Casy,* the Supreme Court extended the *Baxstrom* principle to a sex offender committed under a Wisconsin statute to incarceration for treatment beyond his maximum sentence without the due process protection afforded to other civilly committed persons. Comparing the post-sentencing proceedings in *Humphrey* to those in *Baxstrom,* the Court held that Wisconsin could not deny Humphrey a jury trial simply because it had decided to process him under its Sex Offender Act rather than its Mental Health Act. Thus the Court once again refused to acknowledge a previous involvement with the criminal law as justification for differences in commitment and treatment procedures and standards.

Finally, in *Jackson v. Indiana*[11] the Court considered allegations of constitutional violations in the case of a mentally defective deaf mute who had been committed to an Indiana state mental institution as incompetent to stand trial. Theon Jackson functioned at the level of a preschool child, and could not read, write, or otherwise communicate except through limited sign language. Expert testimony had demonstrated that it was unlikely he would ever improve to the point of trial competency. Thus, the finding that he was incompetent was tantamount to a lifetime sentence in a mental institution even though he had never been convicted of a crime.

The Court held that pending criminal charges were insufficient to establish "dangerousness" and that by subjecting Jackson to a more lenient commitment standard and to a more stringent release standard than those applicable to persons not charged with offenses, Indiana had deprived petitioners of equal protection of the laws under the 14th Amendment.

Although the Supreme Court has not yet dealt directly with the issue of the rights of NGIs, lower courts have since applied the *Baxstrom-Humphrey-Jackson* analysis, and as a result, commitment procedures and standards for NGIs have been largely, though not completely, equalized with those for other civil patients in a few states.[12]

Treatment

In its physical appearance, this is much more like a prison than a hospital. In its architectural planning, it disregards the modern psychiatric concept of the therapeutic community. There are bare corridors, bars, iron gates, rows of cells—all the stigmata of punishment rather than treatment. Patients who occupy individual rooms are locked out of them during the day and have no opportunity to withdraw for privacy. Patients in wards have a reasonable amount of mobility from one area of the hospital to another, although security precautions are in evidence everywhere. . . . Externally, the plant has a misleadingly attractive appearance.

Internally, despite its dehumanizing attributes, it is well maintained and well equipped and might be characterized as a sanitary dungeon.[13]

Unfortunately, the above description by the California Supreme Court of Atascadero State Hospital which houses California's "criminally insane," is applicable to many of the maximum-security mental hospitals throughout the country in which most NGIs are housed. For example, a New York federal court has similarly described Matteawan State Hospital as a place "more likely to drive men mad than to cure the 'insane'."[14] (However, NGIs may no longer be confined in Mattawan, a correctional facility, but must be committed to a civil hospital as a result of a Court of Appeals decision.[15]) And it has been said of Bridgewater State Hospital in Massachusetts that "except for . . . uniformed guards, locked wards, and . . . seclusion rooms, Bridgewater offers little."[16] Indeed, barred cells, guard stations, and a prison-like environment are standard fare in these institutions. In an atmosphere where patients should be developing a sense of self-esteem and identity, abasements and degradation abound. For example, NGIs housed in New Jersey's forensic hospital are routinely hand-cuffed with hands bound to a belt around the waist in a dehumanizing manner whenever they must leave the grounds for a court appearance.

Some states confine all NGIs in maximum-security institutions, located in isolated corners of the state, distant from patients' relatives and friends. These institutions offer generally inferior treatment in terms of staff-patient ratios and consequent lack of psychotherapy and training programs. In addition, maximum security "hospitals" are likely not only to have physical plants which stress security rather than treatment, but to have rules and regulations more suitable for prisons than for treatment facilities. Typically, correspondence, telephone calls, and visitors are monitored, home visits are not permitted, and even grounds privileges and access to outdoor recreation are severely limited.

The conditions under which most NGIs are housed stand in stark contrast to those under which most other civil mental patients are confined. Non-NGI civil patients are usually afforded gradually progressive pass privileges as they are able to demonstrate greater responsibility. Home passes and visits are usually permitted. Telephone calls and correspondence are not likely to be limited. The patients are generally hospitalized near their homes, facilitating visits by friends and relatives. Chains, handcuffs, and barred cells are usually not in use. In other words, although locked wards are present in most mental hospitals, security is not given the primary emphasis.

It is not surprising that statistics demonstrate that NGIs are hospitalized for far longer periods than other civil patients,[17] the duration more likely to be related to the seriousness of the criminal act than to the patient's improvement within the hospital. An especially egregious example of this practice is the unwritten "ten-year rule" whereby patients at California's Atascadero State Hospital who have been acquitted of murder by reason of insanity are not considered for release or transfer for ten years. Similarly, patients charged with serious assaults are not released for 3 years after their symptoms abate.

Clearly, this penal philosophy has no place in a therapeutic environment. It is just as likely that the patient who commits a serious criminal act did so during an acute schizophrenic break which will respond quickly to medication, as it is that nonviolent but bizarre symptoms of the regularly committed civil patient will respond quickly to chemotherapy. An approach to release which relies on the underlying criminal act rather than on the patient's psychiatric condition may even be antitherapeutic, since, after an optimum time in a hospital, patients may regress or become "institutionalized." Thus, prolonging hospitalization is often detrimental rather than helpful.

Medical experts, courts, and legal commentators agree that security institutions sacrifice therapeutic standards and are likely to contribute to longer terms of confinement for patients. According to Weihofen,[19] "There is no way of reconciling these two functions [keeping patients securely locked up and treating them]. The therapeutic ideal calls for allowing patients more and more responsibility for their own actions and judgments, with correlative diminishing restrictions and controls, which inevitably means accepting greater or less security risk."[18]

Both equal protection and due process dictate that NGIs be afforded treatment identical to that of other mental patients. How a patient's commitment originated should in no way dictate the treatment available to him. The security risk a patient represents at any one point in time should be the sole criterion determining whether he must be lodged in a maximum security facility. It is just as inappropriate, and unconstitutional, to presume the necessity for maximum security confinement for NGIs as it is to presume that confinement is necessary in the first place. Under no circumstances should an acquitted patient be lodged in a facility operated by penal authorities.

Recent developments in mental health law make questionable the continued failure to provide treatment to NGIs in accordance with the dictates of their psychiatric condition. These developments include the emerging doctrine of right to treatment, the application of the 8th Amendment proscription against cruel and unusual punishment to hospitalization of the mentally ill, and the expanding restrictions placed upon the use of maximum-security institutions by the requirements of due process of law.

The Right to Treatment

The right to treatment was first judicially adopted in 1967 by the District of Columbia Court of Appeals in the case of an NGI, Charles Rouse. Although the decision[19] was couched in statutory terms, strong dicta indicated that a lack of treatment would violate the due process, equal protection, and the cruel and unusual punishment clauses of the Constitution. Four years after the *Rouse* decision, *Wyatt v. Stickney*[20] first pronounced a constitutional right to treatment. Lower-court cases proclaiming the right to treatment now abound,[21] although the United States Supreme Court has refused to recognize this right unequivocally, stating that there was no reason on the facts of the case presented to it to decide "whether mentally insane persons dangerous to themselves or to others have a right to treatment. . .[22]

Not only should adequate treatment be afforded NGIs whether or not they are in maximum security institutions, but it should be equal to that made available to other state mental patients. This means that no method of therapy should be denied a patient on the basis of his NGI status. Thus, unless the individual's condition is such that he is not an appropriate candidate for such treatment, he should receive grounds privileges, passes, conditional release, outpatient treatment, outdoor exercise, and whatever else is suitable for him at a particular time. It also means that he should not be placed in a maximum security hospital unless his condition requires it. Judicial decisions have begun to adopt this position.

The Proscription Against Cruel and Unusual Punishment

The failure of mental institutions to treat NGIs according to their medical needs subjects them to cruel and unusual punishment in violation of the 8th Amendment both in the traditional respect of imposing extreme punishment and under the more recently announced theory of punishing for status. Clearly, the prohibition applies not only where the abusive conduct is designated "punishment" but also where it is labelled "treatment" or considered by the administering authorities to be for the benefit or improvement of an individual's condition. For example, in both Rhode Island and Texas, federal courts have found that even if juvenile delinquents were being confined solely for rehabilitative purposes rather than punishment *per se,* the 8th Amendment would still be applicable to the conditions of confinement.[23] It has also been applied in New York to juveniles confined as nonconvicted persons in need of supervision[24] and in both Calfornia and New York to sexual psychopaths serving indefinite sentences.[25] Similarly, it has been applied to persons hospitalized for mental illness and mental disability.[26]

Since an NGI may not be mentally ill at the time of acquittal or may regain mental health shortly thereafter, his prolonged incarceration in a mental hospital may constitute cruel and unusual punishment because of the mental anguish that will occur from confinement with the mentally ill. If the NGI is in fact mentally ill, failure to provide him with all the treatment modalities appropriate to his condition would constitute punishment for the status of being an NGI, a condition entered innocently and involuntarily. This, too, would violate the proscription against cruel and unusual punishment.

Restrictions on the Use of Maximum Security Institutions

A number of courts have specifically decried the paucity of treatment opportunities available in maximum security mental hospitals. Generally, the cases elucidate two legal principles. First, penal institutions are inappropriate *per se* for placement of civil patients including NGIs. Second, maximum security nonpenal mental hospitals constitute appropriate placement only when they are the least restrictive alternative and when this fact has been determined by appropriate due process procedures.

Release

Of all the circumstances affecting an acquitted patient's existence, none is more unfair or diverges farther from the norms applicable to other committed patients than the procedures and standards controlling his release. Even where courts and legislatures espouse the ideas that NGIs should receive appropriate treatment and that NGIs should, by virtue of their acquittal, be beyond the pale of criminal punishment, somehow this is forgotten whenever the release of an NGI is proposed.

The reluctance of courts to free patients who have been considered "dangerous" has been described in picturesque terms by Judge David Bazelon:[27]

"(D)angerousness" is a many splendored thing. Unless muzzled by discriminating analysis, it is likely to weigh against nominally competing considerations the way a wolf weighs against a sheep in the same scales: even if the sheep is heavier when weighed separately, somehow the wolf always prevails when the two are weighed together. Keeping dangerousness on a taut leash is especially difficult where there is danger of murder, since the danger is admittedly grave and since its improbability, which theoretically discounts its gravity, is exceedingly difficult to quantify.

Moreover, once a man has shown himself to be dangerous, it is all but impossible for him to prove the negative that he is no longer a menace.

This reflex action against freeing acquitted patients has engendered a conflict between release procedures and standards applied to NGIs and those applied to other civil patients. Although statutes in nearly every state permit an administrative discharge by the hospital director when he believes a patient no longer requires hospitalization, about half of the states require court orders for discharge of NGIs. Furthermore, the burden of proof may be heavier and the standards for release more stringent for NGIs. The procedure for release is often more cumbersome, involving the prosecutor or district attorney and the same judge who signed the commitment order. In addition, NGIs may be denied discharge through periodic review and conditional discharge, avenues open to other patients.

The complexities involved in obtaining release usually ensnare the patient to such a degree that release is unduly delayed and sometimes prevented altogether. The literature recites some recent examples. A Missouri NGI acquitted of murder, had spent the subsequent 14 years hospitalized. A hearing was held at which the hospital recommended a conditional release to an out-patient facility, but despite unanimous psychiatric testimony that the patient had been psychosis-free and without need of medication for 7 years, the appellate court affirmed denial of the conditional release. In so doing, it glossed over the patient's stable state and his lengthy stay in a minimum-security environment, choosing instead to emphasize two minor incidents which had occurred during his many years at the hospital. In one of these he had obtained drugs after a close friend had stopped visiting him; in the other, he had obtained some alcohol. Nothing untoward occurred as a result of either of these episodes, but the court held that the patient had not met his burden of showing that he was free of a dangerous mental disease, even though he no longer suffered from the illness which had caused his hospitalization. In a second case, an appellate court upheld a jury's refusal to release a patient after 7 years of hospitalization despite testimony by three psychiatrists that the patient was no longer "insane" and despite the fact that the patient had only to sustain his position by a preponderance of the evidence. The only witnesses produced by the state were a psychiatrist who had not seen the patient since his trial 6 or 7 years earlier and a police officer who testified that he believed the patient had not changed since the time of his trial. According to the dissent in a third case, a patient was virtually condemned to a life sentence by the court's decision denying release because he had failed to show beyond a reasonable doubt that he would not drink again. The patient had not been psychotic for the 19 months during which he had been hospitalized. Rather, he was diagnosed as having a schizoid personality. He had completed the alcoholic treatment course offered at the hospital, had attended group therapy, had gotten along well with other patients and staff, and had been granted grounds privileges. Two doctors testified that he should be discharged and none recommended otherwise, but the court stated that there was no "guarantee" that he would not drink if released.

These examples demonstrate that courts are often swayed more by the past criminal act than the patient's mental condition. The acknowledgment in all three examples that the patients were not mentally ill at the time of the hearings which denied their release (although some were diagnosed as having personality disorders) signals the presence of preventive detention. Each example also demonstrates an unreasonable retention in custody of an NGI through mechanisms which are more procedurally complex or standards more difficult to meet than those applied to other patients. For example, an administrative discharge, had it been available, would have freed all three patients.

These examples reveal two major hurdles to discharge for NGIs. First, defendants who should never enter the mental health system at all are fed into it by the criminal courts. This group of patients includes those with psychopathic personalities or other behavior or personality disorders. Since such persons never display the severe symptoms of the psychoses, and are unlikely to respond significantly to treatment, they are likely to be in the unfortunate position at any point in time of petitioning for release but evidencing little or no improvement. They may be considered "dangerous," yet not "mentally ill." Second, patients are denied discharge by being refused access to the simplified, less stringent standards and mechanisms available to other civil patients. Thus, their constitutional right to equal protection of the laws is infringed.

Who Should Be Acquitted as an NGI?

The question of who should be considered so seriously mentally ill as to qualify for acquittal on grounds of insanity has been answered by courts in inconsistent ways. All too often the judicial answer has depended upon a particular psychiatrist's definition of "mental illness." Some psychiatrists faced with this question abdicate all responsibility by taking the position that if the diagnosis appears in the *Diagnostic and Statistical Manual of the American Psychiatric Association* the condition is a "mental illness." Some maintain that only psychoses qualify for such a label, and a few respond that no mental condition is an "illness."[28] Wherever the line is drawn, it is an artificial one and courts too often blindly adopt the testifying psychiatrist's demarcation.

The absurdity of this approach is illustrated by the description of two trials. At the first, three Saint Elizabeth psychiatrists testified that the defendant, a sociopath with no psychosis, was not mentally ill, and he was convicted. Then, in a second trial, less than one month later the Saint Elizabeth staff, reflecting a reversal in their internal policy, testified that sociopathy was a mental illness. As a result, the second defendant was acquitted on insanity grounds. The inconsistency resulted in a reversal of the conviction of the first defendant,[29] whereas the second trial result was affirmed.[30]

Unfortunately, since most statutes lack guidelines, many judges feel they have no choice but to adjudicate psychopaths mentally ill if the expert testimony has so indicated. Hence, persons who are properly diagnosed as having only psychopathic or other personality disorders are often acquitted of criminal behavior on insanity grounds and committed as mentally ill and dangerous. Following the acquittal, such courts often admit that the elements of mental illness are lacking, yet continue confinement of the patients as "dangerous."

Judge David Bazelon produced one of the best analyses of the problem in his partial dissent in *United States v. Alexander,*[31] where a defendant pleaded insanity based on his "rotten social background" which he said had conditioned him to respond to racial insults in a violent and involuntary manner. The defendant argued that his upbringing had brought about an "abnormal condition of his mind" tantamount, in terms of resulting behavior, to that of a schizophrenic who acts irrationally. Arguing that under the present state of the law the defendant should have been allowed a more lenient jury instruction regarding this defense, Judge Bazelon went on to consider four options in cases such as this, none of which he considered completely satisfying.

First, he said, narrow limits could be imposed on the responsibility defense so that such a defendant could not use it, thus assuring that he would be imprisoned if convicted. For example, the line could be drawn at psychosis. Second, he could be acquitted for lack of responsibility, and then freed as not mentally ill, although possibly dangerous. Third, a "vaguely therapeutic" rationale for hospitalization could be sought, justifying confinement after acquittal. Fourth, he could be confined in exclusive reliance on his predicted dangerousness, although this would constitute "unadorned preventive dentention." Unfortunately, the fourth alternative is too frequently opted for today, sometimes colored by option three. Choices three and four are the least desirable for, among other problems, they raise the specter of lengthy commitments to mental hospitals for persons not mentally ill or unable to respond to any treatment.

If the public cannot agree to the early or immediate release of an NGI, the use of the insanity defense should be restricted to persons with serious mental illnesses who are in need of treatment. Defense attorneys, prosecutors, and courts cannot continue to condone the use of the insanity defense as a tool in a plea bargain to rid themselves of burdensome caseloads and then expect mental hospitals to function inappropriately as preventive detention centers for persons not mentally ill. Psychiatrists and defense lawyers should be educated to the fact that they are not, in today's world, serving their clients by advancing the insanity plea when their clients are not mentally ill.

Constitutional Considerations

Jackson v. Indiana[32] held that subjecting an accused individual found incompetent to stand trial to a more stringent release standard than that applicable to others not charged with a crime would violate the 14th Amendment.

Following the Supreme Court's lead, three recent cases have held constitutionally intolerable the concept of separate and more stringent release procedures for NGIs. *Reynolds v. Neill*[33] struck down a Texas statute which required an acquitted patient to apply for release to the committing court and obtain a jury determination that he was no longer in need of protective confinement. Other patients could be released at any time by the hospital director under no set standard. In *People v. McQuillan,*[34] the Michigan Supreme Court held that statutory provisions denying NGIs access to civil release procedures, including administrative release by the hospital superintendent, were without a rational basis offending the equal protection clause. Finally, *Wilson v. State*[35] held that release of NGIs must be on the same footing as release of other patients by virtue of the equal protection mandate.

The mechanisms most frequently employed to frustrate release of acquitted patients are unavailability of administrative discharge; a prerequisite of discharge approval by hospital authorities before access to court can be obtained; a higher burden of proof and a more stringent standard of release; participation of prosecutor or attorney general and the committing judge at any release hearing; denial of conditional release procedures; and denial of periodic review.

Various reasons have been suggested for the requirement of judicial discharge of an NGI. First, it has been argued that the combined judgment of court and psychiatrists is better than that of either standing alone and affords greater protection to the public. The problem here is that where the court and psychiatrists are at odds with each other, the court may merely override unanimous psychiatric testimony. Some courts have indicated that it is improper for a judge to retain a patient in the face of unanimous psychiatric testimony favoring his release. If unanimous pro-release testimony is presented, the judge must either order his discharge or appoint still other experts to examine him.[36]

A further problem arising from mandatory court involvement which may unduly retard release of well patients, is the confusion which courts often evidence over certain psychiatric terms. For example, in *State v. Maik*,[37] the New Jersey Supreme Court not only required that the "underlying illness" be cured before release, an unrealistic goal in most cases, but coined a new psychiatric term "neutralization," which it distinguished somehow from "remission." The New Jersey Psychiatric Association criticized the opinion as unworkable, and the new word as without any understandable meaning.[38] *97 N.J.L.J. 327 (1974). Maik* has since been overruled.[39]

Although, to be sure, fewer patients are released by this double-barrier system, the interests of the patient are totally ignored. It has also been suggested that psychiatrists faced with overcrowded and understaffed facilities would release patients too soon. In view of the present-day concern of psychiatrists with malpractice liability, however, and the low percentage of NGIs in hospital populations, it is unlikely that psychiatrists would see in this group of patients a solution to overcrowded conditions. On the other hand, some administrative release critics argue that psychiatrists, acting alone without court approval, would hold onto patients longer than necessary, fearful of making a bad guess concerning mental state. Experience shows that more often the courts frustrate realistic expectations of release than do the psychiatrists. But if in a particular case a psychiatrist were to retain a patient after the time of his recovery, the patient could still seek release by a writ of habeas corpus. Another reason advanced for requiring a judicial discharge is that demanding a medical release would interfere with the doctor-patient relationship. However, it is surely just as likely that this relationship would be adversely affected if a patient knows that his doctor will be testifying against him in court. Finally, it has been argued that, like the matter of commitment, release is a legal issue which is most appropriately resolved in the courts. But it must be remembered that the legal issues in commitment and release are not the same. The first involves deprivation of liberty requiring due-process safeguards, principally a judicial hearing. The latter involves restoration of liberty, in which court intervention is not required unless liberty is not restored.

All of the above reasons ignore the fact that other patients are routinely discharged in nearly every state by hospital personnel when their mental condition is such that hospitalization is no longer necessary. Among the categories of "dangerous" patients who may be discharged by the hospital administrator without application to a court are patients who are civilly committed under standards of dangerousness based on recent overt behavior and patients under criminal indictment who have been converted to civil status pursuant to *Jackson v. Indiana*.[40]

The above reasons also ignore the imposing barrier to appropriate medical care which is erected by the necessity for court approval for release or even transfer to less restrictive facilities. Good psychiatric practice requires flexibility dependent on the patient's condition at a given time. If court intervention is necessary at each treatment juncture, the benefits of treatment responsive to the patient's needs may well be lost. However, only three courts have mandated administrative discharges in states which allow them for other mental patients,[33-35] whereas other courts are still finding that a rational basis exists for different release requirements.[41]

Another source of discrimination against NGIs is the practice in many states of treating release proceedings as a continuation of the criminal case which brought the patient into the mental health system initially. Even the title of the cases reflects the thinking about them: "State versus. . ." or "People versus. . ." rather than "In re. . . ." Thus the judge who sat at the patient's criminal trial and possibly decided the matter of his commitment, is also likely to be the judge who hears petitions for his release.

Additionally, since the case is considered criminal in nature, the prosecutor or district attorney is usually a participant in the release hearing, although he would not have a voice in the release of other patients. Statutes of many states call for notice to him, whether release is sought by the patient through a statutory route or by habeas corpus. It seems clear that if NGIs are to be considered "civil" patients, as this paper proposes, they should be free of interference by the criminal justice system at the time of their release hearing.

Conditional release is an important treatment tool, particularly in the case of many NGIs, because it affords the hospital doctors an opportunity to control and monitor a patient's behavior as restrictions on his freedom are gradually lifted, allowing them to form a more educated opinion on the patient's suitability for absolute discharge. Its use should be available for NGIs, as for other patients, although many states do not provide it for the former group. Even where it is available, it is often abused by judges who use it to regulate every aspect of a patient's life outside the institution. Only conditions directly related to maintaining a patient's mental health are proper.

One last avenue to release is periodic judicial review. It is the most effective method of insuring that no patient is hospitalized beyond the period that his mental condition warrants. Clearly, where periodic review is available to other patients, equal protection requires that it also be available to NGIs. Due process is also a sound basis for requiring periodic reviews for NGIs, for no other method so well assures that the nature and duration of the confinement are rationally related to its purpose of curing mental illness.

REFERENCES

1. For example, Chase v. Kearns, 278 A.2d 132 (Me. 1971).

2. For example, Orencia v. Overholser, 163 F.2d 763 (D.C. Cir. 1947).

3. For example, Lynch v. Overholser, 369 U.S. 705, 715 (1962).

4. For example, State v. Allan, 166 N.W.2d 752 (Iowa 1969).

5. For example Ragsdale v. Overholser, 281 F.2d 943 (D.C. Cir. 1960).

6. Ragsdale v. Overholser, 281 F.2d 943, 947 (D.C. Cir. 1960).

7. Baxstrom v. Herold, 383 U.S. 107 (1966).

8. State v. Krol, 68 N.J. 236, 344 A.2d 289 (1975).

9. Weihofen X: Institutional treatment of persons acquitted by reason of insanity. *tex law rev* 38: 849, 855, 1960, Weihofen X: Treatment of insane prisoners, *Univ. Ill Law Forum* 524, 530 (960); Steadman H., Keveles G.: The community adjustment and criminal activity of the Baxstrom patients: 1966–1970. *Am J Psychiatry* 129:311, 1972.

10. Humphrey v. Cady, 405 U.S. 504 (1972).

11. Jackson v. Indiana, 406 U.S. 715 (1972).

12. For example, Bolton v. Harris, 395 F.2d 642 (D.C. Cir. 1968); Wilson v. State, 259 Ind. 375, 287 N.E.2d 875 (1972); State *ex rel.* Kovach v. Schubert, 64 Wis. 2d 612, 219 N.W.2d 341 (1974), *appeal dismissed*, 419 U.S. 1117, *cert. denied*, 419 U.S. 1130 (1975); State v. Krol, 68 N.J. 236, 344 A.2d 289 (1975); People v. Lally, 19 N.Y. 2d 27, 224 N.E. 2d 87, 277 N.Y.S. 2d 654 (1966); People v. McQuillan, 392 Mich. 511, 221 N.W. 2d 569 (1974); Reynolds v. Neill, 381 F. Supp. 1374 (N.D. Tex. 1974), *vacated sub nom.* Sheldon v. Reynolds, 422 U.S. 1050 (1975); Wilson v. State, 259 Ind. 375, 387 N.E. 2d 875 (1972).

13. People v. Burnick, 14 Cal. 3d 306, 319, 535 P.2d 352, 121 Cal. Rptr. 488, 496 (1975), quoting *Observations and Comments,* based on a survey by the California Medical Association, 21, Jan. 18, 1965.

14. United States *ex rel.* Von Wolfersdorf v. Johnston, 317 F. Supp. 66, 67 (S.D. N.Y. 1970).

15. Kesselbrenner v. Anonymous, 33 N.Y. 2d 161, 305 N.E. 2d 903, 350 N.Y.S. 2d 889 (1973).

16. Nason v. Superintendent of Bridgewater State Hospital, 353 Mass. 604, 609, 233 N.E.2d 908, 911 (1968).

17. Morris G.: The confusion of confinement syndrome extended: The treatment of mentally ill "Non-Criminal Criminals" in New York, *Buffalo Law Rev* 18:393, 394, 1969; Morris G.: "Criminality" and the Right to Treatment, *Univ Chicago Law Rev* 36:784, 790–791, 1969; Lewin T.: Disposition of the irresponsible: Protection following commitment, *Mich Law Rev* 66:721, 728–732, 1968; see also Rubin S: *Psychiatry and the Crim Law* 47: (1965).

18. Weihofen X: Institutional treatment of persons acquitted by reason of insanity. Tex Law Rev 38:853, 1960.

19. Rouse v. Cameron, 373 F.2d 451 (D.C. Cir. 1967).

20. 325 F. Supp. 781 (M.D. Ala. 1971), *aff'd sub nom.* Wyatt v. Aderholt, 503 F.2d 1305 (5th Cir. 1974).

21. For example, Burnham v. Dept. of Public Health, 503 F.2d 1319 (5th Cir. 1974), *cert. denied,* 422 U.S. 1057 (1975); Davis v. Watkins, 384 F. Supp. 1196 (N.D. Ohio 1974); Welsh v. Likins, 373 F. Supp. 487 (D. Minn. 1974); Stachulak v. Coughlin, 364 F. Supp. 686 (N.D. Ill. 1973); Kesselbrenner v. Anonymous, 33 N.Y. 2d 161, 305 N.E. 2d 903, 350 N.Y.S. 2d 889 (1973).

22. O'Connor v. Donaldson, 422 U.S. 563, 573 (1975).

23. Inmates of Boys' Training School v. Affleck, 346 F. Supp. 1354, 1366 (D.R.I. 1972); Morales v. Turman, 364 F. Supp. 166, 173 (E.D. Tex. 1973).

24. For example, Lollis v. New York State Dept. of Soc. Serv., 322 F. Supp. 473 (S.D.N.Y. 1970), *modified,* 328 F. Supp. 1115 (S.D.N.Y. 1971).

25. People v. Feagley, 14 Cal. 3d 338, 535 P.2d 373, 121 Cal. Rptr. 509 (1975); People *ex rel* Kaganovitch v. Wilkins, 23 App. Div. 2d 178, 259 N.Y.S.2d 462 (1965).

26. For example, Knecht v. Gillman, 488 F.2d 1136 (8th Cir. 1973); Rozecki v. Gaughan, 459 F.2d (1st Cir. 1972); New York Association for Retarded Children v. Rockefeller, 357 F. Supp. 752 (E.D.N.Y. 1973).

27. Covington v. Harris, 419 F.2d, 617, 627 (D.C. Cir. 1969).

28. Szasz T: *The Myth of Mental Illness,* rev. ed. New York, Harper & Row, 1974.

29. Blocker v. United States, 274 F.2d 572 (D.C. Cir. 1959).

30. Overholser v. Leach, 257 F.2d 667 (D.C. Cir. 1958), *cert. denied,* 359 U.S. 1013 (1959).

31. United States v. Alexander, 471 F.2d 923, 957 (D.C. Cir. 1973).

32. Jackson v. Indiana, 406 U.S. 715 (1972).

33. Reynolds v. Neill, 381 F. Supp. 1374 (N.D. Tex. 1974) *vacated on other grounds sub nom.* Sheldon v. Reynolds, 422 U.S. 1050 (1975).

34. People v. McQuillan, 392 Mich. 511, 221 N.W.2d 569 (1974).

35. Wilson v. State, 259 Ind. 375, 287 N.E.2d 875 (1972).

36. United States v. McNeill, 434 F.2d 502, 514–15 (D.C. Cir. 1970) (Bazelon, J., concurring); State v. Carter, 64 N.J. 382, 406, 316 A.2d 449, 462 (1974).

37. State v. Maik, 60 N.J. 203, 218–219, 287 A2d 715, 723 (1972).

38. *NJ Law J* 97:327, 1974.

39. State v. Krol, 68 N.J. 236, 265–66, 344 A.2d 289, 305 (1975).

40. Jackson v. Indiana, 406 U.S. 715 (1972).

41. For example, United States v. Ecker, II, No. 75-1074 (D.C. Cir. Apr. 2, 1976); State v. Carter, 64 N.J. 382, 316 A.2d 449 (1974) (Clifford J., concurring and dissenting); Bolton v. Harris 395 F.2d 642 (D.C. Cir. 1968); State v. Clemons, 110 Ariz. 79, 513 P.2d 324 (1973).

Suggestions for Further Reading

Forensic Commitments

Bendt, R. H., et al. "Incompetency to Stand Trial: Is Psychiatry Necessary?" *American Journal of Psychiatry* 130 (1973):1288–1289.

Brady, John P., and Brodie, H. Keith. *Controversy in Psychiatry.* Philadelphia: W. B. Saunders, Co., 1978, Ch. 22.

Competency to Stand Trial and Mental Illness. Rockville, Maryland: National Institute of Mental Health, 1973.

Cooke, G., et al. "Factors Affecting Referral to Determine Competency to Stand Trial." *American Journal of Psychiatry* 130 (1973):870–875.

Doson, D., and Robey, A. "Amnesia and Competency to Stand Trial." *American Journal of Psychiatry* 130 (1973):588–592.

Geller, Jeffrey L., and Lister, Eric M. "The Process of Criminal Commitment for Pretrial Psychiatric Examination: An Evaluation." *American Journal of Psychiatry* 135 (1978):530–60. See especially the bibliography on pp. 59–60.

German, June R., and Singer, Anne C. "Punishing the Not Guilty: Hospitalization of Persons Acquitted by Reason of Insanity." *Psychiatric Quarterly* 49 (1977):238–254.

Graber, Glenn C., and Marsh, Frank H. "Ought a Defendant Be Drugged to Stand Trial?" *Hastings Center Report* 9 (1979):8–10. See critical response in Vol. 9, No. 5, pp. 4, 45.

Hess, J. H., and Thomas, H. "Incompetency to Stand Trial: Procedures, Results, and Problems." *American Journal of Psychiatry* 119 (1963):713–720.

Klerman, Gerald, and Dworkin, Gerald. "Case Studies in Bioethics: Can Convicts Consent to Castration?" *Hastings Center Report* (October 1975):17–19.

Kirschner, Barry. "Constitutional Standards for Release of the Civilly Committed and Not Guilty by Reason of Insanity." *Arizona Law Review* 20 (1978):233–278.

McGarry, A. L. "The Fate of Psychotic Offenders Returned for Trial." *American Journal of Psychiatry* 127 (197):1181–1184.

Menninger, Karl. "The Future of Criminal Law." *Reflections* 3 (1968):40–51.

"Mental Health and Human Rights: Report of the Task Panel on Legal and Ethical Issues." *Arizona Law Review* 20 (1978):125–133.

Morawetz, Thomas. *The Philosophy of Law.* New York: Macmillan, 1980, Ch. 4.

Morris, Grant H. "'Criminality' and the Right to Treatment.' *University of Chicago Law Review* 36 (1969):784–801.

Pendelton, Linda. "Treatment of Persons Found Incompetent to Stand Trial." *American Journal of Psychiatry* 137 (September 1980):1098–1100.

"Psychiatry and the Courts." Special section in *American Journal of Psychiatry* 126 (October 1969):519–550.

Robey, Ames. "Criteria for Competency to Stand Trial: A Checklist for Psychiatrists." *American Journal of Psychiatry* 122 (1965):616–622.

Shapiro, Michael H., and Spece, Roy G., Jr. *Bioethics and Law.* St. Paul: West Publishing Co., 1981, Chs. 6, 7.

Steadman, Henry, and Cocozza, J. *Careers of the Criminally Insane: Excessive Social Control of Deviance.* Lexington, Massachusetts: Lexington Books, 1974.

Szasz, Thomas S. "The Insanity Plea and the Insanity Verdict." *Temple Law Quarterly* 40 (1967):271–282.

Wexler, David B. *Mental Health Law: Major Issues.* New York: Plenum Publishing Co., 1980.

Wilkins, Leslie T. "Putting 'Treatment' on Trial." *Hastings Center Report* 5 (February 1975):35–48.

Winick, Bruce J. "Psychotropic Medication and Competence to Stand Trial." *American Bar Foundation Research Journal* (Summer 1977):769–816. A thorough examination and defense of chemical competency.

Rationality, Freedom, Responsibility and Criminal Insanity

Allen, R. C., et al. *Mental Impairment and Legal Incompetency.* Englewood Cliffs, New Jersey: Prentice Hall, Inc., 1968.

Arrington, Robert L. "Practical Reason, Responsibility, and the Psychopath." *Journal for the Theory of Social Behavior* 9 (March 1979):71–89.

Aubert V., and Messinger, S. "The Criminal and the Sick." *Inquiry* 1 (1958): 137–160.

Audi, Robert. "Moral Responsibility, Freedom, and Compulsion." *American Philosophical Quarterly* 11 (1974):1–14.

Brody, Baruch A., and Engelhardt, H. Tristram, Jr. *Mental Illness: Law and Public Policy.* Boston: D. Reidel, 1980.

Dennett, D. C. "Mechanism and Responsibility." In Honderich, Ted, ed. *Essays on Freedom of Action.* London: Routledge & Kegan Paul, 1973.

Edwards, Rem B. *Freedom, Responsibility and Obligation*. The Hague: Martinus Nijhoff, 1969.

Ennis, Bruce J., and Emery, Richard D. *The Rights of Mental Patients*. New York: Avon Books, 1978, Ch. V.

Fingarette, Herbert. "Criminal Insanity and Criminal Responsibility." *Humanities* 9 (May 1973):153–171.

———. "Insanity and Responsibility." *Inquiry* 15 (1972):6–29.

———. *The Meaning of Criminal Insanity*. Berkeley: University of California Press, 1972.

———. "Responsibility." *Mind* 75 (1966):58–74.

Fingarette, Herbert, and Hasse, Ann Fingarette. *Mental Disabilities and Criminal Responsibility*. Berkeley: University of California Press, 1979.

Flew, Antony. *Crime or Disease*. London: Macmillan, 1973.

Gardner, Martin R. "The Myth of the Impartial Psychiatric Expert—Some Comments Concerning Criminal Responsibility and the Decline of the Age of Therapy. *Law and Psychology Review* 2 (1976):99–118.

Gaylin, Willard. "Skinner Redux." *Harper's* (October 1973):48–56.

Globus, Gordon G. "On 'I': The Conceptual Foundations of Responsibility." *American Journal of Psychiatry* 137 (April 1980):417–422.

Glover, Jonathan. *Responsibility*. New York: Humanities Press, 1970.

Halleck, Seymour L. "The Psychiatrist and the Legal Process." *Psychology Today* 2 (February 1969):25–28.

Hart, H. L. A. *Punishment and Responsibility: Essays in the Philosophy of Law*. New York: Oxford University Press, 1968.

Hoffman, Martin. "The Idea of Freedom in Psycho-Analysis." *International Journal of Psycho-Analysis* 45 (1964):579–583.

Immergluck, Ludwig. "Determinism-Freedom in Contemporary Psychology: An Ancient Problem Revisited." *American Psychologist* 19 (1964):270–281.

Isenberg, Morris. "Responsibility and the Neurotic Patient." *American Journal of Psychoanalysis* 34 (1974):43–50.

Kaplan, Leonard V. "The Mad and the Bad: An Inquiry into the Disposition of the Criminally Insane." *The Journal of Medicine and Philosophy* 2 (1977): 244–304. See his excellent bibliography on pp. 300–304.

Kittrie, Nicholas N. *The Right to Be Different: Deviance and Enforced Therapy*. Baltimore: The Johns Hopkins Press, 1971.

Knight, Robert P. "Determinism, 'Freedom,' and Psychotherapy." *Psychiatry* 9 (1946).

Lewy, Ernst. "Responsibility, Free Will, and Ego Psychology." *International Journal of Psycho-Analysis* 42 (1961):260–270.

Margolis, Joseph. *Psychotherapy and Morality*. New York: Random House, 1966, Chs. 4 and 5.

May, Rollo. "Will, Decision and Responsibility: Summary Remarks." *Review of Existential Psychology and Psychiatry* 1 (1961):249–259.

Menkiti, I. A. "Criminal Responsibility and the Mentally Ill." *The Journal of Value Inquiry* 14 (Fall & Winter 1980):181–194.

Menninger, Karl. *The Crime of Punishment.* New York: Viking Press, 1968.

Moore, Michael S. "Mental Illness and Responsibility." *Bulletin of the Menninger Clinic* 39 (July 1975):308–328.

Neville, Robert. "Where Do the Poets Fit In?" *Hastings Center Report* 1 (1971): 6–8. A critique of Skinner.

Robitscher, Jonas. "Medical Limits of Criminality." *Annals of Internal Medicine* 73 (1970):849–851.

Robitscher, Jonas, and Williams, Roger. "Should Psychiatrists Get Out of the Courtroom?" *Psychology Today* 11 (December 1977):85ff.

Skinner, B. F. *Beyond Freedom and Dignity.* New York: Alfred A. Knopf, Inc., 1971.

Szasz, Thomas S. *Law, Liberty and Psychiatry.* New York: Macmillan, 1963.

———. "The Moral Dilemma of Psychiatry: Autonomy or Heteronomy." *American Journal of Psychiatry* 121 (1964):521–528.

Tancredi, Laurence R. *Legal Issues in Psychiatric Care.* New York: Harper & Row, 1975, pp. 2–10 and 78–86.

Torrey, E. Fuller. *The Death of Psychiatry.* Radnor, Pennsylvania: Chilton Book Co., 1974, Ch. 6.

Walton, Douglas. "Philosophical Perspectives on the Insanity Defense." *Human Context* 7 (1975):546–560.

10. Deprivation and Coercion in Custodial Care and Deinstitutionalization

Introduction

What quality of life and of medical care is available to mental hospital patients, and how do these compare to what would be available to them on the outside? The meaningless routines and nontherapeutic environment of understaffed and underfinanced custodial care institutions are well described in the following article by Martha R. Fowlkes. The institution of the seventies described in her essay was by no means one of the "snake pits" of thirty years ago, but it still represents a low mark against which more modern and progressive institutions may measure their degree of progress. Unfortunately, despite all efforts at reform, many institutions providing little more than minimal custodial care are still to be found. Mental illness is not a high status, high priority illness like cancer or heart disease; and our society is unwilling to spend the necessary money for mental health care or to fund research in this area.

Institutionalization of persons alleged to be mentally deficient or disturbed reached its peak in the United States during the late 1950s and early 1960s. By 1980 the patient population in mental hospitals had been reduced by more than two-thirds as a result of a nationwide emphasis on returning mental patients back to "the community," which has turned out in practice to be any place (including other kinds of institutions) outside mental hospitals.

What really lies behind the emphasis on deinstitutionalization? What factors best explain it? Doubtless the introduction of new, powerful, and effective drugs in the mid-fifties was an important factor in revolutionizing the care and maintenance of psychiatric patients both inside and outside of mental institutions. Doubtless also the anti-psychiatric crusaders who so persistently called attention to the often horrible living conditions and flagrant violations of the moral and civil rights of mental hospital patients had a significant consciousness raising effect. Also, we came to realize more and more that the hospitals were being used and abused as warehouses and dumping grounds for unwanted people who had no business being there in the first place.

Before we pride ourselves too heartily in our moral advancement and in the efficaciousness of moral and legal ideals, we should explore the possibility that the most effective impetus underlying deinstitutionalization has actually been economics. Although incredibly cheap by comparison with other forms of hospitalization, public mental hospitals do cost the taxpayers a good bit of money. The desire to save taxpayers' money, or at least make them believe this is happening, has been a significant if not the most potent factor underlying deinstitutionalization.

There is something very deceptive about the patient population and the financial statistics of deinstitutionalization. As for the patients, we should certainly not leap to the unwarranted conclusion that the hundreds of thousands of persons released from mental hospitals in the past ten years or more are now living independently and are actively enjoying all the freedoms of democracy and the amenities of middle class existence. As the article by Jonathan F. Borus points out, much *de*institutionalization has actually been *re*institutionalization in nursing homes, smaller community mental health centers and hospitals, group homes, foster homes, cheap welfare hotels, missions and flop houses, and in some cases jails, prisons, and reformatories. The push for deinstitutionalization has also coincided with a concerted effort to separate the mentally ill from the mentally retarded; thousands of persons released from mental hospitals have been promptly reinstitutionalized in newly built facilities for the mentally retarded. When institutionalization reached its peak in the late fifties and early sixties one percent of our population was institutionalized. Now, after the deinstitutionalization emphasis has run its course, the figure still stands at one percent.

The economic statistics are extremely misleading as well. The new kinds of institutions into which former mental hospital patients are being shifted also cost money, but the federal government will pay the bills through Medicare and Medicaid in nursing homes, psychiatric units of general hospitals, and for an initial period of funding in regional mental health centers, whereas city, county, and state governments must pay for public mental hospitals. The real game of deinstitutionalization seems to be that of transferring mental patients into programs that federal funds will finance. This permits state governors and legislators to call attention to enormous savings in state tax dollars, while hoping all the while that their local electorate will be too obtuse to realize that the taxpayers are still paying the bills even after the burden has been shifted to the federal level.

Deinstitutionalization may result in real savings to the states if patients are returned to live with family or friends, though even here the federal government is paying much of the bill through SSI (Supplemental Security Income) checks. Many patients try to exist "independently" on the $268 or more per month (a 1981 figure that increases slightly each year) that such checks provide by living in run down welfare hotels or foster homes. In return for such a sum, these residences must provide the basic necessities (food, lodging, and fuel) and still attempt to make a reasonable profit. Obviously, the quality of service that these limited funds will buy is low indeed; and it is no small wonder that many patients would prefer mental hospitals to the diminished quality of life that deinstitutionalization offers. The article by Walter B. Simon deals with the variety of perfectly good reasons which many mental hospital patients have for wanting to remain where they are or to return after a short taste of frustrating freedom. Though many lawyers and antipsychiatrists find the thought unthinkable, there are thousands of mental patients, "crazy but not stupid," who review their realistic options and choose hospitalization. Attention is usually focused on the intense coercion to which mental patients are subjected when they are admitted to the hospital; but the era of deinstitutionalization has brought equally intense and questionable coercion to bear upon the discharge process. If it is a morally objectionable violation of rational autonomy to institutionalize persons against their will, why is it not equally objectionable to deinstitutionalize them against their will? Should they be coerced to assume responsibility for managing their own lives when they do not wish to be autonomous? If the state has spent years creating institutional dependence, has it not incurred an obligation to support what it has created when institutional life is preferred to freedom? How much pressure should be exerted to persuade those individuals to go who do not wish to leave, especially those with passive, dependent personalities who find institutionalization so appealing. Have the taxpayers any right against those few "freeloaders" on the system who are capable of functioning outside public hospitals but who repeatedly "act out" to forestall dismissal or regain admission? What quality of life and of medical care are such persons entitled to receive at public expense? Mental health professionals now have to answer such difficult questions every working day. To date, society has provided them with no clear guidelines for their decisions.

Martha R. Fowlkes

Business as Usual — At the State Mental Hospital

Despite official policy and professional emphasis to the contrary, the custodial mental hospital continues to exist as a major form of state-provided mental health care. In this paper, one such institution, "New England State Hospital,"[1] is described, and the various features of hospital organization that sustain a system of custodial care are discussed. Although the custodial hospital offers little to its patients, its persistent survival can be explained by the number of non-patient vested interests that are well served by the state hospital, precisely in its existing custodial form. The case study of New England State Hospital suggests that reform of state mental institutions depends less on a programmatic formulation of desired changes than on an understanding of the structured resistance to such changes.

It is common knowledge that the custodial state mental hospital is obsolete. From a variety of sources — whether Wiseman's notorious and unsettling film *Titticut Follies,* Kesey's popular novel *One Flew Over the Cuckoo's Nest,* or the sociological studies of Goffman (1961), Dunham and Weinberg (1960), Belknap (1956), and others — comes overwhelming evidence of the failure of such institutions to provide personalized care or active rehabilitative treatment. In a major address in 1963, President Kennedy condemned the "cold mercy of custodial isolation" and urged an end to the practice of confining patients "in an institution to wither away." Congress followed suit by enacting the Mental Retardation and Community Mental Health Centers Act in the same year. Certainly it would be impossible to find any authority in the field of mental

From *Psychiatry* 38 (1975):55–64. Copyright © 1975 by The William Alanson White Psychiatric Foundation, Inc. Reprinted by permission of the publisher and the author.

health care who would have a kind word for the custodial care of the traditional large-scale state mental hospital. Mental health professionals are everywhere being trained in new multidisciplinary approaches and community rehabilitation. Indeed, a growing number of psychiatrists, following the lead of Szasz (1961), are rejecting the notion of mental illness altogether and are openly critical of the utilization of conventional medical solutions for what they view as a nonmedical problem.

Szasz notwithstanding, the real issue in the past decade has not been the abolition but the reform of the state mental hospital. In this connection custodial forms of care have been conceptually, professionally, and officially rejected. Yet in reality, the custodial institution lives on as a dominant, if not *the* dominant, form of state-provided mental health care. In spite of a noticeable decline in the resident population of the nation's state mental institutions in the last half decade, there nonetheless remain over half a million residents in state facilities for the mentally disabled. To be sure, a few of these facilities have made the transformation from custodial to therapeutic and community-oriented care,[2] and most recently a series of "right to treatment" lawsuits have attempted to establish minimally acceptable guidelines for patient care and treatment in the state hospitals of a number of regions across the country.[3] There is little doubt, however, that most state facilities continue essentially unaltered, maintaining dismally low standards of care and treatment, oblivious to the brave new world of mental health care.[4] In the following description of a state hospital I will attempt to indicate why changes that seem obviously desirable seldom occur.

New England State Hospital

The enduring custodial character of the state hospital is well exemplified by the case of New England State Hospital. Established well over 100 years ago, the hospital has in years past housed a peak population of up to 2000 patients. At present there are some 100 patients resident at any given time, one-third of whom are geriatric. Probably two-thirds of all the hospital's patients are "chronic," that is, permanent or long-term residents or regular returnees to the hospital.

New England State Hospital, which serves an area comprising several counties, is situated on hundreds of acres of state land in a sparsely populated part of a small town. The original hospital building, which houses half of all the patients, is a gloomy, fortress-like structure with barred windows. Inside, tiny rooms once intended for single occupancy are now double bedrooms; beds are also lined up in rows against the walls of vast rooms originally meant for use as solariums and infirmaries. Furnishings are sparse, air is close, paint is peeling, and the urine and disinfectant smells of the decades have soaked into walls and floors and mingle to make a permanent stench. Within each major residential unit, patients live in wards, each ward a segment of a hierarchical structure representing degrees of so-called wellness or illness. The traditional locked wards for those the hospital considers the worst of its patients are very much in evidence and contain provisions for restraints and seclusion.

Although occasional happenings of a sensationalist nature are often associated with mental hospitals, the true picture of hospital life is relentlessly passive and inert. For patients on the back or locked wards, life means being locked in, locked up, or tied down. Life on these wards is literally in a perpetual state of suspended animation. Patients elsewhere in the hospital who are less deteriorated, or who are more "manageable" through the heavy use of drugs, have more freedom and are seemingly more active in a physical sense. However, the quality of the activity is aimless and repetitive and is prompted by no particular motivation or encouragement to do anything or go anywhere. People travel incessantly the same route day after day; others stare vacantly at (frequently unfocused) television pictures, or pace the floor, or rock ceaselessly back and forth, or repeat gestures and phrases for hours on end, or sit, or sleep.

Though many patients work regularly at jobs throughout the hospital (it is essential for the maintenance of the hospital that the patients do chores), futility is built into occupations that typically carry with them no pay or promotion or any real appreciation.[5] Occasional movies, dances, a few athletic events, and some sparsely available occupational therapy provide diversions for those who wish to participate. But even those patients who make a relatively busy routine for themselves have no purpose to their busy-ness. They have simply settled into an essentially passive hospital life in a more active way than some others.

Despite the dreariness of the living conditions and the rare instances of brutality, the single most outstanding fact about life in this mental hospital (and the one with the most consequence to patients) is that *nothing ever happens.* The people there as patients have no sense of being there for a purpose, as one would go to a general hospital, say, for an appendectomy and recovery period and then go back to rejoin the outside world. The longer the period of a patient's residence the greater the loss of time perspective. For some the passage of time seems to have become virtually meaningless, marking neither the accomplishment of individually significant tasks or routines in the short run, nor a steady progression toward the achievement of specified ends in the long run. In the mental hospital people just are, that is all, and the hospital is merely custodian of their existence.

The prevailing custodial emphasis of New England State Hospital, however, is not necessarily the product, as is often popularly thought, of patients who are universally so disturbed or helpless as to make the custodial approach inevitable. Rather, the custodial emphasis is sustained by quite specific and predominating features of hospital culture and organization. These same features also operate to make unlikely the introduction of change, or to make unlikely the possibility that change will be successful once introduced.

The Admissions Process

The custodial process is set in motion by hospital admissions policies and procedures. Admission to the hospital occurs primarily as a technical-legal process. Persons are admitted indiscriminately, whether voluntary, physician-referred, or court-referred. The hospital administrators seldom exercise their prerogative to evaluate the qualitative need or reasons for admission, because they believe they might either offend referring parties or prompt a would-be patient to sue the hospital for dereliction of its duties. Either possibility could jeopardize good public relations.

Because the hospital absorbs virtually all comers, outside doctors and agencies often have little sense of what the resources and facilities of the hospital actually are. One local doctor, believing that New England State Hospital performed electric shock treatments, had been referring patients to the hospital for that purpose for some time. The hospital admitted them all, though shock treatments have been discontinued for years.

Lacking a clear sense of treatment goals and what it is trying to accomplish in general for its patients, the hospital does not find it necessary to formulate any meaningful criteria for admission over and above those required by law. In true "chicken and egg fashion," the lack of criteria for admission creates a highly diverse patient population, whose needs and problems are so varied that it becomes nearly impossible for the hospital to formulate overall treatment goals. Within the hospital are to be found alcoholics, drug addicts, persons being examined in connection with court charges, retarded and otherwise organically brain-damaged persons, the elderly and infirm, persons undergoing marital or life adjustment or even post-operative crises, teen-age runaways, and finally persons whose confusion, hallucinations, and disassociated speech obviously indicate a psychotic state. With this kind of admixture of patients, the easiest course for the hospital is to minimize the individuality and variety of patient problems, and to emphasize instead the lowest common denominators of patient needs—food, shelter, and sedation with drugs to ensure cooperative behavior.

Professional Marginality

Although active treatment and rehabilitation programs could be provided for even such a large and diverse patient population, in none of its ranks does the hospital have the professional competency to do so. All but one of the twenty-odd clinical doctors who staffed the various units of the hospital were foreign-born, foreign-trained, and unlicensed, and have little or no psychiatric training. These doctors, by their failure to meet prevailing medical standards and to pass the general medical examinations for foreign doctors, are *legally* unfit and incompetent to enter the mainstream of American medicine and to engage in private medical practice. Yet the state has permitted their indefinite practice in the state mental hospitals. A recent state ruling that would require even these doctors to demonstrate some minimal competence in the basic sciences and English language has been predictably greeted with defensive, self-righteous outrage, by the older doctors especially, who stand to lose their undemanding, relatively well-paid (considering their lack of qualifications), housing-provided niche in the hospital hierarchy.

Aside from their basic medical and psychiatric ineptitude, these doctors generally speak and understand English only poorly and are without the awareness of American culture and social life that would permit understanding of a patient's life situation or background. One doctor, for example, became very confused about why a newly admitted patient was so worried about money, when she had said her husband was a photographer. What the woman had actually said, however, was that her husband was on *welfare*. The doctors often view mentally disturbed behavior with the hostility and contempt that derive from their own unexamined cultural and class biases, and they may be quite patrician in their demeanor with patients.

The professional qualifications of other staff members are comparably weak. Attendants need not even have a high school diploma to qualify for work. Licensed Practical Nurses far outnumber the better trained and educated Registered Nurses. As recently as the spring of 1971, about two-thirds of a social work staff of twenty had only a BA degree. The psychology department numbered more advanced degrees and professional credentials among its members, but the senior psychologist could always be counted on to offer extremely cynical commentary whenever discussion in meetings turned to possibilities for change in the hospital. He once wrote an article in his professional field on the impossibility of doing treatment with mental hospital patients!

The patient, then, is a victim of the limited qualifications of the staff and receives only limited care at their hands. Doctors define their roles very narrowly to include only those functions which they are quite certain they can perform. Therefore, they will interview patients and register diagnoses for legal record-keeping purposes, but the interview is not meant to suggest a doctor-patient relationship, nor does the diagnosis imply a program of treatment. Social workers have traditionally been at the service of both the hospital record room and the doctors, for whom they are expected to gather odds and ends of facts, necessary to complete various patient records but usually socially and psychologically irrelevant.

The nursing role is reduced to its most fundamental and traditional level— that is, simply taking care of people. A "good" patient is one who is easy to care for and have around. Such a patient also becomes a display model of behavior for all other patients. For example, the head nurse on a ward called attention to a pitiful, severely retarded, docile, grinning young man. "He's so good," she said. "We wish all of our patients were like this." (Here, indeed, is proof of the nonfictional nature of Kesey's "Big Nurse," in *One Flew Over the Cuckoo's Nest.*) Of course, a more alert, more capable patient quickly learns to suppress those characteristics which might indicate a greater sense of self-interest and more potential for mental health lest he become a nuisance to the nursing staff. The regression and inertia of the custodial patient becomes the norm.

The Medical Model

Particularly in the context of a staff of poorly qualified physicians, the hierarchical organization of personnel along the lines of the medical model—according to which the doctor not only is in charge but also has unquestioned and unquestionable authority—further fragments and minimizes patient care. Echoing the unimaginative approach of the doctors to whom they are subordinate, personnel in all other departments also function within narrow limits, performing mostly of-the-moment compartmentalized tasks. There is little communication or interrelationship between the various departments. As there is no comprehensive treatment program for an individual patient, there is little incentive for one department to have any interest in or knowledge of what another department might be doing on a patient's behalf. Doctors sometimes discharge patients without informing or consulting any of the other professionals involved.

The doctors are at the top of a status hierarchy that ranks all other jobs as beneath the doctors' in importance and prestige. It is the job of the nonphysician staff simply to complement the "expertise" of the doctors, rather than to make integral contributions of their own to patient care. It is not only lack of money which prevents available job blocs for additional registered nurses from being filled; it is also the lack of encouragement for the well-trained nurse to use her talents in interesting and innovative ways. Similarly, although a new director of social service has been able to hire a number of professionally trained social workers, they can have little impact in a system where their talents are not put to maximum use nor their skills respected. The idea that a social worker might take an active clinical and diagnostic role was greeted with derisive laughter by doctors and psychologists alike in one meeting.

The doctors jealously guard their authority, knowing possibly how little they are respected by other staff members, who frequently make disparaging remarks about them. They also display great resistance to shared professional contributions to patient care, as the following indicates (the reference is to an experimental admissions screening program begun by the social service department and is taken from a letter written by one of the hospital doctors to the local paper):

(Social workers) spend six months or so in an office next to the admissions room eagerly awaiting the proper time to pounce upon the . . . patient with a barrage of prepared social questions, becoming oblivious for an hour or more of his medical and mental needs. And after the patient is thus traumatized . . . the patient is thus released to the doctor.

Schools of social work everywhere will surely be astonished by this news that a patient's mental and medical needs are entirely unrelated to his social self!

Leadership as Public Relations

The hospital administrators themselves do not lead; they simply oversee the *status quo*. Although the superintendent and his two assistants are licensed doctors and trained psychiatrists, they assumed a consultant role, rather than an ongoing active clinical role, in the hospital. All three men are in their sixties and obviously have a vested interest in maintaining their good standing with the state department of mental health until the time of their retirement. They take no issue with the hospital as custodial facility and have no aspirations for it to be otherwise. Nor do they judge it possible to alter the custodial emphasis.

There is great administrative sensitivity to how the hospital appears to the public, and the administrators seem to be primarily concerned with promoting good public relations rather than patient care *per se*. When a group of concerned citizens requested a tour of the hospital, the supervisor ordered all patients normally kept in restraint or seclusion to be released for the period of the visit. Fresh paint on the normally dingy walls of the ward heralded a guided tour for the visiting committee of the state mental health association, who had come to evaluate hospital conditions. Outside donation of clothes is no longer permitted, lest the community think the hospital is not meeting patient needs.

Official statements emphasize the hospital as residential rather than treatment facility and call attention to the improvement of current living conditions over those of the past. When a controversy arose over the numbers of unlicensed physicians in state mental hospitals, the supervisor of New England State Hospital skillfully diverted attention from the real issue of the quality of patient care by threatening that the hospital might have to close and neglect its patients if he lost his staff of doctors through their mere inability to pass exams. Not long afterward the local paper printed a full-page-complete-with-pictures report of progress, comfort, and dedication at New England State Hospital.

The hospital and the semi-rural communities and small urban areas that it serves coexist peacefully. Local people seem to regard the hospital as meeting their needs in a suitably benign and low-keyed manner. They note with appreciation, for example, the recreational use they are permitted of a parcel of hospital land. As volunteers and participants in local mental health organizations, they are gratified to assist the much touted, well-intentioned work of the hospital. During the debate about accreditation of doctors, local public response was supportive of the hospital generally and sympathetic specifically to the doctors, who were clearly seen as underdogs.

From the administrative point of view, the duty of the hospital is to be the waiting receptacle for anyone who comes its way by whatever route. Patients are to be duly admitted, processed, housed, and maintained. Discharge has no specified qualitative meaning. Patients leave when the length of stay required by the admitting paper is up, or a voluntary patient decides to leave, or a family takes a relative home in its custody. The overriding concern of the administrators with regard to any or all parts of this cycle is to comply with all legal requirements and to avoid scandal. Some social workers have attempted to gain placement elsewhere for long-term patients who no longer require hospitalization. Many relatives of such patients, however, have clearly stated their wish that their patient-kin remain where they are. The administration is reluctant to intervene lest the hospital become a target of the families' anger.

Resistance to Change

The administrators have only a passive acceptance of change. Although staff members are not particularly encouraged to try out new ideas or programs, they are usually given indifferent permission to do so on their own motivation. Any changes, of course, require that the formal authority of the doctors and administration is left intact and legal requirements are not interfered with. But attempts to individualize and humanize the system of patient care are outside the scope of the official definition of patient care. While such efforts may be tolerated, therefore, they are not facilitated by any structural changes which would ensure the shared concern and communication necessary for those efforts to be permanently successful.

The experimental admissions program, undertaken in 1971 by the social service department, is a case in point. It was an attempt to replace previous automatic, rubber-stamped procedures with support, advice, and, if possible, referral elsewhere for the person seeking admission. For those finally admitted, the intention was to emphasize helpful involvement with both patient and family from the beginning, and to collect information pertinent to eventual diagnosis and treatment.

It quickly became clear that screening patients had little meaning, when most doctors and hospital administrators had no real interest in formulating specific guidelines for admission and did not wish to hear social service suggestions in that regard. There was also nowhere to go with painstakingly gathered data, when doctors were unresponsive to its use for their understanding or diagnosis of a patient. Significantly, the program was openly welcomed only by the one clinical doctor who happened to be a fully trained psychiatrist.

Like the experimental admissions program, other efforts to broaden the scope of patient care invariably have an idiosyncratic base rather than a structural one and consequently meet with similarly qualified success. The years since 1971 have seen the introduction of a program of behavioral modification on one of the back wards, the provision of in-hospital legal services, and the establishment of an incentive community to aid in the resocialization of 60 chronic patients. In none of these cases, however, was the change suggested or initiated by either the hospital administrators or medical staff, and in two of the three instances, the impetus for change originated outside the hospital altogether, with professionals who wished to establish training opportunities for students. In the face of varying degrees of official indifference, the continued existence of such programs rests mainly on the amount of time and energy that a few individuals are able to give to them.

Even the most dedicated individual efforts, however, are not sufficient to do the job these programs were intended to do, for they exist at arm's length from the ongoing system of patient care; they leave untouched the core structure of custodial care, which tends by its very functioning to weaken the objectives of the new programs. The behavioral modification program, for example, does not involve the ward personnel, who continue to carry out their duties in routine custodial fashion. Thus, the behavioral modification approach receives none of the reinforcement or follow-through necessary to build its effectiveness. In the case of the legal services program, insofar as patients know of its availability, they find their way to legal advice on their own. Only rarely has a staff member referred a patient to the service, and then only with regard to a purely private matter. While not prohibited from doing so, patients are not encouraged by physicians, social workers, or other staff to use the legal service to seek clarification of the legal terms of their own admission and commitment to and discharge from the hospital.

It is far too soon to make any general statement about the long-range success of the incentive community in preparing patients for, and placing them in, living and work settings outside of the hospital. Undoubtedly the incentive community (which receives its own federal funds) actually benefits in many ways by its almost total isolation from the rest of the patient and staff community. But to some degree the potential of the incentive community depends on the potential of the patients referred for participation from the regular hospital wards. Referrals are supposed to reflect a qualitative evaluation of a patient's readiness and capacity to accept the increased responsibility entailed by the resocialization process. The consulting psychologist for the incentive community mentions the problem of inappropriate referrals—patients who are shuttled off into the incentive community less because of their ability to participate than because it is a convenient way to reduce the census population of a given ward. Once again signs of the familiar pattern of cross-purposes at work!

Expectations of Patient Families

Patients and patient families are hardly in a position to offer any criticism of the hospital as it is. For persons with limited ability to pay, New England State Hospital, costing less than $15 a day, is the only care available. Frequently lacking the knowledge with which to judge the quality of hospital care, families are reassured that the care at New England State Hospital is the only care possible. "Your boy is so sick, you'd better sign this paper so we can keep him here (another few weeks) (indefinitely)." I think here of the mother who mentioned that her daughter had been badly bruised in the hospital and said resignedly, "They told me she was hard to handle."

The rigid medical diagnostic approach used by the hospital no doubt conveys the impression to families that mental illness is a sort of irreversible disease entity and leads to rather low expectations of what can be done for a patient in the first place. Thus if a patient has to make frequent return trips to the hospital, as many do, it is not because the hospital might have done a better job of treatment or aftercare planning. It is rather because mental illness is always there and prone to act up, and when it does, it is the accepted rule of the hospital to take care of the patient until symptoms abate.

Families themselves often seek to relieve a host of family tensions by seeking admission for a family member whose behavior is particularly disturbed or disturbing. When they visit their patient-relative in the hospital, they are relieved to see that he or she is calmer or more "normal," the result usually of heavy doses of chlorpromazine or other drugs. Seldom are they concerned with the means used to bring about the change or with how durable or deep the change is. In any case, it is the patient who is expected to change. Hospitalization encourages a focus on the behavior of the patient alone, and spares other family members the need for consideration of their own interactive behavior with the patient and even possible contributions to his problems. Ex-patients whose behavior at home is not as compliant as a family might wish can be readmitted to the hospital as punishment. One woman came with the necessary papers to admit her ex-patient husband, who had evidently been having an affair with a neighbor. The wife didn't like this at all and decided he "must be getting sick again"!

There is no doubt that a more questioning and assertive group of families and patients could motivate the hospital to better safeguard patient interests. For example, a well-educated, once-affluent woman of professional background was admitted to the hospital by her relatives because it was inexpensive and geographically convenient for them. She challenged furiously everything about the hospital, from cleanliness to diagnosis to her own civil rights. Although her refusal to fit in easily with regular hospital routine made her a "problem" case in the eyes of the staff, the fact is that the level of hospital care rose to meet her needs and expectations. She was soon taken out of her restraints and moved to a more open ward, visited by an outside doctor and lawyer upon her request, and permitted to leave the hospital before her required length of stay was technically over. More important, she escaped being permanently committed, as her relatives had wished her to be, because the doctors in charge frankly admitted that she would raise too many objections, and it was unlikely that they could make the psychotic diagnosis "stick."

Custodial Care—Who Benefits?

Now it is easy enough to postulate the kinds of changes needed if mental health care is actually to accomplish anything on behalf of its patients, in contrast to the custodial process discussed above. Much reform could take place within the existing hospital setting that would personalize patient care and facilitate treatment. Ideally the large-scale state institutions would be closed down altogether and replaced, say, by the less removed, more intimate, active settings of day-care centers, foster homes, half-way houses, psychiatric wards in general hospitals, and, of course, greatly expanded outpatient services in community mental health centers. Finally, even those persons whose disabilities are apparently permanent and who are consequently in need of ongoing custodial care surely deserve more cheerful, less stowed-away existences. This utopian state of affairs, of course, presupposes an underpinning of both widespread community concern and generous financial support.

But all that this is really saying is that patient interests ought to be central to mental health care. Indeed, if they were, custodial institutions such as New England State Hospital would long ago have ceased to exist. The explanation for their continued survival, as well as their resistance to change, is to be found in the many vested interests of nonpatient persons and groups, which are well served by the state mental hospital, precisely in its existing custodial form. From a sociological point of view, a New England State Hospital is quite functional — for everyone but its patients (cf. Gans, 1971). The interests served by each custodial facility as an individual institution are manifest in the very organization of the hospital itself as it has been discussed here:

(1) For the community and region, a large state hospital that admits all comers creates the illusion that all local mental health care needs are being met, thus eliminating the need for the tedious and unwelcome business of local planning and spending for mental health care.

(2) For the small town especially, a large-scale custodial mental institution offers employment to many people. As a service, the hospital creates no jarring discrepancy between itself and the often traditional character of other community institutions (education, politics, and the like).

(3) For hospital administrators, the safest route to status, job security, and pensions lies in the maintenance of the *status quo* and the promotion of good public relations.

(4) For poorly qualified, even incompetent professionals, otherwise unavailable jobs exist to which are attached income security, benefits, and at least hospital-defined status and power.

(5) For the hospital staff, custodial care is the easiest form of care.

(6) For a family, the hospital acts as stabilizer when the behavior of one of its members has become annoying or burdensome.

Furthermore, as part of an entire system of mental health care, the state institution undoubtedly receives continual support and reinforcement for its custodial operation from an even broader and more pervasive set of public and professional self-interests than those enumerated above:[6]

(1) For the general hospital and the general public, the state hospital conveniently eliminates the disturbed and disturbing from its midst.

(2) For many outside psychiatrists and other clinical professionals, the hospital siphons off the least affluent and least attractive of the mentally disturbed, whom they would prefer not to serve anyway.

(3) For a state department of mental health, the choice of hospital administrators is more easily made on a utilitarian basis of, say, seniority than on the

more complicated and uncertain basis of suitability for implementing specific formulated goals for patient care.

(4) For a state legislature, custodial care often appears to be the cheapest way, on a short-run, annual budget basis, of providing for a population doubly stigmatized by mental illness and lack of financial resources.

(5) Finally, for a whole society, the public mental hospital reassuringly clarifies matters by officially separating "them" from "us." Persons on the "outside" thus come to develop a sense of their own comparative well-being and a conviction of the rightness and stability of their own ways of life.

The apparent contradiction of the continuing existence of a New England State Hospital in an era dedicated to mental health reform is, thus, more easily understood. For the successful outcome of any decision to supersede custodial care with genuinely therapeutic help is necessarily dependent on two further decisions: to shape mental health policy around the interests of patients, rather than the claims of nonpatients; to design mental health services that reflect, in their own organization and procedures, the increased humanity and involvement of all concerned, rather than considerations of mere expediency. In a time when many pressing social problems clamor for attention and priority, it is perhaps not surprising that the public—legislators, taxpayers, and professionals alike—often chooses the path of least resistance in allowing the problem of mental health care to remain "out of sight, out of mind"—neatly packaged in the form of the custodial institution.

NOTES

I appreciate the comments and advice of Fred A. Kramer, Department of Political Science, University of Massachusetts, and Ely Chinoy, Department of Sociology and Anthropology, Smith College.

1. The name of the hospital is a pseudonym. The author was a member of the social service department of the New England State Hospital from the fall of 1970 to June 1971. Close contact has been maintained with the hospital since that time, and to the best of my knowledge the facts and interpretations contained in this paper remain valid.

2. For a discussion of a somewhat fortuitous shift from custodial to therapeutic care at one state mental hospital, see Robert Clurman, "The Patients Can Walk Out Any Time at Bronx State Mental Hospital," *N.Y. Times Magazine*, April 2, 1972, pp. 14*ff.*

3. With regard to the impact of the "right to treatment" lawsuits, Mechanic (1973) notes that their effect is likely to be more quantitative than qualitative: ". . . standards referring to a humane physical and social environment are more amenable to court action than those pertaining to individualized treatment regimens" (p. 23).

4. For an evaluation of present conditions and number of residents in state facilities for the mentally disabled, see the following articles in the *N.Y. Times*: ". . . Hope for Neglected in Mental Institutions," March 26, 1972, p. 35; "New Hope for the Retarded . . . ," June 11, 1972, pp. 1*ff.*

5. The right of mental patients to receive pay and social security and other employment benefits in return for the work they do in the state hospitals is an issue that has been raised in the courts, both in conjunction with the "right to treatment" suits and separately. As yet, however, no such guidelines are in effect for the patients of New England State Hospital.

6. Additional support for these concluding points may be found variously in the following writings: Cumming and Cumming (1957); Hollingshead and Redlich (1958), see especially Part 4; Coles (1964); Cumming (1967); Scheff (1967), see especially articles by Mechanic and Szasz.

REFERENCES

Belknap, I. *Human Problems of a State Mental Hospital;* McGraw-Hill, 1956.

Coles, R. "Psychiatrists and the Poor," *Atlantic Monthly,* July 1964, pp. 102–106.

Cumming, E. "Allocation of Care to the Mentally Ill, American Style," in M. N. Zald (Ed.), *Organizing for Community Welfare;* Quadrangle Books, 1967.

Cumming, E., and Cumming, J. *Closed Ranks;* Harvard Univ. Press, 1957.

Dunham, H. W., and Weinberg, S. K. *The Culture of the State Mental Hospital;* Wayne State Univ. Press, 1960.

Gans, H. "The Uses of Poverty: The Poor Pay All," *Social Policy* (1971) 2(2):20–24.

Goffman, E. *Asylums;* Doubleday, 1961.

Hollingshead, A. B., and Redlich, F. C. *Social Class and Mental Illness;* Wiley, 1958.

Kennedy, J. F. *Mental Illness and Mental Retardation, Presidential Message;* Govt. Printing Office, 1963.

Kesey, K. *One Flew Over the Cuckoo's Nest;* New Amer. Library, 1962.

Mechanic, D. "The Right to Treatment: Judicial Action and Social Change," paper presented at Conference on Right to Treatment, Dept. of Clin. Psychology, Univ. of Mass., Amherst, 1973.

Scheff, T. J. *Mental Illness and Social Processes;* Harper & Row, 1967.

Szasz, T. J. *The Myth of Mental Illness;* Dell, 1961.

Jonathan F. Borus

Deinstitutionalization of the Chronically Mentally Ill

Deinstitutionalization of the mentally ill has become the predominant public mental-health policy in most states. This policy has been supported by a curious political marriage of liberals, who decry the custodial-level care in state mental hospitals, and conservatives, who see the closing of expensive public institutions as an easy way to save tax dollars. Deinstitutionalization has been effected by discharging long-term inpatients from state hospitals and making it increasingly difficult to admit new patients. Over the past decade, it has resulted in the shift of the primary locus of clinical care in the public sector from traditional inpatient settings to community-based outpatient facilities.

The peculiar historical intertwining of mental-health care and government accounts for the fact that this major change in the delivery of care resulted from sociopolitical as well as clinical considerations. Since colonial times, the care of the mentally ill and the protection of the community from disturbance by them have been responsibilities of the state and local governments. Successively located over the years in jails and almshouses, state hospitals, and outpatient community-mental-health centers (CMHCs), a separate public delivery system dependent on the political process has been maintained for mental-health care. The persistence of this separate system to the present day stems not only from the paucity of insurance coverage for private treatment but also from the chronic and often debilitating nature of severe mental illnesses such as schizophrenia, affective disorders, and organic mental syndromes.

It is the nature of the political process to foster oversimplification of

From *New England Journal of Medicine* 305 (1981):339–342. Reprinted by permission of the publisher and the author.

complex issues so that a single solution can be advocated that will overcome the inertia inhibiting major change in governmental policy or practice. Deinstitutionalization was the political solution proposed in response to professional requests in the 1960s for major improvements in state-hospital care and for the development of public treatment facilities for the mentally ill in the community.[1] In support of this solution, a number of unproved and often conflicting wishful assumptions or fantasies about deinstitutionalization have been presented to the public as facts. This paper discusses five of these fantasies and contrasts them with the clinical realities of deinstitutionalization during the past decade.

Fantasies and Facts

Mental Hospitals Are Harmful and Are Not Needed

Some advocates of deinstitutionalization espouse the wishful assumption that severe mental illnesses do not exist and that the so-called chronically mentally ill primarily have iatrogenic disabilities secondary to confinement in a mental hospital.[2,3] The difficulty with this fantasy is that it disregards the evidence that genetic linkages, differential responses to pharmacologic agents, or organic disorders can define discrete types of disabling mental illness.[4] In addition, it ignores the fact that although a regressive, custodial inpatient milieu can further debilitate these patients, the affective and cognitive symptoms associated with psychotic illness are usually evident before hospitalization and are often the cause for it.

Despite these contradictory facts, this assumption has been used to justify plans to phase out state hospitals. In support of such plans, two factors are cited: the success in cutting the public-mental-hospital census in the past 25 years by over 70 per cent (from 559,000 patients in 1955 to approximately 150,000 today)[5] and the clinical observation that many patients who were previously kept in mental hospitals can be effectively treated as outpatients with psychoactive medication, with or without brief stabilizing hospitalization in general hospitals or CMHCs. However, such plans falsely assume that important societal functions now undertaken by public mental institutions — specifically, care and asylum for the most severely ill and protection of the public from them — can be shifted to community facilities.[6] Experience over the past decade has shown that some patients continue to need mental-hospital settings because of the severity of their behavioral disorders. Such violent, incompetent, or suicidal patients cannot survive in the community and are unsuited for inpatient units in a general hospital or CMHC because they require long-term care in a secure facility for their own protection and that of society.[7] In addition, less severely disturbed patients who are admitted to general-hospital or CMHC inpatient units and who require the temporary security of a locked unit or an extended stay beyond the usual 30-day limit for stabilization are often discharged back to the community before improvement occurs. Without the availability of mental hospitals as backup for public-sector patients, the pressure on acute-care units to free up beds causes a revolving-door syndrome of repeated hospitalizations, each of which is too brief to bring the patient's illness under control.[8]

The political motive underlying the notion that mental hospitals are necessarily harmful is revealed by the lack of opposition to private hospitals that are not dependent on public funding. Many private mental hospitals have locked and long-term units. Neither politicians nor the public view them as harmful or custodial facilities because, unlike state hospitals, they have adequate resources to provide active treatment. The rush to close "harmful" institutions also ignores the growing evidence that many patients discharged from state hospitals have been "transinstitutionalized" to nursing homes and penal institutions.[9,10] It has yet to be demonstrated that either of these settings offers better treatment or custodial care for the mentally ill than do state hospitals.

Outpatient Treatment Is What the Chronically Mentally Ill Really Need

Deinstitutionalization has also been promoted under the assumption that state-hospital care for the less fortunate can be replaced by outpatient psychiatric care that is similar to the private therapy available to patients of means. Unfortunately, differences in resources, scale, and mandate prevent this extrapolation from rich to poor. CMHCs, today's publicly subsidized alternative to private outpatient care, suffer from inadequate funding and unstable staffing (especially of psychiatrists), too large a service responsibility (75,000 to 200,000 citizens per service area), and a mandate that prohibits refusal to treat anyone from their area.[11] Although appropriate outpatient treatment in CMHCs has decreased the need of many patients for institutional care,[12] the marginal funding given CMHCs reinforces the reality that the public will not support the same quality of services for poor patients as the rich can purchase.

This fantasy also assumes that the numerous needs for care that are met by a residential institution can be satisfied solely by outpatient psychiatric treatment. The state hospital took responsibility not only for mental-health care but also for the patient's housing, food, finances, medical care, medications, work activities, and social relations.[13] The deinstitutionalized patient's limited abilities to cope are often overwhelmed when he or she is forced to seek these types of care from multiple, uncoordinated community agencies.[14] Many CMHCs have devoted their limited resources to helping the chronically ill obtain such needed treatment and supportive services. Other CMHCs have ignored this costly task and have preferred to use their resources to treat a much larger group of less severely ill people. The wishful notion that these patients will require such supportive services only for a transitional period as they move from the hospital to independent community life is not supported by the data, which show that the chronically mentally ill need ongoing care to maintain a reasonable level of function.[15,16] Without continuously available services, most of these patients' conditions deteriorate, and they either require rehospitalization or lead isolated, marginal lives in the community that are similar to life in state hospitals' "back wards."[15-17]

The Public Wants Deinstitutionalization

This fantasy hinges on the assumption that the patient and the patient's family and neighbors prefer that treatment take place in the community. In fact, some patients in state hospitals resist leaving the institution that has taken care of them, albeit at a sub-standard level, for many years. Life in the community requires patients to struggle to get basic needs met, and with the scarcity of low-cost housing, the number of homeless patients carrying their worlds around in shopping bags has noticeably increased. Emergency-room clinicians witness daily the desperate attempts of the chronically ill to circumvent the restrictive admissions policies of public hospitals with repeated and often increasingly destructive demonstrations of their need to be admitted when they cannot cope in the community.

Families have often had considerable difficulties with the patient before hospitalization, and thus they hesitate to reassume the psychological and financial burdens of living with their disturbed relative. This stressful task for the family appears to be better tolerated when mental-health professionals provide them with direct support[18]; however, studies to determine the long-term effects on the lives of family members, specifically on the development of young children living with a psychotic relative, have not been reported.

Finally, communities often fear that increased violence and socially disruptive behavior will result from the deinstitutionalization of the mentally ill. Although some exceptional communities have organized impressive efforts to reintegrate these patients, others have used restrictive zoning and legal measures to attempt to prevent large numbers of the chronically ill from living in the area. Citizens may abstractly agree that it is a good idea to return the patient to the community, but few want any to live on their own block. As a result of such sentiment, most group-living facilities for deinstitutionalized patients end up in a community's least attractive neighborhoods to avoid arousing citizens' resistance.[19]

Deinstitutionalization Will Cost Less

The pivotal political assumption that appears to have motivated deinstitutionalization is that state tax dollars would be saved by closing state hospitals and by the resultant decreased cost of providing mental-health services for the chronically ill patients in the community. The fact is that state mental-health budgets have increased over the past decade with inflation and with the continued need to fund both institutional and community care. Although antiquated state hospitals are expensive to heat and maintain, they have proved to be politically difficult to close. Government workers' unions and rural towns whose economies depend on their state hospitals have fought the loss of jobs and the changes that are required to close hospitals and to shift staff to community settings.[20,21] Since deinstitutionalization has been advocated as a cost-saving measure, politicians have been reluctant to allocate sufficient additional resources to improve the institutions and to ensure that adequate community-based programs are in place when patients arrive.

Even though studies to date have not demonstrated direct savings from treating the chronically ill in the community,[19,22] state governments have continued to push deinstitutionalization because it yields them relative savings by shifting some of the fiscal burden onto the federal and local governments. The states have "passed the buck" to the federal government, which provides Supplemental Security Income and Medicaid payments to the severely ill when they are not institutionalized, and to local governments, which must bear the costs of providing additional community services (e.g., those of police, emergency medical workers, and mental-health professionals) to handle the needs of disorganized patients.[5,9,22]

"Someone Else" Is Ultimately Responsible (to Blame) for the Care of These Patients

In the past, state and local governments were held responsible for their hospitals' dismal conditions, which, despite geographic isolation, were intermittently brought to the public's attention by the media, causing great political embarrassment. Although the unmet needs of the chronically ill living in the community are more visible with deinstitutionalization, their care has become diffused among so many agencies that it is unclear whom to hold responsible.[8]

As it has become apparent that the political act of deinstitutionalization alone will not solve the multiple problems of these patients, the states have tried to assign the responsibility (and blame) for community care to the federal government and the CMHC program that it initiated in 1963. In this political shell game, the federal government reminds the states that federal CMHC funding was always designated as "seed money" to stimulate the development of community-based services and was never intended to replace the states' historic responsibility for the mentally ill.[23] Private insurers claim that their subscribers will not support the costs of extended mental-health coverage, and a national health insurance that might support services for the chronically ill remains a distant possibility.

New Initiatives

Two new political initiatives are aimed at clarifying responsibility for the conduct and costs of care of deinstitutionalized patients. Stemming from the findings of the President's Commission on Mental Health, the recently passed Mental Health Systems Act (P.L. 96-398) will provide federal grants to help the chronically mentally ill function outside institutions. The act authorizes appropriation of $48 million for the 1982 fiscal year to state mental-health authorities and CMHCs, which will take responsibility for coordinating services for the chronically ill and upgrading the skills of the staff who work with them.

Considering the size of the problem, the authorized funding for this initiative seems minuscule: the Massachusetts Department of Mental Health alone spends over four times that amount annually on the chronically ill. In addition, it appears doubtful that the conservative new administration and Congress will support even that inadequate funding level. Like past federal mental-health initiatives, this act offers only time-limited seed money to the states, without assuming long-term programmatic or fiscal responsibility. The Mental Health Systems Act, therefore, represents an incremental step that could bolster current services and improve the quality of community-based care systems; it is so limited in size and scope, however, that it cannot solve the vast and expensive problems of the chronically ill.

A second initiative, occurring at the state level, has been the effort to "privatize" the care of the mentally ill. In Massachusetts, for example, both inpatient and outpatient care are being contracted to private non-profit providers, who are not bound to the state delivery system's fiscal inflexibility, civil-service regulations, and union demands. It is hypothesized that private agencies can deliver better and more efficient clinical care than the state can. In addition, these agencies are eligible to recoup third-party reimbursements — less readily available to public providers — which can help support the costs of care. Although this plan inventively aims to create a one-class care system that can better support itself, the basic responsibility for financing this system will remain with the state. Since many of the services required to support the chronically ill are not reimbursable by insurers, the success or failure of privatization will be determined by the willingness of the state to underwrite these final costs. It is questionable whether political administrators and legislators are likely to be any more reliable in funding the increasing costs of care under contract to private providers than they were in funding the state's own delivery system directly.

Politics and Patient Care

The political process has condensed the complex issues of caring for the chronically mentally ill into a single problem, the state hospital, with a single solution, the policy of deinstitutionalization. This policy has replaced the prior political solution, under which institutional care of the mentally ill in the state hospitals was the predominant approach for over a century. To clinicians, it is obvious that patients with chronic mental disorders have substantive illnesses requiring diverse treatment and supportive services in both the hospital and the community. Predictably, deinstitutionalization has helped patients for whom prolonged hospitalization was inappropriate treatment and has hurt patients whose needs for care cannot be met in the community. Clearly, the choice of care should be determined by the clinicians' treatment decisions about individual patients rather than by political policy that indiscriminately dictates any single alternative.

The decade of deinstitutionalization has provided many positive byproducts. In their attempts to help very sick patients, mental-health professionals have learned much about the clinical care of the chronically mentally ill in the community. Innovative model programs, most of which have been supported by special funding from the National Institute of Mental Health, have demonstrated that with discriminate evaluation of the strengths and needs of the individual patient, adequate resources, designated responsibility for care, long-term provision of services, professional flexibility, and public support, many patients can lead reasonable lives outside institutions.[12,15,24]

The limited ability to generalize and reproduce these model programs nationwide is in large part due to the public's enduring unwillingness to pay for high-quality care for the mentally ill. The custodial-level funding that politicians allocated to state hospitals over the years accurately reflected this limited public support; deinstitutionalization has shown that without sufficient resources, simply changing the locus of bad care will not create good care. Since provision of the many high-quality treatment alternatives that the severely ill require is an expensive proposition, it is even less likely to receive broad support in these times of fiscal restraint. Without adequate treatment resources, mental patients can be expected to become more disturbingly visible and bothersome to our communities. It is to be hoped that reinstitutionalization will not be the next "new" political solution, for no single "inexpensive" remedy will alleviate the suffering or adequately serve the complex needs of the chronically mentally ill.

REFERENCES

1. Joint Commission on Mental Illness and Health. Action for mental health. New York: Basic Books, 1961.
2. Szasz TS. The myth of mental illness. Am Psychol. 1960; 15:113–8.
3. Rosenhan DL. On being sane in insane places. Science. 1973; 179:250–8.
4. Snyder SH. Biological aspects of mental disorder. New York: Oxford University Press, 1980.
5. Toward a national plan for the chronically mentally ill: report to the Secretary by the Department of Health and Human Services Steering Committee on the Chronically Mentally Ill, December 1980. Rockville, Md.: Department of Health and Human Services, 1981. (DHHS publication no. (ADM)81-1077).
6. Bachrach LL. Deinstitutionalization: an analytical review and sociological perspective. Washington, D.C.: Government Printing Office, 1976. (DHEW publication no. (ADM)76-351).

7. Lamb HR, Goertzel V. The demise of the state hospital—a premature obituary? Arch Gen. Psychiatry. 1972; 26:489-95.
8. Rieder RO. Hospitals, patients, and politics. Schizophrenia Bull. 1974; 11:9-15.
9. Sharfstein SS, Turner JEC, Clark HW. Financing issues in the delivery of services to the chronically mentally ill and disabled. In: Talbott JA, ed. The chronic mental patient: problems, solutions, and recommendations for a public policy. Washington, D.C.: American Psychiatric Association, 1978:137-50.
10. Swank GE, Winer D. Occurrence of psychiatric disorder in a county jail population. Am J Psychiatry. 1976; 133:1331-3.
11. Borus JF. Issues critical to the survival of community mental health. Am J Psychiatry. 1978; 135:1029-35.
12. Hansell N, Willis GL. Outpatient treatment of schizophrenia. Am J Psychiatry. 1977; 134: 1082-6.
13. Borus JF, Hatow E. The patient and the community. In: Shershow JC, ed. Schizophrenia: science and practice. Cambridge: Harvard University Press, 1978:171-96.
14. Returning the mentally disabled to the community: government needs to do more (report to Congress by the Comptroller General of the United States, January 7, 1977). Washington, D.C.: General Accounting Office, 1977.
15. Stein LI, Test MA. Alternative to mental hospital treatment. I. Conceptual model, treatment program, and clinical evaluation. Arch Gen Psychiatry. 1980; 37:392-7.
16. Davis A, Dinitz S, Pasamanick B. Schizophrenics in the new custodial community. Columbus, Ohio: Ohio State University Press, 1974.
17. Lamb HR, Goertzel V. The long-term patient in the era of community treatment. Arch Gen Psychiatry. 1977; 34:679-82.
18. Creer C, Wing J. Living with a schizophrenic patient. Br J Hosp Med. 1975; 14:73-82.
19. Kirk SA, Therrien ME. Community mental health myths and the fate of former hospitalized patients. Psychiatry. 1975; 38:209-17.
20. Greenblatt M, Glazier E. The phasing out of mental hospitals in the United States. Am J Psychiatry. 1975; 132:1135-40.
21. Becker A, Schulberg HC. Phasing out state hospitals—a psychiatric dilemma. N Engl J Med. 1976; 294:255-61.
22. Weisbrod BA, Test MA, Stein LI. Alternative to mental hospital treatment. II. Economic benefit-cost analysis. Arch Gen Psychiatry. 1980; 37:400-5.
23. Weiner RS, Woy JR, Sharfstein SS, Bass RD. Community mental health centers and the "seed money" concept: effects of terminating federal funds. Community Mental Health J. 1979; 15:129-38.
24. Turner JEC, TenHoor WJ. The NIMH community support program: pilot approach to a needed social reform. Schizophr Bull. 1978; 4:319-44.

Walter B. Simon

On Reluctance to Leave
the Public Mental Hospital

It is usually considered to be a good and desirable thing for all parties concerned that a hospitalized person should prefer to live outside a hospital and
give up his patient status as soon as possible. This is particularly true of
patients in a public mental hospital.[1] Discussions of this topic are often couched
more in moral or emotional terms than in objective ones, and a patient's lack
of desire to leave the hospital is usually considered "bad." I shall suggest here
that certain patients may have rational reasons for wanting to remain at a hospital beyond the time considered appropriate by the staff, that this is particularly true of the socioeconomically inadequate patient, and that the problem
of the chronic patient can be solved only by an explicit recognition of the realistic difficulties such patients would encounter once out of the hospital.

To prefer staying in a public mental hospital rather than go back to the
"outside" is sometimes attributed to internal causes (the illness) and sometimes
thought to be the result of external causes (institutionalization). The latter
notion has resulted in great efforts in recent years to shorten the hospital stay
of patients. Either conception implies that there is something irrational,
inappropriate, or wrong about a patient's desire to stay longer than the staff
considers necessary.

In discussing whether or not it may be desirable for a patient to stay in a hospital, a minimum of six factors should be considered: (1) The type of hospital
concerned; (2) those maladaptive characteristics of the patient usually considered to be evidence of psychopathology; (3) those maladaptive characteristics

From *Psychiatry* 28 (1965):145–156. Copyright © 1965 by The William Alanson White Psychiatric
Foundation, Inc. Reprinted by permission of the publisher and the author.

usually considered to be evidence of social incompetence;[2] (4) the patient's place in the socioeconomic structure; (5) what the patient is apt to gain or lose; and (6) what others (relatives, neighbors, the police, the courts, and so on) are apt to gain or lose. The present discussion will deal with limited aspects of these factors solely in relation to the public mental hospital.

The Acute Unit: Its Patients and Its Functions

"Acute hospital unit" is usually synonymous with "admission service." All, or almost all, newly admitted patients are assigned to this unit. It should be added here that "newly admitted" as administratively defined may mean any of the following: (1) A person never having been seen by a professional person concerning mental problems; (2) a person referred, or committed, by a professional person but little, if at all, known by him; (3) a person known to a nonmental health professional (nonpsychiatric physician, teacher, and so forth) and referred or committed by him; (4) a person known to and referred or committed by a mental health professional; (5) a person having been at a mental health clinic where he has been exposed to one or more professionals; (6) a person who has been in another mental hospital at some earlier time; (7) a person directly transferred from another hospital (that is, he arrives as a patient); (8) a person who has been in the same hospital (that is, he is well-known to the staff: "We know *him*"). These are the steps to chronic patient-hood, from the point of view of admission to a mental hospital. People with the higher numbers in this catalogue usually have been through some or all of the previous steps.

Patients in an acute unit are thus heterogeneous from the point of view of initial onset of illness, ranging from those completely new to the mental patient role to those only too well acquainted with it. Similarly, patients in the acute unit range over the gamut of psychiatric diagnoses. Thus, being a patient in an acute unit does not necessarily mean being acutely disturbed. With the exception of the transfer group, usually comprising only a small percentage of new admissions,[3] the one characteristic all these patients have in common is that all of them lived outside a mental hospital for at least a short period immediately prior to entering this hospital. For many of these patients, this also meant that they managed to get along in society, if not well, at least marginally.

After a patient has been in the acute unit for several days to several months, he is transferred to the chronic unit. The exact time varies with the policy of a particular hospital, the number of new admissions that need be accommodated at a particular time (that is, the bed capacity of the admission ward), and how well the patient gets along with the staff and with his fellow patients.[4] Since many patients remain in the hospital for rather brief periods of time and never leave the admission service,[5] to quite an extent the *discharge* part of a public hospital's statistics refers to the turnover of the admissions unit. From this, it follows that the discharge records of mental hospitals which provide only short-term care and those whose patients for various reasons (administrative policy, monetary cost, and so on) stay for only a brief period would be more comparable to the discharge rate of the public hospital's acute unit than to the discharge rate of the entire public hospital.

In most hospitals, the major therapeutic efforts, particularly those involving psychotherapy, are concentrated on patients in the acute unit. The main watchwords are to "get the patients out," and to "get the patients well." These two aims are not always consistent with each other. Sometimes a few additional weeks or months might be helpful in changing a patient's outlook on life, and perhaps that of his relatives; a very brief hospitalization may be quite useless.[6] In some situations, outpatient care would be preferable, if available; in other situations, temporary separation from the patient's surroundings may be the most important element leading to recovery. This would involve the isolation of a person from circumstances that are unpleasant, or that offer problems which are difficult or impossible to solve.[7] This is the "asylum" or "retreat" function of the hospital.

While such isolation is often desirable, long hospitalization usually would be quite inappropriate, even if the facilities of the hospital are adequate or better.[8] The balancing of the benefits to be derived from a somewhat longer stay with the dangers of institutionalization requires a decision in each individual case. Among the factors to be considered are the needs of the patient and of his relatives, the particular setting, and the availability of treatment personnel.

An Example of the Retreat Function: The Lower-Class
Dissatisfied Housewife

The importance of temporary separation is well illustrated by one sizable group of patients — the lower-class dissatisfied housewife. Many of these women enter a hospital with complaints of depression or anxiety; some would be considered neurotic, some psychotic. These women usually are unable or unwilling to do the housework and take care of the children. An important positive aspect of their hospitalization is that it removes them from a life situation seen as boring and not self-fulfilling; frequently they also feel their efforts as not being properly appreciated. The positive role of hospitalization for this group may be similar to the more well-to-do woman's vacation in the country, fling in the city, weekly bridge game, and so on. On the negative side, the price paid by these women is a certain degree of anxiety and depression — that is, suffering. Their husbands frequently blame them for going to the hospital to avoid their housewifely responsibilities. While many of these husbands have their own problems, there frequently is more than a modicum of truth in their accusations. Mental health professionals often tend to accuse such husbands of "lack of understanding" or of "being paranoid," without taking cognizance of the core of truth involved. Whether or not these women should be hospitalized may hinge more upon ethical or practical considerations than upon psychopathological ones; *Should* the wife have a respite from work? *Could* she keep on managing? Unless early therapeutic intervention has prevented such a configuration from even occurring, the required change in family dynamics often calls for time. Usually, a change of attitude is required of the spouse, as well as of the patient. At any rate, hospitalization here involves the patient's leaving a more-or-less intolerable situation. "Improvement" means that the patient is ready to go home and face it again; "cure" would mean that the family situation had changed sufficiently to prevent circumstances from becoming intolerable again. If the family situation is insoluble, the patient, after a succession of admissions and discharges, may remain in the hospital and become a chronic patient.

The Verbal Therapies in the Public Mental Hospital

It is the lack of treatment personnel that results in many of the failings and much of the disrepute of these public hospitals. Usually, the amount of psychotherapeutic attention at these hospitals is minimal. It has to be recognized even here that the situation is not merely due to hospital deficiencies in manpower and facilities. Psychotherapists tend to choose the "better" patients. Hollingshead and Redlich's comments are illuminating here.

> We are not sure what attributes a good patient must have, but they include sensitivity, intelligence, social and intellectual standards similar to the psychiatrist's, a will to do one's best, a desire to improve one's personality and status in life, youth, attractiveness, and charm. Rarely will such standards be admitted by psychiatrists. On the contrary, psychiatrists claim that the selection for treatment is based purely on psychiatric criteria. . . .[9]

This often results in a bias *against* the patient from the lower social classes, and a bias *for* patients with the same outlook or from the same class as the therapist.[10] It is also clear that the choice of the upper-class patient for psychotherapy is due not only to the attitude of therapists but also to that of patients. More of the lower-class patients tend to deny the need for hospitalization, tend to acknowledge only physical symptoms, and tend not to be verbally facile.[11] Moreover, there is the suspicion on the part of many mental health professionals, confirmed by some evidence, that many lower-class patients have very little use for verbal therapy.[12]

Two types of strategies have been suggested to deal with the patient who is disinterested in psychotherapy. One is the use of patience, perseverance, and so on, in order to "get through" to the patient, and then to commence with the verbal therapy. This is a good approach for some patients, but it is sometimes based on the assumption that psychotherapy is the method of choice for *all* mental patients. Another strategy is not to insist on verbal therapies if there is any indication that other therapies (occupational, industrial, and so forth) might be more appropriate. It could be argued that, for certain patients, such other therapies would not be merely a next best substitute for psychotherapy but the treatment of choice. The proposition that psychotherapy is *always* the best treatment reminds one of Haley's argument about the therapist's one-upmanship.[13] What better way for a verbally adept person to preserve his one-up position than to insist that the only way to mental health (and sometimes freedom) is through talking, particularly when the patient is verbally less adroit! It should be added that this would be no more inappropriate than the insistence of some physicians on the efficacy of physical therapies under all circumstances. Thus, even in the acute unit, treatment should be based on a careful analysis of the patient's condition, his problems, and his environment, and not merely involve a pat application of some standard method, whether this be a psychotherapy, a physiotherapy, an occupational therapy, and so on.[14]

The Chronic Unit: Its Patients and Its Functions

As indicated above, the chronic unit includes patients who have been in a hospital for at least several days and usually for several months. As also noted by other observers, the chronic unit is usually subdivided on a functional basis rather than on a diagnostic one.[15] This involves a coarse classification on the basis of behavior (for example: violent, "sitter," helpful to the nursing staff, and so on), rather than on a medical or scientific basis. A set of conditions in which the functional and scientific criteria tend to coincide are the infirmities of old age. For the present purpose, a chronic mental patient is defined as one who stays in the mental hospital for more than a year after admission.[16] The patients in the chronic unit may then be subdivided into, first, chronic patients proper (hospitalized for at least a year), and, second, a group intermediary between the residents of the acute section and these longer-term patients.

The over-all emphasis of the chronic unit is on custodial care, on the prevention of "psychological atrophy," and on rehabilitation, in more or less that order. Engaging in activities beyond the custodial depends on a hospital's "spirit" (quality of current personnel, tradition, and so on) and on the quantity of its economic and manpower resources.

Since the chronic section is staffed much less intensively than the acute section, a good many patients in the intermediary group are the greatest losers. This intermediary group comprises patients transferred out of the acute unit to make room for new admissions, patients who have difficulties getting along with staff or fellow patients, and others who have been transferred for reasons extraneous to their individual situation. They may well be handicapped by the lack of the more therapeutic atmosphere of the acute section. It is patients of this intermediary group, people who do not "shape up" within a certain time, who often are transferred to public hospitals from the teaching and research hospitals, from the receiving hospitals, and from private hospitals. One might hypothesize that to the extent that a waste of manpower exists, it involves primarily certain insufficiently or improperly treated members of this group.

The Geriatric Component and Their Special Needs

The true chronic group probably makes up the largest proportion of the population of a public mental hospital at any one time. It should be kept in mind that a sizable proportion of this group consists of geriatric patients. Many of these older people were first hospitalized at an advanced age, although some grew old in the hospital. For the overwhelming majority, recovery, rehabilitation, and cure would be similar to the normal expectations of other people of their age and background: Retirement, often with inadequate means, and with insufficient opportunity for constructive activity. Not unusually, these patients come to the hospital from nursing homes to which they had been sent (sometimes more, sometimes less willingly) by their relatives or by agencies such as a welfare department. In many cases their condition prevents their being adequately cared for in their own home by any but the most well-to-do families. Others might be able to live at home under average conditions of family care, but their families may be unable or unwilling to expend the effort, the money, or both. Some patients have no immediate family. Thus, a sizable proportion of this geriatric group is unable to live at home; and a public or private institution such as a domiciliary, old age home, rest home, or nursing home is needed. Most of these institutions more or less insist that their residents be reasonably well behaved. If they do not behave, they have to leave. Often, this means being sent to a public mental hospital.

It is as true for elderly patients as it is for other age groups that public mental hospitals have little control over whom they admit.[17] At any rate, many of these people cannot live at home and have to live at public expense. The question is, where? Only the physically more infirm *have* to live at a public hospital; the rest do not require treatment facilities in the ordinary sense of the word. On the other hand, since they do have to stay somewhere, are equal or better facilities available? It is by no means clear whether a good many public or private institutions would give equal or better care. In the current stress on the "hell-hole" aspects of public mental hospitals, the fact that they may give better care than at least some of the alternate facilities is often ignored. This is at times true even of such basics as food, clothing, and shelter. Transfer of patients from a public mental hospital to a less desirable institution could be therapeutic for the hospital rather than for the released patients.[18]

This is not intended as an apologia for the public mental hospitals, but rather to point to some of their social functions. They take care of the indigent or semi-indigent in a marginal, if not an adequate, fashion. To take care of these people in style would be desirable from the point of view of many; one would suspect that to appropriate the requisite money for this would be most undesirable from the point of view of many more!

Hospitalization and the Patient's Limitations

Aside from the geriatric patients, a good many of the chronic patients belong to subgroups of the population characterized by undesirable aspects above and beyond being or having been a mental patient. Such aspects may be subclassified on the basis of their initial occurrence: (1) Those already existing before a particular hospitalization, (2) those appearing during a particular admission, and (3) those that develop only after a particular hospitalization.

Some of the more important limitations existing even *before* the first admission of adult patients are those of intelligence, of schooling, and of occupational skill.[19] For the sake of the present argument, it is immaterial whether any of these limitations are due to genetic factors, to innate factors, to lack of opportunity, or to a combination of these. Nor is it argued that such factors are either the cause or the effect of any mental illness, or that they lead to hospitalization. Rather, it is held that these factors play a role (or act as one of several causes) in *prolonging* hospitalization.

It should also be added that age is important as a catalytic variable. The younger a person is, the more opportunities remain open; the older, the more remote the chances of achieving certain goals. Of course, just because the chances are remote does not mean that it is impossible to realize these goals — just that it is unlikely. In addition, the chances of achieving certain complex, long-range goals may depend upon the sequential achievement of a series of intermediary ones. Serious interference with the nature or with the timing of any of these intermediary goals may play havoc with the achievement of the final goal, or prevent it entirely. It should be emphasized that time and sequence of achievement are equally important for the "normal" person. Thus, to obtain a bachelor's degree after one is 45 is possible but not too likely; to go ahead then with one's studies and earn a doctoral degree is even less likely; the chance of obtaining great wealth or fame in a field entered so belatedly becomes quite remote. The effect of realistic constraints upon a person's "potential for self-actualization" has probably been most clearly sensed by Erikson.[20]

Another important limitation is the chronic patient's lack of social know-how and his consequent difficulties in communicating with other people. Many chronic schizophrenic patients (comprising the major portion of the chronic group) are people who are relatively isolated socially. A large proportion, particularly of the men, are single.[21] Patients whose hospital stay is rather brief tend to have a better premorbid social and sexual adjustment than patients who become chronic.[22] Whether married or not, many patients are hard to get along with—they are "difficult people." While they may want to form better relations with others, they frequently act in such a way as to repel other people.

Limitations and undesirable traits acquired during hospitalization, particularly if it is long, could all be summarized under the heading of a considerable decrease in self-confidence. A major component of this is the complete or partial atrophy of various skills. This is one aspect of institutionalization, and includes the decline in instrumental skills as well as in interpersonal ones. Another aspect of institutionalization is loss of initiative—an excessive reliance on others to plan and furnish such basics as food, shelter, clothing, and other basic requirements of living. To some extent, this is true of inmates of other "total institutions" such as prisons, religious orders, and so on.[23] Frequently, this also applies to "partially institutionalized" persons, such as many members of the regular armed forces, some employees of mental hospitals, and others.

In addition, events may occur outside the hospital which vitally affect the patient and may act as a limitation to him. For example, the death of relatives, in addition to the emotional effect upon the patient, often adds to his objective difficulties in obtaining his release. There may be no one left who is willing to assume responsibility for taking him out of the hospital, or who can provide him with needed economic support. The moving away of relatives may have similar consequences. If his spouse divorces him, this may also add to his objective difficulties, as well as increasing his loneliness and frustration. It is, of course, also true that in some cases events such as death and divorce may have positive consequences: The patient may inherit money, the disappearance of obstructionistic controls may increase his potential freedom of movement, and so on.

Central among negative aspects *after* hospitalization is the patient's own feeling of stigma. Of almost equal importance are such attitudes of the patient's relatives as their reluctance to tolerate his idiosyncrasies, and their anticipation of his renewed failure.[24] The work of Freeman and Simmons and of Lefton and his co-workers indicates that these factors are not quite as crucial as had been previously suggested, and points to the importance of the patient's *self*-expectations and of his symptoms.[25]

Another common problem for released patients is loneliness. This is partly due to some of the limitations already discussed—the patient may lack relatives, or be estranged from those he has, he may never have married or made friends, and he may encounter prejudice against former mental patients. But there are other reasons. Particularly after a long hospitalization, old friendships may be hard to pick up again. The unmarried patient finds that those of his age group are now married; if he attempts to renew old friendships, he probably feels like the proverbial fifth wheel on the wagon. It should be added that nonpatients who have not met the normative expectations of their group are likely to be in the same situation.

It is probably particularly here that the public mental hospital plays a crucial role, since it provides companionship for a great many of the patients.

At the very least, there are *potential* social contacts. For some patients, certain forms of group psychotherapy provide a pleasant form of socializing—like the old army game of griping and talking about getting out. For many chronic patients, the friends or acquaintances made at the hospital are the only ones they have left.

Other services provided by the hospital are many varieties of recreation and individual care. While food, services, and living accommodations are by no means glorious, they are at least tolerable in many hospitals nowadays. For a good many of the patients, at least some of the conditions in the hospital are superior to anything they could expect on the outside. It is certainly not unusual to hear some "wise" patient say that on the salary he could hope to earn on the outside, he would not be able to do many things that he cannot do now in the hospital. Obviously, all this is particularly true of people in modest or poor economic circumstances.

The Rehabilitation Potential of the Chronic Patient

To complicate matters further, a person's ability to obtain a job depends not only upon his own willingness to work and his proficiency in a particular occupation, but on other factors as well. The state of the total labor market, national as well as local, is of crucial importance. In our society, with its increasing demand for higher skills and more schooling, some of the limitations mentioned above are a great handicap.[26] The demand for such limited people is not great, even if they never have been mental patients. Having been a mental patient may tend to decrease their employability, but this may not be the crucial factor, for there is at least anecdotal evidence that former mental patients obtain employment with relative ease in the scarcer occupations, such as the professions. Thus the stigma and even some of the hallmarks of mental illness are not the only handicaps that the mental patient has to overcome to establish and maintain a place for himself outside the hospital. At times they may not even be the major ones. Frequently, patients have a perfectly good reason for lacking self-confidence, even without the stigma—a long history of failure in the economic, social, and sexual areas of life. It would not be much of an exaggeration to describe many people in this portion of the chronic group as belonging to a society of the successless.

Much of the current emphasis on rehabilitation is certainly based on the premise that more is required than the eradication of psychopathology.[27] Still, one wonders if all the implications are faced squarely. Thus, there are some patients whose self-actualizing potential is greatly limited, whose families may be unable or reluctant to help them, whose lot in life would be a harsh one in any case, with little to look forward to. For them, life within a public mental hospital does not have quite the horror that it has for many of the critics of the hospitals. When urged to leave the hospital, a member of this group may answer with the old joke: "I may be crazy but I'm not stupid!" Not too many patients decide this deliberately, although expedient motives are often only too obvious even in patients who are not malingerers in the usual sense. For some of these, one may speculate that manifestations of psychopathology are an indirect demand to be taken care of.[28] Since, no doubt quite necessarily, society looks down on free-loaders, people who have little to look forward to if thrown on their own resources may feel it necessary to convince not only others but themselves that their claim to the sick role is a legitimate one.

These people shy away from freedom and responsibility, and they show little enthusiasm for the marginal existence that would be their lot if they left the hospital. Some feel reluctant to work at the menial jobs they might get outside the hospital because they believe — some rightfully, some wrongly — that they are entitled to something better. The reasons others give for their lack of motivation to leave the hospital may be even less in accord with middle-class norms and expectations. For these people some disposition is required, since they refuse, or are unable, to make adequate provisions for themselves.

It has been argued that not only the therapeutic function but also the custodial function of the public mental hospital should go back to the community.[29] In theory, this is an excellent suggestion. In practice, the problem is similar to the one for the geriatric group discussed above: Is society willing and able to pay for equivalent or better facilities? The fact remains that whether these people are called patients or something else, as long as they are unable to take care of themselves properly, society has to make some provision for them.

Taking all this into consideration, one may hypothesize that a chronic patient's being willing and able to try again depends on the balance of society's help and hindrance before release, on the balance of expected rewards and punishments after release, and on the relation of these factors to the rewards and punishments open to him as a mental patient. To put it somewhat differently, if chronic mental patients are asked, "Do you want to stay here?," many patients would answer, "Yes," either directly or indirectly. This is well known to anyone working with these patients; to others imbued with the "hell-hole" view of the public mental hospital it may seem surprising. To the question, "Should a patient feel that he wants to stay here?," even many people working with these patients will answer, "No." The desire to stay at a hospital or return to it is explained as a sign of perversity, institutionalization, evidence of pathology, and so on. Once one disengages oneself from the preconception that all people want to be free and on their own, the explanation of a patient's desiring to stay becomes quite obvious. It is simply the outcome of the various forces that work in the direction of staying or leaving. If the future on the outside looks very dim, a person may want to stay.

To complicate matters even more, for a patient to admit the possibility of a successful posthospital career involves the claim to certain abilities which might be inconsistent with the inadequacy implied in the sick role. The desire to try to leave might then endanger current security.[30]

Reactions of Well People to Persons Occupying the Sick Role

If a patient prefers staying in a hospital, certain other issues become prominent. In most societies, each adult is supposed to be carrying his part of the burden. Societies may vary in the proportion of invalids (that is, those assigned the sick role) they can tolerate, but any society has its limits. Thus, sanctions are required to prevent overuse of the sick role. The prejudice against mental patients is one aspect of this.[31] It may be added that this is true even if one subscribes to some reductionistic theory of mental illness—be it physiologic, biochemical, or genetic. Social sanctions affect judgments of what is normal and what is deviant; they need not affect the *development* of the deviant behavior.

It is of interest in this connection that the loudest outcry about prejudice against the mental patient is often made by people who express great surprise, indignation, and repugnance when they hear of a patient's wanting to remain in a public mental hospital. This attitude is another aspect of these same sanctions.

Other Factors Influencing Reluctance

The Well Person's Denial of These Sanctions

Certain aspects of the humane treatment of the mental patient—admonitions to treat him as if he were normal—may be hypothesized as a denial of such sanctions. To the extent that the mental patient acts normally, he certainly should be treated accordingly. The anticipation of trouble may lead to the occurrence of trouble.[32] On the other hand, if a patient or former patient *does* act inappropriately, ignoring this may be as much or more for the benefit of the onlooker than for the benefit of the patient. It usually involves a pained, awkward attitude which is more harmful to the patient than would be an attitude of outright awareness.

The admonition to treat the abnormal as normal is a contradiction in terms. It involves certain paradoxes, both for the patient and for the onlooker. The patient finds that certain of his actions are treated differently from similar actions of a normal person. Some peculiarities of his are treated as if they were normal actions. If the patient is not aware of what is odd about his actions, an attitude of denial on the part of others may prevent him from realizing how oddly he acts; at best, he will not realize what specific aspect affected the onlooker. This makes it more difficult for such patients to learn about the effect they have on their environment and to improve it; that is, it interferes with the reality-testing function. If the patient is more or less aware of his oddities, an onlooker's studiedly acting as if he were not noticing implies that the patient is not responsible for his behavior, that he can't help it. As Parsons has pointed out, this is one component of the sick role.[33] It is also a component of the role of the child. It involves help and protection but also the often patronizing attitude that the person cannot be responsible for himself. It is thus one of the factors leading to infantilizing in general and institutionalization in particular.[34]

The Decrease of Expectations

The decrease of expectations often advocated as a way of helping a mental patient presents a somewhat similar problem. Temporarily, this may be a worthy measure with certain people. In the long run, it merely confers second-class citizenship. Freeman and Simmons have presented some arguments that the decrease of expectations is not necessarily helpful to the patient.[35] This attitude can easily lead to excessive infantilizing with a consequent lack of realization of potential. It is felt that admonitions to "get a job done," without trying to ascertain what is interfering with performance any more than one would with a nonpatient, can often lead to better performance than an exhaustive study of causes. A studied ignoring of implicit or explicit excuses based on the tune, "Have pity on me, I'm just a poor patient," often works wonders. One might add that such a callous approach is not easy for those who are trained to look for dynamics, to act in the humane tradition, and to avoid hurting a patient's feelings. Certainly a patient should not be hurt, but one can be more blunt and expect more than is often implied. It seems preferable to treat the patient not as an irresponsible child but as an agent more or less responsible for his own fate. It will then be found that many patients can perform on a much higher level than has been thought. As indicated above, this also involves the realization that there are limitations to the rehabilitation of persons — not because they are patients but because everyone has limitations, and because whatever a person's potential may have been, the possibilities of self-realization tend to decrease over time.

The Patient's Reality Testing

It may be objected that the approach suggested in the preceding paragraph contradicts what has been said earlier concerning the patient's inertia, his clinging to the security of the hospital, and so on.[36] So it does. It is my feeling that this contradiction is merely another version of the dilemmas encountered in the treatment of schizophrenics.[37] By denying the reality of the chronic patient's difficulties or by implying that no quandary exists about his leaving the hospital, one will never make him want to leave the hospital. But by admitting the reality of certain difficulties and conditions which face him, one may be able to cajole and persuade him to leave the hospital and try living in the community again.

Concluding Comments

In the public mental hospital, the aim of the acute service is to help the patient get back to the community in serviceable fashion, as soon as possible. In a good many instances, hospitalization could and should have been prevented entirely. As has been pointed out, *long* hospitalization should be avoided in any case. In some situations, particularly those involving certain acutely ill persons, and possibly those which present an unsolvable problem, the temporary removal of a person from his home may be unavoidable. Whether placement in a public mental hospital, voluntary or involuntary, is the best disposition is another matter. Various types of asylums, halfway houses, and quasi jails may do just as well, depending on the particular circumstances.

The chronic group, on the other hand, usually is institutionalized already. The emphasis is on keeping the person more or less intact and preventing him from getting worse. Many of these people are greatly handicapped and often can expect many difficulties outside the hospital unless they are given considerable help before and after leaving. A good many do not want to leave. Many of them could live in some nonhospital "asylum." The basic difficulty for many is not that they are incurably or hopelessly ill, but rather that they are too limited to deal with the problems of life, particularly the socioeconomic ones, in our society. Thus, the aim of the hospital should not be to cure them but to rehabilitate (that is, train or retrain) them. Those who cannot be retrained, either because of their own limitations or those of the hospital, *will have to be taken care of somewhere.* This is also the implication of sending patients to rest homes, foster homes, nursing homes, and so on. In other words, those who sound the clarion call to eradicate mental illness and clear out the hospitals must face the *current* reality of the inadequate person who has to be taken care of by someone.

I have also pointed out that for various reasons a certain number of persons want to continue to enjoy whatever benefits the public mental hospital has to offer. Social sanctions are required to keep this number reasonably small. Thus, any attempt to treat this type of mental patient as normal is doomed to failure. For one thing, it involves a logical paradox: The deviate is not normal. For another, prejudices against the mental patient are part of society's method of preventing an excessively large number of invalids.

I do not claim that these remarks apply to all hospitalized mental patients. Nor do I claim that many of those patients to whom it does apply might not want to leave the hospital. Rather, I hold that many of the latter group are unwilling or unable to pay the price in effort and responsibility. In order to deal with some of these problems of the hospitalized mental patient, I feel that those in the mental health professions have to face up to what many of them already know—that a patient may have perfectly sensible reasons for staying in or returning to a hospital. Once this is realized, discussions with patients can be conducted on a somewhat more rational basis. Even so, it may not always be easy to work with such patients. To paraphrase Eissler, the patients cannot forgive our success in life, while we cannot forgive their self-indulgence and lack of responsibility.[38]

NOTES

1. In using the term, public mental hospital, I refer to state hospitals and veterans neuropsychiatric hospitals, but not to teaching and research hospitals even though state run.

2. See Leslie Phillips and Edward Zigler, "Social Competence: The Action-Thought Parameter and Vicariousness in Normal and Pathological Behaviors," *J. Abnormal and Social Psychology* (1961) 63:137–146; and "Role Orientation, the Action-Thought Dimension, and Outcome in Psychiatric Disorder," *J. Abnormal and Social Psychology* (1964) 68:381–389. See also Edward Zigler and Leslie Phillips, "Social Effectiveness and Symptomatic Behaviors," *J. Abnormal and Social Psychology* (1960) 61:231–238; and "Social Competence and Outcome in Psychiatric Disorder," *J. Abnormal and Social Psychology* (1961) 63:264–271.

3. Some large cities have public receiving hospitals which keep patients for a limited period of time and then send them to a "regular" state hospital if continued hospitalization is required. Such a state hospital would get many transfers, but a transfer here would be somewhat similar to the shifts from the acute to the chronic units of the average state hospital.

4. For a study of transfers, see Robert Sommer and Gwyneth Witney, "The Chain of Chronicity," *Amer. J. Psychiatry* (1961) 118:111–117.

5. For example, in the Massachusetts State Hospitals, about 75 percent of new admissions stay less than 90 days; of newly admitted patients with a psychotic diagnosis, about 50 percent leave within 90 days. See Mass. Dept. of Mental Health (Division of Medical Statistics and Research), *Discharges to Community From 12 DMH Mental Hospitals Considered as a Unit, by Time in Hospital Before Discharge, Sex and Category of Psychiatric Diagnosis, 1957 and 1960;* Boston, Dept. of Mental Health, 1962.

6. See the comments on "the fear of psychiatric hospitalization as a destructive power," in Alfred H. Stanton, "Milieu Therapy and the Development of Insight," PSYCHIATRY (1961) Suppl., 24:19–29.

7. See Fred Pine and Daniel Levinson, "A Sociopsychological Conception of Patienthood," *Internat. J. Social Psychiatry* (1961) 7:106–122. B. W. Murphy, "Some Interpersonal Processes and Situations Delaying Discharge from a Psychiatric Institute," *Diseases Nervous System* (1951) 12: 273–277.

8. See Nathaniel S. Lehrman, "Follow-up of Brief and Prolonged Psychiatric Hospitalization," *Comprehensive Psychiatry* (1961) 2:227–240.

9. August Hollingshead and Fredrick Redlich, *Social Class and Mental Illness;* New York, Wiley, 1958; p. 192.

10. See Hollingshead and Redlich, in footnote 9, pp. 300–302. Robert Kahn and Max Pollack, "Sociopsychological Factors Affecting Therapist-Patient Relationships," pp. 155–168, in *Psychoanalysis and Human Values,* edited by Jules H. Masserman; New York, Grune & Stratton, 1960. Robert A. Moore, Elissa P. Benedek, and John G. Wallace, "Social Class, Schizophrenia and the Psychiatrist," *Amer. J. Psychiatry* (1963) 120:149–154.

11. See Hollingshead and Redlich, in footnote 9; pp. 344–351. See Moore, Benedek, and Wallace, in footnote 10.

12. See, for instance, Bernard Stotsky, "How Important Is Psychotherapy to the Hospitalized Psychiatric Patient," *J. Clin. Psychology* (1956) 12:32–36.

13. Jay Haley, "The Art of Psychoanalysis," *Etc.* (1958) 18:190–200.

14. See S. M. Miller and Elliot G. Mishler, "Social Class, Mental Illness and American Psychiatry," *Milbank Memorial Fund Quart.* (1959) 37:174–199. Jerome D. Frank, "The Dynamics of the Psychotherapeutic Relationship," PSYCHIATRY (1959) 22:17–39.

15. See, for instance: Ivan Belknap, *Human Problems of a State Mental Hospital;* New York, McGraw-Hill, 1956; Ch. 8. Erving Goffman, *Asylums: Essays on the Social Situations of Mental Patients and Other Inmates;* Garden City, N.Y., Doubleday Anchor Books, 1961; p. 361.

16. The one-year mark seems to be an important turning point; Clausen and Kohn report that "status as of one year after admission to the hospital was a good index of status five years after admission." John A. Clausen and Melvin L. Kohn, "Social Relations and Schizophrenia: A Research Report and a Perspective," pp. 295–320, in *The Etiology of a Schizophrenia,* edited by Don D. Jackson; New York, Basic Books, 1960. Sommer and Witney, and some of the authors they refer to, use the *two*-year mark to define chronicity (see footnote 4).

17. This is particularly true of state hospitals, which usually have to admit anyone sent there by the courts, by the police, by physicians, and so on. Veterans hospitals are in a similar position as far as "service-connected" patients are concerned.

18. Walter B. Simon, "A Skeptic's View of the Mental Illness Game, Or, an Old State Hospital Hand's Jaundiced Look at Progress," *Mental Hygiene* (1965) 49:69–73.

19. One report does not find that these variables discriminate those patients who stayed 90 days from those who stayed longer; see James Lindeman, George W. Fairweather, Gideon B. Stone, and Robert S. Smith, "The Use of Demographic Characteristics in Predicting Length of Neuropsychiatric Hospital Stay," *J. Consulting Psychology* (1959) 23:85–89. Zigler and Phillips found an "index of social competence" to be related to length of stay in the hospital (see footnote 2, 1961), and, in what appears to be a reanalysis of their 1961 data, report a less clear-cut relation between competence and outcome (see footnote 2, 1964).

20. Erik H. Erikson, "Identity and the Life Cycle," *Psychol. Issues* (1959), No. 1; *Childhood and Society;* New York, Norton, 1950; pp. 61–63, 219–234.

21. See Amerigo Farina, Norman Garmezy, and Herbert Barry III, "Relationship of Marital Status to Incidence and Prognosis of Schizophrenia," *J. Abnormal and Social Psychology* (1963) 67: 624–630.

22. Leslie Phillips, "Case History Data and Prognosis in Schizophrenia," *J. Nervous and Mental Disease* (1953) 117:515–525.

23. See Erving Goffman, in footnote 15; pp. 3–124.

24. Referring particularly to long-term neurotics who had been of great economic and emotional expense to the family, Kubie discusses the intensity of the deferred hopes of the family and the difficulty, if not impossibility, for the former patient to repay such debts. This is less true for the group here under consideration. Lawrence S. Kubie, "The Challenge of the Partial Cure," *J. Chronic Diseases* (1959) 9:292–297.

25. Howard E. Freeman and Ozzie G. Simmons, *The Mental Patient Comes Home;* New York, Wiley, 1963; p. 49. Mark Lefton, Shirley Angrist, Simon Dinitz, and Benjamin Pasamanick, "Social Class, Expectations, and Performance of Mental Patients," *Amer. J. Sociology* (1962) 68: 79–87. See also Marjorie P. Linder and David Landy, "Post-Discharge Experience and Vocational Rehabilitation Needs of Psychiatric Patients," *Mental Hygiene* (1958) 42:29–44.

26. Robert M. Frumkin, "Occupation and Major Mental Disorders," pp. 136–160, in *Mental Health and Mental Disorder,* edited by Arnold M. Rose; New York, Norton, 1955.

27. For instance, see Linder and Landy, in footnote 25.

28. For the conception of symptoms as communication, see Kenneth L. Artiss, "The Symptom as an Informative and Communicative Device," pp. 9–39, in *The Symptom as Communication in Schizophrenia,* edited by Kenneth L. Artiss; New York, Grune & Stratton, 1959. See also Thomas S. Szasz, *The Myth of Mental Illness;* New York, Hoeber-Harper, 1961; p. 187.

29. Joint Commission on Mental Illness and Health, *Action for Mental Health;* New York, Basic Books, 1961; pp. 48–49.

30. For an excellent discussion of this and other dilemmas of the mental patient, see Kai T. Erikson, "Patient Role and Social Uncertainty—A Dilemma of the Mentally Ill," PSYCHIATRY (1957) 20:263–274.

31. One may speculate that many aspects of this prejudice against mental patients have a realistic basis. See Walter B. Simon, "The Effect of Stereotypes on Interpersonal Judgments," unpublished paper, 1963.

32. Concerning the "self-fulfilling prophecy," see Robert K. Merton, *Social Theory and Social Structure* (revised enlarged edition); Glencoe, Ill., Free Press, 1957; pp. 421–436.

33. Talcott Parsons, *The Social System;* Glencoe, Ill., Free Press, 1951; pp. 436–438.

34. On the ethics of helpfulness and helplessness, see Thomas S. Szasz, *The Myth of Mental Illness;* New York, Hoeber-Harper, 1961; pp. 183–203.

35. See Freeman and Simmons in footnote 25; pp. 197, 204.

36. See also Maxwell Jones, *The Therapeutic Community;* New York, Basic Books, 1953; pp. 53–54, 159–160.

37. See Kurt R. Eissler, "Limitations to the Psychotherapy of Schizophrenia," *Psychiatry* (1943) 6:381–391.

38. See footnote 37.

Suggestions for Further Reading

Deinstitutionalization

Arnhoff, Franklyn N. "Social Consequences of Policy Toward Mental Illness." *Science* 188 (1975):1277–1281.

Bachrach, Leona. *Deinstitutionalization: An Analytical Review and Sociological Perspective.* Washington, D.C.: National Institute of Mental Health, 1976.

———. "Is the Least Restrictive Environment Always the Best?" *Hospital and Community Psychiatry* 31 (February 1980):97–103.

Bakal, Yitzak, ed. *Closing Correctional Institutions.* Lexington, Massachusetts: Lexington Books, D. C. Heath and Co., 1973.

Bassuk, Ellen L., and Gerson, Samuel. "Deinstitutionalization and Mental Health Services." *Scientific American* 238 (February 1978):46–53.

Borus, Jonathan F. "Deinstitutionalization of the Chronically Mentally Ill." *The New England Journal of Medicine* Vol. 305 (August 6, 1981):339–342.

Bradley, Valerie. *Deinstitutionalization of Developmentally Disabled Persons: A Conceptual Analysis and Guide.* Baltimore: University Park Press, 1978.

Braun, Peter, et al. "Overview: Deinstitutionalization of Psychiatric Patients, A Critical Review of Outcome Studies." *American Journal of Psychiatry* 138 (June 1981):736–749.

"Deinstitutionalization: What Went Wrong." Special issue of *Hospital and Community Psychiatry* 30 (September 1979).

Dowart, Robert A. "Deinstitutionalization: Who Is Left Behind?" *Hospital and Community Psychiatry* 31 (May 1980):336–338.

Fairweather, G. E., et al. *Community Life for the Mentally Ill.* Chicago: Aldine Publishing Co., 1969.

"Institutionalization." In Reich, Warren T., ed. *Encyclopedia of Bioethics* Vol. II. New York: The Free Press, 1978, pp. 779–784.

Jones, M. *The Therapeutic Community.* New York: Basic Books, 1953.

Kaplan, Leonard V. "State Control of Deviant Behavior: A Critical Essay on Scull's Critique of Community Treatment and Deinstitutionalization." *Arizona Law Review* 20 (1978):189–232.

Klerman, Gerald L. "Better But Not Well: Social and Ethical Issues in the Deinstitutionalization of the Mentally Ill." *Schizophrenia Bulletin* 3 (1977): 617–631.

Lamb, H. R. "What Did We Really Expect from Deinstitutionalization?" *Hospital and Community Psychiatry* 32 (February 1981):105–109.

Lamb, H. R., and Goertzel, V. "Discharged Mental Patients—Are They Really in the Community?" *Archives of General Psychiatry* 24 (1971):29–34.

Linn, Margaret W., et al. "Hospital vs. Community (Foster) Care for Psychiatric Patients." *Archives of General Psychiatry* 34 (January 1977):78–83.

Martin, Denis V. "Institutionalization." *The Lancet* 269 (1955):1188–1190.

Ozarin, Lucy D., and Sharfstein, Steven S. "The Aftermaths of Deinstitutionalization, Problems and Solutions." *Psychiatric Quarterly* 50 (1978):128–132.

Penn, N., et al. "The Dilemma of Involuntary Commitment: Suggestions for a Measurable Alternative." *Mental Hygiene* 53 (1969):4–10.

Polak, Paul R. "Debathtubization: A Modern Fable." *American Journal of Orthopsychiatry* 48 (July 1978):396–397.

Reich, Robert. "Care of the Chronically Mentally Ill—A National Disgrace." *American Journal of Psychiatry* 130 (August 1973):911–912.

Reich, Robert, and Siegal, Lloyd. "Psychiatry Under Siege: The Chronic Mentally Ill Shuffle to Oblivion." *Psychiatric Annals* 3 (1973):37–55.

Robbins, Edwin, and Robbins, Lillian. "Charge to the Community: Some Early Effects of a State Hospital System's Change of Policy." *The American Journal of Psychiatry* 131 (June 1974):641–645.

Robitscher, Jonas. *The Powers of Psychiatry.* Boston: Houghton Mifflin, 1980.

Rothman, David J. "Decarcerating Prisoners and Patients." *Civil Liberties Review* 1 (1973):8–30.

Scull, Andrew. *Decarceration, Community Treatment and the Deviant: A Radical View.* Englewood Cliffs, New Jersey: Prentice-Hall, Inc., 1977.

Simon, W. B. "On Reluctance to Leave the Public Health Hospital." *Psychiatry* 28 (1965):145–156.

Stein, L. I., et al. "Alternative to Mental Hospital Treatment." *Archives of General Psychiatry* 37 (April 1980):392–412.

Whitmer, Gary E. "From Hospitals to Jails: The Fate of California's Deinstitutionalized Mentally Ill." *American Journal of Orthopsychiatry* 50 (January 1980):54–64.

Williams, Roger M. "From Bedlam to Chaos: Are They Closing the Mental Hospitals Too Soon?" *Psychology Today* 10 (May 1977):124ff.

Wills, David P., ed. Special issue on deinstitutionalization, *Milbank Memorial Fund Quarterly/Health and Society* 57 (Fall 1979).

Wolpert, Julian, and Wolpert, Eileen R. "The Relocation of Released Mental Hospital Patients into Residential Communities." *Policy Sciences* 7 (1976): 31–51.

Quality of Care and Quality of Life

Bartlett, F. L. "Institutional Peonage: Our Exploitation of Mental Patients." *Atlantic* 214 (1964):116–119.

Blatt, B. "The Dark Side of the Mirror." *Mental Retardation* 6 (1968):42–44.

Blatt, B., and Mangel, C. "Tragedy and Hope of Retarded Children." *Look* 41 (1967):96–99.

"Conference Report: Handling the Violent Patient in the Hospital." *Hospital and Community Psychiatry* 29 (July 1978):463–467.

Goffman, Erving. *Asylums*. New York: Doubleday and Co., 1961.

Katz, Michael, and Zimbardo, Philip. "Making it as a Mental Patient." *Psychology Today* 10 (April 1977):122–126.

Stone, Michael H. "Management of Unethical Behavior in a Psychiatric Hospital Staff." *American Journal of Psychotherapy* 29 (July 1975):391–401.

Suchotliff, Leonard C., et al. "The Struggle for Patients' Rights in a State Hospital." *Mental Hygiene* 54 (April 1970):230–240.

Tancredi, Laurence R., et al. *Legal Issues in Psychiatric Care*. New York: Harper & Row, 1975, Part IV.

Vail, D. G. *Dehumanization and the Institutional Career*. Springfield, Illinois: Charles C. Thomas, 1966.

Wielgus, K. "Custodial and Therapeutic Patient Relationships." *Ethics in Science and Medicine* 3 (July 1976):71–94.

"Work and Institutional Peonage." Special issue of *Hospital and Community Psychiatry* 27 (February 1976).

Contributors

Teodoro Ayllon, Ph.D., is professor of psychology and special education at Georgia State University, Atlanta.

David Avery is assistant professor of psychiatry at the Harbor View Medical Center in Seattle, Washington.

William T. Blackstone, Ph.D. (1931–1977), was professor of philosophy and chairman of the Division of Social Sciences at the University of Georgia. His principal areas of interest were ethics and political philosophy. He was also president of the American Society for Value Inquiry.

Christopher Boorse, Ph.D., is associate professor of philosophy at the University of Delaware, Newark.

Jonathan F. Borus, M.D., practices psychiatry at the Massachusetts General Hospital (Boston) and is on the faculty of the Harvard Medical School.

Peter R. Breggin, M.D., P.A., is a psychiatrist in Bethesda, Maryland, and author of *The Psychology of Freedom* (Prometheus Books, 1980).

Stephan L. Chorover, Ph.D., is professor of psychology at the Massachusetts Institute of Technology.

Rem B. Edwards, Ph.D., is professor of philosophy at the University of Tennessee, Knoxville.

H. Tristram Engelhardt, Jr., Ph.D., M.D., is senior research scholar at the Kennedy Institute Center for Bioethics at Georgetown University, Washington, D.C.

Herbert Fingarette, Ph.D., is professor of philosophy at the University of California, Santa Barbara.

Martha R. Fowlkes, Ph.D., is currently a teacher in the Department of Sociology and Anthropology at Smith College.

June Resnick German, J.D., was supervising attorney for the Mental Health Information Service, First Judicial Department, New York.

Robert W. Gibson, M.D., 105th president of the American Psychiatric Association, is medical director of Sheppard and Enoch Pratt Hospital in Towson, Maryland.

Glenn C. Graber, Ph.D., is professor of philosophy at the University of Tennessee, Knoxville, and a clinical associate in medical ethics at the University of Tennessee Center for the Health Sciences/Knoxville Units.

David F. Greenberg, Ph.D., is associate professor of sociology at New York University.

Toksoz B. Karasu, M.D., is a professor of psychiatry at Albert Einstein College of Medicine at Bronx Municipal Center.

Gerald L. Klerman, M.D., is a psychiatrist at the Massachusetts General Hospital (Boston) and a professor of psychiatry at Harvard Medical School.

Charles W. Lidz, Ph.D., is assistant professor, Department of Psychiatry, School of Medicine, and Department of Sociology, University of Pittsburgh and the Western Psychiatric Institute and Clinic.

Joseph M. Livermore, L.L.B., is professor of law at the University of Arizona College of Law in Tucson.

A. Louis McGarry, M.D., is medical director of the Division of Forensic Services and professor of psychiatry at the State University of New York, Stony Brook.

Ruth Macklin is associate clinical professor of community health at Albert Einstein College of Medicine, Yeshiva University.

Carl P. Malmquist, M.D., M.S., is professor of psychology and child development at the University of Minnesota. He is also psychiatric consultant to Hennepin County (Minnesota) District.

Vernon H. Mark, M.D., is associate professor of surgery at Harvard Medical School and director of neurosurgery at Boston General Hospital. With psychiatrist Frank R. Ervin, Mark coauthored *Violence and the Brain* (Harper, 1970).

Frank H. Marsh, J.D., Ph.D., was associate professor of philosophy at Old Dominion University, where he taught bioethics and philosophy of law. He now holds a joint appointment in medicine and philosophy at the University of Colorado, Denver.

Paul E. Meehl, Ph.D., is professor of psychology, College of Liberal Arts; professor of clinical psychology, Department of Psychiatry, Medical School, University of Minnesota.

Alan Meisel, J.D., is assistant professor, School of Law and Department of Psychiatry, School of Medicine, University of Pittsburgh and the Western Psychiatric Institute and Clinic.

Michael S. Moore, J.D., is professor of law at the University of Southern California, Los Angeles.

Rosalind Pollack Petchesky, Ph.D., is assistant professor of political and social theory at Ramapo College.

Jonas Robitscher, J.D., M.D. (1920—1981), was director of the National Institute of Mental Health Program "Social-Legal Uses of Forensic Psychiatry," University of Pennsylvania. At the time of his death, he was Henry R. Luce Professor of Law and the Behavioral Sciences at Emory University Schools of Law and Medicine.

Loren H. Roth, M.D., M.P.H., assistant professor, Department of Psychiatry, School of Medicine, and director of the Law and Psychiatry Program, University of Pittsburgh and the Western Psychiatric Institute and Clinic.

Peter Sedgwick, Ph.D., is professor of politics at the University of Leeds in W. Yorkshire, England.

Saleem A. Shah, Ph.D., is chief of the Center for Studies of Crime and Delinquency, National Institute of Mental Health.

Walter B. Simon, Ph.D., is a psychologist at Norwich Hospital, Norwich, Connecticut.

Anne C. Singer, J.D., was assistant deputy advocate, New Jersey Department of the Public Advocate.

Thomas S. Szasz, M.D., is professor of psychiatry at the State University of New York, Upstate Medical Center, Syracuse. He has written many articles and books on the subject of psychiatric treatment. His impressive list of books includes: *The Myth of Mental Illness* (1961), *Law, Liberty, and Psychiatry* (1963), *The Ethics of Psychoanalysis* (1965), *Ideology and Insanity* (1970), *The Manufacture of Madness* (1970), *The Theology of Medicine* (1977), and *Sex by Prescription* (1980).

Elliot S. Valenstein, Ph.D., is professor of psychology and neuroscience at the University of Michigan. He has served as chief of a neurophysiology section of the Walter Reed Institute of Research in Washington, D.C.; as a staff member of the Fels Research Institute in Yellow Springs, Ohio; and has taught at Antioch College and the University of California, Berkeley. He is the author of *Brain Control: A Critical Examination of Brain Stimulation and Psychosurgery* (Wiley-Interscience, 1973).

Robert M. Veatch, Ph.D., is currently professor at the Kennedy Institute of Ethics, Georgetown University, Washington, D.C.